Heart Failure

Heart Failure

Second Edition

Edited by

Marc J. Semigran MD
Massachusetts General Hospital, Boston, MA, USA

Jordan T. Shin MD, PhD
*Cardiovascular Research Center,
Massachusetts General Hospital,
Boston, MA, USA*

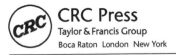

CRC Press
Taylor & Francis Group
Boca Raton London New York

CRC Press is an imprint of the
Taylor & Francis Group, an **informa** business

CRC Press
Taylor & Francis Group
6000 Broken Sound Parkway NW, Suite 300
Boca Raton, FL 33487-2742, USA

First issued in paperback 2019

© 2013 by Taylor & Francis Group, LLC
CRC Press is an imprint of Taylor & Francis Group, an Informa business

No claim to original U.S. Government works

Typeset by Exeter Premedia Services Pvt Ltd., Chennai, India

ISBN-13: 978-1-4200-7699-8 (hbk)
ISBN-13: 978-0-367-38053-3 (pbk)

**Visit the Taylor & Francis Web site at
http://www.taylorandfrancis.com**

**and the CRC Press Web site at
http://www.crcpress.com**

Contents

Contributors   VIII

Preface   XI

PART I: CELLULAR AND MOLECULAR BASIS FOR HEART FAILURE

1. **A brief primer on the development of the heart**   1
   Serge Gregoire and Sean M. Wu

2. **The genetics of dilated and hypertrophic cardiomyopathies**   9
   Calum A. MacRae

3. **Molecular signaling networks underlying cardiac hypertrophy and failure**   31
   Gerald W. Dorn II

4. **Excitation–contraction coupling in the normal and failing heart**   43
   Mattew Coggins, Bernhard Haring, and Federica del Monte

5. **Myocardial energetics and metabolism in the failing heart**   64
   Joanne S. Ingwall

6. **Animal models of heart failure**   78
   William Carlson

PART II: PATHOPHYSIOLOGY OF HEART FAILURE

7. **Ventricular remodeling and secondary valvular dysfunction in heart failure progression**   95
   Kibar Yared and Judy Hung

8. **Neurohormonal and cytokine activation in heart failure**   119
   Dennis M. McNamara

9. **Cardiomyopathies in the adult**   137
   Richard Rodeheffer

10. **Water and salt: The cardiorenal syndrome**   160
    Maria Rosa Costanzo

PART III: THE DEMOGRAPHICS, DIAGNOSIS, AND MONITORING OF HEART FAILURE

11.   **The clinical syndrome of heart failure**   208
      Thomas DiSalvo and Jordan Shin

12.   **Clinical profiles and bedside assessment**   240
      Lynne Warner Stevenson

13.   **Prognosis in heart failure**   252
      J. Susie Woo and Wayne C. Levy

14.   **Biomarkers in heart failure**   264
      Ravi V. Shah and Thomas J. Wang

15.   **Noninvasive imaging modalities for the evaluation of heart failure**   278
      Kimberly A. Parks, Malissa J. Wood, Ian S. Rogers, and Godtfred Holmvang

16.   **Role of invasive monitoring in heart failure: Pulmonary artery catheters in the post-ESCAPE era**   313
      W. H. Wilson Tang and Gary S. Francis

PART IV: THE MEDICAL TREATMENT OF CLINICAL HEART FAILURE

17.   **Conventional therapy of chronic heart failure: Diuretics, vasodilators, and digoxin**   320
      G. William Dec

18.   **Conventional therapy of chronic heart failure: Beta-adrenergic blockers**   330
      G. William Dec

19.   **Angiotensin receptor blockers for heart failure**   341
      George V. Moukarbel

20.   **Anticoagulation in systolic heart failure**   353
      Ronald S. Freudenberger

21.   **Role of mineralocorticoid receptor antagonists in patients with heart failure**   365
      Mara Giattina and Flora Sam

22.   **Treatment of heart failure with preserved ejection fraction**   377
      Barry A. Borlaug

23.   **Cardiac resynchronization therapy**   388
      William T. Abraham

24. **Management of atrial and ventricular arrhythmias in heart failure** 401

Usha Tedrow and William G. Stevenson

25. **Ultrafiltration for the management of volume overload** 427

Bradley A. Bart

26. **Heart failure and palliative care** 445

Joshua M. Hauser and Robert O. Bonow

PART V: MOLECULAR AND BIOLOGIC THERAPIES

27. **Gene therapy for heart failure** 457

Stefan P. Janssens

Index *475*

Contributors

William T. Abraham, MD The Ohio State University Heart Center, Division of Cardiovascular Medicine, Columbus, OH, USA

Bradley A. Bart, MD Hennepin County Medical Center, University of Minnesota, Minneapolis, MN, USA

Robert O. Bonow, MD, MS Center for Cardiovascular Innovation, Northwestern University Feinberg School of Medicine, Chicago, IL, USA

Barry A. Borlaug, MD Division of Cardiovascular Diseases, Department of Medicine, The Mayo Clinic, Rochester, MN, USA

William D. Carlson, MD, PhD Advanced Heart Failure and Cardiac Transplant, Massachusetts General Hospital, Boston, MA, USA

Mattew Coggins, MD Cardiovascular Institute, Beth Israel Deaconess Medical Center, Boston, MA, USA

Federica del Monte, MD, PhD Cardiovascular Institute, Beth Israel Deaconess Medical Center, Boston, MA, USA

Thomas DiSalvo, MD Vanderbilt University School of Medicine, Nashville, TN, USA

Gerald W. Dorn II, MD Center for Pharmacogenomics, Washington University, St. Louis, MO, USA

Gary S. Francis, MD University of Minnesota, Cardiovascular Division, Minneapolis, MN, USA

Ronald S. Freudenberger, MD Division of Cardiology, Medical Director, Heart & Vascular Center, Lehigh Valley Health Network, Allentown, PA, USA

Mara Giattina, MD Boston Medical Center, Boston, MA, USA

Serge Gregoire, MD Cardiovascular Research Center, Massachusetts General Hospital, Boston, MA, USA

Bernhard Haring, MD Cardiovascular Institute, Beth Israel Deaconess Medical Center, Boston, MA, USA

Joshua M. Hauser, MD Northwestern University Medical School, Chicago, IL, USA

Judy Hung, MD Department of Medicine, Division of Cardiology, Massachusetts General Hospital, Harvard Medical School, Boston, MA, USA

Joanne S. Ingwall, PhD Brigham and Women's Hospital, Harvard Medical School, Boston, MA, USA

Stefan P. Janssens, MD, PhD   Division of Cardiovascular Diseases, Gasthuisberg University Hospital, University of Leuven, Belgium

Wayne C. Levy, MD   Division of Cardiology, University of Washington, Seattle, WA, USA

Calum A. MacRae, MD   Cardiology Division, Brigham & Women's Hospital, Boston, MA, USA

Dennis McNamara, MD   Heart Failure Section, University of Pittsburgh Medical Center, Pittsburg, PA, USA

George V. Moukarbel, MD   Division of Cardiovascular Medicine, Brigham and Women's Hospital, Harvard Medical School, Boston, MA, USA

Kimberly A. Parks, MD   Cardiac Transplantation, Massachusetts General Hospital, Boston, MA, USA

Richard J. Rodeheffer, MD   Mayo Clinic, Rochester, MN, USA

Maria Rosa Costanzo, MD, FAHA, FACC   Edward Hospital Center for Advanced Heart Failure, Naperville, IL, USA

Flora Sam MD, FACC, FAHA   Boston University School of Medicine, Whitaker Cardiovascular Institute, Boston, MA, USA

Ravi V. Shah, MD   Department of Medicine, Cardiology Division, Massachusetts General Hospital, Harvard Medical School, Boston, MA, USA

William G. Stevenson, MD   Cardiovascular Division, Brigham and Women's Hospital, Boston, MA, USA

J. Susie Woo, MD   Division of Cardiology, University of Washington, Seattle, WA, USA

Usha B. Tedrow, MD, MSc   Arrhythmia Unit, Cardiovascular Division, Brigham and Women's Hospital, Boston, MA, USA

Thomas J. Wang, MD   Department of Medicine, Cardiology Division, Massachusetts General Hospital, Harvard Medical School, Boston, MA, USA

Lynne Warner Stevenson, MD   Section of Advanced Heart Disease, Brigham and Women's Hospital and Harvard Medical School, Boston, MA, USA

G. William Dec, MD   Massachusetts General Hospital, Harvard Medical School, Boston, MA, USA

W. H. Wilson Tang, MD   Heart and Vascular Institute, Cleveland Clinic, Cleveland, OH, USA

Malissa J. Wood, MD   Harvard Medical School, Boston, MA, USA

Sean M. Wu, MD   Massachusetts General Hospital, Boston, MA and Harvard Stem Cell Institute, Cambridge, MA, USA

Kibar Yared, MD   Department of Medicine, Division of Cardiology, Massachusetts General Hospital, Harvard Medical School, Boston, MA, USA

Godtfred Holmvang, MD   Cardiology Division, Department of Medicine, and Department of Radiology Massachusetts General Hospital, Boston, MA, USA

Ian S. Rogers, MD, MPH   Instructor, Cardiovascular Medicine, Stanford University, Division of Cardiovascular Medicine

Preface

Since the publication of the First Edition of this text, heart failure has grown as a health care problem in both developed and developing countries, with both an increase in the number of patients and greater awareness of the disease among clinicians. Progress in our understanding of the cellular mechanisms of cardiac dysfunction has occurred, and contributions from the areas of developmental biology and regulation of cell survival continue to inform strategies to prevent and treat heart failure. During the past five years, our appreciation for the role of extracardiac organs in the pathophysiology of heart failure has increased, particularly changes in pulmonary and systemic vascular function, gas exchange in the lungs, and in the central nervous system.

In response to the advances in our understanding of the biology of cardiac function and pathophysiology of the heart failure syndrome, the treatment of heart failure has also evolved. Although several new pharmacotherapies have entered late-stage clinical trial since the publication of the First Edition of this text, perhaps the greatest advance has been in the development of devices to treat heart failure, such as resynchronization therapy, ultrafiltration, and mechanical circulatory support. In addition to improving cardiovascular function, these devices also are capable of providing feedback to clinicians and patients that allow them to respond to changes in circulatory physiology and optimization of treatment.

In order to inform the reader of recent progress in our understanding of the pathophysiology and treatment of heart failure, significant additions have been made to each of the sections of the text. Part I, "Cellular and Molecular Basis for Heart Failure" has been revised to include a chapter covering the relevance of developmental biology to the pathophysiology of cardiac dysfunction, including a discussion of the recurrence of expression of fetal genes in the adult with heart failure. A chapter describing animal models of heart failure has been added. The latter chapter provides particular insight into the debate regarding pharmacologic manipulation of the alterations that occur in cardiomyocyte substrate utilization. The second section of the text, "Pathophysiology of Heart Failure," now contains chapters describing recent advances in the understanding of alterations of renal sodium and water excretion that occur in heart failure. A third section, "The Demographics, Diagnosis, and Monitoring of Heart Failure" has been newly added to the text. Chapters in this section describe the classic methods of clinical diagnosis of heart failure as well as the utility of newer imaging modalities that identify the causes and severity of cardiac impairment. It is now recognized that the major cause of hospitalization in heart failure patients is the occurrence of acute decompensated heart failure, and repeated admissions leads to the progression of myocardial and end-organ dysfunction. In response, diagnostic methods have recently been developed to identify the physiologic and neurohormonal changes that precede decompensation. The effective utilization of this information to guide modification of therapy is discussed in this section, as are advances in the use of biomarkers to guide the diagnosis and treatment of heart failure.

The second half of the book focuses on the treatment of heart failure. The first section of this half, "The Medical Treatment of Clinical Heart Failure," reviews the current state of the art of pharmacologic therapies. Challenges remain in the pharmacologic treatment of the disease, yet there are promising advances in the development of agents that address novel targets in the vasopressin and adenosine signaling pathways as well as of immune system modulators and type 5 phosphodiesterase inhibitors. Also discussed in this section are agents for acute decompensated heart failure that target the "cardiorenal" syndrome as defined in Part II. New to this section from the previous edition is a discussion of medical device therapies, such as resynchronization therapy and ultrafiltration. This leads to a discussion of surgical heart failure therapy, and the last section of the text looks to the future, with an update of the progress in gene and cell-based therapies that have been recently made.

The editors of this Edition of *Heart Failure* gratefully acknowledge the work of the authors and editors that preceded them, as they set a high standard for clarity and scientific rigor in the previous edition. It is hoped that the readers of the Second Edition find it to be an informative resource guiding further investigation and care of the patient with heart failure.

1

A brief primer on the development of the heart

Serge Gregoire and Sean M. Wu

INTRODUCTION

Despite tremendous efforts and investments in heart failure research, current therapies are inadequate to reduce the societal burden of this disease. Cardiac transplantation provides the only durable therapy in the long term. However, only a small fraction of the patients are eligible to receive this treatment. Advances in cell-based therapies have raised exciting prospects for new treatments. To realize this promise we need a greater understanding of the mechanisms involved in cardiac cell lineage commitment and differentiation. Embryonic cardiogenesis provides the most appropriate context to study the developmental transition from a multipotent undifferentiated stem cell to a differentiated cardiomyocyte. A greater understanding of the logic of heart formation will accelerate the translation of promising cell-based therapies from bench to bedside and reduce the burden of this disease.

FORMATION OF THE CARDIAC CRESCENT

During vertebrate development, the multichambered heart is the first identifiable organ to form. Cardiac cells are derived from the developing mesoderm, which is formed during gastrulation when epiblast cells ingress through the primitive streak. The cardiogenic mesoderm cells migrate anterolaterally during gastrulation and they remain uncommitted to a cardiac fate because mesodermal progenitor cells marked by the expression of mesoderm posterior 1 (MesP1) contribute to the muscle of the head, neck, and heart. Once these cells have given rise to the anterolateral mesoderm, they adopt a crescent-shaped structure, the *cardiac crescent*, and become irreversibly committed to the cardiac lineage (Fig. 1.1A). The expression of a number of key cardiac transcription factors in the cardiac crescent has been described, including homeodomain (e.g., Nkx2.5 and islet-1 (Isl-1)), GATA (e.g., GATA-4), and T-box transcription factors (1–3). The relationship of the cardiac, vascular, and endothelial population of cells in the heart is not clear, but recent studies suggest that they are all derived from a common cardiovascular progenitor during embryonic development (4–6). Recent studies have also shown that MesP1+ cells contribute to all of the main cell lineages in the heart, namely, cardiomyocytes, smooth muscle, endothelial, and epicardial cells, and may represent such common cardiovascular progenitor cells (7).

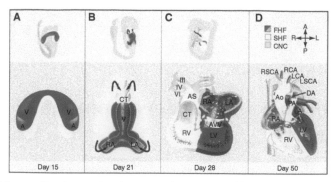

Figure 1.1 Mammalian heart development. (**A**) The cardiogenic mesoderm cells migrate anterolaterally during gastrulation. Once these cells have given rise to the anterolateral mesoderm at about day 15 (ED7.0 in mouse), the FHF cells adopt a crescent-shaped structure, the cardiac crescent, in the anterior region of the embryo. The SHF cells are located medial and dorsal to the FHF. (**B**) Following midline fusion (ED8.0 in mouse day 21 in human), the cardiac crescent generates a tubular structure consisting of an outer myocardial layer and an inner endocardial layer. Moreover, the SHF cells, which lie dorsal to the linear heart tube, begin to migrate (arrows) into the anterior and posterior ends of the tube to form the right ventricle, CT, and part of the atria (A). (**C**) At day 28 in human (ED 8.5 in mouse), rightward looping of the heart tube results in the first asymmetric event in the developing embryo and assigns the right–left identity of the cardiac chambers. Following looping, CNC cells migrate (arrow) into the OFT. This leads to the septation of the OFT and patterns the bilaterally symmetric aortic arch arteries (III, IV, and VI). (**D**) Subsequently, contribution of the CNC cells to the endocardial cushions leads to the septation of the ventricles, atria, and AVV. Mesenchymalization of the endocardial cushions leads to the formation of the aortopulmonary septum and segregation of the systemic and pulmonary ventriculoarterial connections. Proliferation and specification of endocardial cushion cells result in mature valvular structures. Finally, the four-chambered heart is connected to the pulmonary trunk and aorta, which ensures the proper pulmonary and systemic circulation of blood after birth. *Abbreviations*: Ao, aorta; AS, aortic sac; AVV, atrioventricular valves; CNC, cardiac neural crest; CT, conotruncus; DA, ductus arteriosus; FHF, first heart field; LA, left atrium; LCA, left carotid artery; LSCA, left subclavian artery; OFT, outflow tract; PA, pulmonary artery; RSCA, right subclavian artery; RCA, right carotid artery; SHF, second heart field; V, ventricle; LV, left ventricle; RA, right atrium. *Source*: Adapted from Ref. 11.

FORMATION OF THE VENTRICLES

Following midline fusion, the cardiac crescent generates a tubular structure consisting of an outer epithelial myocardial layer and an inner endothelial cell layer, known as the endocardium (Fig. 1.1B) (8). A layer of extracellular matrix, called the cardiac jelly, is found between these two layers and provides the supportive environment for the formation of cardiac valves and trabecular myocardium. This linear heart tube is attached to the embryo proper through the dorsal mesocardium, which marks the separation between right and left sides of the heart tube. Rightward looping of the heart tube results in the first asymmetric event in the developing embryo and assigns the right–left identity of the cardiac chambers (Fig. 1.1C). The left–right asymmetry observed at this stage is mediated by the expression of Sonic hedgehog and Nodal in the lateral mesoderm (9). These signals are interpreted by Pitx2, which further activates asymmetric chamber development (10). Through combinatorial interactions between T-box (e.g., Tbx2, 3, 5, and 20) (11), GATA, and NK transcription factors, chamber-specific developmental events begin to take place. The expression of

Hand1 appears to be specifically required for the formation of the left ventricle (LV), whereas Hand2 is expressed in both ventricles but required only for the development of the right ventricle (RV) (12,13). The addition of cells to the growing poles of the heart tube results in further elongation and looping of the tubular heart (14).

Although initially thought to develop from a single pool of cardiac crescent cells, recent data have established that the right and left ventricles develop from two distinct populations of progenitor cells. The first heart field (FHF) progenitors are derived from the splanchnic mesoderm and give rise to the early heart tube. These cells contribute to the LV, the atria, and the atrioventricular canal. FHF progenitor cells express transcription factors, such as Nkx2.5, Hand1/2, and Tbx5 and 20, but this expression is not exclusive because some are also expressed in the second heart field (SHF) (15). Tbx5, the most specific FHF marker, is expressed in the cardiac crescent, the heart tube, and the developing atria and the LV (16). Genetic deletion of Tbx5 in mice leads to LV hypoplasia and defects in cardiac inflow tract reminiscent of human Holt–Oram syndrome (17).

The SHF progenitor cells can be identified at the cardiac crescent stage by their anatomic location dorsal and medial to the FHF progenitor cells in the cardiac crescent. The SHF progenitor cells express Isl-1, Foxh1, and Fgf 8 and 10 (15), colonize the arterial pole region of the developing heart (18), and give rise to the myocardium of the RV, interventricular septum, and the outflow tract (OFT) (19,20). Progenitors from the SHF express Isl-1, which is essential for the development of the OFT, RV, and the inflow region (21). Addition of SHF cells to the developing heart occurs in two phases. An initial contribution gives rise to the myocardium of the RV and the proximal OFT. A second phase of contribution produces the myocardial wall of the distal OFT region and the smooth muscle cells of the ascending aortic arch and pulmonary trunk (5). The addition of SHF cells to the distal portion of the OFT requires Tbx1 (22). Indeed, deletion of Tbx1 in mice leads to pathologic phenotypes consistent with human DiGeorge syndrome characterized by cardiovascular and craniofacial defects (23). Expression of FGF8 from the developing endoderm is also required for the formation of the OFT, as its absence leads to double-outlet RV or persistent truncus arteriosus (24).

Following the formation of primitive right and left ventricles, cells within these chambers actively express Nkx2.5, Tbx5, and GATA-4 to activate gene expression in a cooperative fashion. Expression of contractile and sarcomeric proteins is enhanced by mechanical loading exerted by the pulsatile blood flow within the heart resulting in further chamber hypertrophy. Locally expressed Tbx2 and 3 compete with Tbx5 to repress transcription in the nonchamber regions, including the inflow tract, the atrioventricular canal, and the OFT. Finally, the Neuregulin-1/ErB2 pathway is crucial for the formation of the trabeculation of the ventricular myocardium via a mechanism that remains to be elucidated (25).

FORMATION OF THE ATRIA

The left and right atrial precursor cells are located caudally and on the laterodorsal surface of the heart tube. These atrial precursors proliferate rapidly and migrate rostrally toward the arterial pole to form the atrial chambers. Cells from the primary atrial septum (a.k.a. septum primum) proliferate and migrate toward the atrioventricular cushions to partition the common atrial chamber into the right and left atria. Subsequently, the endocardial cushion expands both rostrally and caudally to generate the second atrial septum (a.k.a. septum secundum) and the membranous portion of the ventricular septum, respectively. The first molecular evidence for a biologic difference between the right and left atria is the left atrial-specific expression of Pitx2. Indeed, genetic studies in mice have shown that Pitx2 is an essential transcription factor for left atrial development (26).

Cells in the developing atria are mostly derived from the FHF with some contributions from cells in the SHF (21). Indeed, progenitor cells in the SHF contribute to cells at the inlet pole of the common atrium (27). Mice mutant for Nkx2.5 show severe cardiac abnormalities, including absence of the atria (28). Moreover, Isl1 expression at the venous pole provides an explanation for the atrial and atrioventricular septation defects observed in Isl-1 mutant mice (29). Mice lacking the nuclear receptor CoupTFII or Tbx5 lack atrial myocytes (17,30). Retinoid acid signaling is necessary for the atrial precursor cells to initiate atrial morphogenesis (31). Moreover, the requirement (or participation) of Gridlock, Foxc1 and 2, and Sox 7 and 18 in atrial specification has been reported (32–36).

The entry of blood cells from the systemic vessels into the atria is mediated by the left and right horns of the sinous venosus. The left sinus horn connects with the left superior caval vein, and the right sinus horn interfaces with the right superior caval vein. As development progresses, the left superior caval vein regresses, resulting in the formation of the oblique vein. The remnant of the left sinus horn becomes the coronary sinus emptying into the right atrium. Therefore, all the systemic venous tributaries terminate in the right atrium. The venous valves demarcate the junction between the portion of the right atrium derived from the systemic veins and the remainder of the atrial chamber. The left atrium is connected to the pulmonary veins at the corners of the atrial roof (37). It has been shown that the proximal pulmonary vein is derived from atrial cardiomyocytes based on the expression of cardiac sarcomeric proteins and electrophysiologic analysis. This sleeve of myocardium is in electromechanical continuity with cardiomyocytes of the left atrium and has recently been recognized as a common source of atrial tachyarrhythmia. Normally, the origin of the septum primum places the pulmonary vein within the left atrium. In rare circumstances when the septum primum is improperly formed, the left superior pulmonary vein will drain into the right atrium, resulting in anomalous pulmonary venous return. This condition is frequently associated with a primum atrial septal defect.

FORMATION OF THE OUTFLOW TRACT

The OFT is derived from two cell sources. Cells from the SHF populate the proximal OFT and become contiguous with the smooth muscle cells of the aortic arches (Fig. 1.1C). This occurs via epithelial-to-mesenchymal transformation followed by invasion of neurocrest-derived cells from the pharyngeal mesenchyme. This mesenchymalization of the endocardial cushion leads to the formation of the aortopulmonary septum and segregation of the systemic and pulmonary ventriculoarterial connections (38). Concurrently, the aortic arch vessels undergo massive remodeling such that the connection of the aortic OFT with the left fourth arch artery results in the formation of the definitive aortic arch. The developing pulmonary trunk, on the other hand, is in continuity with the artery of the left sixth arch forming the eventual pulmonary artery. Interestingly, the expression of vascular growth factors, such as PDGF and VEGF are required for the asymmetric remodeling of the left fourth and sixth arch arteries (39). Furthermore, reduced blood flow through the right fourth and sixth arch arteries leads to their eventual regression (39).

FORMATION OF THE CORONARY VESSELS

The epicardium is derived from the proepicardial organ, a structure lying adjacent to the venous tributaries of the embryonic heart. Through an epithelial-to-mesenchymal transformation, the epicardium-derived cells (EPDCs) acquire the capacity to migrate and invade the myocardium to give rise to the smooth muscle cells of the coronary arteries as well as the interstitial fibroblasts (Fig. 1.1B, C). Based on lineage tracing studies in chick, the origin of endothelial cells in the coronary vessels was previously thought to arise from epicardial cells as well (40). This view has been challenged as Cre-LoxP-based analysis of epicardial cell derivatives failed to show their contribution to coronary endothelial cells (41). Besides their physical contribution, the EPDCs provide critical signaling mediators, such as FGFs and retinoid acid, for the development of the myocardium (42,43). The secretion of FGFs by epicardial cells also regulates growth and differentiation of smooth muscle cells of the coronary vessels. Moreover, the EPDCs facilitate the entry of cells from the coronary artery plexus within the myocardium into the root of the proximal aorta (44).

FORMATION OF THE VALVES

Valvular defects account for approximately 30% of all cardiovascular malformations (45). During embryogenesis heart valves arise from the AVC and the OFT regions. Endocardial cells in this area undergo endothelial-to-mesenchymal transition mediated by reciprocal signaling events between the endocardium and the myocardium activating, in part, the transforming growth factor-beta (TGFβ) pathway. These molecular events lead, eventually, to the formation of the endocardial cushions. Cells in the cushion differentiate into fibrous tissues that serve as the primordial valve–forming cells and the membranous septa. BMP 2 and Sox 9 expression is required for the proliferation and specification of endocardial cushion cells into mature valvular structures (46). Moreover, transcription factor such as NF-ATc and mediator of BMP signaling such as Smad6 are required for proper valve formation (47). As the forming valves begin to mature, they decellularize progressively and the remaining tissue becomes quite fibrous-like with characteristic of proteins from the cartilage. The three layers of the remaining valve, namely, fibrosa, spongiosa, and atrialis, are composed of collagen, proteoglycan, and elastin, respectively (48).

The left side of the atrioventricular canal (AVC) becomes incorporated into the definitive left atrium as the vestibule of the mitral valve. Similarly, the right side of the AVC is incorporated into the right atrium to form the vestibule of the tricuspid valve. Fusion of cells of the endocardial cushion with the epicardial-derived mesenchyme leads to the interruption of the continuity between atrial and ventricular myocardium.

FORMATION OF THE CONDUCTION SYSTEM

All embryonic cardiomyocytes of the early developing heart possess intrinsic pacemaker activity. Pacemaking impulses are evoked at the posterior inflow tract (sinus venosus and atrium) well before heart begins beating (49). These impulses spread anteriorly and unidirectionally toward the OFT. However, following specialization, dominant pacemaker activity is found at the sinoatrial node (SAN), which resides at the junction of the right atrium and the superior caval vein. This node contains specialized cells that repolarize faster than other immature cardiomyocytes, hence driving the initiation of depolarization.

The origin of the conduction system [e.g., atrioventricular node (AVN) and Purkinje fiber] cells is incompletely understood. The available evidence suggests that they arise from cardiomyocyte precursors (50). Pitx2 suppresses the development of atrial cardiomyocytes into sinoatrial node-like cells in the left atrium (51). HCN4 is expressed in the SAN and plays an important role in the pacemaking activity of the SAN (52). Nkx2.5 suppresses HCN4 and Tbx3 in noncardiac conduction cells (51). Based on this observation, it was suggested that Nkx2.5 prevents the SAN phenotype from invading the atria or the atrial phenotype invading the SAN (51). The region that retains its continuity with the AVC becomes the AVN and the bundle of His (53). When the heart begins to loop, the AVN delays the impulse from the SAN, thereby generating independent contractions of the atrial and ventricular chambers. The atrial and ventricular chambers are also electromechanically separated by the interposed AVC. Nkx2.5 is expressed in the AVN, but not in the SAN (54). This suggests difference in their mechanisms of formation and perhaps functions.

Besides the SAN and the AVN, the conduction system possesses ventricular components, the Purkinje system. These include the atrioventricular bundle of His and the left and right bundles branches. The components of the Purkinje system are believed to originate from a subset of cardiomyocytes surrounding the developing coronary arteries in response to endothelin-1 (55). The ventricular conduction system accounts for the rapid spread of the electrical impulses from the AVN to the apex. It was recently shown that the development of the ventricular components of the conduction system depend on a molecular pathway including Nkx2.5, Tbx5, and Id2 (56). Indeed, Id2 is downstream of Nkx2.5 and Tbx5 and promotes conduction system differentiation in the ventricles. Moreover, the arterial beds seem to play a role in the differentiation of the conduction cells of the Purkinje fibers (55). Finally, the endothelin-1 signaling pathway has been shown to play an important role for Purkinje fiber differentiation (57–59).

DEVELOPMENTAL CARDIOGENESIS AND THERAPEUTIC IMPLICATIONS

Despite tremendous advances in our knowledge of heart development, the goal of mammalian heart regeneration remains elusive. The exciting discoveries in stem cell biology coupled with a system-based approach to explore cardiac cell lineage commitment and differentiation will provide a more comprehensive understanding of the key regulatory networks involved in mammalian cardiogenesis. This knowledge will be critical for our future success in stem/progenitor cell-mediated cardiac repair and for the identification of promising therapeutic avenues, like the creation of a bioartificial heart (60). The use of cardiac cells derived from pluripotent stem cells or from endogenous cardiac stem cells provides much optimism for the hope that one day heart failure can be prevented or even reversed with novel gene or cell-based therapy (61–63).

REFERENCES

1. Bodmer R. The gene tinman is required for specification of the heart and visceral muscles in drosophila. Development 1993; 118: 719–29.
2. Komuro I, Izumo S. Csx: a murine homeobox-containing gene specifically expressed in the developing heart. Proc Natl Acad Sci USA 1993; 90: 8145–9.
3. Lints TJ, Parsons LM, Hartley L, Lyons I, Harvey RP. Nkx-2.5: a novel murine homeobox gene expressed in early heart progenitor cells and their myogenic descendants. Development 1993; 119: 419–31.
4. Kattman SJ, Huber TL, Keller GM. Multipotent flk-1+ cardiovascular progenitor cells give rise to the cardiomyocyte, endothelial, and vascular smooth muscle lineages. Dev Cell 2006; 11: 723–32.
5. Moretti A, Caron L, Nakano A, et al. Multipotent embryonic isl1+ progenitor cells lead to cardiac, smooth muscle, and endothelial cell diversification. Cell 2006; 127: 1151–65.
6. Wu SM, Fujiwara Y, Cibulsky SM, et al. Developmental origin of a bipotential myocardial and smooth muscle cell precursor in the mammalian heart. Cell 2006; 127: 1137–50.
7. Saga Y, Kitajima S, Miyagawa-Tomita S. Mesp1 expression is the earliest sign of cardiovascular development. Trends Cardiovasc Med 2000; 10: 345–52.
8. DeRuiter MC, Poelmann RE, VanderPlas-de Vries I, Mentink MM, Gittenberger-de Groot AC. The development of the myocardium and endocardium in mouse embryos. Fusion of two heart tubes?. Anat Embryol (Berl) 1992; 185: 461–73.
9. Capdevila J, Vogan KJ, Tabin CJ, Izpisua Belmonte JC. Mechanisms of left-right determination in vertebrates. Cell 2000; 101: 9–21.
10. Harvey RP. Patterning the vertebrate heart. Nat Rev Genet 2002; 3: 544–56.
11. Srivastava D. Making or breaking the heart: from lineage determination to morphogenesis. Cell 2006; 126: 1037–48.
12. Srivastava D, Cserjesi P, Olson EN. A subclass of bHLH proteins required for cardiac morphogenesis. Science 1995; 270: 1995–9.
13. Srivastava D, Thomas T, Lin Q, et al. Regulation of cardiac mesodermal and neural crest development by the bHLH transcription factor, dHAND. Nat Genet 1997; 16: 154–60.

14. Kelly RG, Buckingham ME. The anterior heart-forming field: voyage to the arterial pole of the heart. Trends Genet 2002; 18: 210–16.

15. Buckingham M, Meilhac S, Zaffran S. Building the mammalian heart from two sources of myocardial cells. Nat Rev Genet 2005; 6: 826–35.

16. Bruneau BG, Logan M, Davis N, et al. Chamber-specific cardiac expression of Tbx5 and heart defects in Holt-Oram syndrome. Dev Biol 1999; 211: 100–8.

17. Bruneau BG, Nemer G, Schmitt JP, et al. A murine model of Holt-Oram syndrome defines roles of the T-box transcription factor Tbx5 in cardiogenesis and disease. Cell 2001; 106: 709–21.

18. Kelly RG, Brown NA, Buckingham ME. The arterial pole of the mouse heart forms from Fgf10-expressing cells in pharyngeal mesoderm. Dev Cell 2001; 1: 435–40.

19. Verzi MP, McCulley DJ, De Val S, Dodou E, Black BL. The right ventricle, outflow tract, and ventricular septum comprise a restricted expression domain within the secondary/anterior heart field. Dev Biol 2005; 287: 134–45.

20. Waldo KL, Kumiski DH, Wallis KT, et al. Conotruncal myocardium arises from a secondary heart field. Development 2001; 128: 3179–88.

21. Cai CL, Liang X, Shi Y, et al. Isl1 identifies a cardiac progenitor population that proliferates prior to differentiation and contributes a majority of cells to the heart. Dev Cell 2003; 5: 877–89.

22. Xu H, Morishima M, Wylie JN, et al. Tbx1 has a dual role in the morphogenesis of the cardiac outflow tract. Development 2004; 131: 3217–27.

23. Baldini A. DiGeorge syndrome: the use of model organisms to dissect complex genetics. Hum Mol Genet 2002; 11: 2363–9.

24. Abu-Issa R, Smyth G, Smoak I, Yamamura K, Meyers EN. Fgf8 is required for pharyngeal arch and cardiovascular development in the mouse. Development 2002; 129: 4613–25.

25. Smith TK, Bader DM. Signals from both sides: control of cardiac development by the endocardium and epicardium. Semin Cell Dev Biol 2007; 18: 84–9.

26. Ai D, Liu W, Ma L, et al. Pitx2 regulates cardiac left-right asymmetry by patterning second cardiac lineage-derived myocardium. Dev Biol 2006; 296: 437–49.

27. Galli D, Dominguez JN, Zaffran S, et al. Atrial myocardium derives from the posterior region of the second heart field, which acquires left-right identity as Pitx2c is expressed. Development 2008; 135: 1157–67.

28. Lyons I, Parsons L M, Hartley L, et al. Myogenic and morphogenetic defects in the heart tubes of murine embryos lacking the homeo box gene Nkx2-5. Genes Dev 1995; 9: 1654–66.

29. Snarr BS, O'Neal JL, Chintalapudi MR, et al. Isl1 expression at the venous pole identifies a novel role for the second heart field in cardiac development. Circ Res 2007; 101: 971–4.

30. Pereira FA, Qiu Y, Zhou G, Tsai MJ, Tsai SY. The orphan nuclear receptor COUP-TFII is required for angiogenesis and heart development. Genes Dev 1999; 13: 1037–49.

31. Xavier-Neto J, Shapiro MD, Houghton L, Rosenthal N. Sequential programs of retinoic acid synthesis in the myocardial and epicardial layers of the developing avian heart. Dev Biol 2000; 219: 129–41.

32. Herpers R, van de Kamp E, Duckers HJ, Schulte-Merker S. Redundant roles for sox7 and sox18 in arteriovenous specification in zebrafish. Circ Res 2008; 102: 12–15.

33. Kokubo H, Miyagawa-Tomita S, Nakazawa M, Saga Y, Johnson RL. Mouse hesr1 and hesr2 genes are redundantly required to mediate Notch signaling in the developing cardiovascular system. Dev Biol 2005; 278: 301–9.

34. Kume T, Jiang H, Topczewska JM, Hogan BL. The murine winged helix transcription factors, Foxc1 and Foxc2, are both required for cardiovascular development and somitogenesis. Genes Dev 2001; 15: 2470–82.

35. Seo S, Fujita H, Nakano A, et al. The forkhead transcription factors, Foxc1 and Foxc2, are required for arterial specification and lymphatic sprouting during vascular development. Dev Biol 2006; 294: 458–70.

36. Zhong TP, Rosenberg M, Mohideen MA, Weinstein B, Fishman MC. Gridlock, an HLH gene required for assembly of the aorta in zebrafish. Science 2000; 287: 1820–4.

37. Anderson RH, Brown NA, Moorman AF. Development and structures of the venous pole of the heart. Dev Dyn 2006; 235: 2–9.

38. Waldo KL, Hutson MR, Stadt HA, et al. Cardiac neural crest is necessary for normal addition of the myocardium to the arterial pole from the secondary heart field. Dev Biol 2005; 281: 66–77.

39. Yashiro K, Shiratori H, Hamada H. Haemodynamics determined by a genetic programme govern asymmetric development of the aortic arch. Nature 2007; 450: 285–8.

40. Mikawa T, Gourdie RG. Pericardial mesoderm generates a population of coronary smooth muscle cells migrating into the heart along with ingrowth of the epicardial organ. Dev Biol 1996; 174: 221–32.

41. Cai CL, Martin JC, Sun Y, et al. A myocardial lineage derives from Tbx18 epicardial cells. Nature 2008; 454: 104–108.
42. Lavine KJ, Yu K, White AC, et al. Endocardial and epicardial derived FGF signals regulate myocardial proliferation and differentiation in vivo. Dev Cell 2005; 8: 85–95.
43. Merki E, Zamora M, Raya A, et al. Epicardial retinoid X receptor alpha is required for myocardial growth and coronary artery formation. Proc Natl Acad Sci USA 2005; 102: 18455–60.
44. Eralp I, Lie-Venema H, DeRuiter MC, et al. Coronary artery and orifice development is associated with proper timing of epicardial outgrowth and correlated fas-ligand-associated apoptosis patterns. Circ Res 2005; 96: 526–34.
45. Supino PG, Borer JS, Yin A, Dillingham E, McClymont W. The epidemiology of valvular heart diseases: the problem is growing. Adv Cardiol 2004; 41: 9–15.
46. Lincoln J, Kist R, Scherer G, Yutzey KE. Sox9 is required for precursor cell expansion and extracellular matrix organization during mouse heart valve development. Dev Biol 2007; 305: 120–32.
47. Srivastava D, Olson EN. A genetic blueprint for cardiac development. Nature 2000; 407: 221–6.
48. Lincoln J, Lange AW, Yutzey KE. Hearts and bones: shared regulatory mechanisms in heart valve, cartilage, tendon, and bone development. Dev Biol 2006; 294: 292–302.
49. Kamino K. Optical approaches to ontogeny of electrical activity and related functional organization during early heart development. Physiol Rev 1991; 71: 53–91.
50. Mikawa T, Hurtado R. Development of the cardiac conduction system. Semin Cell Dev Biol 2007; 18: 90–100.
51. Mommersteeg MT, Hoogaars WM, Prall OW, et al. Molecular pathway for the localized formation of the sinoatrial node. Circ Res 2007; 100: 354–62.
52. Stieber J, Hofmann F, Ludwig A. Pacemaker channels and sinus node arrhythmia. Trends Cardiovasc Med 2004; 14: 23–8.
53. Wessels A, Vermeulen JL, Verbeek FJ, et al. Spatial distribution of "tissue-specific" antigens in the developing human heart and skeletal muscle. III. an immunohistochemical analysis of the distribution of the neural tissue antigen G1N2 in the embryonic heart; implications for the development of the atrioventricular conduction system. Anat Rec 1992; 232: 97–111.
54. Jay PY, Harris BS, Maguire CT, et al. Nkx2-5 mutation causes anatomic hypoplasia of the cardiac conduction system. J Clin Invest 2004; 113: 1130–7.
55. Hyer J, Johansen M, Prasad A, et al. Induction of Purkinje fiber differentiation by coronary arterialization. Proc Natl Acad Sci USA 1999; 96: 13214–18.
56. Moskowitz IP, Kim JB, Moore ML, et al. A molecular pathway including Id2, Tbx5, and Nkx2-5 required for cardiac conduction system development. Cell 2007; 129: 1365–76.
57. Kanzawa N, Poma CP, Takebayashi-Suzuki K, et al. Competency of embryonic cardiomyocytes to undergo Purkinje fiber differentiation is regulated by endothelin receptor expression. Development 2002; 129: 3185–94.
58. Pennisi DJ, Rentschler S, Gourdie RG, Fishman GI, Mikawa T. Induction and patterning of the cardiac conduction system. Int J Dev Biol 2002; 46: 765–75.
59. Takebayashi-Suzuki K, Yanagisawa M, Gourdie RG, Kanzawa N, Mikawa T. In vivo induction of cardiac Purkinje fiber differentiation by coexpression of preproendothelin-1 and endothelin converting enzyme-1. Development 2000; 127: 3523–32.
60. Ott HC, Matthiesen TS, Goh SK, et al. Perfusion-decellularized matrix: using nature's platform to engineer a bioartificial heart. Nat Med 2008; 14: 213–21.
61. Segers VF, Lee RT. Stem-cell therapy for cardiac disease. Nature 2008; 451: 937–42.
62. Takahashi K, Tanabe K, Ohnuki M, et al. Induction of pluripotent stem cells from adult human fibroblasts by defined factors. Cell 2007; 131: 861–72.
63. Yu J, Vodyanik MA, Smuga-Otto K, et al. Induced pluripotent stem cell lines derived from human somatic cells. Science 2007; 318: 1917–20.

2

The genetics of dilated and hypertrophic cardiomyopathies

Calum A. MacRae

The conceptual framework of cardiovascular disease has changed rapidly since the advent of cardiac catheterization and echocardiography. As novel techniques improve our ability to objectively assess coronary or ventricular anatomy, to define cardiac physiology and, with the advent of magnetic resonance imaging (MRI), to noninvasively assess tissue characteristics so our perception of the nature of many conditions has evolved (1,2).

Pathologic studies had characterized ventricular dilatation and hypertrophy as distinctive adaptive responses of the myocardium to volume or pressure overload (Fig. 2.1). These processes were thought to represent initial homeostatic responses that led to maladaptive physiology, and ultimately heart failure. The application of new diagnostic tools enabled systematic studies of the natural history of myocardial disease. In many instances there was no evidence of an antecedent valvular lesion or myocardial injury (2,3). These early descriptions of cardiomyopathy also recognized familial cases, and the concept of primary myocardial disease emerged. Despite these insights, the majority of cardiomyopathies were thought to result from occult acquired insults, a perception that persists to this day for some forms. Work in animal models of abnormal myocardial loading and myocardial infarction, all subsequently confirmed in humans, established the fundamental pathways of hypertrophy and of ventricular remodeling in response to acquired insults. The substantial variation in individual responses implicated inherited contributions to myocardial pathophysiology irrespective of the primary mechanisms.

The promise of identifying the causal genes underlying primary forms of myocardial dysfunction or variation in responses to acquired injury fueled the tremendous expansion in the application of genetic approaches in cardiomyopathies that has occurred in the last two decades. Using human and model system genetics, great strides have been made in our understanding of the pathophysiology of both ventricular dilatation and hypertrophy. Although molecular diagnostics may yet be several years from impacting day-to-day clinical practice, genetic testing is on the horizon and the interdependence of clinical cardiology and molecular genetics is already evident. This chapter will outline the evolving relationship between molecular genetics and clinical investigation, emphasizing the role of our current knowledge in the diagnosis and management of the major adult cardiomyopathies.

GENETIC METHODS

In any disease the presence of a major genetic effect has implications, not only for molecular studies of the etiology of the disorder, but also for the design and interpretation of

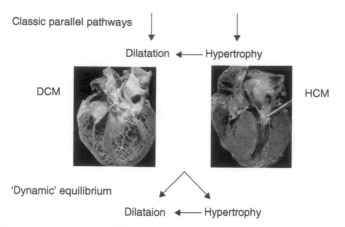

Classic parallel pathways

Dilatation ◄——— Hypertrophy

DCM   HCM

'Dynamic' equilibrium

Dilataion ◄——— Hypertrophy

Figure 2.1 The classic view of HCM and DCM as discrete biologic pathways has been challenged by recent molecular genetic studies, although the physiologic profiles are clearly distinct. Hypertrophy is known to progress to dilatation in many situations, including in some familial cardiomyopathies. However, a single mutation in different individuals within the same family may cause hypertrophy or dilatation, as a result, it is presumed, of genetic or environmental modifiers. Understanding the mechanisms favoring the development of hypertrophy or dilatation will help in the dissection of acquired forms of ventricular remodeling. *Abbreviations*: DCM, dilated cardiomyopathy; HCM, hypertrophic cardiomyopathy.

studies of its diagnosis and management. These clinical inferences are often relevant long before the intricacies of the molecular pathways are understood. To place the clinical and molecular insights in context, some background on the vocabulary and techniques used in genetic analysis is useful (Table 2.1).

Familial Aggregation

Although in some instances the genetic nature of cardiomyopathy is obvious, in many cases the symptomatic individuals represent only a subset of those carrying the underlying trait. Large families with a clear family history of the disease may be the exception rather than the rule, even when a condition is highly heritable. The expression of the phenotype may require additional genetic or environmental factors, or may vary stochastically (Fig. 2.1). To gain an objective sense of how important genetic factors might be in any given form of heart disease, systematic studies of familial aggregation and lineal transmission are necessary (4). There are several ways of crudely estimating the degree of heritability, the most common of which is a simple sibling recurrence risk. A detailed assessment of the mode and magnitude of any heritable component requires more complex segregation analysis using multiple families. The genetic basis for hypertrophic cardiomyopathy (HCM) was obvious from simple inspection (3,5,6), but it required systematic analysis of a first-degree relative to detect the large heritable contribution to dilated cardiomyopathy (DCM) (7).

Genetic Linkage

Genetics has proved to be a powerful tool to define causal mechanisms in biology, not because of some unique property of DNA, but rather because of the magnitude of the underlying effect in Mendelian genetic disorders and the development of techniques to map the underlying genes using the segregation of genetic markers with affection status through families (8). In many situations where disease genes have been cloned, the risk to

Table 2.1   Basic Genetic Terminology

Allele	Any one of the sequence variants of a particular gene.
Genome	The complete DNA sequence of an organism.
Haplotype	A series of sequence variations that are linked together on a single chromosome.
Introns and exons	Genes are initially transcribed as continuous sequences, but only some segments (the exons) of the resulting messenger RNA molecules contain information that encodes the gene's protein product. The intervening regions between exons (the introns), are excised (or spliced) from the RNA to generate the final RNA from which the protein is translated.
Messenger RNA (mRNA)	Following the initial transcription from a gene of a continuous RNA molecule, this molecule is then processed in a number of ways, including splicing to generate the final messenger RNA, which is then translated by the cell's machinery into a protein.
Mutation	Any variation in sequence from a reference state.
Phenotype	The complete set of characteristics of an organism including morphology and function.
Proteome	The complete repertoire of proteins encoded by a genome.
SNP	Most of the variation in DNA sequence between individual members of a population is the result of changes in single nucleotides. These polymorphisms are known as SNPs.
Transcription	The copying of a gene's DNA into RNA.
Translation	The synthesis of a protein from the information encoded in a messenger RNA.

Abbreviation: SNP, *single-nucleotide polymorphism.*

first-degree relatives is several hundred times that in the general population. The theory behind proving causality using genetics closely parallels Koch's postulates in infection—another situation where an abnormal genome is responsible for a disease. If there is a large genetic effect, given the way in which DNA is transmitted to the next generation, it is possible to define a segment of mutated DNA, which when transmitted is sufficient to cause the phenotype in question. This specific segment of DNA can potentially be isolated, and be shown to be distinct from the normal sequence at that location. Finally, the mutated gene, if introduced into a normal organism, should be capable of causing the disease phenotype. Clearly the literal fulfillment of these criteria is not feasible in humans, but the methods of human molecular genetics allow very similar logic to be applied (Table 2.2).

If the DNA of family members can be screened to identify those segments of the genome that are consistently transmitted with the phenotype, then the causative gene can be mapped. The development of panels of informative markers, polymorphic between individuals, made such genetic linkage analyses possible. These anonymous markers allow individual DNA segments to be followed as they pass through a family, defining their relationship (or lack of relationship) with the disease. Using a panel of markers that "scans" the entire genome with even one sufficiently large family with a given genetic disease it is possible to define a minimal location for the disease, and ultimately to identify the causal mutation (9). The passage, or segregation, of a phenotype through a single lineage is the

Table 2.2   Criteria for Defining a Causal Mutation—Discrimination from a Polymorphism

I. *The "mutation" should segregate perfectly with disease*

The sequence anomaly must be present in all the affected individuals and absent from all the
  unaffected individuals. Ideally, two independent means should be used to confirm that this is the
  case. The best statistical support for this segregation is an LOD or logarithm of the odds score
  (also used in anonymous mapping studies), which estimates the likelihood of random
  co-segregation as a function of the number of informative events.

II. *The "mutation" should not be present in a normal population*

Rare polymorphisms may be overrepresented in any given large family. These polymorphisms may
  have functional significance, yet not be responsible for disease. For example, null alleles have been
  described for many genes including that encoding the beta-cardiac myosin heavy chain, but when
  present in the heterozygous state may be of no import. It is necessary to screen a large normal
  population for any putative mutation to ensure that it is not simply an incidental polymorphism.

III. *The "mutation" should effect substantial change on the gene sequence*

There should be indirect evidence that the mutation will have a biologic effect. This may be
  obvious for some mutations, which disrupt the sense of the entire coding sequence of the gene.
  Other mutations will have more subtle effects, changing only a single amino acid residue. The
  confirmation of these substitutions as disease causing may require additional studies, such as
  comparative sequence analyses (with the same gene in other species, or similar genes in the same
  species, to see if a particular residue is highly conserved), *in vitro* structure function analysis or
  in vivo genetic analyses.

IV. *The introduction of the "mutation" should be sufficient to cause disease*

There should be direct evidence that the mutation has a biologic effect. The ultimate proof of
  causality lies in the demonstration that the simple addition of the mutation is sufficient to
  recapitulate the disease. This is usually done in genetic model organisms, but the specific
  knock-in of a point mutation (the most common mutation calls in human disease) is rarely
  performed. Often a causal role is inferred from transgenic expression of a mutant gene or from
  knock-out of the gene. The demonstration of disease in association with a *de novo* mutation in
  humans is the logical equivalent.

hallmark of a genetic trait (4). Segregation also allows other features that track with the
classic phenotype to be identified, informing the investigator about relationships between
apparently incidental clinical findings (Figs. 2.1 and 2.2) (10).

Clinical Diagnosis and Genetic Mapping

It is impossible to separate human molecular genetics from clinical assessment, especially in the study of cardiovascular disorders. The final chromosomal disease interval is
defined in terms of recombinants, that is, individuals whose phenotypes and genotypes
are discordant as a result of inferred chromosomal recombination between the marker
and the disease-causing mutation. The definition of recombinant events is thus completely
dependent on the clinical phenotype (8,9). Given the central role of the phenotype in
mapping and cloning a disease gene, it is conventional to adopt conservative criteria for
assigning positive and negative affection status in human molecular genetics. It is much
better to define an individual as unknown, than to attempt molecular studies with the
wrong diagnosis. The need to exclude equivocal family members has restricted positional
cloning efforts to very large kindreds with highly penetrant forms of disease. This has
also led to difficulties identifying the genes underlying disorders where there are any
genetic or environmental modifiers. The closer a genetic marker is located to the disease-
causing mutation, the fewer recombinants are evident at that marker, until ultimately the
disease-causing mutation itself should segregate perfectly with the phenotype.

Relating Genotype to Phenotype - Variable Expressivity

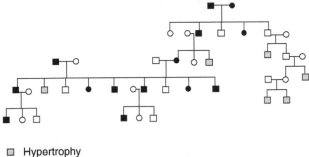

☐   Hypertrophy

■   Sudden death

Figure 2.2 Only the systematic assessment of family members of affected probands reveals the true genetic architecture of a syndrome, which may be very homogeneous as in some of the cardiomyopathies, or highly heterogeneous as in this example from a study of atrial fibrillation.

Positional Cloning

Once a minimal disease interval has been defined by genetic mapping, the techniques of positional cloning are used to identify all the genes within this interval and to screen these genes for mutations (8). The ability to grow, in yeast or bacterial artificial chromosomes, long segments of several hundred thousand base pairs of human DNA, allows large stretches of a human chromosome to be cloned in an overlapping set of such segments. This "contig" of human DNA clones can then be manipulated, and eventually sequenced to define the disease gene. Importantly, the cloning of the mutated gene does not require any *a priori* assumptions regarding the mechanism of disease. This lack of dependence on previous hypotheses has resulted in the discovery of truly novel pathways, and is particularly powerful in complicated disorders with multiple manifestations (11). The completion of the Human Genome project ensures that no matter how large the final disease locus, it is possible to rapidly identify the genes within the final interval (12). This has expedited the cloning of disease genes, and broadened the scope of positional cloning projects to include progressively smaller families with less penetrant diseases (13).

Genetic Association Studies

Not all phenotypes segregate in large families and so other genetic techniques have been developed, which do not use transmission probability, but instead rely on simple association of genotypes with phenotypes within a population (4,14). These studies are qualitatively different from linkage analyses, but have proliferated in recent years (15,16). Genetic association studies have many limitations (17,18). By their nature they are biased in favor of small population-wide effects, so that in the face of etiologic heterogeneity even major genetic effects might be missed. A second major problem is population stratification, which results in spurious association of a polymorphism with disease, simply because both the disease and the unlinked sequence variant are found in the same population subgroup. This can be partly addressed by replicating the findings in large study cohorts drawn from genetically distinct populations. The prior probability that any observed effect is a result of the specific polymorphism(s) studied is usually extremely low, resulting in an unacceptably high false-positive rate (through Bayesian inference). Importantly, because of the absence of segregation information inherent in these studies, it also is impossible to causally relate specific variants or a definitively bounded segment of DNA to a phenotype. The phenotype in question may result from variations in linked genes, in so-called dysequilbrium with the tested polymorphism. These issues would, at least in part, be dealt with by using extended haplotypes of markers in large populations.

Many of these problems are minimized by the use of genome-wide association studies with very rigorous statistical thresholds and robust replication in further cohorts. Nevertheless, several issues remain, most of which are relevant to the study of the cardiomyopathies. The simultaneous identification of multiple novel loci with very small effect sizes has outstripped our ability to evaluate these loci. In addition, many of the most successful studies to date have explained only a small proportion of the heritability. The cost of increasing the size (and power) of many human disease cohorts for secondary analyses of loci of borderline statistical significance and for exploring gene–gene or gene–environment interactions is prohibitive. These findings also confirm that etiologic hetero-geneity must be resolved if genetic studies are to realize their full power. The overall consensus remains that genetic association studies may be extremely difficult to interpret even when carried out in an exemplary fashion, for conditions where there is evidence of very large genetic effects. Ultimately, such approaches may be useful in the detection of disease modifiers.

Locus and Allelic Heterogeneity

Our ability to distinguish discrete pathologic processes, and to undertake genetic analy-sis of these phenotypes is limited by the resolution of current diagnostic techniques. Mutations in many different genes may give rise to very similar phenotypes, a phenom-enon known as genetic heterogeneity. This situation is compounded by the fact that inherited cardiac conditions often result in premature mortality, so that common founder mutations are rare. Virtually every HCM family whose disease results from abnormality of a specific sarcomeric contractile protein has a different mutation (so-called allelic heterogeneity) (11). This degree of heterogeneity also exists for most other Mendelian cardiac conditions where there are "selection" pressures operating against mutations in the causal genes (19). Importantly, subtle differences in the clinical manifestations between mutated genes may not be detectable until genetic studies have been completed (19), and "pure" populations studied.

Modifiers of Simple Traits

Any clinician who has cared for families with monogenic forms of cardiomyopathy will have been struck by the range of clinical manifestations within a single family, in which the primary genetic abnormality is identical in each affected individual. While some of this variable expressivity represents our limited understanding of the phenotype itself, some of the variation is the result of modifier genes or of environmental factors (20). The discovery of such modifier loci or environmental agents is a major focus of current research. If we cannot discern these modifiers in the context of a simple disease caused by a single major gene we will have tremendous difficulty understanding more complex situations where multiple genes interact (4,14).

USING GENETICS IN CLINICAL PRACTICE

Genotypic information is not yet of any utility in patient management. However, clinical genetic analyses have the ability to inform patient care long before the genes for all the inherited cardiomyopathies have been cloned. The application of clinical genetic princi-ples in the diagnosis and management of inherited heart disease will be outlined, before details of the molecular basis of specific disorders are discussed.

Family-Based Diagnosis

The presence of a definitive diagnosis of HCM or DCM in a first-degree relative dramatically changes the implications of any cardiovascular evaluation. For example, minor electrocardiogram (ECG) abnormalities are viewed in a different light in the context of a family history of HCM than if there were no such history (21). In some cases the definitive diagnosis in a particular patient is only clear from the integrated evaluation of multiple individuals within the same family. This is increasingly recognized in families in which several "discrete" phenotypes, such as DCM and arrhythmogenic right ventricular cardiomyopathy, co-segregate. Only the complete evaluation of the entire kindred would allow all of these important features to be detected. The ethical implications of family-based diagnosis remain to be fully explored, but informed consent is critical if the data from multiple individuals are to be collected.

Diagnosis—History

The history often offers evidence that the presenting condition results from an inherited diathesis. Cardiomyopathy patients may have had subtle evidence of disease from an early age. Functional limitations are often attributed to respiratory illness, but it is usually possible to discern other features of the underlying disease. Comparison of exercise capacity at various ages with that of peers is useful in the evaluation of symptoms, such as muscle pains or syncope. The presence of other premature medical disorders suggests specific conditions (Tables 2.3 and 2.4).

A comprehensive family history is an integral part of every patient encounter, but is particularly important in the diagnosis and management of adult cardiomyopathies. In addition to defining the basic structure of the family, it is vital to define in as much detail as is possible any cardiac conditions (or even potential cardiac conditions) in first- or second-degree relatives. Probands will often be unaware of subtle distinctions between cardiac diseases, and many affected relatives of cardiomyopathy patients may be mislabeled as other cardiac conditions, such as valvular heart disease or myocardial infarction. Once the basic family structure is defined, and an overview of any inherited traits is obtained, the actual symptoms, age of onset, specific treatments [e.g., diuretics, pacemakers, implantable cardioverter defibrillators (ICDs), surgery] and modes of death for every member of the nuclear family should be elicited. Specific enquiry regarding extracardiac phenotypes, including skeletal or other myopathies, peripheral sensory or motor neuropathy, and premature diabetes or liver disease, is recommended. On many occasions a family history is not appreciated, simply because the potential connection between different phenotypes is not explicitly considered (22).

It is important to remember that other apparently unrelated disorders or events may in fact represent *formes frustes* of the same primary abnormality (Fig. 2.2). Thus, for example, atrial fibrillation in a young relative of a patient with cardiomyopathy is likely a manifestation of the same gene defect, and an unexplained motor vehicle accident may represent an undetected sudden death (23). The family history also allows some sense of the mode of inheritance to be obtained (Fig. 2.2). A careful family history must also be a prominent feature in any follow-up visits. Patients will often have gleaned much additional family history from interactions with relatives since the initial patient encounter. Indeed, empowering the patient to obtain such information should be a goal of the initial encounter.

Clinical Evaluation

The physical examination and subsequent clinical investigation of any cardiomyopathy patient are also heavily influenced by the genetic basis of the major syndromes. The examination should look for general morphologic abnormalities, such as facial or other

Table 2.3 Major Adult Dilated Cardiomyopathy Loci

Locus	Inheritance Mode	Disease Gene	Specific Clinical Features	References
1q21 CDCD-1	AD	Lamin A/C	AVB, LGMD, CMT	(47)
1q31 CMD-1D	AD	Cardiac troponin T		(55)
2q14-22 CMD-1H	AD	Unknown		(79)
2q31 CMD-1G	AD	Titin		(80)
2q35 CMD-1I	AD	Desmin	RCM, inclusion myopathy	(81)
3p21 CDCD-2	AD	SCN5A	AVB	(46,82)
4q12	AR	β-Sarcoglycan		(83)
5q33 CMD-1L	AD/AR	δ-Sarcoglycan		(84)
6p24	AR	Desmoplakin	ARVC, wooly hair	(85)
6q12-16 CMD-1K	AD	Unknown	Possibly allelic with AFib	(86)
6q22 CMD-1P	AD	Phospholamban		(87)
6q23 CDCD-3	AD	Unknown	AVB, LGMD	(88)
6q23-24 CMD-1J	AD	EYA-4	Sensorineural hearing loss	(89,90)
9q13	AD	Unknown		(91)
10q21-23	AD	Vinculin		
10q21-23	AD	Unknown	Possibly allelic with AFib	(92)
10q22-23	AD	LIM domain binding 3		(93)
10q25	AD	RBM20	Fibrosis, SCD	(94)
11p15 CMD-1M	AD	CSRP3		(56)
11p11	AD	MYBP-C		(95)
12p12 CMD-1O	AD	ABCC9		(96)
14q12 CMD-1S	AD	β-Cardiac myosin heavy chain (MYH7)		(55)
15q14 CMD-1R	AD	α-Cardiac actin	Co-segregating FHC	(53)
19q13	AD	Myotonin	Anticipation, AVB, arrhythmia	(26)
19q13	AD	TNNI3		(97)
Xp21	X-Linked	Dystrophin		(48)
Xq28	X-Linked	Emerin	AVB, humeroperoneal MD	(51)

Notes: This table does not include some putative DCM disease genes where the absence of segregation or functional data precludes definitive attribution of causality. In addition, some contiguous loci may be allelic, but there is insufficient information to determine this at present. *Abbreviations*: AD, autosomal dominant; AFib, atrial fibrillation; AR, autosomal recessive; AVB, atrioventricular block; CMT, Charcot–Marie–Tooth; FHC, familial hypertrophic cardiomyopathy; LGMD, limb-girdle muscular dystrophy; MYBP-C, myosin-binding protein-C; MD, muscular dystrophy; RCM, restrictive cardiomyopathy; SCD, sudden cardiac death.

Table 2.4 Hypertrophic Cardiomyopathy Loci

Locus	Inheritance Mode	Disease Gene	Specific Clinical Features	References
1q31	AD	Cardiac troponin T	Hypertrophy may be less marked	(98)
3p	AD/AR	Myosin light chain 3 kinase	Midcavity/PAP muscle hypertrophy	(70)
7q36	AD	PRKAG2	Glycogen storage AVB, WPW	(71)
9	AR	Frataxin	Ataxia	(78)
11p15	AD	Muscle LIM protein		(99)
11p11	AD	MYBP-C	Often later onset disease	(100)
14q12	AD	MYH7 and MYH 6		(66)
15q14	AD	α-Cardiac actin	Co-segregating DCM	(69)
15q22	AD	α-Tropomyosin		(98)
19q13	AD	Cardiac troponin I	Co-segregating RCM	(101)
20q13	AD	Myosin light chain kinase	Midcavity/PAP muscle hypertrophy	(70)
Xq24	X-linked	LAMP2	Lysosomal storage, SCD	(102)

Abbreviations: AD, autosomal dominant; AR, autosomal recessive; AVB, atrioventricular block; DCM, dilated cardiomyopathy; MYBP-C, myosin-binding protein-C; MYH, myosin heavy chain; PAP, papillary; PRKAG2, adenosine monophosphate-activated protein kinase gamma-2 subunit; RCM, restrictive cardiomyopathy; WPW, ventricular pre-excitation.

dysmorphism, midline defects, cutaneous anomalies, or the typical features of disorders, such as myotonic dystrophy (24). Several forms of cardiomyopathy are associated with myopathy involving extraocular muscles, the limb girdles, or other muscle groups. The evidence of a skeletal myopathy may be subtle, such as a mild scoliosis or distorted pedal architecture. Finally, it is important also to exclude tendon contractures, ataxia, peripheral neuropathy, and other neurological disorders. Cardiomyopathy is by definition a diagnosis of exclusion, and potentially reversible specific heart muscle diseases, such as coronary artery disease, glycogen storage disorders, hemochromatosis, and dysthyroid heart disease should be formally eliminated (25).

Once appropriate permission has been obtained, objective data from other family members are extremely helpful in the diagnosis and management of adult cardiomyopathies. The direct examination of at-risk family members often will be useful in making a diagnosis in equivocal cases. Pathognomonic components of the phenotype, including extracardiac features, may only be present in a limited subset within the family. Objective phenotypic assignment is especially helpful in inferring the mode of inheritance (24). Evidence of any mode of inheritance other than autosomal dominant substantially changes the differential diagnosis in any cardiomyopathy (Tables 2.3 and 2.4). Mitochondrial inheritance is usually seen in the context of left ventricular hypertrophy (LVH), whereas X-linked and recessive syndromes are most often seen with DCM, though Friedreich's ataxia is one recessive cause for myocardial hypertrophy. Progressive changes in the severity of a phenotype from one generation to the next, known as anticipation or reverse anticipation depending on the direction, are characteristic of triplet repeat expansion disorders, such as myotonic dystrophy (26). The study of extended families offers a unique opportunity to investigate patient cohorts with remarkably homogeneous etiologies (27). In a family with a highly penetrant Mendelian disease, an identical etiology may reasonably be inferred for each affected individual, and the key features of the specific disorder evaluated in exquisite detail. The potential of even a moderate size of family for molecular genetic analysis is remarkable, and referral to specialized centers for such studies should be considered (25,28).

Prognosis

The remarkable range of clinical outcomes, even within a single kindred, complicates the clinical management of both DCM and HCM (29–31). There are families where multiple members have died suddenly or required transplantation, and others where the disease is little more than an incidental echocardiographic finding. Initial studies of the presentation, natural history, and clinical physiology of the cardiomyopathies were based on highly selected series from large national referral centers. Subsequent series from regional centers have attempted to redress the balance. However, the major biases implicit in inherited disease have not been addressed in most studies. Without knowing the extent to which individuals (particularly phenotypic outliers) are related, or the contributions of specific families to the overall cohort, it is impossible to begin to interpret even simple studies.

The identification of the underlying gene defects led to the hope that molecular diagnostics would revolutionize risk stratification. Preliminary work has suggested that specific mutations may be associated with high rates of adverse outcome, but these studies by necessity include multiple members from each family. Contradictory results have emerged from both clinical and molecular studies (32,33). The extent of genetic heterogeneity, the large size of the genes involved, and the high rates of new mutation have slowed the arrival of genotype–phenotype studies based on serial probands. Understanding the distinctive contributions of the primary mutation, familial modifiers and therapeutic interventions will require novel statistical methods to robustly extract information from extended families (20,34).

In the absence of rigorous, objective techniques to attribute risk to specific mutations, the effect of the same mutation in different generations of the same family remains a reasonable (albeit imperfect) index of both the likely natural history of the disease and of the prognosis in an individual patient. Family members share not only the same causative mutation but also much of their genetic background, environment, and experiences. A complete family history and evaluation offers a sense of the range of expressivity of a particular genetic defect. It may be difficult to get any real overview of how a condition behaves in a small family, but in larger kindreds clear patterns of natural history sometimes emerge. It is usually possible to assess the penetrance, any major effects of gender and other features, such as anticipation in larger families. At the very least these data are helpful in genetic counseling of potential parents.

The integration of such imperfect data with similarly skewed results from heterogeneous clinical cohorts is, unfortunately, the current state of the art. Dogmatic overinterpretation of both types of data is widespread. In most instances the disparate results seen between studies reflect the underlying etiologic heterogeneity of the study cohorts as much as any true biologic differences. Large series of probands are being genotyped by several groups, but the routine clinical use of genotyping will have to await new sequencing methods (35). The rate of new mutations, and the fact that modifiers may significantly affect risk is also stimulating novel approaches to defining prognosis using proteomics or functional assays.

Asymptomatic affected relatives are another group that might benefit from screening (28). The risk of complications, including death, is not clearly related to symptoms.

There are therapies for both DCM and HCM, some of which are proved to reduce mortality. Systematic screening has been recommended for prognostic reasons in "at-risk" asymptomatic relatives of probands with both DCM and HCM (25). Although there are no objective data to support any form of screening, if undertaken in specialist centers with appropriate counseling, it is reasonable in the context of active research programs.

Management

The management of the cardiomyopathies has also proved to be difficult to study empirically. Once again the literature contains many equivocal or contradictory studies, and consensus is often lacking. This situation reflects the rarity of many of the conditions, aggregation of heterogeneous populations, and ultimately the failure to deal with familial confounders.

In the face of these uncertainties, clinical decisions must be based on what limited information is available, and, as outlined above, much of that information is likely to come from the extended family of the patient. Management strategies often must be tailored to the individual family, and their previous experiences with the disease. For example, despite the lack of support from randomized controlled trials, it is difficult not to implant an ICD in an affected young adult whose siblings have died suddenly from HCM. The history of any disease within extended kindreds is usually firmly embedded in the family psyche, and this may also require management approaches that extend far beyond the individual patient. Family meetings and counseling have a role, and involvement with a research group with long-term positive goals can be extremely helpful in engaging individuals who may have withdrawn from dealing with their disease.

SPECIFIC DISORDERS—DILATED CARDIOMYOPATHY
Definitions and Clinical Features

The diagnostic criteria for DCM have evolved little since the earliest definitions of idiopathic cardiomegaly were first proposed when the exclusion of ischemic or valvular causes of heart failure became possible (2). The most evolved current definition of DCM dates from a NIH conference, and highlights the lack of positive diagnostic features (36). Despite being "a diagnosis of exclusion," several key attributes of the syndrome seem remarkably consistent across a wide variety of studies. The histologic abnormalities seen are almost invariably those of a myocardial dystrophy, with rather patchy myocyte loss, inflammatory infiltrates, and hypertrophy of remaining myocytes. There are several typical modes of clinical presentation. These include an acute left ventricular failure syndrome in younger adults, often associated with an upper respiratory prodrome, classic congestive biventricular heart failure, and sudden cardiac death (37). Increasingly, individuals with asymptomatic left ventricular dysfunction are recognized. Interestingly, the families of probands with overt DCM are enriched not only for DCM, but also for asymptomatic borderline left ventricular enlargement or depression of contractile shortening (38). These phenotypes are presumed to represent *formes frustes* of DCM in carriers of the mutant gene. There is evidence that these individuals have active myocardial disease, and that some progress to DCM, but the precise relationship to overt DCM remains unclear (39).

The possibility that some subtle phenotypes represent early forms of DCM is particularly attractive in the context of the evidence from randomized controlled trials for the efficacy of several drug regimens in asymptomatic left ventricular dysfunction (40). These data, combined with the need to identify gene carriers in the genetic analysis of any pedigree has led to the evolution of less stringent diagnostic criteria for the diagnosis of DCM in the context of a family history (41). Several extracardiac phenotypes are known to be associated with DCM, and may prove more reliable than subtle cardiac criteria for the diagnosis of gene carriers in a genetic study. It is important to recall that while these criteria may be useful for specialized clinical or molecular studies they have not been validated formally in studies of clinical management. Long-term studies of these subclinically affected family members have also described a substantial number of individuals whose echocardiograms revert to normal (42). The concept is emerging of a genetically determined predisposition to DCM, in the context of a range of common myocardial insults. The variability of progression to overt cardiac disease may be the result of distinctive environmental exposures, modifier genes, or other unknown stochastic factors. In any event, it is clear that the data available at present do not allow easy prognostication from any specific subclinical marker. Hopefully, as our understanding of the etiology of DCM increases the mechanism for these variations will be uncovered, and it will prove possible to identify those who will develop clinically significant disease, and to institute appropriate preventive measures.

Etiology of DCM

As a consequence of several clinical and pathologic features of the disease, a large proportion of DCM was thought to represent the sequelae of previous viral myocarditis (43). Many cases present with a history of upper respiratory tract symptoms or a vague systemic inflammatory prodrome, and there are often patchy inflammatory infiltrates in myocardial biopsy specimens. Although viral myocarditis undoubtedly may result in persistent ventricular dysfunction, the process is usually associated with reversible abnormalities. Furthermore, there is evidence that even when associated with such an acute prodrome, DCM is the result of a process that has been active for many years, suggesting that this symptom complex is secondary, perhaps to pulmonary or hepatic congestion (44). Several drugs and other environmental toxins, including alcohol, are known to cause cardiomyopathy through a variety of mechanisms. Similarly, specific nutritional deprivations, such as selenium deficiency or beri-beri, occasionally cause heart failure. Autoimmune diseases have been reported to cluster with DCM, and circulating autoantibodies are found in many patients, but primary immunologic abnormalities have been difficult to identify (45). It was in the context of such conflicting hypotheses that genetic studies became attractive.

Clinical Genetics

Even in the earliest descriptions of DCM, an inherited basis was suspected from the occasional observation of extended families. Michels et al. studied the role of genetic factors in DCM by systematically evaluating the first-degree relatives of probands with DCM for evidence of the same disease (7). There was evidence of DCM in 25% of "at-risk" first-degree relatives. Subsequent work from other investigators has confirmed the prevalence of DCM in relatives and demonstrated that when subclinical phenotypes are included, up to 40% of DCM probands have affected relatives (38). These findings, in the context of the successes of positional cloning approaches in HCM and other syndromes, led to an explosion in the number of genetic studies in DCM. Initial anticipation of early etiologic insights in DCM has been tempered by the consistent finding of small kindreds with relatively few definitively affected individuals (30). Autosomal dominant patterns of inheritance predominate. The large numbers of individuals with subclinical disease have complicated linkage analyses and are one important reason for the high ratio of mapped loci to cloned genes (Table 2.3). The structure of the families seen in DCM undoubtedly reflects some real biologic attribute of the syndrome, but what this is remains unclear.

Genetic Mapping

Genetic linkage studies have identified at least 20 loci at which DCM is a prominent component of the phenotype. Many genetic loci are represented by only a single published family (Table 2.3). These data suggest a high degree of genetic heterogeneity, as seen in HCM. The detection of any allelic heterogeneity will require the identification of the responsible genes at these loci. The genetic heterogeneity is only partly reflected in clinical or phenotypic heterogeneity (30,41). At least two general patterns of disease have been identified, each of which may represent a distinct etiologic pathway. There are several recessive or X-linked muscular dystrophies that are associated with significant cardiomyopathy, often disproportionate to the extent of the skeletal involvement (30,41). The second phenotypic group is represented by families with autosomal dominant atrioventricular conduction block, intraventricular conduction disease, and DCM. These appear to be manifestations of a syndrome, which may also include arrhythmogenic right ventricular cardiomyopathy, or in some cases, limb-girdle muscular dystrophy (30,46,47). Even these clinical entities themselves are known to be genetically heterogeneous. The vast majority of DCM families are small kindreds with two or three clearly affected individuals in a distribution consistent with autosomal dominant inheritance, with no obvious extracardiac features.

Molecular Genetics and Pathophysiology

The genes responsible for several forms of DCM have been identified, and investigation of the basic mechanisms of disease has been initiated. These genes belong to several different gene families, with at present no unifying theme to unite them.

Dystrophin and Associated Proteins

The cloning of the dystrophin gene responsible for Duchenne and Becker variants of muscular dystrophy, both of which have significant cardiac involvement, suggested this protein and other members of the dystrophin-associated glycoprotein complex (DGC) as potential candidates for other forms of DCM. So far only occasional families with X-linked DCM have been directly linked to mutations in the dystrophin gene, and other recessive cardiomyopathies have been found to result from mutations in the sarcoglycan genes (48,49). Several screens of multiple affected probands have effectively excluded this protein complex as a common cause of DCM when unselected for mode of inheritance.

Mutations in this pathway are presumed to cause DCM through the role of the large dystroglycan-associated glycoprotein complex in the structural integrity of the link between cytoskeleton and extracellular matrix. However, work by Coral-Vazquez et al. implicating the DGC in membrane cycling, aggregation of signaling molecules into local, functionally important, clusters, and in adenoviral pathobiology suggests a more complicated picture. Secondary abnormalities of the smooth muscle, affecting the circulation, have also been implicated in both skeletal myopathy and cardiomyopathy (50).

Nuclear Membrane Proteins

The discovery of mutations in the lamin A/C gene in families with conduction disease and DCM suggested that such nuclear membrane proteins may represent a distinct pathway in cardiomyopathy (47). These results built on the demonstration of a very similar cardiac phenotype with mutations in emerin, another nuclear membrane protein (51). While it is possible that this pathway results in DCM through defects in the mechanical integrity of the nucleus, the biologic functions of these genes are only beginning to be understood. Interestingly, lamin A/C is widely expressed, yet the diverse phenotypes associated with mutations in this gene appear to be tissue specific. Several other loci exist where the discrete phenotypes of conduction disease and DCM co-segregate. The cloning of mutated genes at these loci will add further potential pathway members and may elucidate the mechanisms of disease in this subset (52).

Cytoskeletal and Sarcomeric Proteins

Given the specialized role of cardiac myocytes, and the adaptation of the cytoskeletal apparatus in the sarcomere, many of these genes became candidates in the search for the causes of DCM (53). The screening of large numbers of probands for mutations in the cardiac actin gene resulted in the identification of mutations in a very small fraction of these patients. Subsequent screening of series of probands has only confirmed the extreme rarity of actin mutations as causal factors in DCM (54). Interestingly, mutations in other sarcomeric protein genes, previously implicated in hypertrophic disease, have now been shown to cause DCM (55,56). Truncating mutations in the titin gene have been directly implicated as the cause of around 30% of cases. These genes potentially implicate several pathways in the development of DCM, including contractile dysfunction, inefficient energetics, and myocardial sensing of stretch or other stimuli (57,58).

Myotonic Dystrophy

Occasionally, myotonic dystrophy will present with DCM or conduction disease as a prominent component, although it is unusual for this to be the case throughout a single pedigree. The mutated gene appears to be a protein kinase, but the mutation, an expanded triplet repeat in the 3' untranslated region of the coding sequence, may also affect transcription of neighboring loci through the effects on splicing (26). This triplet repeat is unstable as it is transmitted meiotically, and so disease will often become more severe with each progressive generation, a phenomenon known as anticipation. The mechanism by which the mutation results in cardiomyopathy is unknown, but abnormal levels or localization of the myotonin kinase have been hypothesized.

Splicing Factors

Recent work in both animal models and human genetics has implicated mutations in a splicing factor, known as RNA Binding Motif protein 20 (RBM20), in as many as 5–10% of patients with DCM. There is some evidence that mutations in this gene may be more common in families where sudden death is prominent, and that in some of these families extensive interstitial and subendocardial cardiac fibrosis may be common. Interestingly, this splicing factor appears to be required for the transition from fetal-to-adult isoforms for many proteins of diverse functions (sarcomeric, cytoskeletal, metabolic, transmembrane transport) within the heart. Whether this pathway is a true mechanistic link between inherited and acquired forms of heart failure remains to be seen, but understanding the regulation of the fetal gene program will undoubtedly shed insight into all forms of ventricular dysfunction.

Disease Models

The identification of the causal human genes in DCM offers a definitive starting point for the generation of true disease models. The production of genetically modified organisms bearing the cognate mutations allows investigators to unravel the mechanisms of cardiomyopathy from the initial insult through to the final phenotype (11). Insights may also travel in the opposite direction with model organism phenotypes implicating previously unsuspected genes as candidates for DCM (56). Importantly, such inferences require confirmation through human molecular work, as null mutants or tissue-specific transgenics may not reflect any naturally occurring human genotype. For example, mouse models of DGC-related DCM confirmed initial hypotheses suggesting that force transmission is somehow disrupted, but importantly have also revealed many other pathways that may be involved in the abnormal myocardial function seen. Clearly, it will be crucial to understand these multiple mechanisms of disease if we are to be able to design specific therapies for primary myocardial disease.

Specific models for other heritable forms of DCM do not yet exist, although there are intense efforts to generate such models, not only in mouse but in larger animals and in smaller screenable organisms, such as the zebrafish and the fruitfly (59). These model systems will enable the detailed pathophysiology of each gene defect to be explored, the causative pathways to be defined, and ultimately allow screening to directly identify modifier loci or novel therapies. The disparate phenotypes already identified in DCM suggest that no single pathway is the sole culprit in this syndrome. The dissection of the fundamental biology of these conditions should illuminate not only such differences, but also the commonalities which may well be shared with acquired forms of heart failure.

HYPERTROPHIC CARDIOMYOPATHY
Definitions and Clinical Features
In the late 1950s, LVH was believed always to represent an adaptive response to some ventricular loading abnormality (2). Investigators began to describe a familial syndrome characterized by syncope, sudden death, and marked LVH at postmortem (60). The presence of severe disorganization of muscle cells and myofibrils were originally thought to be specific to this syndrome; however, Maron et al's work suggests that this may be a matter of degree. The advent of echocardiography and the study of extended families revealed many asymptomatic yet obviously affected individuals (5). Atypical distributions of left or right ventricular hypertrophy may occur, often with particular patterns observed within a family. Importantly, as noted earlier, there may be no hypertrophy, and the ECG can be more sensitive than echocardiography in the context of an extended family (21), although tissue characterization with MRI may ultimately prove definitive.

HCM usually presents during, or after, the adolescent growth spurt, unfortunately often as sudden death. The mechanism of premature sudden death is not always certain. Ventricular arrhythmias undoubtedly are a major factor, yet coronary anomalies, pulmonary embolism, or other mechanisms have also been invoked (29). Nonsustained ventricular tachycardia (VT) is a marker for sudden death risk, but sophisticated assessments of myocardial substrate may be superior, although difficult to apply widely (61). Syncope was a prominent feature of the earliest descriptions of HCM, and a significant cause of confusion with aortic valve disease. Recurrent syncope is one of the most common clinical presentations of HCM, but here too the precise mechanisms remain obscure (29). There are documented peripheral vasomotor abnormalities in many of these patients, although these do not correlate perfectly with clinical events (62). Chest pain is a typical feature, and often quite debilitating. While ischemia is always invoked there are few data to support this as a common mechanism (63). Coronary anomalies should be excluded in those patients with prominent exertional pain. Patchy abnormalities are seen on thallium studies, but other assessments of myocardial blood flow are usually normal (64). The possibility of primary metabolic mismatch has resurfaced in the search for a unifying hypothesis for HCM pathogenesis (see below) (65). Less prevalent clinical features include substantial functional subaortic and intraventricular obstruction, subaortic membranes, and structural mitral valve abnormalities. There is progression to ventricular dilatation and congestive heart failure in a proportion of patients. Despite the high heritability of HCM, little is known of the segregation patterns of any of the clinical features other than echocardiographic variables. Two decades of investigation failed to uncover the etiology of HCM, until the molecular genetic basis of the syndrome was revealed by work from the Seidman laboratory (9,66).

Clinical Genetics
Early descriptions of HCM realized that a large proportion of cases appeared to be familial, with prominent autosomal dominant inheritance. Studies based on less extreme

echocardiographic phenotypes suggested lower rates of familial disease. Systematic family screening now suggests that as many as 90% of cases have evidence of autosomal dominant disease. The remaining, "sporadic," cases may represent true *de novo* mutations in the genes that cause Mendelian forms of the disease, or poorly penetrant forms of the underlying trait (5).

A large proportion of the genetic studies, and the majority of all clinical studies in HCM, are dominated by individuals from pedigrees with severe hypertrophic phenotypes or a high incidence of sudden death. Attempts to redress this balance have concentrated on nonreferral populations, but virtually every study has failed to assess the potential related-ness of individual subjects from a single center. In a condition dominated by Mendelian forms the biases introduced by events or phenotypes in related individuals, genetic founder effects, or other less obvious confounders make many current clinical investigations diffi-cult to interpret. It is not surprising that conflicting data have appeared on the predictive value of most clinical indices, including ECG and echocardiographic variables (29). There is an unmet need for proband-based clinical studies (and molecular studies), and the devel-opment of segregation-based approaches to the assessment of clinical risk within families.

Clinical genetic studies identified discrete entities within the HCM syndrome several years prior to the use of molecular analyses. Braunwald's initial description of familial HCM noted several large kindreds with evidence of ventricular pre-excitation and LVH (Fig. 2.3) (3). In each family these conditions appeared to co-segregate tightly, and subsequent work has shown that pre-excitation, atrioventricular block, and HCM are linked to a specific locus (22). Although pre-excitation or pseudo-pre-excitation are seen with other forms of HCM, sponta-neous heart block has not been reported in other adult-onset families with autosomal inheri-tance. Interestingly, pre-excitation and atrioventricular block are also seen in HCM due to mitochondrial disease (67). Families in which both HCM and DCM co-segregate represent a second distinctive clinical entity. These kindreds contain multiple individuals with either phenotype, and importantly those with DCM do not appear to have progressed from HCM.

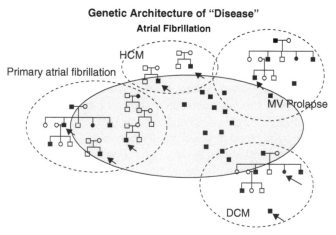

Figure 2.3 Apparently unrelated phenotypes may be mechanistically related from simple clinical observations in extended families. Here left ventricular hypertrophy and ventricular pre-excitation co-segregate in a single pedigree, in a manner consistent with a single auto-somal dominant disorder. The study of individual parts of the pedigree, such as the highlighted nuclear family in which hypertrophy is prominent (enlarged symbols), may give a distorted view of the overall nature of the underlying trait. *Abbreviations*: DCM, dilated cardiomyopathy; HCM, hypertrophic cardiomyopathy; MV, mitral valve.

Although inbred families with heterozygous or more severe homozygous phenotypes have been reported (68), autosomal recessive HCM is uncommon. The most frequent form of recessive ventricular hypertrophy is observed in the context of Friedreich's ataxia, where there is cardiac involvement in the majority of cases. Other situations in which idiopathic cardiac hypertrophy is seen include Noonan's syndrome, and several of the glycogen storage disorders.

Molecular Genetics

HCM is caused by mutations in at least 12 genes, the majority of which encode sarcomeric contractile proteins (11). Although many hundreds of genes have been implicated in experimental forms of LVH, only this group of genes appears to cause human hypertrophic disease. Although there is tremendous variation in the expression of HCM even within a single family, some generalizations about the phenotypes seen with specific genes have emerged. Families with co-segregating HCM and DCM seem to be a particular feature of mutations in the cardiac actin gene on chromosome 15 (69). Focal midcavity and disproportionate papillary muscle hypertrophy are associated with mutations in the myosin light chains (70). The syndrome of massive wall thickening, pre-excitation, and eventual atrioventricular block has been shown to be a result of activating mutations in the PRKAG2 gene (71). In this syndrome the increased wall thickening is due not only to true myocyte hypertrophy, but also to a significant component of inappropriate glycogen storage. Other data have suggested that myosin mutations may be associated with significantly more hypertrophy than troponin mutations (72), and myosin binding protein C mutations may be associated with later onset hypertrophic disease (73,74). Finally, mutations in the cardiac troponin I gene have been associated with families exhibiting both HCM and restrictive cardiomyopathy (75).

Disease Models

Murine models of HCM have been generated and recapitulate many of the features of the human disease (11). There is evidence that the most specific of these models, the Arg-403Gln alpha-cardiac myosin "knock-in" mouse, has significant abnormalities of myocyte cross-bridge cycling. The precise pathways involved have not yet been elucidated, but clearly these mice offer the potential to dissect the fundamental mechanisms of hypertrophy most relevant to human disease. The temptation to invoke a single pathway is strong, but evidence of major genetic modifiers, and discrete hypertrophic disorders with distinctive clinical features suggest otherwise. It is possible even that different mutations in the same gene result in hypertrophy through distinct mechanisms. Inefficient energy utilization may act as an important downstream pathway, and might help reconcile some of the divergent effects of mutations on contractility (76,77). The disease gene in Friedreich's ataxia is a mitochondrial protein, which appears to be a critical player in oxidative stress pathways (78). Many other processes such as sarcomere assembly or cellular transport pathways might also be perturbed, and the systematic study of genetic models will be vital to unraveling the pathophysiology of primary cardiac hypertrophy.

GENETIC TESTING FOR CARDIOMYOPATHY

The last few years have seen tremendous advances in the study of the human cardiomyopathies. The major pathways have been identified in HCM and similar inroads are beginning to be made in DCM. The identification of molecular pathways is the first step in developing a mechanistic understanding of these Mendelian disorders, but also offers the potential for insight into more common types of ventricular remodeling. It is clear that the morphologic classification of the cardiomyopathies that has proved to be so useful for decades will be superceded by a molecular nosology.

There is still much investigation required before molecular diagnostics or prognostics are useful in the management of these disorders. Extremely helpful insights can be gained from simple clinical genetic tools, and these insights may be more immediately applicable than molecular information. Nevertheless, genetic testing for both DCM and HCM is already widely available. The sensitivity and specificity are improving constantly, but remain at a level where molecular diagnosis is often simply not feasible. Allelic and genetic heterogeneity and variable expressivity render prognostication difficult. Negative genetic tests have little value in the presence of overt clinical disease, whereas the majority of "positive" tests have few data to support a definitive causal role. In this setting, management decisions based on the results of genetic testing are fraught with uncertainty, which is already a prominent feature in the management of such patients.

At present, the primary benefit of identifying a causal mutation in a proband is to facilitate screening in family members. A preclinical diagnosis achieved through screening programs can allow initiation of further monitoring programs for disease development, avoidance of high-risk behaviors, and potential implementation of disease-mitigating therapies. Our ultimate desire for tailored prognostication and therapy is probably only to be realized when we can generate phenotypic profiles that can integrate individual genotypic and environmenstal information and yet be common enough to allow accuracy in prediction and classification.

REFERENCES

1. Braunwald E, Bristow MR. Congestive heart failure: fifty years of progress. Circulation 2000; 102(20 Suppl 4): IV14–23.
2. Goodwin JF. Congestive and hypertrophic cardiomyopathies: a decade of study. Lancet 1970; 1: 732–9.
3. Frank S, Braunwald E. Idiopathic hypertrophic subaortic stenosis. Clinical analysis of 126 patients with emphasis on the natural history. Circulation 1968; 37: 759–88.
4. Risch NJ. Searching for genetic determinants in the new millennium. Nature 2000; 405: 847–56.
5. Maron BJ, Nichols PF, Pickle LW, et al. Patterns of inheritance in hypertrophic cardiomyopathy: assessment by M-mode and two-dimensional echocardiography. Am J Cardiol 1984; 53: 1087–94.
6. Greaves SC, Roche AH, Neutze JM, et al. Inheritance of hypertrophic cardiomyopathy: a cross sectional and M mode echocardiographic study of 50 families. Br Heart J 1987; 58: 259–66.
7. Michels VV, Moll PP, Miller FA, et al. The frequency of familial dilated cardiomyopathy in a series of patients with idiopathic dilated cardiomyopathy. N Engl J Med 1992; 326: 77–82.
8. Collins FS. Positional cloning: let's not call it reverse anymore. Nat Genet 1992; 1: 3–6.
9. Jarcho JA, McKenna W, Pare JA, et al. Mapping a gene for familial hypertrophic cardiomyopathy to chromosome 14q1. N Engl J Med 1989; 321: 1372–8.
10. Freimer N, Sabatti C. The human phenome project. Nat Genet 2003; 34: 15–21.
11. Seidman JG, Seidman C. The genetic basis for cardiomyopathy: from mutation identification to mechanistic paradigms. Cell 2001; 104: 557–67.
12. Lander ES, Linton LM, Birren B, et al. Initial sequencing and analysis of the human genome. Nature 2001; 409: 860–921.
13. Ellinor PT, Shin JT, Moore RK, et al. A genetic locus for atrial fibrillation maps to Chromosome 6q12-21. Circulation 2003; 107: 2880–3.
14. Lander ES, Schork NJ. Genetic dissection of complex traits. Science 1994; 265: 2037–48.
15. Marian AJ, Yu QT, Workman R, et al. Angiotensin-converting enzyme polymorphism in hypertrophic cardiomyopathy and sudden cardiac death. Lancet 1993; 342: 1085–6.
16. Candy GP, Skudicky D, Mueller UK, et al. Association of left ventricular systolic performance and cavity size with angiotensin-converting enzyme genotype in idiopathic dilated cardiomyopathy. Am J Cardiol 1999; 83: 740–4.
17. Terwilliger JD, Haghighi F, Hiekkalinna TS, et al. A biased assessment of the use of SNPs in human complex traits. Curr Opin Genet Dev 2002; 12: 726–34.
18. Cardon LR, Bell JI. Association study designs for complex diseases. Nat Rev Genet 2001; 2: 91–9.
19. Keating MT, Sanguinetti MC. Molecular and cellular mechanisms of cardiac arrhythmias. Cell 2001; 104: 569–80.

20. Marian AJ. Modifier genes for hypertrophic cardiomyopathy. Curr Opin Cardiol 2002; 17: 242–52.
21. Ryan MP, Cleland JG, French JA, et al. The standard electrocardiogram as a screening test for hypertrophic cardiomyopathy. Am J Cardiol 1995; 76: 689–94.
22. MacRae CA, Ghaisas N, Kass S, et al. Familial hypertrophic cardiomyopathy with Wolff–Parkinson–White syndrome maps to a locus on chromosome 7q3. J Clin Invest 1995; 96: 1216–20.
23. Gruver EJ, Fatkin D, Dodds GA, et al. Familial hypertrophic cardiomyopathy and atrial fibrillation caused by Arg663His beta-cardiac myosin heavy chain mutation. Am J Cardiol, 1999; 83: 13H–8H.
24. McKusick. Online Mendelian Inheritance in Man, OMIM (TM). McKusick-Nathans Institute for Genetic Medicine. Baltimore, MD Johns Hopkins University. National Center for Biotechnology Information, Bethesda, MD National Library of Medicine 2003.
25. Hunt SA, Baker DW, Chin MH, et al. ACC/AHA guidelines for the evaluation and management of chronic heart failure in the adult: executive summary a report of the American College of Cardiology/American Heart Association Task Force on practice guidelines (committee to revise the 1995 guidelines for the evaluation and management of heart failure): developed in collaboration with the International Society for Heart and Lung Transplantation; endorsed by the Heart Failure Society of America. Circulation 2001; 104: 2996–3007.
26. Mahadevan M, Tsilfidis C, Sabourin L, et al. Myotonic dystrophy mutation: an unstable CTG repeat in the 3' untranslated region of the gene. Science 1992; 255: 1253–5.
27. Leboyer M, Bellivier F, Nosten-Bertrand M, et al. Psychiatric genetics: search for phenotypes. Trends Neurosci 1998; 21: 102–5.
28. Crispell KA, Hanson EL, Coates K, et al. Periodic rescreening is indicated for family members at risk of developing familial dilated cardiomyopathy. J Am Coll Cardiol 2002; 39: 1503–7.
29. Spirito P, Seidman CE, McKenna WJ, et al. The management of hypertrophic cardiomyopathy. N Engl J Med 1997; 336: 775–85.
30. Grunig E, Tasman JA, Kucherer H, et al. Frequency and phenotypes of familial dilated cardiomyopathy. J Am Coll Cardiol 1998; 31: 186–94.
31. Crispell KA, Wray A, Ni H, et al. Clinical profiles of four large pedigrees with familial dilated cardiomyopathy: preliminary recommendations for clinical practice. J Am Coll Cardiol 1999; 34: 837–47.
32. Watkins H, Rosenzweig A, Hwang DS, et al. Characteristics and prognostic implications of myosin missense mutations in familial hypertrophic cardiomyopathy. N Engl J Med 1992; 326: 1108–14.
33. Fananapazir L, Epstein ND. Genotype–phenotype correlations in hypertrophic cardiomyopathy: insights provided by comparisons of kindreds with distinct and identical beta-myosin heavy chain gene mutations. Circulation 1994; 89: 22–32.
34. Blair E, Price SJ, Baty CJ, et al. Mutations in cis can confound genotype–phenotype correlations in hypertrophic cardiomyopathy. J Med Genet 2001; 38: 385–8.
35. Richard P, Charron P, Carrier L, et al. Hypertrophic cardiomyopathy: distribution of disease genes, spectrum of mutations, and implications for a molecular diagnosis strategy. Circulation 2003; 107: 2227–32.
36. Manolio TA, Baughman KL, Rodeheffer R, et al. Prevalence and etiology of idiopathic dilated cardiomyopathy (summary of a National Heart, Lung, and Blood Institute workshop. Am J Cardiol 1992; 69: 1458–66.
37. Braunwald E. Heart Disease: A Textbook of Cardiovascular Medicine. Philadelphia: Saunders, 2001.
38. Keeling PJ, Gang Y, Smith G, et al. Familial dilated cardiomyopathy in the United Kingdom. Br Heart J 1995; 73: 417–21.
39. McKenna CJ. Abnormal cellularity in asymptomatic relatives of patients with idiopathic dilated cardiomyopathy. J Am Coll Cardiol 2003; 41: 709; author reply; 709.
40. Shekelle PG, Rich MW, Morton SC, et al. Efficacy of angiotensin-converting enzyme inhibitors and beta-blockers in the management of left ventricular systolic dysfunction according to race, gender, and diabetic status. a meta-analysis of major clinical trials. J Am Coll Cardiol 2003; 41: 1529–38.
41. Mestroni L, Rocco C, Gregori D, et al. Familial dilated cardiomyopathy: evidence for genetic and phenotypic heterogeneity. Heart Muscle Disease Study Group. J Am Coll Cardiol 1999; 34: 181–90.
42. Mahon NG, Sharma S, Elliott PM, et al. Abnormal cardiopulmonary exercise variables in asymptomatic relatives of patients with dilated cardiomyopathy who have left ventricular enlargement. Heart 2000; 83: 511–17.
43. Kawai C. From myocarditis to cardiomyopathy: mechanisms of inflammation and cell death: learning from the past for the future. Circulation 1999; 99: 1091–100.

44. Csanady M, Högye M, Kallai A, et al. Familial dilated cardiomyopathy: a worse prognosis compared with sporadic forms. Br Heart J, 1995 74: 171–3.

45. Caforio AL, Goldman JH, Haven AJ, et al. Evidence for autoimmunity to myosin and other heart-specific autoantigens in patients with dilated cardiomyopathy and their relatives. Int J Cardiol 1996; 54: 157–63.

46. Olson TM, Keating MT. Mapping a cardiomyopathy locus to chromosome 3p22-p25. J Clin Invest 1996; 97: 528–32.

47. Fatkin D, MacRae C, Sasaki T, et al. Missense mutations in the rod domain of the lamin A/C gene as causes of dilated cardiomyopathy and conduction-system disease. N Engl J Med 1999; 341: 1715–24.

48. Towbin JA, Hejtmancik JF, Brink P, et al. X-linked dilated cardiomyopathy: molecular genetic evidence of linkage to the Duchenne muscular dystrophy (dystrophin) gene at the Xp21 locus. Circulation 1993; 87: 1854–65.

49. Melacini P, Fanin M, Duggan DJ, et al. Heart involvement in muscular dystrophies due to sarcoglycan gene mutations. Muscle Nerve 1999; 22: 473–9.

50. Coral-Vazquez R, Cohn RD, Moore SA, et al. Disruption of the sarcoglycan–sarcospan complex in vascular smooth muscle: a novel mechanism for cardiomyopathy and muscular dystrophy. Cell 1999; 98: 465–74.

51. Bione S, Maestrini E, Rivella S, et al. Identification of a novel X-linked gene responsible for Emery–Dreifuss muscular dystrophy. Nat Genet 1994; 8: 323–7.

52. Hutchison CJ. Lamins: building blocks or regulators of gene expression?. Nat Rev Mol Cell Biol 2002; 3: 848–58.

53. Olson TM, Michels VV, Thibodeau SN, et al. Actin mutations in dilated cardiomyopathy, a heritable form of heart failure. Science 1998; 280: 750–2.

54. MacRae CA. Genetics and dilated cardiomyopathy: limitations of candidate gene strategies. Eur Heart J 2000; 21: 1817–19.

55. Kamisago M, Sharma SD, DePalma SR, et al. Mutations in sarcomere protein genes as a cause of dilated cardiomyopathy. N Engl J Med 2000; 343: 1688–96.

56. Knoll R, Hoshijima M, Hoffman HM, et al. The cardiac mechanical stretch sensor machinery involves a Z disc complex that is defective in a subset of human dilated cardiomyopathy. Cell 2002; 111: 943–55.

57. Towbin JA. The role of cytoskeletal proteins in cardiomyopathies. Curr Opin Cell Biol 1998; 10: 131–9.

58. Chien KR. Genotype, phenotype: upstairs, downstairs in the family of cardiomyopathies. J Clin Invest 2003; 111: 175–8.

59. Xu X, Meiler SE, Zhong TP, et al. Cardiomyopathy in zebrafish due to mutation in an alternatively spliced exon of titin. Nat Genet 2002; 30: 205–9.

60. Watkins H, Seidman CE, MacRae C, et al. Progress in familial hypertrophic cardiomyopathy: molecular genetic analyses in the original family studied by Teare. Br Heart J 1992; 67: 34–8.

61. Saumarez RC, Slade AK, Grace AA, et al. The significance of paced electrogram fractionation in hypertrophic cardiomyopathy: a prospective study. Circulation 1995; 91: 2762–8.

62. Counihan PJ, Frenneaux MP, Webb DJ, et al. Abnormal vascular responses to supine exercise in hypertrophic cardiomyopathy. Circulation 1991; 84: 686–96.

63. Elliott PM, Kaski JC, Prasad K, et al. Chest pain during daily life in patients with hypertrophic cardiomyopathy: an ambulatory electrocardiographic study. Eur Heart J 1996; 17: 1056–64.

64. Nagata S, Park Y, Minamikawa T, et al. Thallium perfusion and cardiac enzyme abnormalities in patients with familial hypertrophic cardiomyopathy. Am Heart J 1985; 109: 1317–22.

65. Ashrafian H, Redwood C, Blair E, et al. Hypertrophic cardiomyopathy: a paradigm for myocardial energy depletion. Trends Genet 2003; 19: 263–8.

66. Geisterfer-Lowrance AA, Kass S, Tanigawa G, et al. A molecular basis for familial hypertrophic cardiomyopathy: a beta cardiac myosin heavy chain gene missense mutation. Cell 1990; 62: 999–1006.

67. Casali C, d'Amati G, Bernucci P, et al. Maternally inherited cardiomyopathy: clinical and molecular characterization of a large kindred harboring the A4300G point mutation in mitochondrial deoxyribonucleic acid. J Am Coll Cardiol 1999; 33: 1584–9.

68. Ho CY, Lever HM, DeSanctis R, et al. Homozygous mutation in cardiac troponin T: implications for hypertrophic cardiomyopathy. Circulation 2000; 102: 1950–5.

69. Mogensen J, Klausen IC, Pedersen AK, et al. Alpha-cardiac actin is a novel disease gene in familial hypertrophic cardiomyopathy. J Clin Invest 1999; 103: R39–43.

70. Poetter K, Jiang H, Hassanzadeh S, et al. Mutations in either the essential or regulatory light chains of myosin are associated with a rare myopathy in human heart and skeletal muscle. Nat Genet 1996; 13: 63–9.

71. Blair E, Redwood C, Ashrafian H, et al. Mutations in the gamma(2) subunit of AMP-activated protein kinase cause familial hypertrophic cardiomyopathy: evidence for the central role of energy compromise in disease pathogenesis. Hum Mol Genet 2001; 10: 1215–20.

72. Varnava A, Baboonian C, Davison F, et al. A new mutation of the cardiac troponin T gene causing familial hypertrophic cardiomyopathy without left ventricular hypertrophy. Heart 1999; 82: 621–4.

73. Niimura H, Bachinski LL, Sangwatanaroj S, et al. Mutations in the gene for cardiac myosin-binding protein C and late-onset familial hypertrophic cardiomyopathy. N Engl J Med 1998; 338: 1248–57.

74. Maron BJ, Niimura H, Casey SA, et al. Development of left ventricular hypertrophy in adults in hypertrophic cardiomyopathy caused by cardiac myosin-binding protein C gene mutations. J Am Coll Cardiol 2001; 38: 315–21.

75. Mogensen J, Kubo T, Duque M, et al. Idiopathic restrictive cardiomyopathy is part of the clinical expression of cardiac troponin I mutations. J Clin Invest 2003; 111: 209–16.

76. Witt CC, Gerull B, Davies MJ, et al. Hypercontractile properties of cardiac muscle fibers in a knock-in mouse model of cardiac myosin-binding protein-C. J Biol Chem 2001; 276: 5353–9.

77. Mukherjea P, Tong L, Seidman JG, et al. Altered regulatory function of two familial hypertrophic cardiomyopathy troponin T mutants. Biochemistry 1999; 38: 13296–301.

78. Campuzano V, Montermini L, Molto MD, et al. Friedreich's ataxia: autosomal recessive disease caused by an intronic GAA triplet repeat expansion. Science 1996; 271: 1423–7.

79. Jung M, Poepping I, Perrot A, et al. Investigation of a family with autosomal dominant dilated cardiomyopathy defines a novel locus on chromosome 2q14-q22. Am J Hum Genet 1999; 65: 1068–77.

80. Gerull B, Gramlich M, Atherton J, et al. Mutations of TTN, encoding the giant muscle filament titin, cause familial dilated cardiomyopathy. Nat Genet 2002; 30: 201–4.

81. Li D, Tapscoft T, Gonzalez O, et al. Desmin mutation responsible for idiopathic dilated cardiomyopathy. Circulation 1999; 100: 461–4.

82. Olson TM, Michels VV, Ballew JD, et al. Sodium channel mutations and susceptibility to heart failure and atrial fibrillation. JAMA 2005; 293: 447–54.

83. Barresi R, Di Blasi C, Negri T, et al. Disruption of heart sarcoglycan complex and severe cardiomyopathy caused by beta sarcoglycan mutations. J Med Genet 2000; 37: 102–7.

84. Tsubata S, Bowles KR, Vatta M, et al. Mutations in the human delta-sarcoglycan gene in familial and sporadic dilated cardiomyopathy. J Clin Invest 2000; 106: 655–62.

85. Norgett EE, Hatsell SJ, Carvajal-Huerta L, et al. Recessive mutation in desmoplakin disrupts desmoplakin-intermediate filament interactions and causes dilated cardiomyopathy, woolly hair and keratoderma. Hum Mol Genet 2000; 9: 2761–6.

86. Sylvius N, Tesson F, Gayet C, et al. A new locus for autosomal dominant dilated cardiomyopathy identified on chromosome 6q12-q16. Am J Hum Genet 2001; 68: 241–6.

87. Schmitt JP, Kamisago M, Asahi M, et al. Dilated cardiomyopathy and heart failure caused by a mutation in phospholamban. Science 2003; 299: 1410–13.

88. Messina DN, Speer MC, Pericak-Vance MA, et al. Linkage of familial dilated cardiomyopathy with conduction defect and muscular dystrophy to chromosome 6q23. Am J Hum Genet 1997; 61: 909–17.

89. Schonberger J, Levy H, Grunig E, et al. Dilated cardiomyopathy and sensorineural hearing loss: a heritable syndrome that maps to 6q23-24. Circulation 2000; 101: 1812–18.

90. Schonberger J, Wang L, Shin JT, et al. Mutation in the transcriptional coactivator EYA4 causes dilated cardiomyopathy and sensorineural hearing loss. Nat Genet 2005; 37: 418–22.

91. Krajinovic M, Pinamonti B, Sinagra G, et al. Linkage of familial dilated cardiomyopathy to chromosome 9. Heart Muscle Disease Study Group. Am J Hum Genet 1995; 57: 846–52.

92. Bowles KR, Gajarski R, Porter P, et al. Gene mapping of familial autosomal dominant dilated cardiomyopathy to chromosome 10q21-23. J Clin Invest 1996; 98: 1355–60.

93. Vatta M, Mohapatra B, Jimenez S, et al. Mutations in Cypher/ZASP in patients with dilated cardiomyopathy and left ventricular non-compaction. J Am Coll Cardiol 2003; 42: 2014–27.

94. Brauch KM, Karst ML, Herron KJ, et al. Mutations in ribonucleic acid binding protein gene cause familial dilated cardiomyopathy. J Am Coll Cardiol 2009; 54: 930–41.

95. Daehmlow S, Erdmann J, Knueppel T, et al. Novel mutations in sarcomeric protein genes in dilated cardiomyopathy. Biochem Biophys Res Commun 2002; 298: 116–20.

96. Bienengraeber M, Olson TM, Selivanov VA, et al. ABCC9 mutations identified in human dilated cardiomyopathy disrupt catalytic KATP channel gating. Nat Genet 2004; 36: 382–7.

97. Carballo S, Robinson P, Otway R, et al. Identification and functional characterization of cardiac troponin I as a novel disease gene in autosomal dominant dilated cardiomyopathy. Circ Res 2009; 105: 375–82.

98. Thierfelder L, Watkins H, MacRae C, et al. Alpha-tropomyosin and cardiac troponin T mutations cause familial hypertrophic cardiomyopathy: a disease of the sarcomere. Cell 1994; 77: 701–12.

99. Geier C, Perrot A, Ozcelik C, et al. Mutations in the human muscle LIM protein gene in families with hypertrophic cardiomyopathy. Circulation 2003; 107: 1390–5.

100. Watkins H, Conner D, Thierfelder L, et al. Mutations in the cardiac myosin binding protein-C gene on chromosome 11 cause familial hypertrophic cardiomyopathy. Nat Genet 1995; 11: 434–7.

101. Kimura A, Harada H, Park JE, et al. Mutations in the cardiac troponin I gene associated with hypertrophic cardiomyopathy. Nat Genet 1997; 16: 379–82.

102. Arad M, Maron BJ, Gorham JM, et al. Glycogen storage diseases presenting as hypertrophic cardiomyopathy. N Engl J Med 2005; 352: 362–72.

3

Molecular signaling networks underlying cardiac hypertrophy and failure

Gerald W. Dorn II

BASIC CONCEPTS OF HYPERTROPHY AND HEART FAILURE

The past three decades have witnessed a revolution in our understanding of the molecular determinants of the cardiac stress response leading to hypertrophy and heart failure. The genesis of currently held concepts was delineation of complex signaling pathways initiated by neurohormones or growth factors that cause, modify, and antagonize cardiac hypertrophy. This chapter provides an overview of some of these findings.

Cardiac hypertrophy and heart failure represent, respectively, the beginning and end of the cardiac response to injury or hemodynamic stress. The most common form of cardiac injury in the United States is myocardial infarction (MI) (1,2). Of approximately 500,000 annual deaths from MI, a half of the victims succumb weeks or months after the acute event from progressive ischemia-related heart failure or its complications. Reactive hypertrophy occurs after MI, but is not sufficient in quantity or quality to compensate for the loss of infarcted myocardium. The other major cause of clinical heart failure is not acute injury, but rather chronic, unremitting hemodynamic overload from poorly controlled hypertension (1,3). Here, cardiac hypertrophy is the early response, and the progression to dilated cardiomyopathy can take decades. Thus, hypertrophy and heart failure represent a temporal continuum of response to virtually all forms of cardiac injury.

It is essential to recognize that the term cardiac "hypertrophy" is ambiguous in that it describes: (*i*) a clinical condition (abnormally increased electrocardiographic or echocardiographic cardiac enlargement) that is a well-established independent risk factor for death (4–6); (*ii*) a process of organ growth in response to increased physiologic demand; and (*iii*) the cellular response of cardiac myocyte enlargement accompanied by characteristic re-expression of embryonic cardiac genes and contractile (7). "Hypertrophy" is not typically used to describe normal developmental cardiac growth, as occurs during the juvenile "growth spurt," because this is not an abnormal response (8). The natural history of clinical cardiac hypertrophy is that it ultimately progresses to heart failure, a multifactorial clinical syndrome defined in nonmechanistic terms as any condition where the heart does not provide adequate cardiac output to meet the physiologic needs of the organism (9). Hearts with systolic failure tend to have dilated chambers and thin-walled ventricles as a result of cell and chamber remodeling (9,10). Mechanistically, the hallmark of decompensated or failing hearts is the loss of viable functioning cardiac myocytes and their replacement by fibrotic tissue (11–13). The characteristic gene expression profile of heart failure includes the expression of atrial and brain natriuretic peptides (7), and measuring plasma concentrations of brain natriuretic peptide (BNP), which has been widely accepted as a useful clinical biomarker of heart failure (14).

Neurohormonal pathways are activated in both acute and chronic cardiac stress, and play critical roles in the ensuing maladaptation. During acute MI, intense pain and decreased cardiac output activate the sympathetic nervous system. Sympathetic catecholaminergic signaling enhances contractility of the noninfarcted myocardium by stimulating inotropic β-adrenergic receptors, and supports blood pressure by stimulating vasoconstrictor α-adrenergic receptors. Although these actions have immediate benefits, they also acutely increase myocardial oxygen demand, and therefore potentially expand the area of ischemic damage (15). Furthermore, circulating and locally released neurohormones directly stimulate cardiomyocytes to undergo hypertrophy via signaling pathways delineated in detail below. Thus, pathologic hypertrophy of cardiac myocytes in noninfarcted myocardium is a consequence of compensatory neurohormonal mechanisms that are initiated in the acute infarction period (16). Similar neurohormonal pathways are activated under conditions of chronic hemodynamic stress, that is, pressure overload from hypertension or aortic valvular stenosis. Consequently, the typical clinical course of both infarcted and hypertensive hearts is of acute functional compensation followed by chronic progressive left ventricular dilatation, and transitioning from an ellipsoidal to a spherical geometry. Ultimately, the changes result in diminished systolic performance and overt heart failure (17,18).

THE EVOLUTION OF HEART FAILURE THERAPEUTICS TARGETING NEUROHORMONAL SIGNALING

It is ironic that modern concepts of cardiac pathophysiology echo ancient Galenic principles of humoral imbalance in health and disease. In today's medicine, the "humors" include the neurohormones epinephrine, norepinephrine, and angiotensin, and restoring humoral imbalance is achieved with pharmacologic receptor blockade or synthesis inhibition (rather than blood letting) (19–21). Epinephrine and norepinephrine stimulate vasoconstrictor α-adrenergic receptors and inotropic β-adrenergic receptors. Angiotensin II is an even more powerful vasoconstrictor, and a potent hormonal stimulus for cardiac myocyte hypertrophy. Each of these vasoconstrictor neurohormones also stimulates cardiac hypertrophy (22,23). Therefore, their secretion in an effort to compensate for decreased cardiac output in heart failure not only increases blood pressure, but further increases hemodynamic stress and directly stimulates the pathologic hypertrophy response (Fig. 3.1). The double-edged sword of neurohormonal stimulation in heart failure has only been fully appreciated over the past two decades (24), prior to which the standard approach for treating heart failure was to stimulate neurohormonal signaling.

The rationale for clinical trials of *pharmacologic neurohormonal activation* in heart failure was developed after two important experimental observations: First, in the early 1960s, Braunwald and Gaffney noted that failing myocardium had markedly lower norepinephrine levels than normal hearts, that is, an "insufficiency of catecholamines" (25,26). Concomitantly, the first clinical experiences with β-adrenergic receptor blockers showed that large doses of propanolol caused acute exacerbation of heart failure symptoms, suggesting a requirement for catecholamines in functional compensation of failing myocardium (27,28). Accordingly, recommended clinical practice at the time included strict avoidance of β-adrenergic blockers and administration of agents (parenteral catecholamines and type I phosphodiesterase inhibitors) that increased adrenergic signaling. The unfortunate result of this well-intended approach was iatrogenic arrhythmic sudden death (29–31) and worsening heart failure due to catecholamine cardiomyopathy (32,33).

The failure of clinical therapeutics designed to increase adrenergic signaling, taken together with a more complete understanding of the role of the overall neurohormonal axis

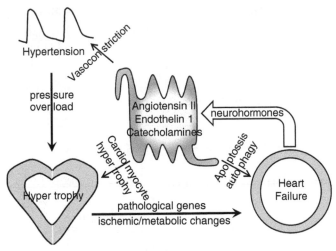

Figure 3.1 Depiction of the multiple effects of neurohormones in cardiac disease. Hypertrophic neurohormones stilmulate receptors (*middle*) that couple to vasoconstrictor responses in the vasculature and increase blood pressure, to hypertrophic responses on cardiac myocytes that contribute to cardiac hypertrophy, and to adverse transcriptional and metabolic responses that predispose to cardiomyocyte death and the transition to dilated and failing hearts. Heart failure itself stimulates neurohormone release, thereby perpetuating a vicious downward functional spiral.

in heart failure (34,35), prompted a re-evaluation of catecholamine therapy in favor of trials employing the reciprocal approach of *pharmacologic neurohormonal inhibition*. In the 1980s, large-scale clinical trials with β-adrenergic receptor antagonists in heart failure showed striking mortality benefits with few adverse consequences when therapy was initiated at low doses and under conditions of close clinical monitoring (36–41). Similar mortality benefit was observed when angiotensin II signaling was inhibited with angiotensin-converting enzyme (ACE) inhibitors (42–44). Modern therapeutics therefore target each of the critical neurohormonal pathways in heart failure with, in addition to β-blockers and ACE inhibitors, angiotensin receptor blockers (45) and aldosterone antagonists (46,47). The theoretic construct that was developed to integrate and explain these clinical and basic findings is called the **Neurohormonal Theory** (24,48), which states that a primary cardiac insult that decreases heart function initiates a vicious cycle wherein local and systemic release of inotropic and vasoconstricting hormones provides immediate circulatory support, but ultimately contributes to worsening of cardiac function (maladaptation) through direct toxic effects on the myocardium (Fig. 3.1).

NEUROHORMONAL SIGNALING PATHWAYS THAT REGULATE HYPERTROPHY

Pathologic hypertrophy is caused by any of a number of partially redundant neurohormonal pathways that activate parallel hypertrophy signaling effectors (49–51). In brief, multiple agonist-receptor pairs, such as those for angiotensin II, endothelin, and catecholamines, produce pathologic hypertrophy through activation of signaling pathways coupled to the heterotrimeric GTP-binding protein, Gq. A critical role for Gq pathways in hypertrophy was unambiguously demonstrated when forced gain or loss of Gq signaling was found to regulate the size of cultured neonatal cardiomyocytes (52), and further supported by studies utilizing in vivo cardiac-specific transgenic overexpression, dominant

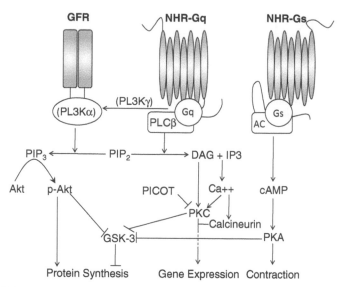

Figure 3.2 Schematic diagram of crosstalk between key cardiac signaling events that promote or antagonize myocardial hypertrophy. (*left, physiological hypertrophy*) Binding of GFR recruits PI3Kα, which phosphorylates membrane PIP2, forming PIP3 that is permissive for Akt activation. Akt stimulates protein synthesis by activating mTOR (not shown) and inhibiting GSK-3, which normally suppresses protein translation. (*center, pathologic hypertrophy*) Binding of angiotensin II, endothelin, or alpha-adrenergic agonists to their cognate Gq-coupled receptors (NHR-Gq) recruits phospholipase Cβ (PLC), which hydrolyzes membrane PIP2 into two products, inositol triphosphate (IP3) that releases calcium (Ca++) from sarcoplasmic reticular stores, and DAG, that activates protein kinase C (PKC). Calcium activates the phosphatase calcineurin and conventional PKC isoforms, both of which regulated hypertrophy gene transcription. PKC plays a role in antihypertrophy signaling as it is inhibited by PICOT, and itself inhibits antihypertrophic GSK-3. Gq-coupled receptors also activate phyisiologic hypertrophy Akt signaling via PI3Kg. (*right, contraction*) Catecholamines bind to Gs-coupled β-adrenergic receptors, activating adenylyl cyclase (AC), and consequently PKA. PKA enhances contractility by improving calcium availability and increasing the sensitivity of contractile proteins to calcium. PKA also can enhance hypertrophy by inhibiting GSK-3. *Abbreviations*: DAG, diacylglycerol; GFR, growth factors to their receptors; GSK-3, glycogen synthase kinase-3; PI3Kα, phsophatidylinositol-3-kinase α; PIP2, phosphatidylinositol-biphosphate; PKA, protein kinase A.

inhibition, and genetic ablation of Gq. Taken together, these studies demonstrated that cardiomyocyte Gq signaling is both necessary and sufficient to produce pressure overload-like hypertrophy (53–55).

Gq and functionally redundant G11 (56,57) activates phospholipase Cβ, which hydrolyzes phosphatidylinositol bisphosphate (PIP2). One of the PIP2 hydrolysis products, inositol triphosphate (IP3), causes release of calcium from intracellular stores, thus increasing cytosolic [Ca^{2+}] and activating the protein phosphatase, calcineurin. Calcineurin then dephosphorylates and promotes nuclear translocation of its target, the NFAT family of transcription factors, which regulate hypertrophic gene expression (58) (Fig. 3.2). The other PIP2 hydrolysis product, diacylglycerol (DAG), activates protein kinase C (PKC) that also regulates hypertrophy genes (49). The PKC family members expressed in myocardium, and which have isoform-specific effects on cardiac growth and contractile function, are the "conventional" DAG- and calcium-dependent PKCα and PKCβ, and the "novel" DAG-dependent but calcium-independent PKCδ and PKCε. Extensive data exist differentiating the specific effects of these individual PKC isoforms in cardiac disease, and have been reviewed in detail elsewhere (49,51).

Pathologic hypertrophy is transduced via Gq-coupled neurohormone receptors, whereas nonpathologic or "physiologic" hypertrophy is stimulated by growth factor receptor tyrosine kinases that activate phosphoinositide-3-kinase (PI3K)/Akt signaling (Fig. 3.2). Insulin-like growth factor (IGF) and growth hormone (GH), which act largely by increasing IGF production, are the major stimuli for both physiologic hypertrophy and normal developmental growth (eutrophy) (59,60). Binding of these and other peptide growth factors to their respective membrane receptors causes receptor dimerization, autophosphorylation, and activation of p110α PI3K. Phosphorylation of PIP2 by PI3K creates PIP3, which recruits the kinase Akt (a.k.a PKB) to plasma membranes. Activated (phosphorylated) Akt then stimulates protein synthesis by activating the mammalian target of rapamycin (mTOR), and by inhibiting antihypertrophic glycogen synthase kinase (GSK). These pathways and their interaction with pathologic hypertrophy signaling have been reviewed in detail (61).

MANIPULATING HYPERTROPHY BY MODIFYING SIGNALING PATHWAYS

The existence of different signaling pathways for pathologic and physiologic hypertrophy, together with the elucidation of distinct molecular and biochemical signatures for exercise-induced and pressure overload hypertrophy, indicate that different forms of hypertrophy result from stress-specific responses. This notion was directly examined by performing functional, histologic, biochemical, and molecular analyses of three forms of intermittent stress: running, swimming, and phasic aortic coarctation (62). Compared to unremitting pressure overload (permanent aortic coarctation), intermittent pressure overload produced functionally compensated concentric hypertrophy with little fibrosis or fetal gene expression, consistent with more physiologic hypertrophy. However, relative myocardial capillary density was pathologically decreased in both intermittent and chronic pressure overload, whereas it was normal in swimming- and running-induced hypertrophy. These studies demonstrate that individual features of pathologic and physiologic hypertrophy can be switched, depending on the nature of the inciting stimulus.

The distinction between pathologic and physiologic hypertrophy is also incomplete at the level of cell signaling pathways: The PI3K/Akt signaling axis is essential to the physiologic hypertrophy response, but overstimulation of the pathway can cause hypertrophy with some pathologic features (63–66). Signaling pathways for pathologic and physiologic hypertrophy can also overlap (49). Membrane PIP2 transmits a signal for physiologic hypertrophy when it is phosphorylated by PI3K, but signals for pathologic hypertrophy when it undergoes hydrolysis by phospholipase C, and different PI3K isoforms are activated by growth factor and neurohormone receptor pathways.

Recently, it has become apparent that hypertrophic signaling is opposed by intrinsic antihypertrophic mechanisms, such as glycogen synthase kinase (GSK3β) (67,68), class II histone deacetylases (HDACII) (69), phospholipase A2 (70), thioredoxin (71), and caveolin 3 (72). GSK3β inhibits hypertrophy gene expression by regulating the activity of the calcineurin substrate, NFAT (73), and the protein translation initiation factor, eIF2B (74), and HDACII modulates the effects of multiple transcription factors to regulate stress-induced hypertrophy (75). These pathways are constitutively active in normal myocardium, but are suppressed by the reaction to injury or hemodynamic stress, which has the effect of disinhibiting prohypertrophic signaling. Other antihypertrophic pathways that are normally quiescent, such as cAMP early repressor (ICER), MCIP-1, ANP/BNP, SOCS-3, are strongly induced by hemodynamic overload and restrain the hypertrophic response by conventional negative feedback mechanisms (76). Taken together, the existence of multiple pro- and anti-hypertrophic signaling pathways with distinct and dissociable effects suggest that pathologic and physiologic hypertrophy should not be viewed as separate entities, but rather as syndromes of associated features that are distinguishable under conditions of atypical stimulation or by molecular manipulation of signaling pathways. Based on this conceptual paradigm, it has been proposed that pathologic hypertrophy can be therapeutically modified so as to be more "physiologic" through manipulation of growth factor signals that regulate different aspects of the hypertrophy response.

THE CELL BIOLOGY OF CARDIAC DECOMPENSATION

Hypertrophied myocardium has distinct qualities compared with normal myocardium, including expression of fetal contractile protein isoforms, reversion to a preference for fetal metabolic substrates, and re-expression of an entire panel of genes that are essential for proper development of the fetal heart, but seem to have no normal physiologic function in adult hearts (7). At the cellular level, the transition from compensated hypertrophy to dilated cardiomyopathy appears to be related in large part to death of cardiac myocytes and their replacement by fibrotic tissue. In cardiac ischemia myocytes death and replacement fibrosis tend to be focal, whereas they are more diffuse in nonischemic failure (77,78). The loss of cellular contractile units further impairs the pumping function of the heart, and rearrangement or "cell slippage" (79) of remaining cardiomyocytes contributes to ventricular wall thinning and cavity dilation, that is, ventricular remodeling.

As cardiomyocyte dropout is central to the progression from compensated hypertrophy to decompensated heart failure, it is important to understand the mechanisms leading to cell death. Interestingly, there is accumulating information that cardiac myocyte ischemia may be the critical factor, whether the primary stimulus for hypertrophy is ischemic or nonischemic. Under conditions of hemodynamic stress and heart failure, myocardial oxygen demand is decreased while coronary perfusion pressure is decreased. The mismatch between myocardial oxygen demand and supply is exaggerated by cardiac myocyte hypertrophy because increased cell diameter constitutes a greater diffusion barrier to oxygen being carried by adjacent myocardial capillaries (core hypoxia) (80). To fully support hypertrophied myocardium, the coronary microvasculature would need to increase in capacity to a similar degree as the increase in myocyte mass (81). Consistent with the notion that hypertrophied hearts are intrinsically ischemic, some findings have identified angiogenesis signaling pathways in cardiac hypertrophy that are necessary for normal function (82). Furthermore, some studies have found that forced neovascularization of cardiac hypertrophy, achieved through manipulation of angiogenic factors, can benefit hypertrophy and preserve contractile function after pressure overloading (73,83). Taken together, these results indicated that angiogenesis is a critical determinant of cardiac myocyte viability, and that inadequate angiogenesis contributes to the transition of functionally compensated cardiac hypertrophy to dilated and failing cardiomyopathic hearts (84).

NEUROHORMONAL STIMULATION PREDISPOSES TO CARDIOMYOCYTE DEATH

There are multiple mechanisms for cardiac myocyte death in the transition for compensated hypertrophy to heart failure, and the dominant form of cell death varies with physiologic context. Although it is convenient to consider necrosis, autophagy, and apoptosis as separate cellular processes, each can be a form of "programmed cell death," and their signaling mechanisms both overlap and crossregulate. Furthermore, in the intact stressed or injured heart, all three are likely to be happening at the same time in the myocardium.

Cardiac myocyte necrosis in decompensated hypertrophy is largely attributed to the aforementioned "ischemic core" mechanism (80). When the cross-sectional area of a cardiac myocyte surpasses the distance across which oxygen can diffuse down its concentration gradient from adjacent capillaries, mitochondria at the core of the cardiomyocyte becossme ischemic, with resulting diminished ATP generating ability, metabolic shutdown, and death. This ischemic stimulus can also activate autophagy, which is more normally a degradative pathway for turning over large protein complexes and a cell survival mechanism that is activated during starvation. Autophagosome-like cytoplasmic inclusions are commonly observed in hypertrophied myocardium of patients with severe aortic stenosis and heart failure (11,85), possibly because normal protein renewal pathways of the proteasome system are overwhelmed by greatly accelerated protein turnover during hypertrophic remodeling. As a consequence, partially degraded or senescent proteins that would normally be eliminated through the lysosomal system are shunted to an overloaded autophagy pathway, where they accumulate and can contribute to cardiomyocyte death (86,87).

Neurohormone-mediated upregulation of cardiac myocyte apoptosis genes seems to play a more central role in cardiomyocyte death and hypertrophy decompensation (88). Apoptosis is a highly regulated cell response that limits the proliferation of abnormal or damaged cells that are unnecessary or could otherwise produce malignant tumors (89). Cells undergoing apoptosis are distinguished by characteristic nuclear chromatin condensation and nuclear fragmentation that forms dense "apoptotic bodies" (90). Apoptotic cell fragmentation provides for elimination of cell remnants by scavenging mononuclear cells without a widespread inflammatory response that can cause collateral cell damage, and is therefore generally considered to be more desirable than simply letting damaged or redundant cells die a necrotic death. However, since the heart is a tissue without significant regenerative capacity (91), cardiac myocyte apoptosis is necessarily rare, with a reported incidence in normal myocardium of 1/10,000 to 100,000 cardiac myocytes (74). This rate of cardiomyocyte apoptosis increases by orders of magnitude in dilated and ischemic cardiomyopathies (78,92) and cardiac hypertrophy (11), and therefore has the potential to contribute significantly to myocyte dropout in these syndromes (93).

There are two apoptosis signaling pathways, initiated either via death receptor activation or mitochondrial outer membrane permeabilization (Fig. 3.3) (94,95). In the death receptor, or "extrinsic," pathway, extracellular cytokines bind to their membrane receptors, promoting receptor oligomerization and the formation of a death signaling complex containing Fas-associated death domain (FADD)-containing protein. The FADD complex recruits caspase-8 and activates the apoptotic caspase cascade. In contrast, the mitochondrial pathway is activated by intrinsic stimuli that cause pore formation in the outer mitochondrial membrane and permits release of cytochrome c into the cytoplasm. The specific mechanism for mitochondrial outer membrane pore formation (which is distinct from the mitochondrial permeability transition pore that mediates nonapoptotic calcium- and oxidative damage-induced cell death (96) depends on coordinated effects of members of the Bcl2 family of mitochondrial-targeted apoptosis–regulating proteins. The actual pore-forming proteins, Bax and Bak, are recruited to the membrane by proapoptotic BH3-only proteins (e.g., Bad, Bid, Nix, and Bnip3), which are themselves restrained by antiapoptotic Bcl2 members (e.g., Bcl2 and Bcl-xl). Apoptosis signaling is stimulated when developmental or physiologic cues shift the balance between pro- and antiapoptotic Bcl2 family members toward apoptosis, either by transcriptional upregulation (Nix and Bnip3), enzymatic cleavage (Bid), dephosphorylation (Bad), or release from sequestration by antiapoptotic members (PUMA) (reviewed in 97). The resulting mitochondrial pores release cytochrome c that participates in the formation of an "apoptosome" complex, which recruits caspase-9 to initiate the caspase cascade. The end result of caspase

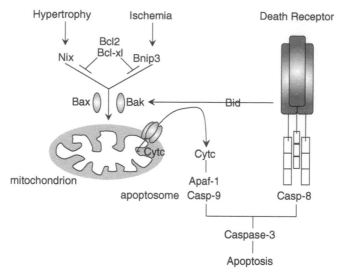

Figure 3.3 Apoptosis signaling pathways in cardiac myocytes. (*left, intrinsic pathway*) Expression of proapoptotic Nix and Bnip3 are increased in hypertrophy and ischemia, respectively. Mitochondrial targeting of these factors facilitates mitochondrial outer membrane permeabilization by Bax and Bak, releasing cytochrome *c* into the cytoplasm, where it complexes in an apoptosome with Apaf-1 and procaspase-9 to activate terminal effector caspase-3. (*right, extrinsic pathway*) Binding of cytokines, such as tumor necrosis factor-α or the Fas ligand, to their receptors recruits procaspase-8, which autoactivates by autolysis, causing cleavage and activation of the terminal apoptotic effector, caspase-3.

activation and proteolysis of caspase-3 targets by either the death receptor or mitochondrial pathways is systematic degradation of intracellular proteins and oligonucleosomal cleavage of DNA.

Hypertrophic signaling is linked to both the death receptor and mitochondrial apoptosis pathways in heart failure. In the death receptor pathway, cytoprotective factors, such as Gp130, potently antagonize death receptor responses. Gp130 is a receptor for interleukin-6 family proteins and has no known function in normal hearts. However, Gp130 is essential for the survival of cardiac myocytes under severe hemodynamic stress as shown by ablation of the Gp130 gene, which after surgical pressure overload, results in massive cardiac myocyte apoptosis leading to dilated cardiomyopathy (98). This experiment not only supports the critical importance of cell survival signaling in hypertrophying hearts, but implies that cell death pathways can be specifically induced in cardiac hypertrophy. Indeed, striking benefits on cardiac remodeling have been observed when prosurvival signaling was favored by artificially increasing the levels of antiapoptotic Bcl2 proteins prior to myocardial injury. Transgenic cardiac overexpression of antiapoptotic Bcl2, or forced expression of antiapoptotic [(apoptosis repressor with caspase recruitment domain (ART)], both decrease myocardial infarct size (99,100). The reciprocal approach of deleting proapoptotic factors, such as pore-forming Bax or its activators Bnip3 or Nix, likewise protects against remodeling after myocardial infarction or pressure overload (101–103). These studies reveal a significant role for apoptosis in the functional decline and geometric remodeling that occur in injured and hemodynamically stressed hearts. As with efforts described above to modify hypertrophy so as to be more "physiological," molecular interference with programmed cell death pathways in cardiac hypertrophy shows promise as a means of preventing the transition to heart failure.

REFERENCES

1. Rosamond W, Flegal K, Furie K, et al. Heart disease and stroke statistics 2008 update: a report from the American Heart association Statistics Committee and Stroke Statistics Subcommittee. Circulation. 2007.

2. Zheng ZJ, Croft JB, Giles WH, Mensah GA. Sudden cardiac death in the United States, 1989 to 1998. Circulation 2001; 104: 2158–63.

3. Levy D, Larson MG, Vasan RS, Kannel WB, Ho KK. The progression from hypertension to congestive heart failure. JAMA 1996; 275: 1557–62.

4. Kannel WB, Gordon T, Offutt D. Left ventricular hypertrophy by electrocardiogram. Prevalence, incidence, and mortality in the Framingham study. Ann Intern Med 1969; 71: 89–105.

5. Levy D, Garrison RJ, Savage DD, Kannel WB, Castelli WP. Prognostic implications of echocardiographically determined left ventricular mass in the Framingham Heart Study. N Engl J Med 1990; 322: 1561–6.

6. Vakili BA, Okin PM, Devereux RB. Prognostic implications of left ventricular hypertrophy. Am Heart J 2001; 141: 334–41.

7. Chien KR, Knowlton KU, Zhu H, Chien S. Regulation of cardiac gene expression during myocardial growth and hypertrophy: molecular studies of an adaptive physiologic response. FASEB J 1991; 5: 3037–46.

8. Dorn GW, Robbins J, Sugden PH. Phenotyping hypertrophy: eschew obfuscation. Circ Res 2003; 92: 1171–5.

9. Diwan A, Dorn GW. Decompensation of cardiac hypertrophy: cellular mechanisms and novel therapeutic targets. Physiology (Bethesda) 2007; 22: 56–64.

10. Carabello BA. Concentric versus eccentric remodeling. Js Card Fail 2002; 8: S258–63.

11. Hein S, Arnon E, Kostin S, et al. Progression from compensated hypertrophy to failure in the pressure-overloaded human heart: structural deterioration and compensatory mechanisms. Circulation 2003; 107: 984–91.

12. Anversa P, Leri A, Beltrami CA, Guerra S, Kajstura J. Myocyte death and growth in the failing heart. Lab Invest 1998; 78: 767–86.

13. Weber KT. Fibrosis and hypertensive heart disease. Curr Opin Cardiol 2000; 15: 264–72.

14. Yancy CW. B-type natriuretic peptides in management of acute decompensated heart failure. Heart Fail Clin 2006; 2: 353–64.

15. Jackson BM, Gorman JH, Moainie SL, et al. Extension of borderzone myocardium in postinfarction dilated cardiomyopathy. J Am Coll Cardiol 2002; 40: 1160–7.

16. St John SM, Pfeffer MA, Moye L, et al. Cardiovascular death and left ventricular remodeling two years after myocardial infarction: baseline predictors and impact of long-term use of captopril: information from the Survival and Ventricular Enlargement (SAVE) trial. Circulation 1997; 96: 3294–9.

17. Fieno DS, Hillenbr HB, Rehwald WG, et al. Infarct resorption, compensatory hypertrophy, and differing patterns of ventricular remodeling following myocardial infarctions of varying size. J Am Coll Cardiol 2004; 43: 2124–31.

18. Shioura KM, Geenen DL, Goldspink PH. Assessment of cardiac function with the pressure-volume conductance system following myocardial infarction in mice. Am J Physiol Heart Circ Physiol 2007; 293: H2870–7.

19. Bristow M. Antiadrenergic therapy of chronic heart failure: surprises and new opportunities. Circulation 2003; 107: 1100–2.

20. Cohn JN, Ferrari R, Sharpe N. Cardiac remodeling–concepts and clinical implications: a consensus paper from an international forum on cardiac remodeling. Behalf of an international forum on cardiac remodeling. J Am Coll Cardiol 2000; 35: 569–82.

21. Gheorghiade M, De Luca L, Bonow RO. Neurohormonal inhibition in heart failure: insights from recent clinical trials. Am J Cardiol 2005; 96: 3L–9L.

22. Simpson P. Norepinephrine-stimulated hypertrophy of cultured rat myocardial cells is an alpha 1 adrenergic response. J Clin Invest 1983; 72: 732–8.

23. Sadoshima J, Izumo S. Molecular characterization of angiotensin II–induced hypertrophy of cardiac myocytes and hyperplasia of cardiac fibroblasts. Critical role of the AT1 receptor subtype. Circ Res 1993; 73: 413–23.

24. Packer M. The neurohormonal hypothesis: a theory to explain the mechanism of disease progression in heart failure. J Am Coll Cardiol 1992; 20: 248–54.

25. Gaffney TE, Braunwald E. Importance of the adrenergic nervous system in the support of circulatory function in patients with congestive heart failure. Am J Med 1963; 34: 320–4.

26. Jr. Braunwald E, Ross J, Kahler R, et al. Reflex control of the systemic venous bed. Effects on venous tone of vasoactive drugs, and of baroreceptor and chemoreceptor stimulation. Circ Res 1963; 2: 539–52.

27. Epstein SE. Clinical and hemodynamic appraisal of beta adrenergic blocking drugs. Ann N Y Acad Sci 1967; 139: 952–67.
28. Stephen SA. Cardiac failure with propranolol. Br Med J 1968; 2: 428.
29. LeJemtel TH, Gumbardo D, Chadwick B, Rutman HI, Sonnenblick EH. Milrinone for long-term therapy of severe heart failure: clinical experience with special reference to maximal exercise tolerance. Circulation 1986; 73, III213–III218.
30. Simonton CA, Daly PA, Kereiakes D, Modin G, Chatterjee K. Survival in severe left ventricular failure treated with the new nonglycosidic, nonsympathomimetic oral inotropic agents. Chest 1987; 92, 118-123.
31. Lubbe WF, Podzuweit T, Opie LH. Potential arrhythmogenic role of cyclic adenosine monophosphate (AMP and cytosolic calcium overload: implications for prophylactic effects of beta-blockers in myocardial infarction and proarrhythmic effects of phosphodiesterase inhibitors. J Am Coll Cardiol 1992; 19: 1622–33.
32. Haft JI. Cardiovascular injury induced by sympathetic catecholamines. Prog. Cardiovasc. Dis 1974; 17: 73–86.
33. Kones RJ. The catecholamines: reappraisal of their use for acute myocardial infarction and the low cardiac output syndromes. Crit Care Med 1973; 1: 203–20.
34. Fowler MB, Bristow MR. Rationale for beta-adrenergic blocking drugs in cardiomyopathy. Am J Cardiol 1985; 55: 120D–4D.
35. Bristow MR, Ginsburg R, Minobe W, et al. Decreased catecholamine sensitivity and beta-adrenergic-receptor density in failing human hearts. N Engl J Med 1982; 307: 205–11.
36. Heilbrunn SM, Shah P, Bristow MR, et al. Increased beta-receptor density and improved hemodynamic response to catecholamine stimulation during long-term metoprolol therapy in heart failure from dilated cardiomyopathy. Circulation 1989; 79: 483–90.
37. Packer M, Bristow MR, Cohn JN, et al. The effect of carvedilol on morbidity and mortality in patients with chronic heart failure. U.S. Carvedilol Heart Failure Study Group. N Engl J Med 1996; 334: 1349–55.
38. CIBIS-II The Cardiac Insufficiency Bisoprolol Study II (CIBIS-II). A romised trial. Lancet 1999; 353: 9.13.
39. The Merit HF Investigators. Effect of metoprolol CR/XL in chronic heart failure: metoprolol cr/xl randomised intervention trial in congestive heart failure (MERIT-HF). Lancet 1999; 353: 2001–7.
40. Hjalmarson A, Goldstein S, Fagerberg B, et al. Effects of controlled-release metoprolol on total mortality, hospitalizations, and well-being in patients with heart failure: the Metoprolol CR/XL Randomized Intervention Trial in congestive heart failure (MERIT-HF). MERIT-HF Study Group. JAMA 2000; 283: 1295–302.
41. Packer M, Coats AJ, Fowler MB, et al. Effect of carvedilol on survival in severe chronic heart failure. N Engl J Med 2001; 344: 1651–8.
42. Davis R, Ribner HS, Keung E, Sonnenblick EH, LeJemtel TH. Treatment of chronic congestive heart failure with captopril, an oral inhibitor of angiotensin-converting enzyme. N Engl J Med 1979; 301: 117–21.
43. Levine TB, Franciosa JA, Cohn JN. Acute and long-term response to an oral converting-enzyme inhibitor, captopril, in congestive heart failure. Circulation 1980; 62: 35–41.
44. The SOLVD Investigators. The SOLVD Investigators Effect of enalapril on survival in patients with reduced left ventricular ejection fractions and congestive heart failure. N Engl J Med 1991; 325: 293–302.
45. Cohn JN, Tognoni G. A randomized trial of the angiotensin-receptor blocker valsartan in chronic heart failure. N Engl J Med 2001; 345: 1667–75.
46. Pitt B, Remme W, Zannad F, et al. Eplerenone, a selective aldosterone blocker, in patients with left ventricular dysfunction after myocardial infarction. N Engl J Med 2003; 348: 1309–21.
47. Pitt B. The role of aldosterone blockade in patients with heart failure. Heart Fail Rev 2005; 10: 79–83.
48. Packer M. Evolution of the neurohormonal hypothesis to explain the progression of chronic heart failure. Eur Heart J 1995; 16(Suppl F): 4.6.
49. Dorn GW, Force T. Protein kinase cascades in the regulation of cardiac hypertrophy. J Clin Invest 2005; 115: 527–37.
50. Frey N, Olson EN. Cardiac hypertrophy: the good, the bad, and the ugly. Annu Rev Physiol 2003; 65: 45–79.
51. Molkentin JD, Dorn II GW. Cytoplasmic signaling pathways that regulate cardiac hypertrophy. Annu Rev Physiol 2001; 63: 391–426.
52. LaMorte VJ, Thorburn J, Absher D, et al. Gq- and ras-dependent pathways mediate hypertrophy of neonatal rat ventricular myocytes following alpha 1-adrenergic stimulation. J Biol Chem 1994; 269: 13490–6.

53. Akhter SA, Luttrell LM, Rockman HA, et al. Targeting the receptor-Gq interface to inhibit in vivo pressure overload myocardial hypertrophy. Science 1998; 280: 574–7.

54. D'Angelo DD, Sakata Y, Lorenz JN, et al. Transgenic Galphaq overexpression induces cardiac contractile failure in mice. Proc Natl Acad Sci U. S. A 1997; 94: 8121–6.

55. Wettschureck N, Rutten H, Zywietz A, et al. Absence of pressure overload induced myocardial hypertrophy after conditional inactivation of Galphaq/Galpha11 in cardiomyocytes. Nat Med 2001; 7: 1236–40.

56. Offermanns S, Zhao LP, Gohla A, et al. Embryonic cardiomyocyte hypoplasia and craniofacial defects in G alpha q/G alpha 11-mutant mice. EMBO J 1998; 17: 4304–12.

57. Offermanns S, Toombs CF, Hu YH, Simon MI. Defective platelet activation in G alphaq)-deficient mice. Nature 1997; 389: 183.186.

58. Molkentin JD, Lu JR, Antos CL, et al. A calcineurin-dependent transcriptional pathway for cardiac hypertrophy. Cell 1998; 93: 215–28.

59. Duerr RL, Huang S, Miraliakbar HR, et al. Insulin-like growth factor-1 enhances ventricular hypertrophy and function during the onset of experimental cardiac failure. J Clin Invest 1995; 95: 619–27.

60. Lupu F, Terwilliger JD, Lee K, Segre GV, Efstratiadis A. Roles of growth hormone and insulin-like growth factor 1 in mouse postnatal growth. Dev Biol 2001; 229: 141–62.

61. Dorn GW. The fuzzy logic of physiological cardiac hypertrophy. Hypertension 2007b; 49: 962–70.

62. Perrino C, Prasad SV, Mao L, et al. Intermittent pressure overload triggers hypertrophy-independent cardiac dysfunction and vascular rarefaction. J Clin Invest 2006; 116: 1547–60.

63. O'Neill BT, Abel ED. Akt1 in the cardiovascular system: friend or foe? J Clin Invest 2005; 115: 2059–64.

64. Condorelli G, Drusco A, Stassi G, et al. Jr. Akt induces enhanced myocardial contractility and cell size in vivo in transgenic mice. Proc Natl Acad Sci USA 2002; 99: 12333–8.

65. Matsui T, Li L, Wu JC, et al. Phenotypic spectrum caused by transgenic overexpression of activated Akt in the heart. J Biol Chem 2002; 277: 22896–901.

66. Shioi T, McMullen JR, Kang PM, et al S. Akt/protein kinase B promotes organ growth in transgenic mice. Mol Cell Biol 2002; 22: 2799–809.

67. Antos CL, McKinsey TA, Frey N, et al. Activated glycogen synthase-3 beta suppresses cardiac hypertrophy in vivo. Proc Natl Acad Sci USA 2002; 99: 907–12.

68. Michael A, Haq S, Chen X, et al. Glycogen synthase kinase-3beta regulates growth, calcium homeostasis, and diastolic function in the heart. J Biol Chem 2004; 279: 21383–93.

69. Zhang CL, McKinsey TA, Chang S, et al. Class II histone deacetylases act as signal-responsive repressors of cardiac hypertrophy. Cell 2002; 110: 479–88.

70. Haq S, Kilter H, Michael A, et al. Deletion of cytosolic phospholipase A2 promotes striated muscle growth. Nat Med 2003; 9: 944–51.

71. Yamamoto M, Yang G, Hong C, et al. Inhibition of endogenous thioredoxin in the heart increases oxidative stress and cardiac hypertrophy. J Clin Invest 2003; 112: 1395–406.

72. Koga A, Oka N, Kikuchi T, et al. Adenovirus-mediated overexpression of caveolin-3 inhibits rat cardiomyocyte hypertrophy. Hypertension 2003; 42: 213–19.

73. Shiojima I, Sato K, Izumiya Y, et al. Disruption of coordinated cardiac hypertrophy and angiogenesis contributes to the transition to heart failure. J Clin Invest 2005; 115: 2108–18.

74. Soonpaa MH, Field LJ. Survey of studies examining mammalian cardiomyocyte DNA synthesis. Circ Res 1998; 83: 15–26.

75. Kong Y, Tannous P, Lu G, et al. Suppression of class I and II histone deacetylases blunts pressure-overload cardiac hypertrophy. Circulation 2006; 113: 2579–88.

76. Hardt SE, Sadoshima J. Negative regulators of cardiac hypertrophy. Cardiovasc. Res 2004; 63: 500–9.

77. Berry JJ, Hoffman JM, Steenbergen C, et al. Human pathologic correlation with PET in ischemic and nonischemic cardiomyopathy. J Nucl Med 1993; 34: 39–47.

78. Olivetti G, Abbi R, Quaini F, et al. Apoptosis in the failing human heart. N Engl J Med 1997; 336: 1131–41.

79. Olivetti G, Capasso JM, Sonnenblick EH, Anversa P. Side-to-side slippage of myocytes participates in ventricular wall remodeling acutely after myocardial infarction in rats. Circ Res 1990; 67: 23–34.

80. Vatner SF. Reduced subendocardial myocardial perfusion as one mechanism for congestive heart failure. Am J.Cardiol 1988; 62: 94E–8E.

81. Hudlicka O, Brown M, Egginton S. Angiogenesis in skeletal and cardiac muscle. Physiol Rev 1992; 72: 369–417.

82. Shiojima I, Walsh K. Regulation of cardiac growth and coronary angiogenesis by the Akt/PKB signaling pathway. Genes Dev 2006; 20: 3347–65.

83. Sano M, Minamino T, Toko H, et al. Ip53-induced inhibition of Hif-1 causes cardiac dysfunction during pressure overload. Nature 2007; 446: 444–8.

84. Dorn GW. Myocardial angiogenesis: its absence makes the growing heart founder. Cell Metab 2007a; 5: 326–7.

85. Schaper J, Froede R, Hein S, et al. Impairment of the myocardial ultrastructure and changes of the cytoskeleton in dilated cardiomyopathy. Circulation 1991; 83: 504–14.

86. Levine B, Klionsky DJ. Development by self-digestion: molecular mechanisms and biological functions of autophagy. Dev Cell 2004; 6: 463–77.

87. Levine B, Yuan J. Autophagy in cell death: an innocent convict? J Clin Invest 2005; 115: 2679–88.

88. Dorn GW. Physiologic growth and pathologic genes in cardiac development and cardiomyopathy. Trends Cardiovasc Med 2005; 15: 185–9.

89. Wyllie AH. Apoptosis (the 1992 Frank Rose Memorial Lecture). Br J Cancer 1993; 67: 205–8.

90. Martelli AM, Zweyer M, Ochs RL, et al. Nuclear apoptotic changes: an overview. J Cell Biochem 2001; 82: 634–46.

91. Oparil S, Bishop SP, Clubb FJ Jr. Myocardial cell hypertrophy or hyperplasia. Hypertension 1984; 6: III38–III43.

92. Narula J, Haider N, Virmani R, et al. Apoptosis in myocytes in end-stage heart failure. N Engl J Med 1996; 335: 1182–9.

93. MacLellan WR, Schneider MD. Death by design. Programmed cell death in cardiovascular biology and disease. Circ Res 1997; 81: 137–44.

94. 94. Crow MT, Mani K, Nam YJ, Kitsis RN. The mitochondrial death pathway and cardiac myocyte apoptosis. Circ Res 2004; 95: 957–70.

95. Foo RS, Mani K, Kitsis RN. Death begets failure in the heart. J Clin Invest 2005; 115: 565–71.

96. Baines CP, Kaiser RA, Purcell NH, et al. Loss of cyclophilin D reveals a critical role for mitochondrial permeability transition in cell death. Nature 2005; 434: 658–62.

97. Strasser A. The role of BH3-only proteins in the immune system. Nat Rev Immunol 2005; 5: 189–200.

98. Hirota H, Chen J, Betz UA, et al. Loss of a gp130 cardiac muscle cell survival pathway is a critical event in the onset of heart failure during biomechanical stress. Cell 1999; 97: 189–98.

99. A., Brocheriou V, Hagege AA, Oubenaissa et al. Cardiac functional improvement by a human Bcl-2 transgene in a mouse model of ischemia/reperfusion injury. J Gene Med 2000; 2: 326–33.

100. Chen Z, Chua CC, Ho YS, Hamdy RC, Chua BH. Overexpression of Bcl-2 attenuates apoptosis and protects against myocardial I/R injury in transgenic mice. Am J Physiol Heart Circ Physiol 2001; 280: H2313–20.

101. Hochhauser E, Kivity S, Offen D, et al. Bax ablation protects against myocardial ischemia-reperfusion injury in transgenic mice. Am J Physiol Heart Circ Physiol 2003; 284: H2351–9.

102. Diwan A, Krenz M, Syed FM, et al. Inhibition of ischemic cardiomyocyte apoptosis through targeted ablation of Bnip3 restrains postinfarction remodeling in mice. J Clin Invest 2007; 117: 2825–33.

103. Diwan A, Wansapura J, Syed FM, et al. Nix-mediated apoptosis links myocardial fibrosis, cardiac remodeling, and hypertrophy decompensation. Circulation 2008; 117: 396–404.

4

Excitation–contraction coupling in the normal and failing heart

Mattew Coggins, Bernhard Haring, and Federica del Monte

THE ELECTRICAL ACTIVITY OF THE HEART

A distinctive feature of the generation of the heartbeat is the plasticity of the action potential (AP) and its pattern at the level of the different specialized cells within the heart (pacemaker cells, conduction system, and working myocytes). At the cellular level, the AP is generated by the coordinated actions of a large number of ion channels. The activation depends on the ion conductance activity of specific voltage-gated ion channels, which mediate rapid, voltage-dependent changes in ion permeability causing a change in the membrane potential. The different complements or densities of channels and pumps determine the differences in the AP characteristics within different cells populating the heart and different myocardial regions. Figure 4.1 shows the AP and the approximate time course of the depolarizing and repolarizing currents carried by the different ion channels in the working myocytes. The AP is classically divided into five phases (Fig. 4.1).

Phase 0

A rapid increase in Na^+ permeability mediated by voltage-sensitive Na^+ channels causing a rapid depolarization during the initial phase of the AP.

Phase 1

A rapid repolarization governed by a transient outward current known as I_{to}. Outward extrusion of K^+ through K^+ channels determines this current. Two separate K^+ channel gene families contribute to the formation of I_{to}:Kv1 (Kv1.4), a member of the shaker family, and Kv4 (Kv4.2 and Kv4.3), members of the shal family, the latter playing a predominant role in the repolarization of the AP in humans. The magnitude of I_{to} varies markedly within the different chambers and walls of the heart. I_{to} density is highest in atrial myocytes and epicardial ventricular myocytes, giving rise to the short AP, and low in endocardial ventricular myocytes.

Phase 2

A slow repolarization phase ensues the plateau of the AP. This phase is characterized by Ca^{2+} entering the cells (I_{Ca}) through L-type Ca^{2+} channels (LTCC). As the phase progresses, repolarization starts by slow inactivation of the L-type Ca^{2+} current and simultaneous activation of the delayed rectifier K currents (I_{KS}), which are mediated by Kv7.1 (KvLQT1) channels and coded by the gene KCNQ1. Mutations in this gene have been described with

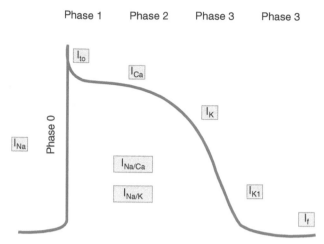

Figure 4.1 Ventricular cardiomyocyte action potential. The figure shows the various phases of the action potential and the corresponding depolarizing and repolarizing currents carried by the different ion channels in the working ventricular cardiomyocytes.

the occurrence of inherited arrhythmias, such as long QT syndrome, short QT syndrome, and familial atrial fibrillation.

Phase 3

Toward the end of the plateau, the rate of depolarization is markedly accelerated by a delayed rectifier current and an inward rectifier current (I_{K1}). Kir2.1 channels, which are encoded by the *KCNJ2* gene have been found essential in the generation of I_{K1}. In human heart failure I_{K1} is downregulated and mutations in Kir2.1 have been associated with Andersen syndrome as well as QT prolongation with ventricular arrhythmias. Also contributing to the depolarization phase are the Na^+/Ca^{2+} exchanger, which further removes Ca^{2+} from the cell and the outward Na^+ currents through the Na^+/K^+ ATPase pump. Altered activity in these channels may contribute to contractile dysfunction and arrhythmogenesis.

Phase 4

This is considered to be the normal resting membrane potential that the cell remains in until excitation by an external electrical stimulus occurs. It coincides with diastole of the chamber of the heart. Spontaneous depolarization during diastole is a normal property of the specialized cells for the conducting system that are the sinoatrial nodal, atrioventricular nodal, and Purkinje cells, but not atrial or ventricular myocytes under normal conditions. It is mainly driven by the hyperpolarization-activated inward current (I_f). I_f is a nonselective cation inward current, which in conjunction with the delayed rectifier current (I_K) that gradually deactivates, favors a net inward current resulting in the depolarization of the cell.

THE CALCIUM SIGNAL—ACTIVATION

In the mammalian heart, the AP-induced depolarization of the cell membrane leads to the opening of cell membrane channels, namely, the voltage-gated LTCC, allowing trans-sarcolemmal influx of calcium ion (Ca^{2+}) into the cell (Fig. 4.2) (reviewed in (1–3)). The LTCC are located in the sarcolemma and (predominantly) within the T-tubule projections and are in proximity to the Ca^{2+} release channels, known as ryanodine receptors (RyRs), located in the membrane of the terminal evagination (terminal cisternae) of the sarcoplasmic reticulum (SR), the major Ca^{2+} storing organelle in the cardiomyocyte. Ca^{2+} entering

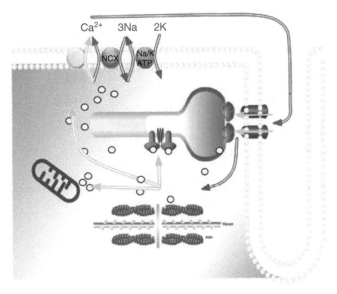

Figure 4.2 Excitation–contraction coupling scheme. Depolarization of the membrane by the action potential leads to the opening of voltage-gated LTCC allowing the entry of a small amount of Ca^{2+} into the cell. Through a coupling mechanism between the LTCC and the SR release channels (RyRs), a larger amount of Ca^{2+} is released activating the myofilaments leading to contraction. During relaxation, Ca^{2+} is re-accumulated back into the SR by the SR Ca^{2+} ATPase pump (SERCA2a) and extruded extracellularly by the sarcolemmal Na^+/Ca^{2+} exchanger. *Abbreviations*: LTCC, L-type calcium (Ca^{2+}) channels; SR, sarcoplasmic reticulum; RyRs, ryanodine receptors.

the cell through a single LTCC can induce the opening of one or a cluster of RyRs resulting in the local release of Ca^{2+} from the SR by the mechanism of Ca^{2+}-induced Ca^{2+} release (CICR) (1–9). The CICR was in the past believed to occur in an all-or-none fashion (Fabiato) (Fig. 4.3A). It is now acknowledged that a discrete activation occurs allowing the recruitment of different numbers of units (couplons) upon various stimulation intensities (Fig. 4.3B).

   From the classical description of the CICR, during membrane depolarization, a large number of LTCC are opened, resulting in a large release of Ca^{2+} from the RyRs, rising cytosolic $[Ca^{2+}]$ from 0.1–0.2 mM to 2–10 mM (Fig. 4.3A). It is now known that a discrete number of LTCC can be progressively opened to activate larger number of RyRs modulating the intensity of the signal (Fig. 4.3B). This amplification of the Ca^{2+} signal is critical for the initiation of contraction, and is dependent on the close association of LTCC and RyR. Groups of 10–25 LTCC and 100–200 RyR occupy focal areas at the junction between the T-tubule and the SR (the junctional cleft) where the space is only 10–20 nm wide (10–12). The grouping of the channels in discrete regions of the membrane has a functional role, which is now described as "local control" of excitation–contraction (E–C) coupling (reviewed in (13,14)). The local $[Ca^{2+}]_i$ in the junctional cleft is established at the onset of the AP by Ca^{2+} entry via LTCC. The resulting SR Ca^{2+} release by groups of 5–20 activated RyRs augments local $[Ca^{2+}]_i$, but because of physical separation this is independent of, and unresponsive to, $[Ca^{2+}]_i$ at neighboring junctions. The independence of Ca^{2+} release from one junction to the next prevents spontaneous Ca^{2+} release events independent of the AP from becoming Ca^{2+} waves, which can lead to uncontrolled electrical activity and arrhythmias (delayed after-depolarizations). Isolated Ca^{2+} release events from a single junction do not affect whole-cell $[Ca^{2+}]_i$ and do not cause activation of the contractile apparatus. In response to an AP, however, about

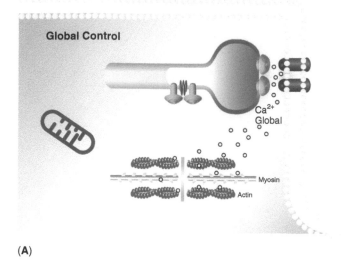

(A)

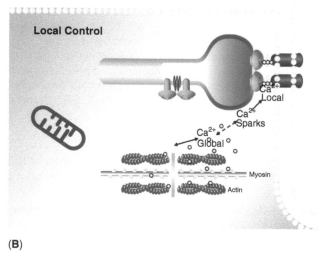

(B)

Figure 4.3   **(A)** global control of CICR. Schematic representation of the classical theory of LTCC to RyRs coupling occur in an all-or-none fashion (Fabiato) now revisited as pictured in **(B)** (local control of CICR) showing that a discrete activation occurs allowing the recruitment of segregated numbers of units (couplons) upon AP stimulation. In the common pool theory the AP activates the LTCC that serves as a trigger to activate the RyRs and Ca^{2+} enters a common pool activating RyRs. In the local control each LTCC–RyRs cluster is independently activated giving rise to elementary release events called "sparks." *Abbreviaions*: AP, action potential; CICR, calcium-induced calcium release; LTCC, L-type calcium (Ca^{2+}) channels; RyRs, ryanodine receptors.

20,000 junctions in a cardiomyocyte are activated nearly simultaneously and the summation of Ca^{2+} release causes a whole-cell Ca^{2+} transient to initiate contraction.

The local control model was lent more credence when, with the advent of confocal microscopy, a unit of Ca^{2+} release was characterized as corresponding to the coordinated opening of groups of RyR (15–28). These signals, termed Ca^{2+} sparks (Fig. 4.4), were first identified as the "elementary events" of spontaneous increases in $[Ca^{2+}]_i$, as detected by laser

Ca²⁺ Sparks

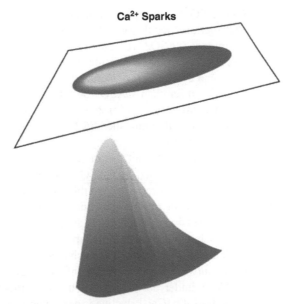

Figure 4.4   Calcium sparks are unitary elements of SR Ca²⁺ release. First described by Cheng in 1999 as elementary events of spontaneous increase in intracellular Ca²⁺, they were detected by laser scanner confocal microscopy and the fluorescent indicator Fluo-3 that. Sparks occur at rest at very low frequency in a stochastic manner and can be produced by the L-type Ca²⁺ channels reflecting the synchronous activation of a cluster of about RyRs at a single junction (local control) following the AP. Signal-averaged Ca²⁺ sparks are registered as line-scan image or surface plot (as schematically represented). The SR Ca²⁺ release takes place at the T-tubules in heart cells.

scanning confocal microscopy (29). Functionally, Ca²⁺ sparks represent Ca²⁺ releases from the SR through the opening of ~10–100 RyRs, based on the ratio of the Ca²⁺ spark current to the RyR single-channel current. Ca sparks are analyzed for their morphology (amplitude, width, and duration), kinetics of rise and decay, and frequency of occurrence. The activity (open probability) of individual RyRs and the number of RyRs recruited during a spark play an important role in the morphology: the more active the Ca²⁺ release channels are, the more Ca²⁺ is released and, as a consequence, the greater the magnitude and frequency of the sparks. Therefore, regulation of RyR activity will have an impact on the size and frequency of Ca²⁺ sparks.

The many metrics of RyR2-mediated SR Ca²⁺release [activation of the channel, sensitivity to $[Ca^{2+}]_i$ and SR Ca²⁺concentration ($[Ca^{2+}]_{SR}$), response to stress, and deactivation following an AP] are regulated by proteins in a complex with RyR (30). The RyR2 homotetramer is associated with a number of proteins, including two SR transmembrane proteins (junctin and triadin), two cytoplasmic proteins (calstabin2, or FKBP12.6, and sorcin), and an SR luminal protein (calsequestrin, CASQ), in addition to its interactions with cytoplasmic kinases [cAMP-dependent protein kinase (PKA) and Ca²⁺/calmodulin–dependent protein kinase (CAMKII)] and phosphatases.

The magnitude of CICR at an individual junction is modulated by $[Ca^{2+}]_{SR}$, an effect that is mediated by CASQ. At high $[Ca^{2+}]_{SR}$, RyR are more sensitive to $[Ca^{2+}]_i$, and a larger fractional release of SR calcium occurs during systole for a given LTCC flux—this is referred to as an increased gain. CASQ is believed to play a central role in SR Ca²⁺-sensing: it acts as a Ca²⁺ buffer, and is associates with the SR surface of RyR and triadin to exert Ca²⁺-dependent regulation (31,32). Studies using both deletion (33) and mutation (34) of the cardiac isoform of CASQ (CASQ2) in mice, however, have shown that additional layers of control exist. After CASQ2 deletion, modulation of CICR by SR calcium was intact (33). Mice engineered to express mutant CASQ2, representing a missense mutation seen in humans with catecholaminergic polymorphic ventricular tachycardia, were found to have reduced expression of CASQ2, and compensatory increases in expression of RyR and SR calreticulin, a less efficient Ca^{2+} buffer than CASQ (34). Despite these compensatory changes, the CASQ-deficient cardiomyocytes (CMs) showed markedly abnormal Ca^{2+} handling under ß-adrenergic stimulation, with diminished SR Ca^{2+} loading, excessive SR Ca^{2+} leak, increased diastolic $[Ca^{2+}]_i$, and arrhythmias.

There is substantial evidence that RyR Ca^{2+} release terminates in response to reduced $[Ca^{2+}]_{SR}$ (35), a process that is likely mediated by CASQ in association with junctin and triadin (31). It is still undetermined, however, whether this mechanism or one involving $[Ca^{2+}]_i$ in the junctional cleft (36) play the more significant role in RyR inactivation.

The regulation of LTCC expression and activity is an area of active research with a bearing on E–C coupling (37–41), but the scope of this chapter does not allow a full discussion. Also of note, the sarcolemmal sodium/calcium exchanger (NCX) can function in "reverse mode," generating an outward current and an influx of Ca^{2+} into the cytosol, although its contribution to $[Ca^{2+}]_i$ under normal conditions is controversial (1,42). The more canonical role of NCX in diastolic $[Ca^{2+}]_i$ decline is described below.

THE CALCIUM SIGNAL—THE EFFECTORS

The release of Ca^{2+} into the myofibrillar space results in myofilament cross-bridge formation and contraction (43–50). The myofilaments are organized in a regular array of thick and thin filaments giving the typical striated appearance of the entire myocyte (Fig. 4.5). Each unit of this striated organization, known as sarcomere, is classically described as composed of one unit of interacting thin and thick filaments.

The thick filaments consist mainly of myosin heavy chains and two pairs of light chains (Fig. 4.5). The "tail" of the molecule is coiled with two myosin heavy chains wound around each other. The "heads" of myosin include the globular region of one myosin molecule and two myosin light chains (46–50). Each myosin head has an ATP-binding area in close proximity to myosin ATPase, which breaks down ATP to release energy for the myofilament sliding. Two myosin heavy chain isoforms exist in human mammalian

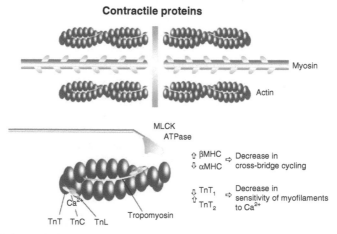

Figure 4.5 Schematic representation of the contractile protein and changes in isoforms of the myofibrillar process that contribute to the failing phenotype.

myocardium, α- and ß-MHC. In human ventricular myocardium only 10–20% is α-MHC while the ß-MHC is more abundant.

The thin filaments are mostly comprised of actin and troponin complex (Tn). Within the sarcomere, the actin polymers intertwine in a helical fashion. At intervals of 385 Å along the thin filaments are a group of three regulatory proteins that constitute the troponin complex carried on a long helical molecule called tropomyosin (Tm). The troponin complex is made up of one molecule each of troponin C, troponin I, and troponin T. The strength of the bond linking troponin I and actin varies depending on the intracellular Ca^{2+} level in turn regulating the actin/myosin interaction.

When the cytosolic Ca^{2+} is low the Tm–Tn complex is positioned in a way that the myosin heads cannot interact with actin. This is due to the bond linking TnI to actin. When cytosolic Ca^{2+} increases, it binds to TnC strengthening the bond between TnC and TnI and weakening the bond linking TnI to actin. This leads to a conformational change of the Tm–TnC complex, which allows the myosin head to interact with actin. When Ca^{2+} binds to TnC it exposes the active site on the thin filament, permitting the myosin head to bind weakly to the actin filaments. Subsequent ATP hydrolysis allows a strong binding of the myosin head to actin and a further shift of the Tm from the actin/myosin groove, which is followed by a power stroke that moves the actin molecule 5–10 nm, locking the myosin head into a rigor state. The myosin head releases ADP and is ready to accept ATP, which starts the cycle again. ATP binding to the myosin head dissociates the thin and thick filaments. This classical model of the activation of the actin/myosin complex by Ca^{2+} binding has been refined in the Geeves–Lehrer three-state model (Fig. 4.6) (51–54). According to this model at rest, Tm is in optimal blocking position (blocked state). With increased

3 Steps model

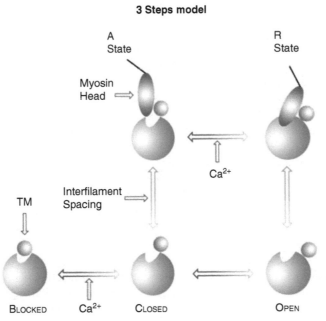

Figure 4.6 The newly proposed three-step model by Geeves–Lehrer of the sequential sensitization of actin–myosin interaction. In absence of Ca^{2+} Tm fully block the myosin-binding site of actin. Upon Ca^{2+} activation Tm partially uncovers the binding site leaving actin in a partially activated state. With Ca^{2+} binding to TnC the weak complex can shift to a higher affinity binding state that can generate the power stroke. *Abbreviation*: Tm, tropomyosin.

cytosolic Ca^{2+}, its binding to TnC leads to partial movement of Tm and to an actin–myosin weak binding (closed state or A state). Further Ca^{2+} increase can strengthen the complex binding state (R state). The A to R transition forces Tm further allowing for the recruitment of more cross-bridges.

In addition to the actin–myosin and troponin–tropomyosin complex, a much more intricate structural network of proteins and intermediate filaments regulates the force generation and transduction as well as the signaling pathways mediating the cell–cell communications and the crosstalk between myocytes and interstitial tissue. Those elements become of particular importance in mediating the response to stretch and increased pressure to the ventricle (hypertrophy and heart failure).

THE CALCIUM SIGNAL—INACTIVATION

Relaxation occurs when Ca^{2+} dissociates from TnC and is either re-accumulated into the SR by the cardiac isoform of the SR/endoplasmic reticulum (ER) Ca^{2+} ATPase (SERCA2a) or extruded outside the cell by the sarcolemmal Na^+/Ca^{2+} exchanger (NCX). The contributions of these mechanisms for lowering cytosolic Ca^{2+} vary among species. In humans ~75% of the Ca^{2+} is removed by SERCA2a and ~25% by NCX, with a small contribution from sarcolemmal Ca^{2+} ATP-ase and mitochondrial uptake. Although these two mechanisms work in concert to induce relaxation, their balanced activity is critical because increased activity of NCX functionally removes Ca^{2+} from the intracellular pool, allowing depletion of the SR Ca^{2+} stores.

SERCA2a transports Ca^{2+} into the lumen of the SR against a Ca^{2+} gradient by an energy-dependent mechanism (one molecule of ATP is hydrolyzed for the transport of two Ca^{2+} ions). The Ca^{2+} pumping activity of SERCA2a is regulated by the small transmembrane protein phospholamban (PL). In its unphosphorylated state, PL inhibits SERCA2a, whereas phosphorylation of PL by PKA at Ser16, by CAMKII at Thr17 or protein kinase C at Ser 10 reverses this inhibition. PL-mediated SR Ca^{2+} reuptake control is finely tuned by a cascade of protein phosphatases and kinases by which a protein phosphatase 1 (PP1) dephosphorylate PL increasing SERCA2a inhibition and in turn is inhibited by the PP1 inhibitor. In the SR, Ca^{2+} cannot be as a free ion and is buffered by a number of proteins such as calsequestrin (CASQ).

REGULATION OF CONTRACTILITY

A number of endogenous and exogenous factors regulate the strength of contraction in CMs.

Hormonal regulation is carried out by:

The ß-adrenergic signaling is the major regulator and controls both the rapid response to changes in contractility requirements as well as the more sustained tone. Catecholamines are the principal chemical mediators of the ß-adrenergic signaling and can be either released locally by the sympathetic nerve terminals or released in the circulation by the adrenal medulla. Circulating and locally released catecholamines bind to membrane receptors (myocardial ß1 and ß2 adrenoreceptors) (Fig. 4.1) and in turn activate adenylyl cyclase through stimulatory G proteins (Gsa), which results in the production of cAMP. Binding of cAMP to the regulatory subunit of PKA triggers a conformational change that allows the catalytic subunits of the enzyme to dissociate and phosphorylate protein substrates at serine and threonine subunits. These sites are present in all proteins regulating the E–C coupling and represent the site of control of the contractile response. Therefore, a complex signaling pathway regulates the response to adrenergic stimulation that includes a number of feedback signaling to synchronize the effectors and shut them off, but also redundancies to respond to potential defect in individual pathways (Fig. 4.7).

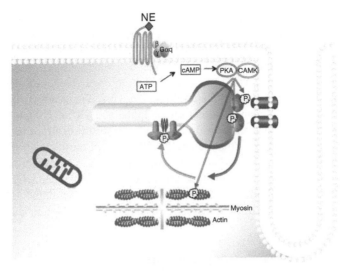

Figure 4.7 Cellular modulators of cardiac contractility. A number of SRs affect Ca^{2+} handling in cardiac myocytes. Agonists through G proteins increase adenyl cyclase activity resulting in cAMP production and activation of PKA leading to phosphorylation of all components of E–C coupling leading to a greater release of calcium from the SR and a faster relaxation: the L-type Ca^{2+} channels, allowing an increase in calcium entry, phosphorylation of phospholamban, increasing SERCA2a activity, and phosphorylation of troponin I decreasing the sensitivity of the myofilaments to Ca^{2+}. *Abbreviation*: SRs, sarcolemmal receptors.

In cardiac cells, PKA phosphorylates

- the LTCC resulting in increased Ca^{2+} entry
- RyR at serine 2808 resulting in increased systolic Ca^{2+} release
- PL at its serine 16 resulting in the release of inhibition of SERCA2a and enhanced Ca^{2+} uptake into the SR
- TnI resulting in enhanced detachment of Ca^{2+} from TnC and improved actin/myosin allosteric interaction.

The overall effects of PKA phosphorylation is to increase the strength of the contraction and enhance relaxation, thereby combining inotropic and lusitropic effects. ß3 receptors are the latest identified adrenergic receptor in the heart and convey an inhibitory function on contractility.

Other hormonally regulated signals are mediated by angiotensin I or endothelin I. Their relative receptors couple to heterotrimeric G proteins: Gq, which activates phospholipase C and inositol triphosphate (IP3) releasing Ca^{2+} from ER stores. Both angiotensin and endothelin receptor activation cause a more modest increase in contractility.

Mechanical regulation involves a frequency-dependent increase in force generation [force–frequency relationship (FFR)] and the length-dependent activation of the myofilaments both contributing to the short-term regulation of contractile strength in the heart. In the human and most mammalian normal heart, increasing heart rate results in enhanced trans -sarcolemmal Ca^{2+} influx secondary to high-frequency–induced recruitment of Ca^{2+} currents, resulting in more Ca^{2+} release from the SR and stronger contraction.

Whereas previously thought to be largely a Ca^{2+}-independent regulatory mechanism linked to the number of crossbridge interactions, the length-dependent activation of the myofilaments is now suggested to be also a function of the reduced distance between actin/mosin active sites, increasing the Ca^{2+} sensitivity of the myofilaments (55).

CHANGES OBSERVED IN HEART FAILURE

In CMs isolated from patients with heart failure, contraction and relaxation exhibit a similar set of abnormalities regardless of the etiology. The same changes were recapitulated in many animal models. Most changes affect sarcolemmal and SR ion channels, pumps, and receptors; signal transduction; expression and Ca^{2+} sensitivity of myofilaments; and the efficiency of metabolic pathways that generate ATP. Some of these changes may be adaptive in the face of the high workload and stress of heart failure and exacerbate the already compromised state. In fact, other than mutations of some of the players, which control E–C coupling (PL) or of the end effectors of the contractile force (myofilaments), the primary mechanism initiating the deleterious cascade of changes described in the failing heart remains unknown.

Action Potential and Repolarizing Currents

Changes in Ca^{2+} handling proteins and channel proteins governing cardiac repolarization have a significant impact on the electrical activity of the failing heart (56,57). Prolongation of the AP duration is a prominent feature of heart failure. Various ionic currents have been shown to be altered in heart failure. The inward rectifier K^+ current (IK1) and the transient outward K^+ current (I_{to}) are significantly reduced in heart failure. Associated with the reduction in I_{to}, there is a decrease in the expression of Kv4.2 and Kv4.3. Other changes in ionic currents are summarized in the side panel of Fig. 4.8. All those changes in ionic current lead to a prolongation in the duration of the AP and increased time of Ca^{2+} influx in the cell.

Calcium Handling—Activation and Inactivation

Abnormal Ca^{2+} cycling is a key component of cardiomyocyte dysfunction (4,44,45,58–68).

Cardiomyocytes isolated from failing human hearts exhibit three important alterations (59,60): (*i*) A decrease in the amplitude of systolic Ca^{2+} transients, (*ii*) an increase in diastolic $[Ca^{2+}]_i$, and (*iii*) a prolonged contraction and relaxation phase (60). This complex

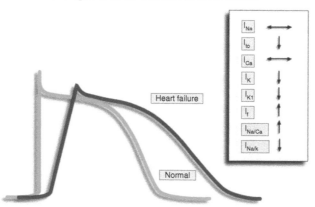

Figure 4.8   Changes in AP in heart failure: In failing hearts, the action potential duration is markedly prolonged and is associated with changes in ionic currents.

disarray can be understood by considering the relative changes in expression and regulation of the cell's Ca^{2+} handling proteins seen in heart failure (Table 4.1) (4,44,45,58,61–68). It must be noted that there are a number of different experimental models of heart failure, as there are distinct clinical etiologies. This discussion will focus on those alterations that appear to be common to the endpoint of impaired E–C coupling.

1. The conductive properties of both LTCCs and RyRs from patients with heart failure, as assayed by voltage clamp, are essentially normal. The mechanism of CICR may be defective, however, as a result of impaired coupling at the junction such that LTCC have a reduced ability to activate adjacent RyR (69,70) (decreased gain). Reduced coupling could be explained by increased width of the junctional cleft or disruption of the T-tubule system resulting in both the mismatch of the two Ca^{2+} channels and an increase in the distance between LTCC and RyRs (Figs. 4.9 and 4.10) (71–76). It is not known whether this abnormality is common to all etiologies of failure.
2. In both failing human hearts and experimental models of heart failure, there is reduced expression of SERCA2a. PL expression and phosphorylation are altered as well (77–79), although there is some disagreement over the net effect on SERCA2 function. Consequently, the $[Ca^{2+}]_i$ transient is reduced secondary to a decrease in the SR Ca^{2+} load and the rising and decaying time is elongated (80–87).
3. Concurrently, there is an increase in Na^+/Ca^{2+} exchanger expression and activity. The enhanced expression of the exchanger has been hypothesized to be compensatory for the reduction of SERCA2a because the Na^+/Ca^{2+} exchanger can operate to bring Ca^{2+} into the cell or extrude it out from the cell. In fact, there is an increase in sensitivity to compounds that produce positive inotropic effects through raised intracellular Na^+, either by inhibiting the Na^+/K^+-ATPase or by opening Na^+ channels, in failing human hearts (83).

These changes initially detected using Ca^{2+}-sensitive ionophores were also lately detectable by confocal microscopy. The Ca^{2+} spark were characterized in explanted failing human hearts as well as different animal models of cardiac hypertrophy and heart failure.

Table 4.1   Summary of Changes in the Expression of E–C Coupling Proteins in the Failing Heart

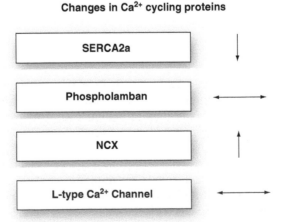

Changes in Ca^{2+} cycling proteins

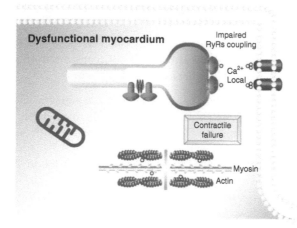

Figure 4.9 Calcium spark is generated by the stochastic opening of the L-type calcium channels and the subsequents activation of RyR2. In the failing heart disruption of the T-tubules architecture contributes to disruption of L-type Ca^{2+} channels to ryanodine receptors with increased distance between the two proteins, thereby decreasing the coupling and release mechanisms.

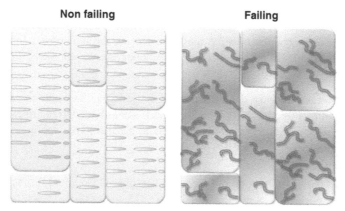

Figure 4.10 Schematic diagram of the T-tubule disorganization in normal and failing myocytes.

Ca^{2+} spark frequency, an index of basal sensitivity to release activation, has been shown to be higher in failing than nonfailing myocytes when SR Ca^{2+} load was matched. Furthermore, in the intact cellular environment the increase in Ca^{2+} spark frequency was assumed to be the primary contributing factor to the elevated diastolic SR Ca^{2+} leak in heart failure.

Finally, there is evidence that diminished SR Ca^{2+} release during heart failure may increase the sensitivity of RyRs to luminal Ca^{2+}, resulting in enhanced spark-mediated SR Ca^{2+} leakage and reduced intra-SR $[Ca^{2+}]$ in turn activating a number of changes in protein synthesis and post-translation modification (beyond the scope of the present chapter). The reasons for the abnormal RyRs behavior are unknown. Disrupted protein–protein interactions within the RyRs complex, altered covalent modification of RyRs, such as phosphorylation, or acquired defects by reactive intracellular metabolites are being discussed.

End Effectors: The Contractile Proteins

A number of abnormalities occur at the level of the contractile proteins in failing myocardium (Fig. 4.5). There is a decrease in the fast isoform of the myosin heavy chain (α-MHC) and an increase in the slower isoform ß-MHC. However, those changes, described in rodents are less relevant in human disease as the ß-MHC is the main isoform found in the normal human heart. Conversely, in nonfailing myocardium, there is one single predominant isoform for troponin T referred to as Troponin T1. A second isoform (Troponin T2) increases substantially in ventricular myocardium of patients with heart failure. These isoform shifts and changes of the contractile proteins have direct consequences on the functional properties of muscle contraction. An increase in ß-MHC results in a decrease in crossbridge cycling rate and an increase in energy conservation because fewer ATP molecules are split. It also leads to slower contraction and relaxation phases, which are characteristic of the failing myocardium. An increase in the expression of Troponin T2 leads to a decrease in the sensitivity of the myofilaments to Ca^{2+} and an abnormal response to agents targeting the myofilaments. Furthermore, a decrease in myosin light chain kinase has been shown and there is a 20–30% reduction in myofibrillar protein content. Finally, it was reported that cardiac myosin-binding protein-C (cMyBP-C), which is an important regulator of cardiac contractility and cardiac output via phosphorylation by PKA after ß-adrenergic stimulation, is less phosphorylated in human and experimental heart failure (88,89).

Force-Frequency

FFR is an important intrinsic regulatory mechanism for rapid changes of cardiac contractility, and hence the result of the interplay between Ca^{2+} handling and contractile response. Under physiologic conditions the FFR in most mammalian ventricular myocardium is positive, that is, a rise in contractile response combined with an increase in the amplitude of Ca^{2+} transients is induced by an elevation of the stimulation frequency at fixed preload. In failing CMs the force–frequency response is negative leading to a decrease in contraction and Ca^{2+} release with increasing frequency. This impaired FFR seems only in part be explainable by the inability of contractile proteins to further increase contractility, but rather a reflection of an altered functional balance between Ca^{2+} reuptake and Ca^{2+} extrusion. In this context, the role of the SR appears to be crucial.

A decrease in SERCA2a activity may contribute significantly to an impaired systolic and diastolic function. Mice studies overexpressing SERCA2a find a positive FFR compared with a flat relationship in the controls. This supports the notion that SERCA2a is key for the induction of a positive FFR. An increase in SERCA2a expression enhances the ability of the SR to store Ca^{2+}, such that more Ca^{2+} is available to be released during each heartbeat at higher stimulation rates (90).

In the failing human ventricular myocardium, SERCA2a activity has been found to be suppressed. Overexpression of SERCA2a in human ventricular myocytes isolated from patients with end-stage heart failure restored the positive FFR, thus strengthening the idea of correlating SERCA2a activity with FFR (91). Additionally, the important role of the SR Ca^{2+} load has been underlined by the finding that the inhibition of SR Ca^{2+} ATPase by thapsigargin abolishes the positive FFR in the nonfailing human ventricular myocytes but has no effect in the failing myocytes. Therefore, no differences in the FFR between nonfailing and failing myocytes can be detected after the inhibition of SR Ca^{2+} ATPase (91–95).

Table 4.2 Summary of Changes in the Expression of Adrenergic Receptors and G-Coupled Second Messengers in the Failing Heart

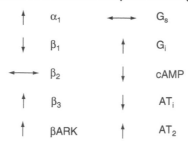

Alterations of membrane receptors in failing hearts

↑	α_1	⟷	G_s
↓	β_1	↑	G_i
⟷	β_2	↓	cAMP
↑	β_3	↓	AT_i
↑	βARK	↑	AT_2

ß-Receptor Signaling

Increased sympathetic tone is the first physiologic response of the heart to reduced cardiac output. The stimulation of the sympathetic nervous system results in phosphorylation of the ECC proteins by PKA. PKA phosphorylation modulates RyR2 function by changing the sensitivity of RyR2 to Ca^{2+} resulting in "leaky" channel as well as dissociation of the stabilizing proteins composing the macromolecular complex.

Chronic hyperactivity of the sympathetic nervous system is one of the first changes described in heart failure and results in the downregulation of ß-AR, ß-AR uncoupling, and an upregulation of the ß-AR kinase (ß-ARK1) (Table 4.2). As a consequence to these molecular changes, there is reduced functional responsiveness to ß-adrenergic agonists and cAMP-dependent inotropic agents. These lead to a reduction in cAMP and consequently inactivation of PKA, and reduced phosphorylation of proteins involved in Ca^{2+} homeostasis as described earlier.

CAMKII Signaling

CAMKII belongs to a family of multifunctional protein kinases that regulate Ca^{2+} homeostasis and are essential for normal cardiac function (96–104). CAMKII expression and activity is found to be increased in failing human myocardium and in many animal models of cardiac hypertrophy and heart failure (105–108). CAMKII is initially activated by binding to calcified calmodulin (Ca^{2+}/CaM), which in turn reorders the structure of the CAMKII molecule by disinhibiting the catalytic domain and exposing the regulatory domain. Excessive CAMKII is involved in many maladaptive cellular events for it has been described to activate hypertrophic genes by phosphorylating class II histone deacetylases (HDACs) and inflammatory reactions by enhanced activity of NF-κB after myocardial infarction. It reportedly amplifies the disruption of intracellular Ca^{2+} homeostasis in heart failure by increasing the opening probability of voltage-gated Ca^{2+} channels and RyRs and has been associated with modulating voltage-gated Ca^{2+} channels and Na+ channels. Finally, CAMKII enfolds proapoptotic signaling during myocardial infarction, excessive catecholamine, angiotensin II exposure, and aortic banding surgery. It could be shown that enhanced adrenergic stimulation results in apoptotic signaling pathways via PKA-independent stimulation of LTCC, and thereby activating CAMKII. This mechanistic link between ß-receptor signaling and CAMKII may contribute to the deterioration of cardiac function in the failing heart. However, the precise adrenergic subtype (possibly ß1) that is responsible for the activation of CAMKII in the heart has not been fully elucidated at this point (98,105,107,109–116).

Architectural Changes

The sarcolemmal membrane of mammalian ventricular CMs is characterized by the presence of invaginations called transverse tubules (T-tubules). T-tubules constitute transverse elements with longitudinal extensions that occur at the Z-line. As mentioned before, some studies have highlighted the role of structural changes in the T-tubule architecture in the disruption of the CICR coupling (73,117,118). Other reported T-tubule restructuring in heart failure might explain the poor coordination of Ca^{2+} release (119,120). In this case, the reorganization of T-tubule cellular structure may produce "rogue" or "orphaned" RyRs that might respond differently to local Ca^{2+} changes. Thus, this concept combines the idea of T-tubule loss resulting in an increasing gap between LTCC and underlying RyRs with dyssynchronous Ca^{2+} release (Figs. 4.9 and 4.10). Observed Ca^{2+} sparks that are not uniformly distributed within heart failure cells and that disappear from areas devoid of T-tubules may reinforce this concept (74,81,121–124).

IMPLICATIONS FOR TREATMENT OF HEART FAILURE

Manipulation of the Ca^{2+} cycling machinery and in the ß-adrenergic signaling pathways second messengers (125–127) in heart failure has met with success (58,61,128–131).

EXCITATION–CONTRACTION COUPLING IN HUMAN STEM/PROGENITOR CELLS

The recognition that heart failure in animals and humans may be successfully targeted with implantation/activation of stem/progenitor cells has raised vivid discussions. Although a comprehensive description of the current potential sources of attempting to replace heart failure tissue is beyond the scope of the present chapter, two sources of cells from which Ca^{2+} handling characteristics have been more systematically addressed will hereby be described because overall, the suitability of stem cell–derived CMs for regenerating cardiac tissue depends, in part, on their contractile characteristics, which in turn are determined by their pattern of excitability, Ca^{2+} handling, and E–C coupling. One source of replacing heart failure tissue is proposed through activation and commitment of quiescent cardiac progenitor cells (CPCs) stored in myocardial niches in the adult heart. Another mean involves the use of CMs derived from human embryonic stem cells (hESCs) followed by implantation into the adult heart.

Cardiac Progenitor Cells

Human cardiac progenitor cells (hCPC) positive for the surface marker c-kit have been examined for their Ca^{2+} handling properties. In these cells, Ca^{2+} oscillations have been identified independently from the presence or absence of extracellular Ca^{2+}. Interestingly, these oscillations that correlate positively with cell growth are regulated by the release of Ca^{2+} from the ER through activation of inositol 1,4,5-triphosphate receptors (IP3Rs) and the reuptake of Ca^{2+} by SERCA2a. Although RyRs have not been detected in c-kit-positive hCPC, IP3Rs and SERCA2a seem to be highly expressed in hCPCs. Furthermore, Na^+/Ca^{2+} (NCX) exchanger, store-operated Ca^{2+} channels, and plasma membrane Ca^{2+} pump have also been found functionally in hCPCs, but an effect on Ca^{2+} oscillations has not been described (132).

Human Embryonic Stem Cells

hESCs can be induced to differentiate *in vitro* into CMs (hESC-CMs). These cells have been shown to express cardiac markers as well as express key Ca^{2+} handling proteins, including SERCA2b, the Na^+/Ca^{2+} exchanger, and RyR2. Furthermore, spontaneous APs, $[Ca^{2+}]_i$ transients, and contractile activity could also be detected. Despite these findings, there is still considerable ongoing discussion as to the fundamental mechanisms of ECC in these cells. This may in part be explainable through the use of hESC-CMs generated and prepared via different methods (e.g., embryoid body differentiation), which can influence the purity of cardiac cells and their maturation. It has been shown that hESC-CMs require Ca^{2+} entry through LTCC and that the (less-developed) SR also contributes to the $[Ca^{2+}]_i$ transient in these cells (133–138). Similar to adult ventricular myocytes, membrane depolarization triggers large L-type Ca^{2+} currents (I_{Ca}) and corresponding whole-cell $[Ca^{2+}]_i$ transients in hESC-CMs, and the amplitude of both I_{Ca} and the $[Ca^{2+}]_i$ transients are graded by the magnitude of the depolarization. Furthermore, Ca^{2+} sparks can be recorded in hESC-CMs. Thus, current evidence supports a model of local control of SR Ca^{2+} release by the I_{Ca} during E–C coupling in hESC-CMs similar to adult CMs (133,135,136). However, some differences in intracellular Ca^{2+} handling of hESC-CMs properties from the adult myocardium were referred to an immature SR capacity. Specifically, it is suggested that hESCM-CMs display $[Ca^{2+}]_i$ transients and contractions, negative FFR, and lack of postrest potentiation. Additionally, in these cells, contraction seems to depend on transsarcolemmal Ca^{2+} influx rather than on SR Ca^{2+} release (137). On the other hand, it was further reported that hESC-CMs do exhibit caffeine- and ryanodine-sensitive SR Ca^{2+} stores, even at early stages. To this point there seems to be increasing evidence in favor of an existence of a functional SR in hESC-derived CMs (133–136,139).

Furthermore, as in c-kit-positive hCPCs IP3-dependent Ca^{2+} signaling seems to play a functional role during cardiac development. Reportedly, IP3R are the first Ca^{2+} release channels expressed in embryos and contribute to the spontaneous activity in mouse ESC-CMs. However, the significance of inositol-1,4,5-trisphosphate (IP3) receptors in hESC-CMs remains to be elucidated (134,140–143).

CONCLUSION

Through the window of ECC, we can get a better understanding of heart failure at the cellular and molecular levels. Abnormal intracellular Ca^{2+} handling seems to be the common pathway that induces a decrease in contractility and a worsening in arrhythmias. Our understanding of the key abnormalities in ionic changes within the cardiac cell in the failing heart may provide new therapeutic strategies for cardiac heart failure.

REFERENCES

1. Bers DM. Cardiac excitation–contraction coupling. Nature 2002; 415: 198–205.
2. Bers DM. Calcium cycling and signaling in cardiac myocytes. Annu Rev Physiol 2008; 70: 23–49.
3. Bers DM, Weber CR. Na/Ca exchange function in intact ventricular myocytes. Ann N Y Acad Sci 2002; 976: 500–12.
4. Gwathmey JK, Slawsky MT, Hajjar RJ, Briggs GM, Morgan JP. Role of intracellular calcium handling in force–interval relationships of human ventricular myocardium. J Clin Invest 1990; 85: 1599–613.
5. Fabiato A. Calcium-induced release of calcium from the cardiac sarcoplasmic reticulum. Am J Physiol Cell Physiol 1983; 245: C1–14.
6. Trafford AW, Diaz ME, Eisner DA. Coordinated control of Cell Ca2+ loading and triggered release from the sarcoplasmic reticulum underlies the rapid inotropic response to increased L-type Ca2+ current. Circ Res 2001; 88: 195–201.
7. Wier WG. Gain and cardiac E–C coupling: revisited and revised. Circ Res 2007; 101: 533–5.
8. Bers DM. Calcium and cardiac rhythms: physiological and pathophysiological. Circ Res 2002; 90: 14–17.
9. Piacentino V 3rd, Weber CR, Chen X, et al. Cellular basis of abnormal calcium transients of failing human ventricular myocytes. Circ Res 2003; 92: 651–8.
10. Carl SL, Felix K, Caswell AH, et al. Immunolocalization of sarcolemmal dihydropyridine receptor and sarcoplasmic reticular triadin and ryanodine receptor in rabbit ventricle and atrium. J. Cell Biol 1995; 129: 673–82.

11. Sommer JR. Comparative anatomy: in praise of a powerful approach to elucidate mechanisms translating cardiac excitation into purposeful contraction. J Mol Cell Cardiol 1995; 27: 19–35.

12. Franzini-Armstrong C, Protasi F, Ramesh V. Shape, size, and distribution of Ca2+ release units and couplons in skeletal and cardiac muscles. Biophys. J 1999; 77: 1528–39.

13. Wier WG, Balke CW. Ca2+ release mechanisms, Ca2+ sparks, and local control of excitation–contraction coupling in normal heart muscle. Circ Res 1999; 85: 770–6.

14. Guatimosim S, Dilly K, Ferno Santana L, et al. Local Ca2+ signaling and EC coupling in heart: Ca2+ sparks and the regulation of the [Ca2+]i transient. J Mol Cell Cardiol 2002; 34: 941.

15. Pratusevich VR, Balke CW. Factors shaping the confocal image of the calcium spark in cardiac muscle cells. Biophys J 1996; 71: 2942–2957.

16. Satoh H, Blatter LA, Bers DM. Effects of [Ca2+]i, SR Ca2+ load, and rest on Ca2+ spark frequency in ventricular myocytes. Am J Physiol. 1997; 272: H657–668.

17. Bonev AD, Jaggar JH, Rubart M, Nelson MT. Activators of protein kinase C decrease Ca2+ spark frequency in smooth muscle cells from cerebral arteries. Am J Physiol. 1997;273: C2090–2095.

18. Satoh H, Hayashi H, Blatter LA, Bers DM. BayK 8644 increases resting calcium spark frequency in ferret ventricular myocytes. Heart Vessels 1997: 58–61.

19. Smith GD, Keizer JE, Stern MD, Lederer WJ, Cheng H. A simple numerical model of calcium spark formation and detection in cardiac myocytes. Biophys J 1998; 75: 15–32.

20. Parrington J, Coward K. The spark of life. Biologist (London) 2003; 50: 5–10.

21. Zhuge R, Fogarty KE, Tuft RA, Walsh JV Jr. Spontaneous transient outward currents arise from microdomains where BK channels are exposed to a mean Ca(2+) concentration on the order of 10 microM during a Ca(2+) spark. J Gen Physiol 2002; 120: 15–27.

22. Shtifman A, Ward CW, Yamamoto T, et al. Interdomain interactions within ryanodine receptors regulate Ca2+ spark frequency in skeletal muscle. J Gen Physiol 2002; 119: 15–32.

23. Gonzalez A, Kirsch WG, Shirokova N, et al. The spark and its ember: separately gated local components of Ca(2+) release in skeletal muscle. J Gen Physiol 2000; 115: 139–58.

24. Gyorke S. Ca2+ spark termination: inactivation and adaptation may be manifestations of the same mechanism. J Gen Physiol 1999; 114: 163–6.

25. Fill M, Mejia-Alvarez R, Kettlun C, Escobar A. Ryanodine receptor permeation and gating: glowing cinders that underlie the Ca2+ spark. J Gen Physiol 1999; 114: 159–61.

26. Imaizumi Y, Ohi Y, Yamamura H, et al. Ca2+ spark as a regulator of ion channel activity. Jpn J Pharmacol 1999; 80: 1–8.

27. Izu LT, Wier WG, Balke CW. Theoretical analysis of the Ca2+ spark amplitude distribution. Biophys J 1998; 75: 1144–62.

28. Keizer J, Smith GD. Spark-to-wave transition: saltatory transmission of calcium waves in cardiac myocytes. Biophys Chem 1998; 72: 87–100.

29. Cheng H, Lederer WJ, Cannell MB. Calcium sparks: elementary events underlying excitation–contraction coupling in heart muscle. Science 1993; 262: 740–4.

30. Bers DM. Macromolecular complexes regulating cardiac ryanodine receptor function. J Mol Cell Cardiol 2004; 37: 417–29.

31. Gyorke I, Hester N, Jones LR, Gyorke S. The role of calsequestrin, triadin, and junctin in conferring cardiac ryanodine receptor responsiveness to luminal calcium. Biophys. J 2004; 86: 2121–8.

32. Gyorke S, Hagen BM, Terentyev D, Lederer WJ. Chain-reaction Ca(2+) signaling in the heart. J Clin Invest 2007; 117: 1758–62.

33. Knollmann BC, Chopra N, Hlaing T, et al. Casq2 deletion causes sarcoplasmic reticulum volume increase, premature Ca2+ release, and catecholaminergic polymorphic ventricular tachycardia. J Clin Invest 2006; 116: 2510–20.

34. Song L, Alcalai R, Arad M, et al. Calsequestrin 2 (CASQ2) mutations increase expression of calreticulin and ryanodine receptors, causing catecholaminergic polymorphic ventricular tachycardia. J Clin Invest 2007; 117: 1814–23.

35. Terentyev D, Viatchenko-Karpinski S, Valdivia HH, Escobar AL, Gyorke S. Luminal Ca2+ controls termination and refractory behavior of Ca2+-induced Ca2+ release in cardiac myocytes. Circ Res 2002; 91: 414–20.

36. Sham JS, Song LS, Chen Y, et al. Termination of Ca2+ release by a local inactivation of ryanodine receptors in cardiac myocytes. Proc Natl Acad Sci USA 1998; 95: 15096–15101.

37. Altamirano J, Bers DM. Effect of intracellular Ca2+ and action potential duration on L-type Ca2+ channel inactivation and recovery from inactivation in rabbit cardiac myocytes. Am J Physiol Heart Circ Physiol 2007; 293: H563–73.

38. Altamirano J, Bers DM. Voltage dependence of cardiac excitation contraction coupling: unitary Ca2+ current amplitude and open channel probability. Circ Res 2007; 101: 590–7.

39. Gao T, Chien AJ, Hosey MM. Complexes of the alpha 1c and beta subunits generate the necessary signal for membrane targeting of class c L-type calcium channels. J Biol Chem 1999; 274: 2137–44.

40. Leach RN, Desai JC, Orchard CH. Effect of cytoskeleton disruptors on L-type Ca channel distribution in rat ventricular myocytes. Cell Calcium 2005; 38: 515–26.

41. Wang H-G, George MS, Kim J, Wang C, Pitt GS. Ca2+/calmodulin regulates trafficking of cav1.2 Ca2+ channels in cultured hippocampal neurons. J. Neurosci 2007; 27: 9086–93.

42. Sipido KR, Maes M, Van de Werf F. Low efficiency of Ca2+ entry through the Na+-Ca2+ exchanger as trigger for Ca2+ release from the sarcoplasmic reticulum: a comparison between L-type Ca2+ current and reverse-mode Na+-Ca2+ exchange. Circ Res 1997; 81: 1034–44.

43. Hajjar RJ, Schwinger RH, Schmidt U, et al. Myofilament calcium regulation in human myocardium. Circulation 2000; 101: 1679–85.

44. Gwathmey JK, Kim CS, Hajjar RJ, et al. Cellular and molecular remodeling in a heart failure model treated with the beta-blocker carteolol. Am J Physiol 1999; 276(5 Pt 2): H1678–90.

45. Gwathmey JK, Liao R, Helm PA, Thaiyananthan G, Hajjar RJ. Is contractility depressed in the failing human heart? [Review] [40 refs]. Cardiovascular Drugs & Therapy 1995; 9: 581–7.

46. Solaro RJ, Varghese J, Marian AJ, Chandra M. Molecular mechanisms of cardiac myofilament activation: modulation by pH and a troponin T mutant R92Q. Basic Res Cardiol 2002; 97: I102–10.

47. Solaro RJ, Montgomery DM, Wang L, et al. Integration of pathways that signal cardiac growth with modulation of myofilament activity. J Nucl Cardiol 2002; 9: 523–33.

48. Martin AF, Phillips RM, Kumar A, et al. Ca(2+) activation and tension cost in myofilaments from mouse hearts ectopically expressing enteric gamma-actin. Am J Physiol Heart Circ Physiol 2002; 283:H642–9.

49. de Tombe PP, Solaro RJ. Integration of cardiac myofilament activity and regulation with pathways signaling hypertrophy and failure. Ann Biomed Eng 2000; 28: 991–1001.

50. Wolska BM, Keller RS, Evans CC, et al. Correlation between myofilament response to Ca2+ and altered dynamics of contraction and relaxation in transgenic cardiac cells that express beta-tropomyosin. Circ Res 1999; 84: 745–51.

51. Lehrer SS, Geeves MA. The muscle thin filament as a classical cooperative/allosteric regulatory system. J Mol Biol 1998; 277: 1081–9.

52. Fuchs F, Wang YP. Sarcomere length versus interfilament spacing as determinants of cardiac myofilament Ca2+ sensitivity and Ca2+ binding. J Mol Cell Cardiol 1996; 28: 1375–83.

53. Gordon AM, Homsher E, Regnier M. Regulation of contraction in striated muscle. Physiol Rev 2000; 80: 853–924.

54. Fuchs F, Smith SH. Calcium, cross-bridges, and the Frank–Starling relationship. News Physiol Sci 2001; 16: 5–10.

55. Irving TC, Konhilas J, Perry D, Fischetti R, de Tombe PP. Myofilament lattice spacing as a function of sarcomere length in isolated rat myocardium. Am J Physiol Heart Circ Physiol 2000; 279: H2568–73.

56. Kaprielian R, Wickenden AD, Kassiri Z, et al. Relationship between K+ channel down-regulation and [Ca2+]i in rat ventricular myocytes following myocardial infarction. J. Physiol 1999; 517(Pt 1): 229–245.

57. Kaprielian R, del Monte F, Hajjar RJ. Targeting Ca2+ cycling proteins and the action potential in heart failure by gene transfer. Basic Res Cardiol 2002; 97: I136–45.

58. del Monte F, Harding SE, Dec GW, Gwathmey JK, Hajjar RJ. Targeting phospholamban by gene transfer in human heart failure. Circulation 2002; 105: 904–7.

59. Gwathmey JK, Copelas L, MacKinnon R, et al. Abnormal intracellular calcium handling in myocardium from patients with end-stage heart failure. Circ Res 1987; 61: 70–6.

60. Beuckelmann DJ, Nabauer M, Erdmann E. Intracellular calcium handling in isolated ventricular myocytes from patients with terminal heart failure. Circulation 1992; 85: 1046–55.

61. del Monte F, Williams E, Lebeche D, et al. Improvement in survival and cardiac metabolism after gene transfer of sarcoplasmic reticulum Ca(2+)-ATPase in a rat model of heart failure. Circulation 2001; 104: 1424–9.

62. DeSantiago J, Maier LS, Bers DM. Frequency-dependent acceleration of relaxation in the heart depends on CaMKII, but not phospholamban. J Mol Cell Cardiol 2002; 34: 975–84.

63. del Monte F, Harding SE, Schmidt U, et al. Restoration of contractile function in isolated cardiomyocytes from failing human hearts by gene transfer of serca2a. Circulation 1999; 100: 2308–11.

64. Despa S, Islam MA, Pogwizd SM, Bers DM. Intracellular [Na+] and Na+ pump rate in rat and rabbit ventricular myocytes. J Physiol 2002; 539: 133–143.

65. Despa S, Islam MA, Weber CR, Pogwizd SM, Bers DM. Intracellular Na(+) concentration is elevated in heart failure but Na/K pump function is unchanged. Circulation 2002; 105: 2543–8.

66. Force T, Hajjar R, Del Monte F, Rosenzweig A, Choukroun G. Signaling pathways mediating the response to hypertrophic stress in the heart. Gene Expr 1999; 7: 337–348.
67. Ginsburg KS, Weber CR, Despa S, Bers DM. Simultaneous measurement of [Na]i, [Ca]i, and I(NCX) in intact cardiac myocytes. Ann N Y Acad Sci 2002; 976: 157–8.
68. Gwathmey JK, Hajjar RJ. Relation between steady-state force and intracellular [Ca2+] in intact human myocardium. Index of myofibrillar responsiveness to Ca2+. Circulation 1990; 82: 1266–78.
69. Gomez AM, Valdivia HH, Cheng H, et al. Defective excitation–contraction coupling in experimental cardiac hypertrophy and heart failure. Science 1997; 276: 800–6.
70. Yue DT. Quenching the spark in the heart. Science 1997; 276: 755–6.
71. He J-Q, Conklin MW, Foell JD, et al. Reduction in density of transverse tubules and L-type Ca2+ channels in canine tachycardia-induced heart failure. Cardiovasc Res 2001; 49: 298–307.
72. Brette F, Orchard C. T-tubule Function in Mammalian Cardiac Myocytes. Circ Res 2003; 92: 1182–92.
73. Balijepalli RC, Lokuta AJ, Maertz NA, et al. Depletion of T-tubules and specific subcellular changes in sarcolemmal proteins in tachycardia-induced heart failure. Cardiovasc Res 2003; 59: 67–77.
74. Song LS, Sobie EA, McCulle S, et al. Orphaned ryanodine receptors in the failing heart. Proc Natl Acad Sci USA. 2006; 103: 4305–4310.
75. Orchard C. T-tubule trouble. J Physiol 2006; 574: 330.
76. Louch WE, Mork HK, Sexton J, et al. T-tubule disorganization and reduced synchrony of Ca2+ release in murine cardiomyocytes following myocardial infarction. J Physiol 2006; 574: 519–33.
77. Haghighi K, Kolokathis F, Pater L, et al. Human phospholamban null results in lethal dilated cardiomyopathy revealing a critical difference between mouse and human. J Clin Invest 2003; 111: 869–76.
78. Minamisawa S, Hoshijima M, Chu G, et al. Chronic phospholamban–sarcoplasmic reticulum. Calcium ATPase interaction is the critical calcium cycling defect in dilated cardiomyopathy. Cell 1999; 99: 313.
79. Schmitt JP, Kamisago M, Asahi M, et al. Dilated cardiomyopathy and heart failure caused by a mutation in phospholamban. Science 2003; 299: 1410–13.
80. Yue DT. Quenching the spark in the heart. Science 1997; 276: 755–6.
81. Lyon AR, MacLeod KT, Zhang Y, et al. Loss of T-tubules and other changes to surface topography in ventricular myocytes from failing human and rat heart. Proc Natl Acad Sci USA. 2009; 106: 6854–9.
82. Kubalova Z, Terentyev D, Viatchenko-Karpinski S, et al. Abnormal intrastore calcium signaling in chronic heart failure. Proc Natl Acad Sci USA 2005; 102: 14104–9.
83. Guatimosim S, Dilly K, Santana LF, et al. Local Ca(2+) signaling and EC coupling in heart: Ca(2+) sparks and the regulation of the [Ca(2+)](i) transient. J Mol Cell Cardiol 2002; 34: 941–50.
84. Domeier TL, Blatter LA, Zima AV. Alteration of sarcoplasmic reticulum Ca2+ release termination by ryanodine receptor sensitization and in heart failure. J Physiol 2009; 587: 5197–5209.
85. Shannon TR, Ginsburg KS, Bers DM. Quantitative assessment of the SR Ca2+ leak–load relationship. Circ Res 2002; 91: 594–600.
86. Lindner M, Erdmann E, Beuckelmann DJ. Calcium content of the sarcoplasmic reticulum in isolated ventricular myocytes from patients with terminal heart failure. J Mol Cell Cardiol 1998; 30: 743–9.
87. Song LS, Pi Y, Kim SJ, et al. Paradoxical cellular Ca2+ signaling in severe but compensated canine left ventricular hypertrophy. Circ Res 2005; 97: 457–64.
88. Sadayappan S, Gulick J, Klevitsky R, et al. Cardiac myosin binding protein-C phosphorylation in a ß-myosin heavy chain background. Circulation 2009; 119: 1253–62.
89. El-Armouche A, Pohlmann L, Schlossarek S, et al. Decreased phosphorylation levels of cardiac myosin-binding protein-C in human and experimental heart failure. J Mol Cell Cardiol 2007; 43: 223–9.
90. Hashimoto K, Perez NG, Kusuoka H, et al. Frequency-dependent changes in calcium cycling and contractile activation in SERCA2a transgenic mice. Basic Res Cardiol 2000; 95: 144–51.
91. del Monte F, Harding SE, Schmidt U, et al. Restoration of contractile function in isolated cardiomyocytes from failing human hearts by gene transfer of SERCA2a. Circulation 1999; 100: 2308–11.
92. Endoh M. Force–frequency relationship in intact mammalian ventricular myocardium: physiological and pathophysiological relevance. Eur J Pharmacol 2004; 500: 73–86.
93. Davia K, Davies CH, Harding SE. Effects of inhibition of sarcoplasmic reticulum calcium uptake on contraction in myocytes isolated from failing human ventricle. Cardiovasc Res 1997; 33: 88–97.
94. Munch G, Bolck B, Brixius K, et al. SERCA2a activity correlates with the force–frequency relationship in human myocardium. Am J Physiol Heart Circ Physiol 2000; 278: H1924–32.
95. Delgado C, Artiles A, Gomez AM, Vassort G. Frequency-dependent increase in cardiac Ca2+ current is due to reduced Ca2+ release by the sarcoplasmic reticulum. J Mol Cell Cardiol 1999; 31: 1783–93.
96. Marx SO, Reiken S, Hisamatsu Y, et al. PKA Phosphorylation dissociates FKBP12.6 from the calcium release channel (ryanodine receptor): defective regulation in failing hearts. Cell 2000; 101: 365–76.

62 HEART FAILURE

97. Wehrens XH, Lehnart SE, Reiken S, et al. Ryanodine receptor/calcium release channel PKA phosphorylation: a critical mediator of heart failure progression. Proc Natl Acad Sci USA 2006; 103: 511–18.
98. Guo T, Zhang T, Mestril R, Bers DM. Ca2+/calmodulin-dependent protein kinase II phosphorylation of ryanodine receptor does affect calcium sparks in mouse ventricular myocytes. Circ Res 2006; 99: 398–406.
99. Lehnart S, Marks AR. Regulation of ryanodine receptors in the heart. Circ Res 2007; 101: 746–9.
100. Benkusky NA, Weber CS, Scherman JA, et al. Intact ß-adrenergic response and unmodified progression toward heart failure in mice with genetic ablation of a major protein kinase a phosphorylation site in the cardiac ryanodine receptor. Circ Res 2007; 101: 819–29.
101. Yang D, Zhu WZ, Xiao B, et al. Ca2+/calmodulin kinase II-dependent phosphorylation of ryanodine receptors suppresses Ca2+ sparks and Ca2+ waves in cardiac myocytes. Circ Res 2007; 100: 399–407.
102. Ai X, Curran JW, Shannon TR, Bers DM, Pogwizd SM. Ca2+/calmodulin-dependent protein kinase modulates cardiac ryanodine receptor phosphorylation and sarcoplasmic reticulum Ca2+ leak in heart failure. Circ Res 2005; 97: 1314–22.
103. MacDonnell SM, Garcia-Rivas G, Scherman JA, et al. Adrenergic regulation of cardiac contractility does not involve phosphorylation of the cardiac ryanodine receptor at serine 2808. Circ Res 2008; 102: 65–72.
104. Bridge JHB, Savio-Galimberti E. What are the consequences of phosphorylation and hyperphosphorylation of ryanodine receptors in normal and failing heart?. Circ Res 2008; 102: 995–7.
105. Ling H, Zhang T, Pereira L, et al. Requirement for Ca2+/calmodulin-dependent kinase II in the transition from pressure overload-induced cardiac hypertrophy to heart failure in mice. J Clin Invest 2009; 119: 1230–40.
106. Gangopadhyay JP, Ikemoto N. Intracellular translocation of calmodulin and Ca2+/calmodulin-dependent protein kinase II during the development of hypertrophy in neonatal cardiomyocytes. Biochem Biophys Res Commun 2010; 396: 515–21.
107. Zhang T, Maier LS, Dalton ND, et al. The deltaC isoform of CaMKII is activated in cardiac hypertrophy and induces dilated cardiomyopathy and heart failure. Circ Res 2003; 92: 912–19.
108. Zhang T, Brown JH. Role of Ca2+/calmodulin-dependent protein kinase II in cardiac hypertrophy and heart failure. Cardiovasc Res 2004; 63: 476–86.
109. Yoo B, Lemaire A, Mangmool S, et al. Beta1-adrenergic receptors stimulate cardiac contractility and CaMKII activation in vivo and enhance cardiac dysfunction following myocardial infarction. Am J Physiol Heart Circ Physiol 2009; 297: H1377–86.
110. Singh MV, Kapoun A, Higgins L, et al. Ca2+/calmodulin-dependent kinase II triggers cell membrane injury by inducing complement factor B gene expression in the mouse heart. J Clin Invest 2009; 119: 986–96.
111. Ai X, Curran JW, Shannon TR, Bers DM, Pogwizd SM. Ca2+/calmodulin-dependent protein kinase modulates cardiac ryanodine receptor phosphorylation and sarcoplasmic reticulum Ca2+ leak in heart failure. Circ Res 2005; 97: 1314–22.
112. Dzhura I, Wu Y, Colbran RJ, Balser JR, Anderson ME. Calmodulin kinase determines calcium-dependent facilitation of L-type calcium channels. Nat Cell Biol 2000; 2: 173–7.
113. Lu J, McKinsey TA, Nicol RL, Olson EN. Signal-dependent activation of the MEF2 transcription factor by dissociation from histone deacetylases. Proc Natl Acad Sci USA 2000; 97: 4070–4075.
114. Anderson ME. CaMKII and a failing strategy for growth in heart. J Clin Invest 2009; 119: 1082–5.
115. Zhu WZ, Wang SQ, Chakir K, et al. Linkage of beta1-adrenergic stimulation to apoptotic heart cell death through protein kinase a-independent activation of Ca2+/calmodulin kinase II. J Clin Invest 2003; 111: 617–25.
116. Sag CM, Wadsack DP, Khabbazzadeh S, et al. Calcium/calmodulin-dependent protein kinase II contributes to cardiac arrhythmogenesis in heart failure. Circ Heart Fail 2009; 2: 664–75.
117. Orchard C, Brette F. T-tubules and sarcoplasmic reticulum function in cardiac ventricular myocytes. Cardiovasc Res 2008; 77: 237–44.
118. Louch WE, Mork HK, Sexton J, et al. T-tubule disorganization and reduced synchrony of Ca2+ release in murine cardiomyocytes following myocardial infarction. J Physiol 2006; 574: 519–533.
119. Benitah JP, Kerfant BG, Vassort G, Richard S, Gomez AM. Altered communication between L-type calcium channels and ryanodine receptors in heart failure. Front Biosci 2002; 7: 263–75.
120. Cannell MB, Crossman DJ, Soeller C. Effect of changes in action potential spike configuration, junctional sarcoplasmic reticulum micro-architecture and altered T-tubule structure in human heart failure. J Muscle Res Cell Motil 2006; 27: 297–306.
121. Salle L, Brette F. T-tubules: a key structure of cardiac function and dysfunction. Arch Mal Coeur Vaiss 2007; 100: 225–30.

122. Gomez AM, Valdivia HH, Cheng H, et al. Defective excitation–contraction coupling in experimental cardiac hypertrophy and heart failure. Science 1997; 276: 800–6.
123. Meethal SV, Potter KT, Redon D, et al. Structure–function relationships of Ca spark activity in normal and failing cardiac myocytes as revealed by flash photography. Cell Calcium 2007; 41: 123–34.
124. Litwin SE, Zhang D, Bridge JH. Dyssynchronous Ca(2+) sparks in myocytes from infarcted hearts. Circ Res 2000; 87: 1040–7.
125. Volkers M, Weidenhammer C, Herzog N, et al. The inotropic peptide ß-arkct improves ß-ar responsiveness in normal and failing cardiomyocytes through gß γ-mediated L-type calcium current disinhibition. Circ Res 2011; 108: 27–39.
126. Rengo G, Lymperopoulos A, Leosco D, Koch WJ. GRK2 as a novel gene therapy target in heart failure. J Mol Cell Cardiol 2011; 50: 785–92.
127. Brinks H, Koch WJ. BetaARKct: a therapeutic approach for improved adrenergic signaling and function in heart disease. J Cardiovasc Transl Res 3: 499–506.
128. Hoshijima M, Ikeda Y, Iwanaga Y, et al. Chronic suppression of heart-failure progression by a pseudophosphorylated mutant of phospholamban via in vivo cardiac rAAV gene delivery. Nat Med 2002; 8: 864–71.
129. Hoshijima M, Knöll R, Pashmforoush M, Chien KR. Reversal of calcium cycling defects in advanced heart failure: toward molecular therapy. J Am Coll Cardiol. 2006; 48: 15–23.
130. Kaye DM, Preovolos A, Marshall T, et al. Percutaneous cardiac recirculation-mediated gene transfer of an inhibitory phospholamban peptide reverses advanced heart failure in large animals. J Am Coll Cardiol 2007; 50: 253–60.
131. Ikeda Y, Hoshijima M, Chien KR. Toward biologically targeted therapy of calcium cycling defects in heart failure. Physiology 2008; 23: 6–16.
132. Ferreira-Martins J, Rondon-Clavo C, Tugal D, et al. Spontaneous calcium oscillations regulate human cardiac progenitor cell growth. Circ Res 2009; 105: 764–74.
133. Zhu WZ, Santana LF, Laflamme MA. Local control of excitation–contraction coupling in human embryonic stem cell-derived cardiomyocytes. PLoS ONE 2009; 4: e5407.
134. Satin J, Itzhaki I, Rapoport S, et al. Calcium handling in human embryonic stem cell-derived cardiomyocytes. Stem Cells 2008; 26: 1961–72.
135. Itzhaki I, Schiller J, Beyar R, Satin J, Gepstein L. Calcium handling in embryonic stem cell-derived cardiac myocytes: of mice and men. Ann N Y Acad Sci 2006; 1080: 207–15.
136. Liu J, Fu JD, Siu CW, Li RA. Functional sarcoplasmic reticulum for calcium handling of human embryonic stem cell-derived cardiomyocytes: insights for driven maturation. Stem Cells 2007; 25: 3038–44.
137. Dolnikov K, Shilkrut M, Zeevi-Levin N, et al. Functional properties of human embryonic stem cell-derived cardiomyocytes: intracellular Ca2+ handling and the role of sarcoplasmic reticulum in the contraction. Stem Cells 2006; 24: 236–45.
138. Kehat I, Kenyagin-Karsenti D, Snir M, et al. Human embryonic stem cells can differentiate into myocytes with structural and functional properties of cardiomyocytes. J Clin Invest 2001; 108: 407–14.
139. Fu JD, Li J, Tweedie D, et al. Crucial role of the sarcoplasmic reticulum in the developmental regulation of Ca2+ transients and contraction in cardiomyocytes derived from embryonic stem cells. FASEB J 2006; 20: 181–3.
140. Rosemblit N, Moschella MC, Ondriasa E, et al. Intracellular calcium release channel expression during embryogenesis. Dev Biol 1999; 206: 163–77.
141. Poindexter BJ, Smith JR, Buja LM, Bick RJ. Calcium signaling mechanisms in dedifferentiated cardiac myocytes: comparison with neonatal and adult cardiomyocytes. Cell Calcium 2001; 30: 373–82.
142. Kapur N, Banach K. Inositol-1,4,5-trisphosphate-mediated spontaneous activity in mouse embryonic stem cell-derived cardiomyocytes. J Physiol 2007; 581: 1113–1127.
143. Mery A, Aimond F, Menard C, et al. Initiation of embryonic cardiac pacemaker activity by inositol 1,4,5-trisphosphate-dependent calcium signaling. Mol Biol Cell 2005; 16: 2414–23.

5

Myocardial energetics and metabolism in the failing heart

Joanne S. Ingwall

ATP is the high-energy phosphate-containing compound directly used for excitation and contraction in muscle cells. Cleavage of the terminal phosphate (a phosphoryl bond) by ATPases [ATP → ADP + inorganic phosphate (Pi)] releases chemical energy that is converted into the work for contraction, ion pumping, and macromolecular synthesis. Because the amount of ATP in the heart is small (~10 mM, enough for only a few beats) compared with demand (as much as 10,000 times greater), the myocardial cell must continually re-synthesize ATP to maintain normal cardiac pump function and cellular viability. Thus the rates of ATP utilization and re-synthesis are very large.

The metabolic machinery used to meet the energy demands of the myocyte without allowing the [ATP] (where [] signifies concentration) to fall is impressive (Fig. 5.1). All pathways re-phosphorylate ADP. ATP re-synthesis by fatty acid oxidation (FAO) in mitochondria is normally sufficient to meet the dynamic demands for chemical energy. Under conditions of high ATP demand, the myocyte uses other pathways to ensure a constant supply of ATP, namely, glycolysis and the phosphotransferase reactions catalyzed by creatine kinase (CK) and adenylate kinase (AK). Phosphoryl transfer between sites of ATP production and utilization occurs by means of metabolic relays via CK, AK, and glycolysis (1–3). The physical association of these metabolic relays with energy-utilizing proteins creates microenvironments whereby phosphoryl groups can be supplied to ATPases without exchange between bulk and local cytosolic pools, improving the efficiency of ATP supply (1–3).

The different pathways for ATP supply have different rates of ATP synthesis: phosphoryl transfer via CK is ~10 times faster than ATP synthesis in mitochondria (~0.7 mM/sec), which is ~20 times faster than glycolysis (4). The relative contributions of these metabolic pathways to overall ATP synthesis changes rapidly in response to changes in fuel supply, hormonal and neural signals, availability of substrates and inhibitors of specific enzyme reactions, and by chemical modification of proteins. During acute increases in work in the normal myocardium, these biochemical pathways rapidly mobilize substrates, such as glycogen (5), influx more glucose (6), and use phosphocreatine (PCr, the primary energy reserve compound in the heart) (7) to support the demand for more ATP. In this way, the *sum* of increased rates of ATP synthesis by the mitochondria, glycolysis, and glycogenolysis and the phosphotransferase reactions matches the *sum* of increased rates of ATP utilization by the sarcomere and ion pumps.

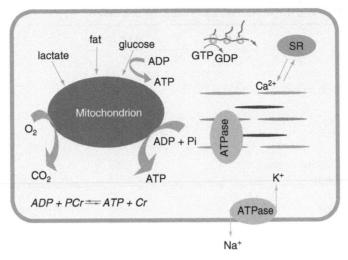

Figure 5.1 The integration of the ATP-synthesizing and ATP-utilizing pathways. The primary ATP-utilizing reactions (shown on the *right*) are actomyosin ATPase in the myofibril, the Ca^{2+}-ATPase in the sarcoplasmic reticulum and the Na^+, K^+-ATPase in the sarcolemma. Also shown is a polypeptide chain representing the requirement of ATP for macromolecular synthesis (in the form of GTP for protein synthesis). The primary ATP-synthesizing pathways (*left*) are oxidative phosphorylation in the mitochondria and the glycolytic pathway. Also shown (*bottom*) is the creatine kinase (CK) reaction, representing the kinases that supply ATP via rapid phosphoryl transfer. *Source*: Redrawn from Ref. 4.

Shown by investigators using many different tools studying the failing human myocardium and a wide variety of animal models of chronic demand overload, it is now known that myocardial metabolism in the failing heart remodels, resulting in a progressive loss of [ATP] and [PCr]. The remodeling is controlled by energy sensors, such as AMP, which lead to changes in phosphorylation state (as well as other chemical modifications) of many proteins for short-term preservation of ATP (8) and by activation of transcription factors that coordinately control long-term remodeling of entire ATP synthesis and utilizing pathways (9,10). There is consensus that in compensated hypertrophy, flux through the CK reaction is lower (11,12), glucose uptake and utilization increase while FAO either remains the same (13,14) or decreases (15,16). In uncompensated hypertrophy and other forms of heart failure, FAO is lower (15–18). Importantly, increases in glucose uptake and utilization are not sufficient to compensate for overall decrease in ATP supply (19,20). Given that the requirement for ATP for all metabolic processes and for cell viability is absolute, there has been renewed interest in the study of ATP and the heart. Some of the many reviews published over the past few years relevant to the energetics of the failing heart are referenced (2,3,5,8,9,21–31).

LOWER [ATP] AND [PCr] IN THE FAILING HEART

Summary: The normal integration of ATP synthesis and ATP utilization is not preserved in the failing myocardium; ATP demand outstrips ATP supply and [ATP] and [PCr] fall.

In the failing human myocardium and in hearts of animal models of end-stage failure, [ATP] is ~30% lower than in normal myocardium (Table 5.1). The fall in [ATP] has been shown in both left and right ventricular myocardium, in widely different species, and due to a variety of etiologies. The rate of fall in [ATP] is progressive, and is due to the loss of the adenine nucleotide pool (32).

Table 5.1 [ATP] and [Cr] in Normal and Failing Myocardium[a]

	ATP (mM)	Cr_{total} (mM)
Animal models		
Control rat (88)	28[b]	–
65% RVH due to monocrotaline supply	18[a]	–
Control dog (32)	10	26
Pacing induced HF	8.0	16
Non-failing TO2 hamster (89)	8.7	21
Failing TO2 hamster	6.4	7.4
Control turkey (90)	8.5	18
Furazolidine DCM	6.5	13.5
Human myocardium		
Normal (11)	10	42
Failing	7.6	15

[a]LV except where indicated.
[b]μmol/g dry weight.
Abbreviations: LVH, left ventricular hypertrophy; RVH, right ventricular hypertrophy; HF, heart failure; DCM, dilated cardiomyopathy.

[PCr] and total [Cr] both fall in hypertrophied and failing myocardium (28,33,34). ^{31}P and ^{1}H NMR spectroscopy have been used to show decreased PCr/ATP and decreased absolute levels of Cr, PCr, and ATP in hypertrophied and failing human myocardium due to a wide variety of etiologies, in complete accord with the large number of large and small animal studies (24,28). Note that because [ATP] also falls in the failing myocardium, the fall in PCr/ATP underestimates the decrease in [PCr]. The decrease in [Cr] occurs earlier, is faster, and occurs to a greater extent than the fall in [ATP] (32). Whereas the fall in [ATP] is not more than ~30%, the decrease in [Cr] (from normal values of 20–45 mM, depending on species) can be as much as 50–70% in severely failing myocardium (24). Cr is not made in excitable tissues, but rather accumulates through the action of the Cr transporter (CrT). Decreased amount of CrT on the sarcolemma explains the decrease in Cr accumulation in the failing myocardium (35–37). Trafficking of CrT to the plasma membrane is regulated by stress, insulin, growth factors, and mammalian target of rapamycin (38).

METABOLIC REMODELING: IMPAIRED ENERGY RESERVE

Summary: Metabolism remodels in the failing heart, leading to a loss in energy reserve and ultimately to a fall in [ATP]. The time line is: decreased energy reserve via CK leading to increase in [ADP] and [AMP], triggering an increase in glycolysis. Although glycolysis increases, glycolytic reserve is limited. ATP synthesis by FAO in mitochondria falls. Thus, metabolic reserve for ATP synthesis by all the major ATP-synthesis pathways in the failing heart is limited.

DECREASED METABOLIC RESERVE VIA CK

Decreased [Cr] coupled with decreased CK activity (V_{max}, primarily activity of the MM–CK and sMtCK isozymes) combine to limit energy reserve via CK in the hypertrophied and failing heart. In animal models of severe heart failure, ~30% and ~60% decreases in CK V_{max} and [Cr], respectively, combine to reduce the unidirectional velocity of the CK reaction (CKvel) by ~70%. Measurement of CKvel using saturation transfer NMR in failing human myocardium demonstrate lower CKvel, by ~50% (12), as predicted from biochemical analysis of the CK system in human myocardium (11) and observed for experimental models (24). Given that the CKvel is nearly an order of magnitude faster than ATP synthesis by any other reaction, the decrease in CKvel of ~50% is a major loss of energy reserve. The decreases in [Cr] and CK V_{max} are reversible (39,40).

There are two consequences of decreased capacity for phosphoryl transfer via CK and AK: increased cost of mechanical work and decreased contractile reserve. This has been shown in otherwise normal rat hearts in which either CK V_{max} or [Cr] was decreased and in a variety of genetically manipulated mouse hearts (41–45). For example, in AK1 null mouse hearts, although flux through the CK reaction and glycolysis increased to compensate for the loss of AK, more ATP per contraction was used in AK-deficient muscle (46). A consequence of the disruption of energy transfer relay via CK within the myocyte is well illustrated by increased electrical vulnerability of the heart caused by failure to supply ATP via CK to the K_{ATP} channel in MM–CK null mouse hearts (47). Hearts from mice unable to synthesize Cr had normal contractile performance at baseline but reduced contractile reserve when challenged with an inotropic agent and increased susceptibility to ischemic injury (43).

A gain-of-function strategy has been used to test whether increasing CrT protein could rescue the cytosolic Cr pool in the failing mouse heart (48). The myocardial Cr pool increased on average twofold but, unexpectedly, the fraction of Cr that was phosphorylated was lower by ~50%, despite normal CK activity. As a consequence of the lower PCr-to-Cr ratio, cytosolic [ADP] increased and the chemical driving force for ATPase reactions, $|\Delta G_{\sim ATP}|$, was lower. These hearts developed left ventricular hypertrophy, dilatation, and contractile dysfunction. This experiment supports a causal relationship between decreased energy reserve and contractile dysfunction.

The observations that increased free [Cr] and decreased [PCr]/[Cr] lead to contractile dysfunction (39,48) raise the question of whether the loss of Cr in the failing heart is compensatory or deleterious (32). The notion that loss of Cr could be compensatory seems counter intuitive. Loss of Cr reduces the velocity of the CK reaction, and thus reduces the primary energy buffer in the heart at a time when overall energy supply is compromised. However, loss of Cr also minimizes the increase in free [ADP] and hence maintains a near normal $|\Delta G_{\sim ATP}|$ required to drive ATPase reactions. Maintaining low cytosolic [ADP] also results in low [AMP], reducing loss of purines from the heart.

A gain-of-function strategy modulating CK activity in normal and failing myocardium has been accomplished using conditional overexpression of MM–CK, the dominant CK isoenzyme, in the mouse heart. Increasing MM–CK activity did not alter contractile function in normal mice but did increase contractile function and improved survival in failing mouse hearts (49). Importantly, showing cause and effect, acute withdrawal of MM–CK activity led to loss of contractile function in these failing mouse hearts.

Based on experiments such as these in animal models showing a relationship between energy reserve via the CK system and contractile reserve of the heart, it seems likely that the decreased energy reserve observed for the human failing heart has a similar functional correlate. The failing heart is "energy starved" with respect to its capacity to rapidly re-synthesize ATP. The energy-poor heart cannot recruit its contractile reserve without expending a disproportionate amount of energy, a nonsustainable condition.

DECREASED METABOLIC RESERVE VIA GLYCOLYSIS

The increase in glucose uptake observed in hypertrophied hearts is explained by increased expression of the insulin-independent glucose transporter GLUT1; expression of the dominant insulin-regulated glucose transporter GLUT4 is decreased (6,50). One mechanism leading to increased glucose uptake and utilization in the hypertrophied myocardium is triggered by the demand for more ATP (Fig. 5.2). Decreases in [PCr] without a concomitant fall in total [Cr], a characteristic of hypertrophied myocardium, lead to increases in [ADP], [AMP], and [Pi]. The increase in [AMP] activates the "low-on-fuel" sensor AMP-activated protein kinase (AMPK) (50,51). The consequences of activating AMPK are to activate proteins in ATP-synthesis pathways (increasing ATP supply) and to decrease the activity of proteins in ATP-consuming pathways (conserving ATP). Key among these are GLUT1 and phosphofructokinase-2 (PFK-2), leading to production of fructose-2, 6-Pi_2, a potent allosteric activator of the rate-limiting protein for glycolysis, PFK (52). Thus, increased ATP demand, manifests as decreased PCr, in the hypertrophied heart signals an increase in glycolytic flux by two coordinate mechanisms: increasing glucose transport (increasing substrate supply) and activating PFK (increasing utilization).

Unlike for control hearts, glucose uptake rates and glycolysis measured in the hypertrophied myocardium of animal models do not increase *further* during work challenge (53,54). Importantly, this limitation in metabolic reserve has also been observed in a group of Class I/II patients with dilated cardiomyopathy (20). These results suggest that the presumably adaptive increase in glycolysis is not sufficient to meet ATP demand. ATP utilization exceeds supply, leading to the inexorable loss of ATP in the failing heart.

Genetic strategies have been used to test whether increasing glucose utilization *further* in a mouse model of pressure overload hypertrophy renders hypertrophied hearts more tolerant to chronic hemodynamic overload (55). Transgenic mice with cardiac-specific

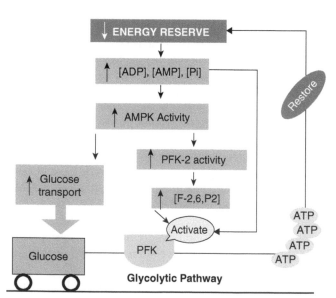

Figure 5.2 Coordinate control of glycolysis by AMPK. In chronic pressure-overload cardiac hypertrophy in the rat, increased ATP demand (signaled as decreased PCr) leads to an increase in glycolytic flux by two coordinate mechanisms: increasing glucose transport (increasing substrate supply) and activating PFK in the glycolytic pathway (increasing utilization), both mediated by AMPK. See text for more explanation. *Abbreviation*: AMPK, AMP-activated protein kinase. *Source*: Reprinted from Ref. 52.

overexpression of GLUT1 were used to increase basal glucose transport in the heart. Comparing transgenic and wild-type hearts subjected to chronic pressure overload, it was found that increasing myocardial glucose uptake protected against the progression to heart failure and improved survival. This study suggests that increasing the capacity for ATP synthesis, in this case via glycolysis, can alter the natural history of heart failure. The GLUT1 overexpressing mouse was also used to rescue mouse hearts deficient in the transcriptional activator peroxisome proliferator-activated receptor α (PPAR-α), which have a threefold decrease in FAO and threefold increase in carbohydrate utilization characteristic of the failing heart (19). PPAR-α null mouse hearts sustained baseline function but not high workloads, had higher than normal MVO_2 yet produced less ATP, and [ATP] fell upon inotropic challenge. PPAR-α null mouse crossed with the GLUT1 overexpresser mouse sustained increased work without losing [ATP], and MVO_2 and ATP synthesis rates returned to normal. These genetic studies suggest that glucose utilization, if sufficiently high, can support and sustain high workload in the failing heart.

DECREASED METABOLIC RESERVE VIA MITOCHONDRIAL ATP SYNTHESIS

O_2 is not limiting in the failing myocardium (56,57), and at least in some models, MVO_2 is increased (32). The increase in MVO_2, however, is not sufficient to prevent the loss of ATP in the failing myocardium.

Genomic and proteomic studies (58,59), as well as measures of enzyme activities, have shown that many proteins involved in fatty acid (FA) transport and utilization are downregulated in failing hearts, contributing to the overall decrease in mitochondrial ATP synthesis. This is under transcriptional and post-transcriptional control (see next section). Experiments using isolated mitochondria, skinned fibers, isolated hearts (27,60) and *in vivo* hearts (56), all support the conclusion that oxidative capacity of mitochondria is reduced in the failing myocardium. Increases in uncoupling proteins (UCPs) (60) as well as increases in reactive O_2 species and NO likely contribute (27,30,61). A decreased capacity of mitochondrial substrate oxidation in the failing heart leads to decreased cardiac efficiency (32).

FA supply for oxidation is decreased in the failing heart (20,62). Utilization of exogenous vs. endogenous FA has been compared in an animal model of pressure overload hypertrophy (15). FAO rates using exogenous FA were near normal in mild to moderate heart failure, but fell as the disease stage progressed. In contrast, endogenous fats (triacylglycerols, TAGs) were not oxidized even in early failure. Importantly, as also noted for a group of Class I/II patients with dilated cardiomyopathy (20), oxidation rates did not increase further for either exogenous or endogenous fats with β-adrenergic challenge.

A potentially important compensatory mechanism for reduced exogenous FAO has been found in an animal model of heart failure due to pressure overload (16). When FAO fell and was uncoupled to tricarboxylic acid (TCA) cycle flux, TCA cycle flux was unexpectedly sustained by use of glycolysis-derived pyruvate through anaplerosis, a pathway that uses pyruvate to supply oxaloacetate downstream from acetyl-CoA in the TCA cycle. Although initially compensatory, because conversion of pyruvate to oxaloacetate via anaplerosis consumes an ATP, this is less efficient than the standard use of pyruvate through the TCA cycle. The increase in energy cost is not likely to be sustainable. This could be one step in the transition from compensatory hypertrophy to failure.

As for the sections on CK and glycolysis, here we present some examples where genetic tools were used to manipulate mitochondrial ATP supply.

The transcriptional co-activator PGC-1α is referred to as a "master regulator," which controls mitochondrial biogenesis and the synthesis of entire metabolic pathways for ATP synthesis. Modeling the observation that PGC-1α is downregulated in hypertrophied and failing heart (63), PGC-1α null mice have been used to define the consequences of reduced PGC-1α on ATP synthesis and contractile reserve in the heart (64). The absence of PGC-1α not only led to reduced gene expression for proteins required for FAO and oxidative phosphorylation (OXPHOS), but their enzyme activities were reduced. Importantly, [ATP] was decreased by ~20%, a large decrease similar to that observed in end-stage failing hearts caused by a variety of physiologic stresses (Table 5.1). Importantly, this was the case despite the presence of PGC-1β, which has many overlapping targets with PGC-1α. PGC-1α null hearts had reduced contractile reserve. Consistent with these defects, PGC-1α null mice subjected to pressure overload progress to failure more rapidly than wild-type hearts (65). Although massive overexpression of PGC-1α led to mitochondrial proliferation to such an extent that the sarcomeres became displaced, leading to cardiomyopathy and heart failure, short-term PGC-1α overexpression reversed contractile dysfunction (66,67), suggesting causative links among PGC-1α expression, mitochondrial biogenesis, ATP synthesis, and contractile performance.

Genetic manipulation in the mouse has identified other players in the control of ATP production. For example, mouse hearts deficient in the gene for mitochondrial transcription factor A (Tfam) developed progressive and rapid mitochondrial dysfunction and had a life span of only 10–12 weeks (68). These hearts demonstrated an early switch in metabolism characterized by downregulation of genes encoding FAO proteins and decreased activities of mitochondrial proteins. The late increase in mitochondrial mass and upregulation of genes important for glycolysis failed to compensate for respiratory chain defects. Importantly, this metabolic remodeling took place early, consistent with cause and consequence. Lending further support to the essential role of ATP production to the failing heart, ablating muscle LIM protein in mice led to regional decreases in mitochondrial density and decreases in PGC-1α (69).

ON THE INTEGRATION OF ATP-SYNTHESIZING PATHWAYS

Mouse transgenesis models have provided important insights into the integration of ATP-synthesizing pathways and how this integration remodels in response to decreases in the major phosphotransferase reaction in the heart, CK. Using mouse hearts deficient in either MM–CK or both MM–CK and sMtCK, experimental and mathematical modeling of metabolite dynamics has been reported (70). For mouse hearts lacking both MM–CK and sMtCK, phosphoryl flux through adenylate kinase, glycolysis and the guanine nucleotide circuit all increased (70). Thus, rearrangements in phosphotransfer and substrate utilization networks compensate for CK deficiency. Extrapolating these results to the failing myocardium, it seems likely that similar compensation occurs during early heart failure, explaining how [ATP] is maintained at values greater than 70% of normal; however, it is not likely than maintaining this new steady state can be sustained and disease progresses.

METABOLIC REMODELING IS UNDER TRANSCRIPTIONAL AND POST-TRANSCRIPTIONAL CONTROL

The past decade has witnessed an explosion of information identifying the molecular links between physiologic and metabolic stimuli and the regulation of gene expression in the heart. Not only have the metabolic targets of specific nuclear receptors and DNA-binding transcriptional activators been identified, but we are also beginning to learn how their signals are amplified and sustained to remodel metabolism. Transcription is activated when transcriptional activators, including PPARs, estrogen receptors (ERRs), retinoid receptors (RXRs), nuclear respiratory factors (NRFs), and MEF-2 form protein–protein complexes with PPAR-γ co-activators, PGC-1α and β, tethering PGC-1s to DNA. When complexed

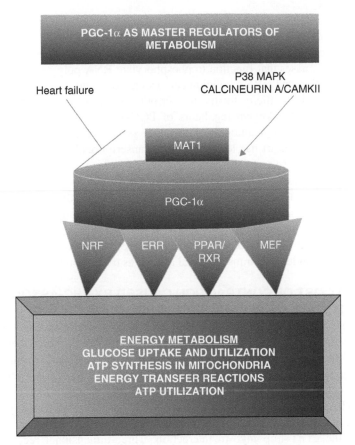

Figure 5.3 PGC-1α as master regulators of cardiac metabolism. Cartoon showing transcriptional activators and co-activators important for long-term molecular remodeling of all aspects of ATP metabolism. MAT1 functions by tethering Cdk7 and cyclin H to PGC-1α, allowing transcription to occur. Each transcriptional family of activators—NRFs, ERRs, PPARs, RXRs, and MEF-2—confers specificity of promoters targeted by PGC-1α, although there is considerable overlap. PGC-1α is activated by p38 MAPK and calcineurin A/CAMKII in response to cold, fasting, and growth stimuli. Importantly, PGC-1α is lower in the failing heart. *Abbreviations*: ERRs, estrogen receptors; NRFs, nuclear respiratory factors; PPARs, peroxisome proliferator-activated receptors; RXRs, retinoid receptors.

with the transcriptional activators, PGC-1s activate genes encoding proteins comprising entire metabolic pathways that control ATP synthesis in mitochondria, phosphoryl transfer, glucose uptake and utilization, and also ATP-utilizing proteins (Fig. 5.3).

The different transcriptional factors confer specificity of PGC-1s for its genomic targets, although substantial overlap exists. For example (71), the ERRα/PGC-1α complex targets a set of promoters common to genes encoding a wide spectrum of energy producing (FA and glucose uptake, β-oxidation, OXPHOS, TCA cycle, electron transport chain), transferring (sMtCK and adenine nucleotide transporter) and utilizing proteins. In hypertrophied ERRα null mouse hearts, genes for ATP synthesis and transfer were all decreased while genes encoding the stress protein BB–CK was increased. These experiments support the notion that the normal ERRα/PGC-1α complex is required to blunt the loss of capacity for ATP synthesis in pressure overload hypertrophy. ERRγ also plays a major role in the metabolic switch from carbohydrate metabolism to oxidative metabolism in the postnatal heart (72). The partial reversal to a nonoxidative phenotype in the hypertrophied and failing hearts is likely under its control as well.

PGC-1s are themselves regulated. Of particular interest here are Cdk9 and Cdk7, cyclin-dependent kinases that function to phosphorylate RNA polymerase II so that transcriptional elongation and mRNA capping can occur. Cdk7 and 9 target PGC-1s, thereby conferring additional specificity for the transcriptional control of ATP synthesizing and utilizing reactions. Other known regulators of PGC-1s in striated muscle include p38 MAPK, calcineurin A/Ca^{2+}/calmodulin–dependent protein kinase and possibly AMPK (10,73,74). The failing heart has lower levels of transcriptional factors and co-activators (31,63,71) and higher levels of Cdk7 and 9 (10,73).

Unlike the impressive progress made understanding the genomic events that control normal and hypertrophic growth and the development of cardiac dysfunction, much less is known about post-transcriptional control. We do know that the notion that there is a 1-to-1 correspondence in the number of mRNA transcripts and the number of functional proteins is not correct. An example is the observation that CK isozyme activity in failing and recovery myocardium is under post-transcriptional as well as transcriptional control (39).

INCREASED COST OF CONTRACTION CAUSED BY FHC-ASSOCIATED MISSENSE MUTATIONS IN SARCOMERIC PROTEINS

It is important to emphasize that although the current focus of most studies of ATP metabolism is on the various pathways for ATP synthesis, the "metabolic driver" is the need for more ATP by the sarcomere and ion pumps. This is well illustrated by studies defining cardiac energetics of hypertrophic cardiomyopathy (HCM) and, in particular, familial hypertrophic cardiomyopathy (FHC). Elegant analyses of changes in protein dynamics caused by FHC-associated missense mutations at residue 92 in the tropomyosin-binding domain of cardiac troponin (cTnT) (75) have shown large mutation-specific differences in dynamics of the cTnT–tropomyosin interaction. Three-dimensional reconstructions of wild-type and R403Q smooth muscle myosin bound to actin showed that, unlike the normal fixed actin–myosin loop interaction, the mutant myosin–actin interaction showed disarray (76). One common consequence of these remarkable changes in structure and dynamics is increased cost of tension development indicated by decreased [PCr] (77–80). These energetic defects are not secondary to hypertrophy, but instead are caused by altered sarcomere structure and function. One consequence of increased cost of contraction is elevated [ADP], known to slow the crossbridge cycle and contribute to diastolic dysfunction (see below) (81,82). The most common phenotype of hearts bearing missense mutations in sarcomeric proteins associated with FHC is diastolic dysfunction; whether the mutation leads to hypertrophy or to systolic dysfunction is variable.

ON CAUSES AND CONSEQUENCES

Even using bioengineered mouse models where only one amino acid or one protein is manipulated, demonstrating causes and consequences in the failing heart is challenging. This is because metabolism is designed to be redundant; failure ensues only when the capacity for all the back-up systems is exhausted. A few examples of "causes and consequences" are given here.

ON CAUSE

Myocyte size, their location, hemodynamic factors and ability to adapt to stress all play important roles leading to altered gene expression in the failing heart. This is illustrated by a study in which cell size and enzyme activities of several proteins known to change in cardiac hypertrophy and failure (so-called fetal enzymes) were measured in myocytes isolated from different regions of hypertensive and nonhypertensive hypertrophied rat hearts (83). The activities of some proteins increased in proportion to myocyte size, whereas others were diluted and still others increased out of proportion to myocyte size. The idea that sustained hemodynamic load causes changes in gene expression in some but not all proteins is also supported by studies showing that the decreases in MM–CK and the mitochondrial CK (sMtCK) isozymes, but not in MB–CK, were reversed in heart failure patients given a ventricular assist device (40) and in an animal model of recovery from severe heart failure (39).

The study linking MM–CK activity and contractile performance in the failing mouse heart using conditional overexpression techniques is a major accomplishment showing that decreased contractile reserve in the failing myocardium can be caused by decreased MM–CK activity. The important next step would be to test whether gain and loss of the mitochondrial isoform of CK, which is severely diminished in heart failure, also correlates with contractile performance (49).

ON CONSEQUENCE

Diastolic dysfunction is a common heart failure phenotype. Of the many causes of diastolic dysfunction, one of them is increased cost of contraction leading to higher [ADP]. The increases in [ADP] in the absence of changes in any of the other known regulators of myofilament function in rat hearts with low CK activity was sufficient to slowdown crossbridge cycling and impair diastolic function (81,82). Thus, the increases in [ADP] secondary to decreased [PCr] observed in hypertrophy and heart failure, including FHC, may contribute to diastolic dysfunction.

A physiologic consequence of decreased capacity to increase ATP synthesis, regardless of etiology, is high risk of acute mechanical failure during an abrupt increase in work state, a hypoxic or ischemic insult, or an arrhythmia. One demonstration of the greater susceptibility of the energy-poor heart to acute stress is the faster rate of loss of systolic performance during zero-flow ischemia in isolated mouse hearts deficient in the MM- and sMtCK genes (84). Another example is shown by studies of myocardial infarction in the rat (85). Myocardial [PCr] and CK reaction velocity were decreased by ~90% and [ATP] by 18% (the heart failure phenotype) in rats by feeding them with the Cr analog β-guanidinoproprionic acid, a competitive inhibitor of CrT and the CK reaction. Unlike control rat hearts who survived acute myocardial infarction, the 24-hour mortality of rats with severely compromised CK–PCr system was 100%.

RESCUING THE FAILING MYOCARDIUM

One clinically relevant lesson to be learned from the study of cardiac energetics is that the failing heart has limited energy reserve and, and while it can increase work, it does so with a higher cost of contraction. This increases susceptibility to arrhythmia and ischemic injury. The clinical observations that patients treated with inotropic drugs that increase ATP utilization have poor long-term outcomes is explained by the lack of energy reserve (21,86). Research into ways of increasing systolic performance or reducing diastolic dysfunction by manipulating sarcomere function without increasing cost of developed tension merits support.

Another rescue strategy seeks to take advantage of the small increase in the ratio of ATP production to O_2 consumed for glucose. Drugs that shift metabolism away from FAO and toward glucose metabolism improve the efficiency of ATP production, but by only a small amount. Drugs that target 3-ketoacyl CoA thiolase (3-KAT), the last enzyme involved in β-oxidation, and CPT-1, which transports FA across the inner mitochondrial membrane, shift metabolism away from FAO (22) and increase glucose utilization. It is possible, however, that both glucose and FA are required for the failing heart (87). This topic merits further investigation.

Direct manipulation of adenine nucleotide and Cr pools has been elusive clinically. Notable in this regard is the report studying experimental right ventricular hypertrophy (88) showing that folate treatment protected against loss of adenine nucleotides and diastolic dysfunction. Folate is a required substrate for *de novo* synthesis of ATP. As folate is both readily available and inexpensive, strategies such as this may be useful in slowing the progression to failure.

In any rational strategy, care should be taken to match intervention with the stage of disease. The different pathways for ATP synthesis are compromised at different times in the evolution of compensated to uncompensated hypertrophy. Loss of energy reserve supported by CK occurs first, and triggers an increase in glycolysis, followed by decreased FAO. Ideally, interventions designed to alter metabolic pathways must be matched to *stage of metabolic dysfunction*, analogous to NYHA classes.

ACKNOWLEDGMENTS

The author wishes to thank Linda Johnson for her assistance. This work was supported in part by research funds from the Department of Medicine, Brigham and Women's Hospital and the National Institutes of Health.

REFERENCES

1. De Sousa E, Veksler V, Minajeva A, et al. Subcellular creatine kinase alterations. implications in heart failure. Circ Res 1999; 85: 68–76.
2. Dzeja PP, Chung S, Terzic A. In: Saks V. ed Molecular system bioenergetics: Energy for life. Weinheim: Wiley–VCH, 2007.
3. Ingwall JS. Transgenesis and cardiac energetics: new insights into cardiac metabolism. J Mol Cell Cardiol 2004; 37: 613–23.
4. Ingwall JS. ATP and the Heart. In: Norwell, MA: Kluwer Academic Publishers, 2002: 3–6.
5. Taegtmeyer H, Wilson CR, Razeghi P, Sharma S. Metabolic energetics and genetics in the heart. Ann N Y Acad Sci 2005; 1047: 208–18.
6. Zhang J, Duncker DJ, Ya X, et al. Effect of left ventricular hypertrophy secondary to chronic pressure overload on transmural myocardial 2-deoxyglucose uptake. a 31P NMR spectroscopic study. Circulation 1995; 92: 1274–83.
7. Bittl JA, Ingwall JS. Reaction rates of creatine kinase and ATP synthesis in the isolated rat heart. a 31p NMR magnetization transfer study. J Biol Chem 1985; 260: 3512–17.
8. Dyck JRB, Lopaschuk GD. AMPK alterations in cardiac physiology and pathology: enemy or ally? J Physiol 2006; 574: 95–112.
9. Finck BN, Kelly DP. PGC-1 coactivators: inducible regulators of energy metabolism in health and disease. J Clin Invest 2006; 116: 615–22.
10. Sano M, Izumi Y, Helenius K, et al. Menage-a-trois 1 is critical for the transcriptional function of PPAR-γ coactivator 1. Cell Metab 2007; 5: 129–42.
11. Nascimben L, Ingwall JS, Pauletto P, et al. Creatine kinase system in failing and nonfailing human myocardium. Circulation 1996; 94: 1894–901.
12. Weiss RG, Gerstenblith G, Bottomley PA. ATP flux through creatine kinase in the normal, stressed, and failing human heart. Proc Natl Acad Sci USA 2005; 102: 808–13.
13. Degens H, de Brouwer KF, Gilde AJ, et al. Cardiac fatty acid metabolism is preserved in the compensated hypertrophic rat heart. Basic Res Cardiol 2006; 101: 17–26.
14. Lei B, Lionetti V, Young ME, et al. Paradoxical downregulation of the glucose oxidation pathway despite enhanced flux in severe heart failure. J Mol Cell Cardiol 2004; 36: 567–76.
15. O'Donnell JM, Fields AD, Sorokina N, Lewandowski ED. The absence of endogenous lipid oxidation in early stage heart failure exposes limits in lipid storage and turnover. J Mol Cell Cardiol 2008; 44: 315–22.
16. Sorokina N, O'Donnell JM, McKinney RD, et al. Recruitment of compensatory pathways to sustain oxidative flux with reduced carnitine palmitoyltransferase i activity characterizes inefficiency in energy metabolism in hypertrophied hearts. Circulation 2007; 115: 2033–41.
17. Osorio JC, Stanley WC, Linke A, et al. Impaired myocardial fatty acid oxidation and reduced protein expression of retinoid x receptor-alpha in pacing-induced heart failure. Circulation 2002; 106: 606–12.

18. Stanley WC, Recchia FA, Lopaschuk GD. Myocardial substrate metabolism in the normal and failing heart. Physiol Rev 2005; 85: 1093–129.

19. Luptak I, Balschi JA, Xing Y, et al. Decreased contractile and metabolic reserve in peroxisome proliferator-activated receptor-alpha-null hearts can be rescued by increasing glucose transport and utilization. Circulation 2005; 112: 2339–46.

20. Neglia D, De Caterina A, Marraccini P, et al. Impaired myocardial metabolic reserve and substrate selection flexibility during stress in patients with idiopathic dilated cardiomyopathy. Am J Physiol Heart Circ Physiol 2007; 293: H3270–8.

21. deGoma EM, Vagelos RH, Fowler MB, Ashley EA. Emerging therapies for the management of decompensated heart failure: from bench to bedside. J Am Coll Cardiol 2006; 48: 2397–409.

22. Fragasso G. Inhibition of free fatty acids metabolism as a therapeutic target in patients with heart failure. J Clin Pract 2007; 61: 603–10.

23. Gustafsson AB, Gottlieb RA. Heart mitochondria: gates of life and death. Cardiovasc Res 2007; 77: 334–43.

24. Ingwall JS, Weiss RG. Is the failing heart energy starved?. Circ Res 2004; 95: 135–45.

25. Kodde IF, van der Stok J, Smolenski RT, de Jong JW. Metabolic and genetic regulation of cardiac energy substrate preference. Comp Biochem Physiol Part A 2006; 146: 26–39.

26. Marin-Garcia J, Goldenthal MJ. Mitochondrial centrality in heart failure. Heart Fail Rev 2008; 13: 137–50.

27. Murray AJ, Edwards LM, Clarke K. Mitochondria and heart failure. Curr Opin Clin Nutr Metab Care 2007; 10: 704–11.

28. Neubauer S. The failing heart—an engine out of fuel. N Engl J Med 2007; 356: 1140–51.

29. Taha M, Lopaschuk GD. Alterations in energy metabolism in cardiomyopathies. Ann Med 2007; 39: 594–607.

30. Tsutsui H. Mitochondrial oxidative stress and heart failure. Intern Med 2006; 45: 809–13.

31. Ventura-Clapier RF, Garnier A, Veksler V. Energy metabolism in heart failure. J Physiol 2004; 555: 1–15.

32. Shen W, Asai K, Uechi M, et al. Progressive loss of myocardial atp due to a loss of total purines during the development of heart failure in dogs: a compensatory role for the parallel loss of creatine. Circulation 1999; 100: 2113–18.

33. Herrmann G, Decherd M. The chemical nature of heart failure. Ann Intern Med 1939; 12: 1233–44.

34. Ingwall JS. The hypertrophied myocardium accumulates the mb-creatine kinase isozyme. Eur Heart J 1984; 5: 129–39.

35. Boehm E, Chan S, Monfared M, et al. Creatine transporter activity and content in the rat heart supplemented by and depleted of creatine. Am J Physiol Endocrinol Metab 2003; 284: 399–406.

36. Neubauer S, Remkes H, Spindler M, et al. Down regulation of the Na(+)-creatine co-transporter in failing human myocardium and in experimental heart failure. Circulation 1999; 100: 1847–50.

37. Ten Hove M, Chan S, Lygate C, et al. Mechanisms of creatine depletion in chronically failing rat heart. J Mol Cell Cardiol 2005; 38: 309–13.

38. Strutz-Seebohm N, Shojaiefard M, Christie D, et al. Pikfyve in the sgk1 mediated regulation of the creatine transporter slc6a8. Cell Physiol Biochem 2007; 20: 729–34.

39. Shen W, Spindler M, Higgins M, et al. The fall in creatine levels and creatine kinase isozyme changes in the failing heart are reversible: Complex post-transcriptional regulation of the components of the ck system. J Mol Cell Cardiol 2005; 39:537–44.

40. Park SJ, Zhang J, Ye Y, et al. Myocardial creatine kinase expression after left ventricular assist device support. J Am Coll Cardiol 2002; 39: 1773–9.

41. Saupe KW, Spindler M, Hopkins JC, Shen W, Ingwall JS. Kinetic, thermodynamic, and developmental consequences of deleting creatine kinase isoenzymes from the heart. reaction kinetics of the creatine kinase isoenzymes in the intact heart. J Biol Chem 2000; 275: 19742–6.

42. Saupe KW, Spindler M, Tian R, Ingwall JS. Impaired cardiac energetics in mice lacking muscle-specific isoenzymes of creatine kinase. Circ Res 1998; 82: 898–907.

43. ten Hove M, Lygate CA, Fischer A, et al. Reduced inotropic reserve and increased susceptibility to cardiac ischemia/reperfusion injury in phosphocreatine-deficient guanidinoacetate-n-methyltransferase-knockout mice. Circulation 2005; 111: 2477–85.

44. Tian R, Ingwall JS. Energetic basis for reduced contractile reserve in isolated rat hearts. Am J Physiol 1996; 270: H1207–16.

45. Zweier JL, Jacobus WE, Korecky B, Brandejs-Barry Y. Bioenergetic consequences of cardiac phosphocreatine depletion induced by creatine analogue feeding. J Biol Chem 1991; 266: 20296–304.

46. Janssen E, Dzeja PP, Oerlemans F, et al. Adenylate kinase 1 gene deletion disrupts muscle energetic economy despite metabolic rearrangement. EMBO J 2000; 19: 6371–81.

47. Abraham MR, Selivanov VA, Hodgson DM, et al. Coupling of cell energetics with membrane metabolic sensing. integrative signaling through creatine kinase phosphotransfer disrupted by m-ck gene knock-out. J Biol Chem 2002; 277: 24427–34.

48. Wallis J, Lygate CA, Fischer A, et al. Supranormal myocardial creatine and phosphocreatine concentrations lead to cardiac hypertrophy and heart failure: insights from creatine transporter-overexpressing transgenic mice. Circulation 2005; 112: 3131–9.

49. Gupta A, Akki A, Wang Y, et al. Creatine kinase-mediated improvement of function in failing mouse hearts provides causal evidence the failing heart is energy starved. J Clin Invest 2012; 122: 291–302.

50. Tian R, Musi N, D'Agostino J, Hirshman MF, Goodyear LJ. Increased adenosine monophosphate-activated protein kinase activity in rat hearts with pressure-overload hypertrophy. Circulation 2001; 104: 1664–9.

51. Allard MF, Parsons HL, Saeedi R, Wamboldt RB, Brownsey R. AMPK and metabolic adaptation by the heart to pressure overload. Am J Physiol Heart Circ Physiol 2007; 292: 140–8.

52. Nascimben L, Ingwall J, Lorell B, et al. Mechanisms for increased glycolysis in the hypertrophied rat heart. Hypertension 2004; 44: 662–7.

53. Allard MF, Schonekess BO, Henning SL, English DR, Lopaschuk GD. Contribution of oxidative metabolism and glycolysis to atp production in hypertrophied hearts. Am J Physiol 1994; 267: H742–50.

54. Tian R, Abel ED. Responses of GLUT4-deficient hearts to ischemia underscore the importance of glycolysis. Circulation 2001; 103: 2961–6.

55. Liao R, Jain M, Cui L, et al. Cardiac-specific overexpression of GLUT1 prevents the development of heart failure due to pressure-overload in mice. Circulation 2002; 106: 2125–31.

56. Kong SW, Bodyak N, Yue P, et al. Genetic expression profiles during physiological and pathological cardiac hypertrophy and heart failure in rats. Physiol Genomics 2005; 21: 31–42.

57. Arany Z, Wagner BK, Ma Y, et al. Gene expression-based screening identifies microtubule inhibitors as inducers of pgc-1alpha and oxidative phosphorylation. Proc Natl Acad Sci USA 2008; 105: 4721–6.

58. Murray AJ, Cole MA, Lygate CA, et al. Increased mitochondrial uncoupling proteins, respiratory uncoupling and decreased efficiency in the chronically infarcted rat heart. J Mol Cell Cardiol 2008; 44: 694–700.

59. Gong G, Liu J, Liang P, et al. Oxidative capacity in failing hearts. Am J Physiol Heart Circ Physiol 2003; 285: 541–8.

60. Murakami Y, Zhang Y, Cho YK, et al. Myocardial oxygenation during high work states in hearts with postinfarction remodeling. Circulation 1999; 99: 942–8.

61. Sheeran FL, Pepe S. Energy deficiency in the failing heart: linking increased reactive oxygen species and disruption of oxidative phosphorylation rate. Biochemica et Biophysica Acta 2006; 1757: 543–52.

62. Martin M, Gomez MA, Guillen F, et al. Myocardial carnitine and carnitine palmitoyltransferase deficiencies in patients with severe heart failure. Biochemica et Biophysica Acta 2000; 1502: 330–6.

63. Garnier A, Fortin D, Delomenie C, et al. Depressed mitochondrial transcription factors and oxidative capacity in rat failing cardiac and skeletal muscles. J Physiol 2003; 551: 491–501.

64. Arany Z, He H, Lin J, et al. Transcriptional coactivator pgc-1a controls the energy state and contractile function of cardiac muscle. Cell Metab 2005; 1: 259–71.

65. Arany Z, Novikov M, Chin S, et al. Transverse aortic constriction leads to accelerated heart failure in mice lacking PPAR-γ coactivator 1a. Proc Natl Acad Sci USA 2006; 103: 10086–91.

66. Lehman JJ, Barger PM, Kovacs A, et al. Peroxisome proliferator-activated receptor gamma coactivator-1 promotes cardiac mitochondrial biogenesis. J Clin Invest 2000; 106: 847–56.

67. Russell LK, Mansfield CM, Lehman JJ, et al. Cardiac-specific induction of the transcriptional coactivator peroxisome proliferator-activated receptor gamma coactivator-1a promotes mitochondrial biogenesis and reversible cardiomyopathy in a developmental stage-dependent manner. Circ Res 2004; 94: 525–33.

68. Hansson A, Hance N, Dufour E, et al. A switch in metabolism precedes increased mitochondrial biogenesis in respiratory chain-deficient mouse hearts. Proc Natl Acad Sci USA 2004; 101: 3136–41.

69. van den Bosch BJ, van den Burg CM, Schoonderwoerd K, et al. Regional absence of mitochondria causing energy depletion in the myocardium of muscle LIM protein knockout mice. Cardiovasc Res 2005; 65: 411–18.

70. Dzeja PP, Hoyer K, Tian R, et al. Rearrangement of energetic and substrate utilization networks compensate for chronic myocardial creatine kinase deficiency. J Physiol 2011; 589: 5193–211.

71. Huss JM, Imahashi K-i, Dufour CR, et al. The nuclear receptor ERRα is required for the bioenergetic and functional adaptation to cardiac pressure overload. Cell Metab 2007; 6: 25–37.

72. Alaynick WA, Kondo RP, Xie W, et al. ERRγ directs and maintains the transition to oxidative metabolism in the postnatal heart. Cell Metab 2007; 6: 13–24.

73. Sano M, Wang SC, Shirai M, et al. Activation of cardiac cdk9 represses pgc-1 and confers a predisposition to heart failure. Embo J 2004; 23: 3559–69.

74. Puigserver P, Spiegelman BM. Peroxisome proliferator-activated receptor-gamma coactivator 1 alpha (pgc-1 alpha): transcriptional coactivator and metabolic regulator. Endocr Rev 2003; 24: 78–90.

75. Ertz-Berger BR, He H, Dowell C, et al. Changes in the chemical and dynamic properties of cardiac troponin t cause discrete cardiomyopathies in transgenic mice. Proc Natl Acad Sci USA 2005; 102: 18219–24.

76. Volkmann N, Lui H, Hazelwood L, et al. The r403q myosin mutation implicated in familial hypertrophic cardiomyopathy causes disorder at the actomyosin interface. PLoS ONE 2007; 2: e1123.

77. Crilley JG, Boehm EA, Blair E, et al. Hypertrophic cardiomyopathy due to sarcomeric gene mutations is characterized by impaired energy metabolism irrespective of the degree of hypertrophy. J Am Coll Cardiol 2003; 41: 1776–82.

78. He ZH, Bottinelli R, Pellegrino MA, Ferenczi MA, Reggiani C. Atp consumption and efficiency of human single muscle fibers with different myosin isoform composition. Biophys J 2000; 79: 945–61.

79. Javadpour MM, Tardiff JC, Pinz I, Ingwall JS. Decreased energetics in murine hearts bearing the r92q mutation in cardiac troponin t. J Clin Invest 2003; 112: 768–75.

80. Spindler M, Saupe KW, Christe ME, et al. Diastolic dysfunction and altered energetics in the alphamhc403/+ mouse model of familial hypertrophic cardiomyopathy. J Clin Invest 1998; 101: 1775–83.

81. Tian R, Christe ME, Spindler M, et al. Role of mgadp in the development of diastolic dysfunction in the intact beating rat heart. J Clin Invest 1997; 99: 745–51.

82. Tian R, Nascimben L, Ingwall JS, Lorell BH. Failure to maintain a low adp concentration impairs diastolic function in hypertrophied rat hearts. Circulation 1997; 96: 1313–19.

83. Smith SH, Kramer MF, Reis I, Bishop SP, Ingwall JS. Regional changes in creatine kinase and myocyte size in hypertensive and nonhypertensive cardiac hypertrophy. Circ Res 1990; 67: 1334–44.

84. Hopkins J, Miao W, Ingwall J. Paradoxical effects of creatine kinase deletion on systolic and diastolic function in ischemia. Circulation 1998; 98: I–758.

85. Horn M, Remkes H, Stromer H, Dienesch C, Neubauer S. Chronic phosphocreatine depletion by the creatine analogue beta-guanidinopropionate is associated with increased mortality and loss of atp in rats after myocardial infarction. Circulation 2001; 104: 1844–9.

86. Brixius K, Lu R, Boelck B, et al. Chronic treatment with carvedilol improves Ca(2+)-dependent atp consumption in triton x-skinned fiber preparations of human myocardium. J Pharmacol Exp Ther 2007; 322: 222–7.

87. Tuunanen H, Engblom E, Naum A, et al. Free fatty acid depletion acutely decreases cardiac work and efficiency in cardiomyopathic heart failure. Circulation 2006; 114: 2130–7.

88. Lamberts RR, Caldenhoven E, Lansink M, et al. Preservation of diastolic function in monocrotaline-induced right ventricular hypertrophy in rats. Am J Physiol Heart Circ Physiol 2007; 293: H1869–76.

89. Tian R, Nascimben L, Kaddurah-Daouk R, Ingwall JS. Depletion of energy reserve via the creatine kinase reaction during the evolution of heart failure in cardiomyopathic hamsters. J Mol Cell Cardiol 1996; 28: 755–65.

90. Liao R, Nascimben L, Friedrich J, Gwathmey JK, Ingwall JS. Decreased energy reserve in an animal model of dilated cardiomyopathy relationship to contractile performance. Circ Res 1996; 78: 893–902.

6

Animal models of heart failure

William Carlson

Heart failure is the major cause of mortality in Western countries. Medical treatment of heart failure is associated with 50% survival at 5 years. Experimental models are essential for us to better understand the progression of the disease and elaborate new therapy and there are several excellent reviews that have been published in the past (1–4). Heart transplantation, left ventricular (LV) assist devices, artificial hearts, cardiac bioassist techniques, and pharmacologic agents require animal models for testing and optimizing before they are implemented in clinical trials and used as routine treatment in patients. The perfect model of heart failure that reproduces every aspect of the natural disease does not exist. Acute and chronic heart failure models have been developed to reproduce different aspects of the pathophysiology. It is important to understand the strengths and weaknesses of each model to apply them appropriately either to understand the pathophysiology or to test new treatments.

The prevalence of congestive heart failure (CHF) increases with age. It is 1–2% in adults up to age 65 years, 2–3% in those over 65 years, and reaches 5–10% in patients older than 75 years (5). Despite significant improvements in the medical therapy of congestive heart failure, the mortality rate is in excess of 50% after 5 years (5,6). Surgical treatment, including heart transplantation and LV assist devices, has been used to interrupt the progression toward disability and death. Medical therapies have been developed over the past 20 years that can modify the hemodynamic abnormalities that occur and have helped to elucidate pathways that may interrupt the pathophysiology of the underlying cellular and molecular processes.

Heart failure has many underlying causes, and the frequency of the causes have been changing over the last several decades. According to the Framingham Heart Study (5), coronary heart disease was the etiologic factor in 67% of patients with CHF, primary myocardial disease accounted for 20%, and valvular heart disease was the cause in 10%. Regardless of the etiology, the syndrome of advanced heart failure is composed of a complex picture, including altered hemodynamics, disturbed myocardial function, ventricular remodeling, neurohormonal alterations, cytokine activation, and endothelial dysfunction (7–10), leading a final common pathway, which at the cellular level involves apoptosis, a chronic inflammatory process and fibrosis (9,11,12).

Research associated with heart failure has focused on understanding the mechanism of heart failure and the evaluation of different therapeutic modalities (6,8,10). A requirement of all studies on heart failure is an adequate and appropriate model of heart failure in animal models. The ideal model should be able to reproduce each of the aspects of the progression of naturally occurring CHF. However, none of the models available is able to entirely reproduce the abnormalities of CHF. Some models reproduce neuroendocrine changes, whereas others better reproduce the remodeling that occurs during chronic heart failure. Acute models are not going to reproduce the neuroendocrine dysfunction, whereas a chronic model might. Therefore, the appropriate model should be selected to evaluate the specific aspects of heart failure being investigated. Heart failure has been induced in different species using a variety of techniques, including volume overload, pressure overload, fast pacing, myocardial infarction, or with cardiotoxic drugs. Models of genetically induced cardiomyopathy are also available in small animals. Each of these models has its strengths and weaknesses, and understanding the models is important in order to employ the appropriate model for the question being posed.

DIFFERENT ANIMAL SPECIES
Small Animal Models of Heart Failure
Small animal models, such as mice, rats, or rabbits, offer a number of advantages over large animals but also some disadvantages. The animals are relatively inexpensive and easy to obtain. They have a short gestation period and a large sample size can be produced in a relatively short period of time. Because of their small size, they are easy to house. However, the small size makes certain work more difficult. Surgery is more difficult, and imaging such as echocardiography can be a challenge. These models have been used to study long-term pharmacologic interventions, and are frequently used with the endpoint of mortality (13,14). There are, however, several limitations to rat models related to differences in myocardial function, in comparison to the human heart (5). Rat myocardium has a very short activation potential and normally lacks a plateau phase (14). Calcium removal from cytosol is predominantly through the sarcoplasmic reticulum (SR). Calcium and the sodium–potassium exchange activity is less relevant (15,16). Alpha-myosin heavy-chain isoforms predominate in the normal rat myocardium and shift toward the β-myosin isoform with hemodynamic loading or hormonal changes (17). In addition, the resting heart rate of rats is five times that of humans and the force–frequency relationship is the inverse of that in humans (15). Rabbit models are more expensive than rat models but less expensive than large animal models. There are some distinct advantages of the rabbit models over the rat models. Normal rabbit myocardium exhibits some important similarities to the human heart: (*i*) The β-myosin heavy-chain isoform predominates in adult animals, (*ii*) calcium elimination is controlled about 70% by the SR and 30% by the Na^+/Ca^{2+} exchanger, (*iii*) the force–frequency relationship is positive (15,16,18). These factors are important considerations, especially for studying the function of new pharmacologic agents.

Large Animal Models of Heart Failure
Large animal models, such as dogs, goats, sheep, and pigs, facilitate the study of LV function, volume, mass, and hemodynamics more accurately than small animal models, simply because of their size. Chronic instrumentation is easier, the animals tolerate the instrumentation more readily, and errors in measurements are smaller. Drawbacks to the use of large animals are the high cost of procurement, housing, and handling. In the dog models, there are several important relationships that should be considered. The force–frequency relationship evaluated by the slope of the end systolic pressure–volume relationship, E_{max}, has been shown to be positive in autonomically intact awake dogs, as well as during autonomic blockade (18). The β-myosin heavy-chain isoforms predominate in the dog myocardium, as they do in the human myocardium. In addition, the excitation contraction coupling in the myocardium of dogs appears to be similar to that in the human myocardium.

SPECIFIC MODELS OF HEART FAILURE
There are a number of techniques that are used to induce heart failure in the different animals. Some are better at simulating the changes that occur in acute heart failure and others are better at simulating the changes observed in chronic heart failure. Some models can be

combined. The major categories are volume overload, pressure overload, rapid pacing, ischemic injury, toxic injury, and genetically altered models.

VOLUME OVERLOAD
Acute Volume Overload
Acute volume overload is usually produced by an infusion of isotonic fluids or colloids to reproduce the hemodynamics of fluid overload observed in acute or chronic heart failure (19,20). It can be used alone or, commonly, in conjunction with another model of heart failure. In this fashion, volume overload can be used to evaluate myocardial reserve. It has also been used to evaluate hemodynamic parameters of diastolic dysfunction, and systolic dysfunction.

Chronic Volume Overload
Chronic volume overload can be used to induce left- and/or right-sided heart failure with severe ventricular dilation. Surgical techniques commonly used to induce volume overload are the creation of an arteriovenous fistula (carotid artery to jugular vein), and induction of mitral valve regurgitation (21–24). These models produce chronic changes of LV dilation, neurohormonal activation, including the renin–angiotensin–aldosterone system (RAAS) and sympathetic systems (25–27).

Mitral regurgitation can be induced in dogs using a percutaneous procedure. Under general anesthesia, an introducer is placed in the left ventricle through the carotid artery. Flexible rat-tooth forceps inserted through the sheath are used to cut the mitral chordae sequentially. Chordae are cut until the pulmonary capillary wedge pressure increases by 20 mmHg, the cardiac output drops by 50%, and arterial pressure decreases (21). In 3–6 months, mitral regurgitation increases LV end-diastolic volume by 75% and LV stroke volume doubles. LV mass increases, while right ventricular free wall mass remains relatively unchanged (21). This model is associated with myocyte lengthening and the reduction of myocytes contractility. It is commonly used to test medical treatment of heart failure that target hemodynamics. It has also been used to study abnormalities at the cellular level, but they are limited because they do not mimic the complete spectrum of heart failure at a molecular level.

Volume and Pressure Overload in Rabbits
Volume overload, pressure overload, and the combination of both are used to induce heart failure in rabbits. Chronic severe aortic regurgitation in rabbits, created by aortic valve perforation with a catheter, produces LV hypertrophy, followed by systolic dysfunction and heart failure after a period of months (28). Occurrence of heart failure is more consistently and rapidly observed when aortic regurgitation is combined with aortic constriction. In another model, aortic insufficiency is produced by destroying the aortic valve with a catheter introduced through the carotid artery. After 14 days, aortic constriction is performed just below the diaphragm. Heart failure occurs about four weeks after the initial procedure (29,30). Heart failure is associated with alterations in the β-adrenoceptors system similar to those in humans (29). Furthermore, in this model there is inversion of the force–frequency relationship and alteration of postrest potentiation, which closely resembles the situation in the human heart (31). Interestingly, protein and mRNA levels of Na^+/Ca^{2+} exchanger were significantly increased in failing compared with nonfailing animals, whereas SR Ca^{2+}-ATPase was not significantly altered (32). This may indicate that increased transsarcolemmal calcium loss by increased Na^+/Ca^{2+} exchanger activity may decrease calcium availability to contractile proteins and decrease myocardial function even without direct alteration of SR function.

Volume Overload in Goats
Volume overload can also be produced by creating an arteriovenous fistula between the carotid artery and the jugular vein in goats or dogs (33). These models can produce a 50%

increase of the LV end-diastolic volume without increasing end-diastolic pressure (22). This technique has been used in combination with doxorubicin to induce biventricular heart failure (24). Stable ventricular hypocontractility with LV dilation was observed. A higher dose of doxorubicin was associated with more pronounced LV dysfunction and was associated with clinical symptoms of heart failure.

Because this model closely mimics alterations of myocardial function observed in the end-stage failing human myocardium, this model may be well suited to study alterations in excitation–contraction coupling processes occurring during the transition from compensated hypertrophy to failure.

PRESSURE OVERLOAD

Hypertension is associated with an increased risk for the development of heart failure clinically. It is therefore important to consider models of hypertension and ventricular hypertrophy when the evaluation of new treatment of heart failure is tested in an animal model. Models involving an abnormal pressure load have been most useful in the study of the pathogenesis of hypertrophy, subcellular and molecular mechanisms of heart failure, and vascular changes associated with heart failure.

Aortic Banding

Animal models of pressure overload have been produced by supravalvular aortic stenosis with narrowing of the aorta above the valve, inducing a pattern of ventricular strain similar to that of aortic stenosis (34). This model is created by dissecting the ascending aorta free from the pulmonary artery and placing a Dacron patch around the aorta, reducing the diameter of the aorta is reduced by 50% (35). The aortic and LV pressures are then checked to confirm that a 50–60 mmHg systolic pressure gradient has been created. This model produces marked LV hypertrophy, but does not reproduce neurohormonal activation or LV systolic dysfunction, until it has been established for **3–6 months**. It can be combined with acute volume overload to study diastolic dysfunction and has been useful in the study of chronic changes of myocardial fibrosis (36).

PRESSURE OVERLOAD IN RATS AND MICE
Aortic Banding in Rats

Constriction of the aorta above the renal arteries in rats produces LV hypertrophy and subsequently CHF. This model has been used frequently to study LV hypertrophy. After 20 weeks of banding, two distinct groups can be identified: those with and those without reduction in LV systolic pressure (37). Animals with LV hypertrophy and reduced systolic pressures showed an increase in LV volume and reduced ejection fraction (38). Animals in this subgroup showed increased β-myosin heavy-chain mRNA and atrial natriuretic factor mRNA. Plasma catecholamine levels and myocardial renin–angiotensin levels were also found to increase in this subset of animals (39). These models have also been useful in the study of fibrosis and the role of the TGFβ-BMP in controlling fibrosis and the putative endothelial to mesenchymal transition (40).

Systemic Hypertension in Rats

The systemic hypertensive rat is a well-established model of genetic hypertension. The cardiac function fails at 20 months, and more than 50% of the animals have clinical signs of heart failure (41,42). LV geometry and function are altered on echocardiography. Heart failure is characterized by neurohumoral changes and apoptosis. The systemic hypertensive rat is a good model to reproduce hypertension-induced heart failure in humans and to study the transition from hypertrophy to failure (41,42). An advantage of this model is that it does not require surgery and pharmacologic intervention for induction. Another strain of rats with diabetes develops systemic hypertension and heart failure at an earlier age but the presence of diabetes complicates this model (43).

Spontaneous Hypertensive Rats

Spontaneous hypertensive rats (SHR) have been used as a good animal model for the study of hypertension. In this model, LV function is preserved up to about one year of age (44). At 18–24 months, LV dysfunction develops, which includes reduced markers of performance and increased fibrosis. LV geometry is altered on echocardiography (41,42). Those animals with heart failure also show neurohormonal changes. Altered calcium cycling was also observed in this model, although there was no decrease in mRNA of the SR calcium pump, during the transition from compensated hypertrophy to CHF (45,46). There was a significant reduction of myocyte mass that accompanied the transition from stable LV function to CHF and an increase in the number of myocytes undergoing apoptosis was observed. The progression to LV dysfunction was also marked by a significant increase in the expression of genes encoding extracellular matrix. It is worth noting that treatment with the angiotensin-converting enzyme inhibitor, captopril, was associated with a reduction in the number of myocytes undergoing apoptosis (47), suggesting a pivotal role of the RAAS system in apoptosis.

Spontaneous Hypertensive Heart Failure Rats

Selective breeding of spontaneously hypertensive rats that developed CHF before 18 months of age has produced a more malleable animal model of the spontaneously hypertensive rats. Rats that carry a gene *facp* that encodes the defective leptin receptor (SH-HF/Mcc-facp) (48) developed CHF earlier than the traditional spontaneously hypertensive rats. These animals show a progressive increase in plasma renin activity, atrial naturetic peptide, and aldosterone levels. Plasma renin activity levels were independently correlated with cardiac hypertrophy (49).

Aortic Banding in Guinea Pigs

A model of pressure overload in guinea pigs has been developed. These animals have some of the advantages of the rats without some of the disadvantages. Guinea pigs have their aortas banded similar to the procedure used for rats. Eight weeks after the banding of the descending thoracic aorta in guinea pigs, overt heart failure develops in a subgroup of animals (50–52). Myocardial function is altered in a fashion that has some similarities with end-stage failing human myocardium. The force–frequency relationship is blunted in isolated myocytes from failing hearts (50). A decrease in SR-Ca^{2+}-ATPase protein levels and phospholamban protein levels was also observed following eight weeks of banding as compared with an age-matched banded group without clinical signs of heart failure (51). Normal guinea pig myocardium, such as the human ventricular myocardium, contains predominantly the β-myosin heavy chain with small amounts of -myosin. This is shifted completely to β-myosin without any -myosin heavy chain in the hypertrophied and failing hearts (52). These studies show that this guinea pig model has similarities to human heart failure with respect to calcium cycling, myosin isoforms, and myocardial function. This model may have advantages for investigating the transition from cardiac hypertrophy to failure and the alterations in excitation–contraction coupling systems that occur during this transition.

RAPID-PACING MODELS OF HEART FAILURE

Fast pacing of the heart has been used to produce a progressive and reliable model of heart failure in several different animal species (53), including rabbits, dogs, pigs, and sheep (42,54,55).

The most completely studied and characterized models are the dog models. These models have many similarities to the failing human heart and have been extensively used for testing of pharmacologic agents and the pathogenesis of remodeling.

There are several dog models of heart failure produced by rapid pacing. In one model where the right ventricle was paced at rates between 180 and 240 beats per minute, the animals developed heart failure in three to four weeks (56,57). This model produces dilation of the left and right ventricles without hypertrophy (58). It also produces increases in cardiac volume with fluid retention and diastolic dysfunction. It produces time-dependent changes in neurohormonal activation with early elevation of catecholamines, and atrial natriuretic peptide (59–61) then late elevation of renin, angiotensin, aldosterone, endothelin-1, and tumor necrosis factor-alpha (60,62,63). Chronic tachycardia also produced abnormalities in calcium handling and disruption of the extracellular matrix by activation of matrix metalloproteases, gelatinase, and cytokines. Remodeling is accompanied by decreased and delayed systolic LV torsional deformation and loss of early diastolic recoil. In addition, there is a significant reduction in the number of myocytes after fast pacing for only one week. This myocyte loss during fast pacing has been shown to be a result of apoptosis (programmed cell death). Some changes are, however, temporary and after cessation of the stimulation for two to three weeks, systolic and diastolic function of the heart recovered in part (64). Other changes, such as hypertrophy of the ventricular walls and persistence of the ventricular dilation, occur during recovery.

Considerable changes seem to occur in myocyte shape, in cytoskeleton, and in the extracellular matrix. In contrast to findings in human heart failure, collagen content was shown to be decreased and its structure altered, which may result in decreased collagen support (65). Changes in cytoskeleton and extracellular matrix were suggested to be a major factor for ventricular remodeling, and apoptotic cell death was also suggested to play a key role in the development of CHF (66,67). Significant alterations have been observed in the β-adrenoceptor–adenylyl-cyclase system. These include decreased β-adrenergic receptor density (65). Unlike the situation in human heart failure, mRNA levels of adenylyl-cyclase have been shown to be reduced consistent with reduced basal and forskolin-stimulated adenylyl cyclase activity (67).

Consistent with the findings in failing human hearts, force–frequency relationship is blunted or reversed in the rapid-pacing dog model of heart failure (68,69). Altered force–frequency relationship in this model was also observed at the level of the isolated myocyte (70). Increases in preload do not further augment stroke volume suggesting that the Frank–Starling reserve is exhausted under in vivo conditions (71). This model was shown to be associated with malignant arrhythmias and sudden cardiac death, which may be related to prolongation of the action potential (72).

In other models where healthy dogs were subjected to rapid electronic pacing at rates above 200 beats a minute, CHF is also produced within several weeks (64,73,74). This model results in progressive, biventricular chamber dilation after three to four weeks. The animals show a significant decrease in ejection fraction and increased diastolic dysfunction. Cardiac output falls and systemic vascular resistance increases (64,75,76). There are also significant changes in the neurohormonal systems. In these models, there is no significant change in left ventricular mass or LV hypertrophy (64,74). When the pacing is terminated, hemodynamic, volume, and neurohormonal abnormalities, resolved (77). The neuro hormonal activation is time dependent, with early activation of the sympathetic nervous system showing increased plasma catecholamine levels and decreased parasympathetic tone (59,60). Plasma atrial naturetic protein levels are also elevated early after the onset of hemodynamic changes (61). Systemic activation of the renin–angiotensin system is also seen and correlates with progressive LV dysfunction (60,61). Endothelial dysfunction is noted, with decreased nitric oxide-mediated coronary vasodilation, both agonist stimulated and flow stimulated similar to what occurs in patients with heart failure (63).

At the level of the myocardium, contractile force has been shown to be decreased and calcium transients were prolonged (78). These models show that relaxation is impaired in isolated myocytes from failing hearts (79). This may be related to altered expression and function of calcium-handling proteins. Although an earlier report suggested that $SR-Ca^{2+}$-ATPase mRNA levels measured in LV endocardial biopsies at baseline and at the onset of pacing tachycardia-induced failure do not significantly change (80), data indicates that expression of $SR-Ca^{2+}$-ATPase is decreased. Similar to changes that occur in the failing human heart, mRNA and protein levels of SR calcium ATPase are decreased and mRNA and protein levels of the sarcolemmal Na^+/Ca^{2+}-exchanger are significantly increased (81). The latter findings are consistent with measurements showing a decreased activity of the SR calcium pump in mongrel dogs with pacing-induced heart failure and in Doberman pinscher dogs with dilated cardiomyopathy (82). Thus, altered calcium handling may result from reduced SR calcium uptake and accumulation and increased calcium sequestration into the extracellular space. In addition, a decreased number of ryanodine receptors has been suggested (82), and in the pacing tachycardia failure model, $[^3H]$ ryanodine receptor binding has been found to be depressed. This depression occurred as early as one day after pacing and remained at this depressed level up to four to seven weeks of pacing when heart failure was manifest (83). In the same study, dihydropyridine binding was not altered in the failing animals (83). Whether altered myofilament calcium sensitivity contributes to altered myocardial function in this model is not clear (84,85).

Chronic-Pacing Models

By altering the pacing protocol, a chronic model of heart failure has been produced. Several different protocols have been implemented to induce chronic CHF. Rapid pacing at 230 bpm for four weeks, and then 190 bpm for another four weeks, induced heart failure in dogs (86). Severe persistent CHF was confirmed by a number of measurements. Pressure volume loops, hemodynamic parameters, echocardiography, LV mass, and wall stress were all abnormal. Pathologic examinations, plasma atrial natriuretic peptide, and catecholamine levels were also found to be consistent with chronic CHF (86). Most of the systolic and diastolic measurements were abnormal and stable at eight weeks.

These models are well suited for the study of certain aspects of CHF because they do not require major surgical trauma, such as thoracotomy and pericardiectomy, which may interfere with the interpretation of physiologic data. These models have been used to evaluate the progression of heart failure, because they progress over several weeks, allowing sequential observation in a short period of time and have similarities to certain aspects of clinically observed heart failure. They trigger LV dilation and pump failure and the neurohormonal activation, which closely parallels those observed in humans with CHF. However, myocardial ischemia and hypertrophy, which are a common component of the development of CHF, are not present in this model. The severity of the CHF is a function of the stimulus. The severe dilation of both ventricles has been associated with mitral annular dilation and mitral regurgitation, which are major factors in the progression of clinical heart failure (55).

The fast-pacing models have been used for a number of purposes. They have been used to evaluate defects at the cellular and extracellular levels. They have been used to evaluate new pharmacologic strategies. They have also been used to evaluate different surgical interventions that alter remodeling during heart failure and to evaluate the recovery phase after different interventions (87–90). The chronic models that do not have recovery of cardiac function are more appropriate for the evaluation of different therapeutic modalities than the models with recovery of the cardiac function.

The pacing-tachycardia dog model seems to be valuable for studying neurohumoral mechanisms and peripheral circulatory alterations, both of which closely resemble that observed in human heart failure. Furthermore, alterations in myocardial function and molecular changes in calcium-handling proteins underlying altered myocardial function show considerable similarities to the failing human heart. This may allow the study of the transition from a compensated state of LV dysfunction to overt failure with respect to alterations in calcium homeostasis. The model also provides temporal and mechanistic information on LV remodeling and allows the study of pharmacologic interventions to influence the remodeling process. The limitations of the rapid-pacing model include an uncertain pathogenesis, and lack of long-term stability because heart failure is reversible when pacing is stopped. Furthermore, unlike clinical forms of CHF, the development of CHF by chronic rapid pacing is not associated with hypertrophy or increased collagen content. Loss of collagen support may considerably contribute to ventricular remodeling in this model.

The technique of tachycardia pacing to induce heart failure has also been used in pigs and sheep and findings similar to those in dogs have been observed with respect to clinical, hemodynamic, and neurohumoral changes (91–94).

MODELS OF ISCHEMIA AND INFARCTION

The clinical disorder of CHF in the majority of patients is caused by coronary artery disease, producing myocardial infarction or ischemia. Myocardial infarction and ischemia produces LV dysfunction and remodeling, which include changes in geometry, structure, and function. Remodeling, which is initially adaptive, ultimately leads to the clinical entity of heart failure. The mechanism responsible for this deleterious transition from adaptive remodeling to dysfunction is not yet fully understood. It is known that it involves neurohormonal axis, loading conditions of the remaining myocardium, and alteration of the extracellular matrix [2, 3, 4 and 5]. There are a number of animal models that have been developed to study this process. These models employ either a surgical intervention through a thoracotomy to place a ligature around the coronary artery, or a catheterization to perform coronary embolization. Rat models have been extensively studied but have the disadvantages of surgery on small animals and a large variation in the size of the infarct. Canine models have been studied extensively but have the disadvantage that they develop collateral circulation. Porcine, ovine, and rat hearts have a coronary circulation, which is more similar to that of a human heart and have become more popular.

Rat Coronary Ligation Model

Myocardial infarction can be induced following the ligation of a coronary artery in Sprague–Dawley rats and is a widely used model for heart failure (95). Ligation of the left coronary artery results in a myocardial infarction of variable size and the occurrence of overt heart failure after three to six weeks. The heart failure is not uniform and depends on the size of the infarct produced. In animals with a sizable myocardial infarct, the heart will progressively dilate, with reduced systolic function, and increase filling pressures (13,96). Progression of left ventricular dysfunction is associated with neurohumoral activation similar to that seen in patients with CHF. Calcium flux is altered with the decrease in L-type calcium channels. Activation of the renin–angiotensin system is observed, with increased angiotensin-converting enzyme activity in both the left ventricle and the kidney (97). Unfortunately, it is difficult to control the size of the infarct and there is a high mortality in this model. Some studies in Lewis inbred rats have shown a more uniform size of the myocardial infarct produced by ligation of the left coronary artery with a relatively low mortality (98).

Large Animal Models of Infarction

There are several large animal models of heart failure produced by surgical ligation of the left anterior descending coronary artery, a diagonal branch, or the circumflex artery. This model has been used to produce myocardial ischemia or infarction and postinfarction remodeling (99–104). This technique has been used in sheep to produce infarction of the left ventricle (99). After eight weeks, a fall in cardiac output and LV dp/dt is observed with an increase in LV end-diastolic pressure. In this model, the noninfarcted myocardium maintains normal blood flow, whereas the blood flow in the infarcted myocardium is significantly reduced. This model has the advantage that the animals do not develop collateral circulation and do not require repeated infarct. It provides the opportunity to study the border zones of infarcts where there is hypocontractile myocardium, which is normally perfused (105).

Modifications of this model have been produced by ligation of the distal part of the left anterior descending the second diagonal branches of the circumflex coronary artery and ligation of the posterior descending artery. This induces aneurysmal dilation of the left ventricular wall within 4 hours of ligation (102). The aneurysm progresses over the next two months with thinning of the LV wall. Ligation of the second and third oblique branches of the circumflex coronary artery induced an infarction in the posterior wall and the papillary muscle (102). After eight weeks mitral regurgitation develops. Ligation of the second and third marginal branches of the circumflex artery and the posterior descending artery produced a larger infarct of the posterior wall with an infarct of the papillary muscle with severe mitral regurgitation, 1 hour after ligation. These models have been used primarily for the study of hemodynamic alterations and agents that might reduce cellular injury to infarcted tissue.

Canine Models of Ischemia and Infarction

Canine models of myocardial ischemia have the disadvantage that extensive collateral circulation can develop after ligation of a coronary artery in which extensive collaterals reperfuse and salvage ischemic tissue. To palliate this problem, repeated embolization of microspheres at weekly intervals over 10 weeks has been used to decrease the ejection fraction to less than 0.35 (105). Three months after the final microembolization, there are clinical signs of heart failure, with LV dilatation, decreased ejection fraction, and elevated plasma norepinephrine levels (105–107) similar to that observed in humans (108). A decreased number of β-adrenoceptors and L-type calcium channels are also observed three months after the final embolization procedure (109). Furthermore, SR Ca^{2+}-ATPase activity and protein levels were reduced in LV myocardium (110). This model has been used to study the progression from LV dysfunction to heart failure and the influence of pharmacologic interventions (111). It has also been used to evaluate different surgical interventions to treat heart failure (112,113). One major advantage of this model is that varying degrees of LV dysfunction can be regulated by the number of embolic events. The heart failure induced by this model is irreversible but malignant dysrhythmias contribute to high mortality rates.

Ameroid Constrictors

Ameroid constrictors have been used to induce a progressive occlusion of coronary arteries in different species (114–116). Ameroid constrictors are made of hygroscopic casein in a stainless ring. The casein swells after absorption of water from the surrounding tissue, after which fibrous tissue develops around the ameroid constrictor. Placement of ameroid constrictors requires a thoracotomy and dissection of a coronary artery. Multiple ameroid constrictors can be placed around multiple coronary arteries (114,117). The coronary arteries are occluded in three to six weeks with different degrees of collateral circulation (118). In dogs, LV dysfunction develops two months after implantation with different degrees of CHF. This model is useful for the study of collateral circulation (118). Dogs have been known to possess pre-existing extensive collateral circulation, whereas pigs, similar to humans, do not have an extensive network of collaterals (115,117,118). In pigs, delayed occlusion induces a collateral-dependent ischemic bed that can support normal cardiac function.

Coiling/Gelfoam
After surgical exposure of a carotid artery, coils have been placed into the left anterior descending artery of pigs. Gelfoam sponges have been placed within the coil to completely obstruct the coronary artery (119). The coil and the sponges have also been placed at the origin of the second diagonal artery. This technique eliminates the need for a thoracotomy for the placement of a suture around a diagonal branch. Surgical placement of a suture may induce inflammation and development of collateral circulation. Percutaneous transcatheter occlusion of coronary arteries have been facilitated by the development of platinum coils, compatible with magnetic fields.

NATURALLY OCCURRING DILATED CARDIOMYOPATHY
Large-Breed Dogs
Large-breed dogs have been found that develop idiopathic dilated cardiomyopathy around the age of five to seven years (120,121). They frequently have atrial fibrillation or ventricular arrhythmias. Severe LV or biventricular dilation with thinning of the ventricular wall are present, resulting in augmentation of LV wall stress and neurohormonal activation, the hallmark of dilated cardiomyopathy in humans. Progression of the disease leads to CHF in four to six months after onset of the first clinical signs of heart failure (120,122). The dilated cardiomyopathy observed is similar to the idiopathic dilated cardiomyopathy observed clinically (123). In this model there is a 50% survival rate at two to four months making it valuable for mortality studies of new therapeutic strategies (124–126).

Syrian Hamsters
Certain strains of Syrian hamsters develop a cardiomyopathy with moderate compensatory hypertrophy that leads to a dilated cardiomyopathy. This model has been used to study the pathophysiology and treatment of CHF (127–129). Invasive monitoring has been performed to measure LVEDP, dp/dt, tau, and cardiac output in the hamster after femoral cutdown (128). In one model cardiac myolysis develops in hamsters at one month, cardiac hypertrophy in five months, and a dilated cardiomyopathy at eight months. Signs of overt heart failure develop at one year of age. In another strain, ventricular wall thinning is apparent by three months, and heart failure occurs at four months without the development of cardiac hypertrophy (129).

DRUG-INDUCED MODELS OF HEART FAILURE
Doxorubicin
Doxorubicin is a chemotherapeutic commonly used to treat cancer. It has been found to have cardiotoxic effects leading to a dilated cardiomyopathy. The cardiac toxicity is produced by free radicals and lipid peroxidation. These cause changes in lysosomes, sarcolemmas, mitochondria, and SR (130). These changes induce calcium overload, activation of hydrolytic enzymes, and reduction in energy production (131). The reduction in cardiac function is accompanied by the loss of structural integrity.

Doxorubicin cardiotoxicity is dose dependent (132) and has been used to induce heart failure in different animal species—dog, sheep, and goats (23,24,132–134).

Doxorubicin has been delivered by intravenous and intracoronary injections (133,134). Intracoronary injection delivers doxorubicin in a smaller dose producing heart failure without systemic toxicity (133,135). Heart failure produced by doxorubicin is characterized by biventricular enlargement, thinning of the ventricular wall, and reduction of the ejection fraction measured by echocardiography (133,136). An arteriovenous fistula has been used to induce biventricular heart failure in combination with doxorubicin (22–24), which allows the use of a lower dose of doxorubicin and reduces the risk of systemic toxicity.

This model has a direct correlate with the clinical entity of doxorubicin cardiomyopathy and is different form the other more common types of clinical heart failure. It has been used to evaluate different treatment modalities for heart failure. However, the model has several limitations. The degree of LV dysfunction is variable. It is associated with a high incidence of arrhythmia and a high mortality rate. Doxorubicin-induced heart failure is irreversible and progressive. Cellular transplantation, dynamic cardiomyoplasty, and adynamic cardiomyoplasty have been evaluated for the treatment of doxorubicin-induced heart failure (23,134,137).

Propranolol

Propranolol is a β-blocker that has a profound and prolonged negative inotropic effects on cardiac tissue. Intravenous injections at doses of 2–3 mg/kg will induce a significant reduction of mean arterial pressure, cardiac output, LV max dp/dt, E_{max} and LVEF (138–141). Intravenous propranolol injection provides an acute, stable, and predictable model of heart failure. This model does not provide ventricular dilation, which might be a limitation for the testing of cardiac bioassist techniques. It has been used to evaluate cardiomyoplasty, aortomyoplasty, and skeletal muscle (139,140,142,143).

Monocrotaline

Monocrotaline has been used in rats and dogs to induce pulmonary hypertension and subsequent right-sided hypertrophy and failure (144,145). Monocrotaline is a pyrrolizidine alkaloid found in the plant species *Crotalaria spectabilis*. Administration of monocrotaline causes a pulmonary vascular syndrome characterized by proliferative pulmonary vasculitis, pulmonary hypertension, and cor pulmonale (146). Monocrotaline undergoes hepatic transformation from the action of the cytochrome P450 monooxygenase system in the liver to form the monocrotaline pyrrole, which then circulates to the lung parenchyma. The initial injury leads to increased capillary permeability, moderate interstitial edema, fibrosis, macrophage accumulation, modification of pneumocytes II, and alveolar edema (146). The initial injuries result in endothelial degeneration or hyperplasia, hypertrophy of medial smooth muscle, and adventitial edema. These changes result in augmentation of pulmonary vascular resistance and pressure overload of the right ventricle.

In dogs the monocrotaline pyrrole needs to be administered, because the adult dog liver does not possess the enzymatic components necessary to process the monocrotaline to its active metabolite, monocrotaline pyrrole (147).

This model has been used to evaluate neointimal proliferation during pulmonary hypertrophy and its modulation, ventricular hypertrophy, regulation of gene expression, neuroendocrine modulation, and hemodynamic variations with pulmonary hypertension (145). This model has been used in dogs to evaluate cardiopulmonary transplantation with chronic pulmonary hypertension (144).

CONCLUSIONS

A wide variety of animal models of heart failure are available for understanding heart failure and evaluating new treatment modalities. Animal models have been instrumental in elucidating cellular and extracellular mechanisms causing LV dysfunction and remodeling. When heart failure models are induced in small animals, it is important to consider the short biologic periods for pathologic development and functional evaluation. None of the models reproduces completely the progression of the natural disease. Each model has its own strengths and weaknesses. An investigator should choose the model that will best reproduce the aspect of heart failure being studied. Combinations of different models could produce a model that more closely resembles the clinical entity of CHF in patients.

Combinations of different causes of heart failure might provide a new avenue for the understanding of CHF and the development of therapeutic strategies. Because diastolic dysfunction is getting recognized as a risk factor for the development of CHF it could be of value to combine models of diastolic dysfunction with models of myocardial ischemia, for example.

REFERENCES

1. Monnet E, Chacques JC. Animal models of heart failure: what is new? Annal Thoracic Surg 2005; 79: 1445–53.
2. Hasenfuss G. Animal models of human cardiovascular disease, heart failure and hypertrophy. Cardiovasc Res 1998; 39: 60–76.
3. Patten RD, Hall-Porter MR. Small animal models of heart failure development of novel therapies, past and present. Circ Heart Fail 2009; 2: 138–44.
4. Dixon JA, Spinale FG. Large animal models of heart failure: a critical link in the translation of basic science to clinical practice. Circ Heart Fail 2009; 2: 262–71.
5. Ho KKL, Anderson KM, Kannel WB, Grossman W, Levy D. Survival after the onset of congestive heart failure in Framingham heart study subjects. Circulation 1993; 88: 107–15.
6. Redfield MM. Epidemiology and pathophysiology of heart failure. Curr Cardiol Rep 2000; 2: 179–80.
7. Feldman AM, Li YY, McTiernan CF. Matrix metalloproteinases in pathophysiology and treatment of heart failure. Lancet 2001; 357: 654–5.
8. Francis GS, Wilson Tang WH. Pathophysiology of congestive heart failure. Rev Cardiovasc Med 2003; 4: S14–20.
9. McTiernan CF, Feldman AM. The role of tumor necrosis factor alpha in the pathophysiology of congestive heart failure. Curr Cardiol Rep 2000; 2: 189–97.
10. Chen HH, Burnett JC. Natriuretic peptides in the pathophysiology of congestive heart failure. Curr Cardiol Rep 2000; 2: 198–205.
11. Marshall D, Sack MN. Apoptosis: a pivotal event or an epiphenomenon in the pathophysiology of heart failure? Heart 2000; 84: 355–6.
12. Champion HC, Skaf MW, Hare JM. Role of nitric oxide in the pathophysiology of heart failure. Heart Fail Rev 2003; 8: 35–46.
13. Pfeffer MA, Pfeffer JM, Fishbein MC, et al. Myocardial infarct size and ventricular function in rats. Circ Res 1979; 44: 503–12.
14. Sakai S, Miyauchi T, Kobayashi M, et al. Inhibition of myocardial endothelin pathway improves long-term survival in heart failure. Nature 1996; 384: 353–5.
15. Bers DM. Control of cardiac contraction by SR-Ca release and sarcolemmal-Ca fluxes. In: Bers DM, ed. Excitation–contraction coupling and cardiac contractile force. Developments in cardiovascular medicine. vol. 122 Dordrecht, Boston, London: Kluwer Academic Publishers, 1991: 149–70.
16. Pieske B, Maier LS, Weber T, Bers DM, Hasenfuss G. Alterations in sarcoplasmic reticulum Ca2+-content in myocardium from patients with heart failure. Circulation 1997; 96: 199.
17. Swynghedauw B. Developmental and functional adaptation of contractile proteins in cardiac and skeletal muscles. Physiol Rev 1986; 66: 710–71.
18. Hasenfuss G, Mulieri LA, Blanchard EM, et al. Energetics of isometric force development in control and volume-overload human myocardium. Comparison with animal species. Circ Res 1991; 68: 836–46.
19. Shirota K, Huang Y, Kawaguchi O, et al. Functional recovery of the native heart after cardiomyoplasty in sheep with heart failure: passive and dynamic effects of volume loading. Ann Thorac Surg 2002; 73: 849–54.
20. Toyoda Y, Okada M, Kashem MA, Mukai T. Effects of cardiomyoplasty on right ventricular filling during volume loading. Ann Thorac Surg 1998; 65: 1676–9.

21. Young AA, Orr R, Smaill BH, Dell'italia LJ. Three-dimensional changes in left and right ventricular geometry in chronic mitral regurgitation. Am J Physiol 1996; 271: H2689–700.

22. Bolotin G, Lorusso R, Kaulbach H, et al. Acute and chronic heart dilatation model-induced in goats by carotid jugular A-V shunt. Basic Appl Myol 1999; 117: 198–9.

23. Chekanov VS. A stable model of chronic bilateral ventricular insufficiency (dilated cardiomyopathy) induced by arteriovenous anastomosis and doxorubicin administration in sheep. J Thorac Cardiovasc Surg 1999; 117: 198–9.

24. Tessier D, Lajos P, Braunberger E, et al. Induction of chronic cardiac insufficiency by arteriovenous fistula and doxorubicin administration. J Card Surg 2003; 18: 307–11.

25. Dell'Italia LJ. The canine model of mitral regurgitation. Heart Fail 1995; 11: 208–18.

26. Nagatsu M, Zile MR, Tsutsui H, et al. Native beta-adrenergic support for left ventricular dysfunction in experimental mitral regurgitation normalizes indexes of pump and contractile function. Circulation 1994; 89: 818–26.

27. Tsutsui H, Spinale FG, Nagatsu M, et al. Effects of chronic beta-adrenergic blockade on the left ventricular and cardiocyte abnormalities of chronic canine mitral regurgitation. J Clin Invest 1994; 93: 2639–48.

28. Magid NM, Opio G, Wallerson DC, Young MS, Borer JS. Heart failure due to chronic experimental aortic regurgitation. Am J Physiol 1994; 267: H556–62.

29. Gilson N, el Houda Bouanani N, Corsin A, Crozatier B. Left ventricular function and beta-adrenoceptors in rabbit failing heart. Am J Physiol 1990; 258: H634–41.

30. Ezzaher A, Bouanani NEH, Su JB, Hittinger L, Crozatier B. Increased negative inotropic effect of calcium channel blockers in hypertrophied and failing rabbit hearts. J Pharmacol Exp Ther 1991; 257: 466–71.

31. Ezzaher A, Boudanani NEH, Crozatier B. Force-frequency relations and response to ryanodine in failing rabbit hearts. Am J Physiol 1992; 263: H1710–15.

32. Pogwizd SM, Qi M, Samarel AM, Bers DM. Upregulation of Na+/Ca2+-exchanger gene expression in an arrhythmogenic model of nonischemic cardiomyopathy in the rabbit. Circulation 1997; 96: 8.

33. McCullagh WH, Covell JW, Ross J Jr. Left ventricular dilatation and diastolic compliance changes during chronic volume overloading. Circulation 1972; 45: 943–51.

34. Chien SF, Diana JN, Brum JM, Bove AA. A simple technique for producing supravalvular aortic stenosis in animals. Cardiovasc Res 1988; 22: 739–45.

35. Lips DJ, Van der Nagel T, Steendijk P, et al. Left ventricular pressure-volume measurements in mice: comparison of closed-chest versus open-chest approach. Basic Res Cardiol 2004; 99: 351–9.

36. Zeisberg EM, Tarnavaski O, Zeisberg M, et al. Endothelial-to-mesenchymal transition contributes to cardiac fibrosis. Nat Med 2007; 13: 952–61.

37. Feldman AM, Weinberg EO, Ray PE, Lorell BH. Selective changes in cardiac gene expression during compensated hypertrophy and the transition to cardiac decompensation in rats with chronic aortic banding. Circ Res 1993; 73: 184–92.

38. Weinberg EO, Schoen FJ, George D, et al. Angiotensin-converting enzyme inhibition prolongs survival and modifies the transition to heart failure in rats with pressure overload hypertrophy due to ascending aortic stenosis. Circulation 1994; 90: 1410–22.

39. Schunkert H, Lorell BH. Role of angiotensin II in the transition of left ventricular hypertrophy to cardiac failure. Heart Fail 1994; 10: 142–9.

40. Extra Reference on p. 5. LOOK UP.

41. Li Z, Bing OH, Long X, Robinson KG, Lakatta EG. Increased cardiomyocyte apoptosis during the transition to heart failure in the spontaneously hypertensive rat. Am J Physiol 1997; 272: H2313–19.

42. Mitchell GF, Pfeffer JM, Pfeffer MA. The transition to failure in the spontaneously hypertensive rat. Am J Hypertens 1997; 10: 120S–6S.

43. Park S, McCune SA, Radin MJ, et al. Verapamil accelerates the transition to heart failure in obese, hypertensive, female SHHF/Mcc-fa(cp) rats. J Cardiovasc Pharmacol 1997; 29: 726–33.

44. Okamoto K, Aoki K. Development of a strain of spontaneously hypertensive rats. Jpn Circ J 1963; 27: 282–93.

45. Bing OH, Brooks WW, Conrad CH, et al. Intracellular calcium transients in myocardium from spontaneously hypertensive rats during the transition to heart failure. Circ Res 1991; 68: 1390–400.

46. Boluyt MO, O'Neill L, Meredith AL, et al. Alterations in cardiac gene expression during the transition from stable hypertrophy to heart failure. Marked upregulation of genes encoding extracellular matrix components. Circ Res 1994; 75: 23–32.

47. Li Z, Bing OH, Long X, Robinson KG, Lakatta EG. Increased cardiomyocyte apoptosis during the transition to heart failure in the spontaneously hypertensive rat. Am J Physiol 1997; 272: H2313–19.

48. Chua SC Jr, Chung WK, Wu-Peng XS. Phenotypes of mouse diabetes and rat fatty due to mutations in the OB (leptin) receptor. Science 1996; 271: 994–6.

49. Holycross BJ, Summers BM, Dunn RB, McCune SA. Plasma-renin activity in heart failure-prone SHHF/Mcc-facp rats. Am J Physiol 1997; 273: H228–33.

50. Siri FM, Krueger J, Nordin C, Ming Z, Aronson RS. Depressed intracellular calcium transients and contraction in myocytes from hypertrophied and failing guinea pig hearts. Am J Phys 1991; 261: H514–30.

51. Kiss E, Ball NA, Kranias EG, Walsh RA. Differential changes in cardiac phospholamban and sarcoplasmic reticulum Ca^{2+}-ATPase protein levels. Effects on Ca^{2+} transport and mechanics in compensated pressure-overload hypertrophy and congestive heart failure. Circ Res 1995; 77: 759–64.

52. Malhotra A, Siri FM, Aronson R. Cardiac contractile proteins in hypertrophied and failing guinea pig heart. Cardiovasc Res 1992; 26: 153–61.

53. Shinbane JS, Wood MA, Jensen DN, et al. Tachycardia-induced cardiomyopathy: a review of animal models and clinical studies. J Am Coll Cardiol 1997; 29: 709–15.

54. Moe GW, Stopps TP, Howard RJ, Armstrong PW. Early recovery from heart failure: insights into the pathogenesis of experimental chronic pacing-induced heart failure. J Lab Clin Med 1988; 112: 426–32.

55. Timek TA, Dagum P, Lai DT, et al. Tachycardia-induced cardiomyopathy in the ovine heart: mitral annular dynamic three-dimensional geometry. J Thorac Cardiovasc Surg 2003; 125: 315–24.

56. Kashem A, Hassan S, Crabbe DL, Melvin DB, Santamore WP. Left ventricular reshaping: effects on the pressure–volume relationship. J Thorac Cardiovasc Surg 2003; 125: 391–9.

57. Moe GW, Armstrong P. Pacing-induced heart failure: a model to study the mechanism of disease progression and novel therapy in heart failure. Cardiovasc Res 1999; 42: 591–9.

58. Shi Y, Ducharme A, Li D, et al. Remodeling of atrial dimensions and emptying function in canine models of atrial fibrillation. Cardiovasc Res 2001; 52: 217–25.

59. Eaton GM, Cody RJ, Nunziata E, Binkley PF. Early left ventricular dysfunction elicits activation of sympathetic drive and attenuation of parasympathetic tone in the paced canine model of congestive heart failure. Circulation 1995; 92: 555–61.

60. Travill CM, Williams TD, Pate P, et al. Haemodynamic and neurohumoral response in heart failure produced by rapid ventricular pacing. Cardiovasc Res 1992; 26: 783–90.

61. Redfield MM, Aarhus LL, Wright RS, Burnett JC Jr. Cardiorenal and neurohumoral function in a canine model of early left ventricular dysfunction. Circulation 1993; 87: 2016–22.

62. Luchner A, Stevens TL, Borgeson DD, et al. Angiotensin II in the evolution of experimental heart failure. Hypertension 1996; 28: 472–7.

63. Wang J, Seyedi N, Xu XB, Wolin MS, Hintze TH. Defective endothelium-mediated control of coronary circulation in conscious dogs after heart failure. Am J Physiol 1994; 266: H670–80.

64. Armstrong PW, Stopps TP, Ford SE, de Bold AJ. Rapid ventricular pacing in the dog: pathophysiologic studies of heart failure. Circulation 1986; 74: 1075–84.

65. Spinale FG, Holzgrefe HH, Mukherjee R, et al. Angiotensin-converting enzyme inhibition and the progression of congestive cardiomyopathy. Effects on left ventricular and myocyte structure and function. Circulation 1995; 92: 562–78.

66. Liu Y, Cigola E, Cheng W, et al. Myocyte nuclear mitotic division and programmed myocyte cell death characterize the cardiac myopathy induced by rapid ventricular pacing in dogs. Lab Invest 1995; 73: 771–87.

67. Ishikawa Y, Sorota S, Kiuchi K, et al. Downregulation of adenylylcyclase types V and VI mRNA levels in pacing-induced heart failure in dogs. J Clin Invest 1994; 93: 2224–9.

68. Ohno M, Cheng CP, Little WC. Altered left ventricular systolic and diastolic force–frequency relation in heat failure. Circulation 1994; 90: 112.

69. Cheng CP, Noda T, Nozawa T, Little WC. Effect of heart failure on the mechanism of exercise-induced augmentation of mitral valve flow. Circ Res 1993; 72: 795–806.

70. Ravens U, Davia K, Davies Ch, et al. Tachycardia-induced failure alters contracile properties of canine ventricular myocytes. Cardiovasc Res 1996; 32: 613–21.

71. Komamura K, Shannon RP, Ihara T, et al. Exhaustion of Frank–Starling mechanism in conscious dogs with heart failure. Am J Physiol 1993; 265: H1119–31.

72. Pak PH, Nuss HB, Kaab S, et al. Repolarization abnormalities, arrhythmia and sudden death in canine tachycardia induced cardiomyopathy. J Am Coll Cardiol 1997; 30: 576–84.

73. Whipple GH, Sheffield LT, Woodman EG, Theophilis C, Friedman S. Reversible congestive heart failure due to rapid stimulation of the normal heart. Proc New Eng Cardiovasc Soc 1961; 20: 39–40.

74. Wilson JR, Douglas P, Hickey WF, et al. Experimental congestive heart failure produced by rapid ventricular pacing in the dog: cardiac effects. Circulation 1987; 75: 857–67.

75. Ohno M, Cheng CP, Little WC. Mechanism of altered patterns of left ventricular filling during the development of congestive heart failure. Circulation 1994; 89: 2241–50.

76. Kiuchi K, Shannon RP, Sato N, et al. Factors involved in delaying the rise in peripheral resistance in developing heart failure. Am J Physiol 1994; 267: H211–16.

77. Armstrong PW, Gordon WM. The development of and recovery from pacing-induced heart failure. In: Spinale FG, ed. Pathophysiology of tachycardia-inuced heart failure. Armonk, NY: Futura Publishing Company, 1996: 45–59.

78. Perreault CL, Shannon RP, Komamura K, Vatner SF, Morgan JP. Abnormalities in intracellular calcium regulation and contractile function in myocardium from dogs with pacing-induced heart failure. J Clin Invest 1992; 89: 932–8.[ISI][Medline].

79. Zile MR, Mukherjee R, Clayton C, Kato S, Spinale FG. Effects of chronic supraventricular pacing tachycardia on relaxation rate in isolated cardiac muscle cells. Am J Physiol 1995; 268: H2104–13.

80. Williams RE, Kass DA, Kawagoe Y, et al. Endomyocardial gene expression during development of pacing tachycardia-induced heart failure in the dog. Circ Res 1994; 75: 615–23.

81. O'Rourke B, Ling FP, Tomaselli GF, Marban E. Excitation contraction coupling alterations in canine tachycardia-induced heart failure. Circulation 1997; 96: 238.

82. Cory CR, Shen H, O'Brien PJ. Compensatory asymmetry in down-regulation and inhibition of the myocardial Ca^{2+} cycle in congestive heart failure produced in dogs by idiopathic dilated cardiomyopathy and rapid ventricular pacing. J Mol Cell Cardiol 1994; 26: 173–84.

83. Vatner DE, Sato N, Kiuchi K, Shannon RP, Vatner SF. Decrease in myocardial ryanodine receptors and altered excitation–contraction coupling early in the development of heart failure. Circulation 1994; 90: 1423–30.

84. Wolff MR, Whitesell LF, Moss RL. Calcium sensitivity of isometric tension is increased in canine experimental heart failure. Circ Res 1995; 76: 781–9.

85. O'Leary EL, Colston JT, Freeman GL. Maintained length-dependent activation of skinned myocardial fibers in tachycardia heart failure. Circulation 1992; 86: 284.

86. Takagaki M, McCarthy PM, Tabata T, et al. Induction and maintenance of an experimental model of severe cardiomyopathy with a novel protocol of rapid ventricular pacing. J Thorac Cardiovasc Surg 2002; 123: 544–9.

87. Lazzara RR, Trumble DR, Magovern JA. Dynamic descending thoracic aortomyoplasty: comparison with intraaortic balloon pump in a model of heart failure. Ann Thorac Surg 1994; 58: 366–71.

88. Mott BD, Oh JH, Misawa Y, et al. Mechanisms of cardiomyoplasty: comparative effects of adynamic versus dynamic cardiomyoplasty. Ann Thorac Surg 1998; 65: 1039–44.

89. Oh JH, Badhwar V, Mott BD, Li CM, Chiu RCJ. The effects of prosthetic cardiac binding and adynamic cardiomyoplasty in a model of dilated cardiomyopathy. J Thorac Cardiovasc Surg 1998; 116: 148–53.

90. Capouya ER, Gerber RS, Drinkwater DC, et al. Girdling effect of nonstimulated cardiomyoplasty on left ventricular function. Ann Thorac Surg 1993; 56: 867–71.

91. Spinale FG, Fulbright BM, Mukherjee R, et al. Relation between ventricular and myocyte function with tachycardia-induced cardiomyopathy. Circ Res 1992; 71: 174–87.

92. Spinale FG, Hendrick DA, Crawford FA, et al. Chronic supraventricular tachycardia causes ventricular dysfunction and subendocardial injury in swine. Am J Phys 1990; 259: H218–29.

93. Spinale FG, Tomita M, Zellner JL, et al. Collagen remodeling and changes in LV function during development and recovery from supraventricular tachycardia. Am J Physiol 1991; 261: H308–18.

94. Spinale FG, Tempel GE, Mukherjee R, et al. Cellular and molecular alterations in the beta adrenergic system with cardiomyopathy induced by tachycardia. Cardiovasc Res 1994; 28: 1243–50.

95. Kajstura J, Zhang X, Reiss K, et al. Myocyte cellular hyperplasia and myocyte cellular hypertrophy contribute to chronic ventricular remodeling in coronary artery narrowing-induced cardiomyopathy in rats. Circ Res 1994; 74: 383–400.

96. Litwin SE, Katz SE, Morgan JP, Douglas PS. Serial echocardiographic assessment of left ventricular geometry and function after large myocardial infarction in the rat. Circulation 1994; 89: 345–54.

97. Pinto YM, de Smet BG, van Gilst WH, et al. Selective and time-related activation of the cardiac renin–angiotensin system after experimental heart failure: relation to ventricular function and morphology. Cardiovasc Res 1993; 27: 1933–8.

98. Liu YH, Yang XP, Nass O, et al. Chronic heart failure induced by coronary artery ligation in Lewis inbred rats. Am J Physiol 1997; 272: H722–7.

99. Moainie SL, Gorman JH 3rd, Guy TS, et al. An ovine model of postinfarction dilated cardiomyopathy. Ann Thorac Surg 2002; 74: 753–60.

100. Nishina T, Nishimura K, Yuasa S, et al. A rat model of ischemic cardiomyopathy for investigating left ventricular volume reduction surgery. J Card Surg 2002; 17: 155–62.

101. Llaneras MR, Nance ML, Streicher JT, et al. Large animal model of ischemic mitral regurgitation. Ann Thorac Surg 1994; 57: 432–9.
102. Markovitz LJ, Savage EB, Ratcliffe MB, et al. Large animal model of left ventricular aneurysm. Ann Thorac Surg 1989; 48: 838–45.
103. Chachques JC, Duarte F, Cattadori B, et al. Angiogenic growth factors and/or cellular therapy for myocardial regeneration: a comparative study. J Thorac Cardiovasc Surg 2004; 128: 245–53.
104. Horwitz LD, Fennessey PV, Shikes RH, Kong Y. Marked reduction in myocardial infarct size due to prolonged infusion of an antioxidant during reperfusion. Circulation 1994; 89: 1792–801.
105. Pfeffer MA, Braunwald E. Ventricular remodeling after myocardial infarction. Experimental observations and clinical implications. Circulation 1990; 81: 1161–72.
106. Blaustein AS, Hoit BD, Wexler LF, et al. Characteristics of chronic left ventricular dysfunction induced by coronary embolization in a canine model. Am J Cardiovasc Pathol 1995; 5: 32–48.
107. Huang Y, Kawaguchi O, Zeng B, et al. A stable ovine congestive heart failure model. A suitable substrate for left ventricular assist device assessment. ASAIO J 1997; 43: M408–13.
108. Sabbah HN, Stein PD, Kono T, et al. A canine model of chronic heart failure produced by multiple sequential coronary microembolizations. Am J Physiol 1991; 260: H1379–84.
109. Gengo PJ, Sabbah HN, Steffen RP, et al. Myocardial beta adrenoceptor and voltage-sensitive calcium channel changes in a canine model of chronic heart failure. J Mol Cell Cardiol 1992; 24: 1361–9.
110. Gupta RC, Shimoyama H, Tanimura M, et al. SR Ca^{2+}-ATPase activity and expression in ventricular myocardium of dogs with heart failure. Am J Physiol 1997; 273: H12–18.
111. Sabbah HN, Shimoyama H, Kono T, et al. Effects of long-term monotherapy with enalapril, metoprolol, and digoxin on the progression of left ventricular dysfunction and dilation in dogs with reduced ejection fraction. Circulation 1994; 89: 2852–9.
112. Saavedra WF, Tunin RS, Paolocci N, et al. Reverse remodeling and enhanced adrenergic reserve from passive external support in experimental dilated heart failure. J Am Coll Cardiol 2002; 39: 2069–76.
113. Chaudhry PA, Mishima T, Sharov VG, et al. Passive epicardial containment prevents ventricular remodeling in heart failure. Ann Thorac Surg 2000; 70: 1275–80.
114. Hartman JC, Warltier DC. A model of multivessel coronary artery disease using conscious, chronically instrumented dogs. J Pharmacol Methods 1990; 24: 297–310.
115. Harada K, Friedman M, Lopez JJ, et al. Vascular endothelial growth factor administration in chronic myocardial ischemia. Am J Physiol 1996; 270: H1791–802.
116. Chekanov V, Akhtar M, Tchekanov G, et al. Transplantation of autologous endothelial cells induces angiogenesis. Pacing Clin Electrophysiol 2003; 26: 496–9.
117. Firoozan S, Wei K, Linka A, et al. A canine model of chronic ischemic cardiomyopathy: characterization of regional flow-function relations. Am J Physiol 1999; 276: H446–55.
118. Hartman JC, Kampine JP, Schmeling WT, Warltier DC. Actions of isoflurane on myocardial perfusion in chronically instrumented dogs with poor, moderate, or well-developed coronary collaterals. J Cardiothorac Anesth 1990; 4: 715–25.
119. Li RK, Weisel RD, Mickle DA, et al. Autologous porcine heart cell transplantation improved heart function after a myocardial infarction. J Thorac Cardiovasc Surg 2000; 119: 62–8.
120. Monnet E, Orton EC, Salman M, Boon J. Idiopathic dilated cardiomyopathy in dogs: survival and prognostic indicators. J Vet Intern Med 1995; 9: 12–17.
121. Tidholm A, Haggstrom J, Hansson K. Effects of dilated cardiomyopathy on the renin-angiotensin-aldosterone system, atrial natriuretic peptide activity, and thyroid hormone concentrations in dogs. Am J Vet Res 2001; 62: 961–7.
122. Tidholm A, Svensson H, Sylven C. Survival and prognostic factors in 189 dogs with dilated cardiomyopathy. J Am Anim Hosp Assoc 1997; 33: 364–8.
123. Darke PG. Myocardial disease in small animals. Br Vet J 1985; 141: 342–8.
124. Hamlin RL, Benitz AM, Ericsson GF, Cifelli S, Daurio CP. Effects of enalapril on exercise tolerance and longevity in dogs with heart failure produced by iatrogenic mitral regurgitation. J Vet Intern Med 1996; 10: 85–7.
125. Monnet E, Orton EC. Dynamic cardiomyoplasty for dilated cardiomyopathy in dogs. Semin Vet Med Surg (Small Anim) 1994; 9: 240–6.
126. Borenstein N, Chetboul V, Rajnoch C, Bruneval P, Carpentier A. Successful cellular cardiomyoplasty in canine idiopathic dilated cardiomyopathy. Ann Thorac Surg 2002; 74: 298–9.
127. Ikeda Y, Ross J Jr. Models of dilated cardiomyopathy in the mouse and the hamster. Curr Opin Cardiol 2000; 15: 197–201.
128. Ryoke T, Gu Y, Mao L, et al. Progressive cardiac dysfunction and fibrosis in the cardiomyopathic hamster and effects of growth hormone and angiotensin-converting enzyme inhibition. Circulation 1999; 100: 1734–43.

129. Yoo KJ, Li RK, Weisel RD, et al. Heart cell transplantation improves heart function in dilated cardio-myopathic hamsters. Circulation 2000; 102: III204–9.

130. Lee V, Randhawa AK, Singal PK. Adriamycin-induced myocardial dysfunction in vitro is mediated by free radicals. Am J Physiol 1991; 261: H989–95.

131. Gille L, Nohl H. Analyses of the molecular mechanism of adriamycin-induced cardiotoxicity. Free Radic Biol Med 1997; 23: 775–82.

132. Bristow MR, Sageman W, Scott R, et al. Acute and chronic cardiovascular effects of doxorubicin in the dog: the cardiovascular pharmacology of drug-induced histamine release. J Cardiovasc Pharmacol 1980; 2: 487–515.

133. Monnet E, Orton EC. A canine model of heart failure by intracoronary adriamycin injection: hemo-dynamic and energetic results. J Card Fail 1999; 5: 255–64.

134. Cheng W, Justicz AG, Soberman MS, et al. Effects of dynamic cardiomyoplasty on indices of ven-tricular systolic and diastolic function in a canine model of chronic heart failure. J Thorac Cardiovasc Surg 1992; 103: 1207–13.

135. Toyoda Y, Okada M, Kashem MA. A canine model of dilated cardiomyopathy induced by repetitive intracoronary doxorubicin administration. J Thorac Cardiovasc Surg 1998; 115: 1367–73.

136. Christiansen S, Redmann K, Scheld HH, et al. Adriamycin-induced cardiomyopathy in the dog—an appropriate model for research on partial left ventriculectomy? J Heart Lung Transplant 2002; 21: 783–90.

137. Monnet E. Adynamic cardiomyoplasty: effect on cardiac efficiency and contractile reserve in dogs with adriamycin-induced cardiomyopathy. J Card Surg 2002; 17: 60–9.

138. Dell'italia LJ, Blackwell GG, Urthaler F, Pearce DJ, Pohost GM. A stable model of left ventricular dysfunction in an intact animal assessed with high fidelity pressure and cinemagnetic resonance imaging. Cardiovasc Res 1993; 27: 974–9.

139. Fischer EI, Chachques JC, Christen AI, Risk MR, Carpentier AF. Benefits of aortic and pulmonary counterpulsation using dynamic latissimus dorsi myoplasty. Ann Thorac Surg 1995; 60: 417–21.

140. Thomas GA, Hammond RL, Greer K, et al. Functional assessment of skeletal muscle ventricles after pumping for up to four years in circulation. Ann Thorac Surg 2000; 70: 1281–90.

141. Chachques JC, Grandjean PA, Cabrera Fischer EI, et al. Dynamic aortomyoplasty to assist left ven-tricular failure. Ann Thorac Surg 1990; 49: 225–30.

142. Millner RWJ, Burrows M, Pearson I, Pepper JR. Dynamic cardiomyoplasty in chronic left ventricular failure: an experimental failure model. Ann Thorac Surg 1993; 55. 493–501.

143. Cheng W, Avila RA, David BS, et al. Dynamic cardiomyoplasty: left ventricular diastolic compliance at different skeletal muscle tensions. Am Surg 1994; 60. 128–31.

144. Chen EP, Bittner HB, Tull F, et al. An adult canine model of chronic pulmonary hypertension for cardiopulmonary transplantation. J Heart Lung Transplant 1997; 16. 538–47.

145. Werchan PM, Summer WR, Gerdes AM, McDonough KH. Right ventricular performance after monocrotaline-induced pulmonary hypertension. Am J Physiol 1989; 256: H1328–36.

146. Wilson DW, Segall HJ, Pan LC, et al. Mechanisms and pathology of monocrotaline pulmonary toxic-ity. Crit Rev Toxicol 1992; 22: 307–25.

147. Agnoletti G, Cornacchiari A, Panzali AF, et al. Effect of congestive heart failure on rate of atrial natriuretic factor release in response to stretch and isoprenaline. Cardiovasc Res 1990; 24: 938–45.

148. Narayan P, McCune SA, Robitaille PM, Hohl CM, Altschuld RA. Mechanical alternans and the force–frequency relationship in failing rat hearts. J Mol Cell Cardiol 1995; 27: 523–30.

7

Ventricular remodeling and secondary valvular dysfunction in heart failure progression

Kibar Yared and Judy Hung

INTRODUCTION

Heart failure (HF) remains an important public health problem affecting an estimated 5 million people in the United States (1). The prevalence of heart failure is increasing and the number of people discharged each year from hospital with a diagnosis of heart failure is estimated at approximately 1 million (2). In 2008, it is estimated that direct and indirect costs of heart failure in the United States will total \$34.8 billion, representing 8% of the total anticipated budget for cardiovascular diseases (2,3).

As heart disease progresses to heart failure, the heart size increases, cardiac function deteriorates, and symptoms of HF become more evident. This clinical syndrome results from changes to the heart's cellular matrix and molecular components modified by mediators that drive homeostatic control. Ventricular remodeling encompasses many such changes and is defined by the International Forum on Cardiac Remodeling as "the genomic expression resulting in molecular, cellular, and interstitial changes and manifested clinically as changes in size, shape, and function of the heart resulting from cardiac load or injury (4)."

Ventricular remodeling describes structural changes in the left ventricle (LV) in response to chronic alteration in loading conditions. Remodeling can consequently be either physiologic or pathologic (4). Physiologic remodeling is a compensatory change in the dimensions and function of the heart, typically observed in athletes. Pathologic remodeling may occur after myocardial infarction (MI), with pressure overload (hypertension and aortic stenosis), in inflammatory myocardial disease (myocarditis), with idiopathic dilated cardiomyopathy, or with volume overload (valvular regurgitation). Growth and remodeling of the myocardium are the appropriate structural responses to pressure and volume overload that burdens the LV. The myocardial wall performs in response to pressure load in order to normalize wall stress and the ventricle dilates in response to volume load. These remodeling processes in the LV may initially be viewed as compensatory or adaptive and may be critical to support continuing LV function in these situations (5). Eventually, however, these compensatory remodeling changes exert long-term adverse effects on survival. On the other hand, in conditions such as MI and ischemia, and non-ischemic forms of myocarditis and cardiomyopathy, the observed structural changes may be largely maladaptive from the beginning. Accurate assessment of LV ejection fraction (LVEF) and LV volumes are important prognostic indexes of mortality and morbidity (Fig. 7.1).

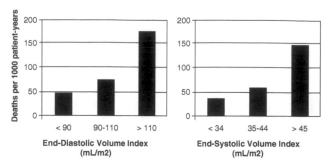

Figure 7.1 The relationship between left ventricular size as assessed by the left ventricular end-diastolic dimension and left ventricular end-systolic dimension following acute myocardial infarction and survival. *Abbreviations*: ml, milliliters; m2, meters squared.

PATHOGENESIS OF VENTRICULAR REMODELING

Remodeling is associated with a number of cellular changes, including myocyte hypertrophy, loss of myocytes due to apoptosis (6–8) or necrosis (9), and fibroblast proliferation (10), and fibrosis (11,12). Although the precise mechanisms of all the pathways and cells involved in LV remodeling remain incomplete, a scenario of the potential mechanisms at the molecular level has been suggested. Both volume and pressure load results in biomechanical stretching of cardiac myocytes. With stretching of myocytes, local production or release of angiotensin II, norepinephrine, and endothelin is augmented. Locally generated angiotensin II plays a role in these processes, in part, via alterations in gene expression (13–16). These neurohormonal changes stimulate myocyte hypertrophy, whereas increases in angiotensin II, aldosterone, and cytokines stimulate collagen synthesis, leading to fibrosis and remodeling of the extracellular matrix (4). Reduced nitric oxide bioactivity contributes to the cellular and interstitial growth because nitric oxide normally serves as an inhibitor of remodeling (17).

The process of ventricular remodeling elicited by MI results in a necrotic segment of myocardium and a surrounding border zone of impaired perfusion (18). After MI, a complex series of progressive adverse effects takes place (Fig. 7.2). First, noncontractile and potentially expanding scar tissue forms in the infarcted zone. Subsequently, this expansion induces a volume load upon the ventricle with an ensuing pressure load (19–21). Further remodeling may occur with additional ischemic insults. Generally, remodeling of the left ventricle, and the consequent fall in ejection fraction (22), is proportional to infarct size (23). The processes involved in postinfarct remodeling include lengthening of cardiomyocytes with resultant myocyte slippage and ventricular wall thinning (23–27). Infarct expansion then occurs (18,24,28,29), followed by an inflammatory response and reabsorption of necrotic tissue (24) leading to scar formation. There is evidence to support continued expansion of the infarct zone (29) may lead to LV deformation and dilation (23,24,29). Alternatively, other studies have shown that left ventricular enlargement is not the result of progressive infarct expansion, but rather is caused by an increase in the length of the remaining contractile tissue (21). Changes in the noninfarcted regions of the myocardium include compensatory myocyte hypertrophy (23,24,27,28), with subsequent excessive accumulation of collagen in the cardiac interstitium (30).

In summary, etiologies for why the ventricle remodels may vary but they share many common pathways in terms of mechanical, biologic, and molecular events. Although cardiac myocytes are thought to be the major target of these events, other components, such as

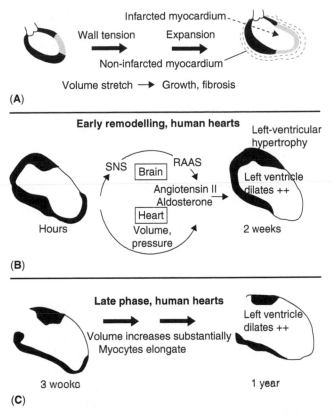

Figure 7.2 **(A)** Simplified overall pattern based on animal models. Schematic demonstrating the potential for substantial remodeling of the infarct zone and increased volume of the noninfarcted zone. Endocardial wall motion of two different human hearts in the early postinfarct phase **(B)** and late postinfarct phase **(C)** derived from contrast ventriculography. Black shading is the extent of preserved movement of endocardial surface in noninfarcted zone. *Abbreviations*: RAAS, renin–angiotensin–aldosterone system; SNS, sympathetic nervous system. *Source*: From Ref. 19.

fibroblasts, collagen, the interstitium, and coronary vasculature, also play an important role in cardiac remodeling. Neurohumoral activation, hemodynamic load, and other factors influence the process of remodeling.

NEUROHORMONAL ACTIVATION

Some have suggested that HF should be viewed as a neurohormonal model, in which HF progresses as a result of the overexpression of biologically active molecules that are capable of exerting deleterious effects on the heart and circulation (31). Compensatory mechanisms, such as activation of the adrenergic nervous system and renin–angiotensin–aldosterone system (RAAS), have so far been described. These are responsible for maintaining cardiac output through increased retention of salt and water, peripheral arterial vasoconstriction, increased myocardial contractility, and activation of inflammatory mediators that are responsible for cardiac repair and remodeling. The important concept that arises from this model is that the overexpression of biologically active molecules contributes to disease progression by virtue of the deleterious effects these molecules exert on the heart and circulation.

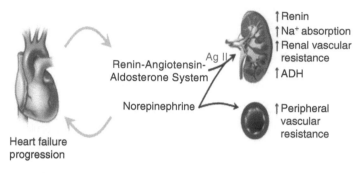

Figure 7.3 Heart failure leads to a release of neurohormonal factors (renin and ADH) and an increase in peripheral vascular resistance through its effects on the renin–angiotensin–aldosterone system and the levels of norepinephrine. These, in turn, act to worsen the progression of heart failure. *Abbreviations*: ADH, antidiuretic hormone; Ag II, angiotensin II.

Neurohormonal activation is an important cause of ventricular remodeling (32–37). Although initially adaptive, neurohormonal activation may be deleterious over long term, in part by contributing to pathologic remodeling (38). Neurohormones such as norepinephrine and angiotensin II are synthesized directly within the myocardium and thus act in both an autocrine and paracrine manner. With HF progression, gradual increases in the release of renin, norepinephrine, and antidiuretic hormone (ADH) occur that are proportional to the severity of the cardiac dysfunction (Fig. 7.3) (35,38). Plasma norepinephrine levels are elevated in HF patients (34,35) and higher levels of norepinephrine, as well as hyponatremia (due to ADH-induced water retention), correlate with a poorer long-term prognosis (33,35,39). Plasma brain natriuretic peptide (BNP) concentrations are also increased in HF patients and correlate with symptom severity and prognosis (40). In contrast to the deleterious effect of angiotensin II and norepinephrine, BNP release from cardiac myocytes in the failing heart may protect against pathologic remodeling (41).

Angiotensin II promotes cardiac remodeling by several mechanisms. The peptide is a potent vasoconstrictor and it also enhances salt and water retention, both of which result in increased pressure and volume load on the LV. These in turn stimulate the development of myocardial hypertrophy, both eccentric (in the case of volume overload) and concentric (pressure overload) in nature. Angiotensin II also causes cardiac myocyte loss due to its direct toxic effects and initiating programmed cell death or apoptosis (42). Studies in humans have shown that angiotensin-converting enzyme (ACE) inhibitors reduce mortality in heart failure by slowing and in some cases even reversing certain parameters of cardiac remodeling (43–45). Both systemic and locally generated angiotensin II seem to participate in this process, acting via alterations in gene expression (13–16). Angiotensin II appears to be an important mediator of the cellular responses to myocardial stretch, with local production by cardiac myocytes (46). In human myocardial tissue, ACE is markedly increased at the edge of the necrotic, scarred zone (47), whereas in an animal model there is increased expression of angiotensin 1 (AT_1) receptor mRNA in noninfarcted, viable areas of the myocardium (48). AT_1 receptors have been identified on cardiac myocytes and human fibroblasts cultured from cardiomyopathic and ischemic hearts (49). Acting through these AT_1 receptors, angiotensin II increases protein synthesis and induces hypertrophy in cardiac myocytes (15,46) and collagen synthesis by fibroblasts (46,50,51) an effect that can be reduced by ACE inhibition (52).

Harada et al. demonstrated that more marked LV enlargement and remodeling occurs in wild-type mice than in AT_{1A} receptor knockout mice following a large MI. In this study, all of the wild-type mice developed HF compared with none of the knockout mice, thus implicating the AT_1 receptor and its downstream actions in cardiac remodeling (48). Further support for this role comes from the observation that transgenic mice with overexpression of the AT_1 receptor limited to the cardiac myocyte develop cardiac hypertrophy and remodeling, even without a change in the systemic blood pressure (52). Animal models have shown that remodeling is minimized or, as in established disease, reversed by blocking the AT_1 receptor with angiotensin II receptor antagonists (53,54). Further evidence of the clinical importance of the role of angiotensin in cardiac remodeling has been demonstrated with the observation that the AT_1 receptor antagonist, valsartan, was equally effective to ACE inhibition with captopril, in preventing mortality and hospitalization for heart failure in patients with a MI complicated by LV dysfunction (55).

Angiotensin II stimulates the release of aldosterone, which may also participate in the remodeling process. Serum levels of aldosterone in heart failure patients are increased up to 20 times compared with normal subjects. During the acute phase of MI, a significant amount of plasma aldosterone is extracted by myocardial cells as blood passes through the coronary circulation and the extracted aldosterone plays an important role in modulating postinfarct LV remodeling (56). The role of aldosterone in the remodeling of the LV was further clarified in a transgenic rat model deficient in brain angiotensinogen and subject to acute coronary artery ligation to produce MI (57). Increases in right and left ventricular diameter, amount of interstitial fibrosis and cardiomyocyte diameter as well as perivascular fibrosis, laminin, and fibronectin (all markers of collagen deposition) were significantly inhibited compared with controls. As well, the concentration of aldosterone in the transgenic rats did not increase, as it did significantly in controls. Clearly, this relative secondary hyperaldosteronism state may contribute to the postinfarction remodeling via stimulation of collagen synthesis by myocardial fibroblasts, and resulting in myocardial hypertrophy and fibrosis (56,58,59). Treatment with agents that compete with the mineralocorticoid receptor (e.g., spironolactone, eplerenone) have demonstrated significantly attenuated myocardial interstitial fibrosis and suppressed transcriptional activity of nuclear factor kappa β and mRNA expression of remodeling-related genes coding for proteins, such as collagen types I and III (60,61).

Other factors that can also contribute to remodeling include endothelin, cytokines (e.g., TNF-α and certain types of interleukins) (62), oxidative stress, matrix metalloproteinases (MMPs), and peripheral monocytosis (63). Potent vasoconstrictor peptides, such as endothelin, are found in elevated concentrations in patients with HF. In an animal model of HF, long-term endothelin blockade was found to impair pathologic remodeling (64,65). Circulating concentrations of TNF-α are increased in patients with HF in proportion to the severity of the disease (36,66). Depression in LV function, cardiac myocyte shortening, and LV dilation, a phenotype observed in experimental and clinical models of heart failure was observed after infusion of pathophysiologically relevant concentrations of TNF-α (67). There is increasing literature on the potential importance of oxidative stress, defined as an imbalance between production of oxygen free radicals and antioxidant defenses, in progressive HF. MMPs contribute to tissue remodeling in a number of disease states (e.g., aortic aneurysm) and have also been implicated in cardiac remodeling (68,69). In animal models, remodeling can be attenuated by inhibition of MMP (70–72). Peripheral monocytosis, which occurs two to three days after an acute MI, reflects monocyte and macrophage infiltration of the necrotic myocardium. A higher peak monocyte level is associated with a larger left ventricular end-diastolic volume and lower LVEF, whereas a peak monocyte count 900/μL independently predicts HF, LV aneurysm formation, and cardiac events (63).

Myocytes themselves are thought to be fundamentally involved in the remodeling process. Altered loading conditions (e.g., increased preload) stretch cell membranes. Located on the cell membrane and responding to deformation of the cell membrane are stretch sensors, examples of which are (*i*) Integrins: a family of transmembrane proteins linking the cytoskeleton to the extracellular matrix; (*ii*) stretch-activated ion channels; (*iii*) Na$^+$/H$^+$ exchangers; and (*iv*) heterotrimeric G proteins (73–77). Although the exact mechanism remains incompletely understood, these stretch sensors, when activated, induce a number of signaling pathways involved in the remodeling process (74). There are three major signaling pathways, which are stretch mediated: (*i*) P13-K dependent signaling; (*ii*) JAK/STAT signaling; and (*iii*) calcium-mediated stretch-activated channels (74,78).

EXTRACELLULAR MATRIX DEGRADATION

The components of the myocardium involved in the remodeling process include the cardiac myocytes and the extracellular matrix (ECM), which provides the scaffolding to maintain normal myocyte architecture. The extracellular matrix is composed of basement membrane proteoglycans and fibrillar collagen, particularly subtypes I and III. Maintenance of myocyte shape, alignment, and architecture is critically dependent on the supporting extracellular matrix. Ross and Borg have demonstrated that the ECM plays an active role in the remodeling process; not only in providing structural support proteins but also as an important interface for cellular signaling. In particular, integrins appear to be critically important in the transduction of extracellular signals as well as being anchors for cellular adhesion in the ECM (79). In response to myocardial injury and decreased contractile function, a number of cellular, biomechanical and humoral factors (particularly cytokines such as TNF-α and interleukin-1) are activated, leading to modulation of MMP activation.

MMPs are an important family of enzymes active in remodeling in several disease states (80,81), and at least 20 different MMPs have been identified and include collagenases, gelatinases, and stromelysins and membrane-type metalloproteinases.

The release and activation of MMPs are mediated by biomechanical factors, as well as neurohormonal (82) and cytokine activation. They, in turn, cause extracellular matrix degradation, which results in the weakening of the myocyte and myofibril scaffolding network. Inevitably, this degradation of the support scaffolding leads to myocyte stretch, with lengthening and thinning of the myocyte and loss of the normal myocyte architecture, so-called myocyte "slippage" (83–87). These changes lead to ventricular thinning and infarct expansion, which may cause increased wall stress and, in turn, promote further remodeling.

FIBROSIS

The myocardium consists of myocytes tethered and supported by a connective tissue network composed largely of fibrillar collagen. Collagen is the major insoluble fibrous protein in the ECM and in connective tissue. A delicate balance of synthesis and degradation by interstitial fibroblasts and MMPs, respectively, is maintained and plays an important role in cardiac remodeling and in the pathogenesis of heart failure, the significance of which has been demonstrated in numerous studies.

In human and animal models of remodeling after MI, collagen synthesis is stimulated by fibroblasts and causes fibrosis of both the infarcted and noninfarcted regions of the ventricle (11,12,88,89). Myocardial collagenase (MMP-1) is usually present in its inactive form in the ventricle and is activated after myocardial injury (90). The activated form may contribute to an increase in chamber dimension and is a possible cause of myocyte slippage, a contributor to chamber remodeling (28). In an animal model of hypertension and HF, the transition from hypertrophy to HF correlated with an increased expression of MMPs (91). In a series of hypertensive patients with HF, those with systolic dysfunction had a lower collagen volume fraction and a higher expression of MMP-1 than those with diastolic dysfunction (92). In this same study, the increases in MMP-1 expression and consequent collagen degradation were directly correlated with end-diastolic volume and inversely correlated with LVEF. Additionally, MMP-9 (gelatinase B) is expressed in great amounts after MI and may be a mediator of collagen accumulation and remodeling. Mice with a targeted deletion of MMP-9 or those given an inhibitor to MMP have reduced collagen accumulation in the infarcted areas and less LV dilation than wild-type or control mice (72,93). Diminished left ventricular remodeling was also seen after MMP inhibition in an animal model of chronic volume overload (70).

BNP is another protein overexpressed in HF. Studies in BNP knockout mice have shown increased cardiac fibrosis in response to ventricular pressure overload, suggesting that the release of BNP from myocytes in the failing heart may provide some protection against pathologic remodeling (41).

ALTERATIONS IN MYOCYTE STRUCTURE AND FUNCTION

Hypertrophy of the surviving myocytes is not only an important adaptive response to loss of contractile function, but also leads to a change in the biologic phenotype of the myocyte. This change is secondary to reactivation of genes that are normally not expressed postnatally. The activation of these fetal genes, the so-called fetal gene program, is also accompanied by decreased expression of a number of genes that are normally expressed in the adult heart (94). Activation of the "fetal gene program" may contribute to the contractile dysfunction that develops in the failing myocyte. The processes that lead to myocyte hypertrophy are complex, involving several cellular signaling pathways. Both mechanical and neurohormonal factors play important roles in stimulating fetal genetic reactivation and subsequent myocyte hypertrophy. The stimuli for the genetic reprogramming of the myocyte include mechanical stretch of the myocyte, neurohormones (norepinephrine, angiotensin II), inflammatory cytokines (TNF, IL-6), other peptides and growth factors (endothelin), and reactive oxygen species (superoxide, nitric oxide). These stimuli occur both locally within the myocardium, where they exert autocrine/paracrine effects, and systemically where they exert endocrine effects. In addition to the signaling pathways mediated by endothelin-1 and MAP kinases, the gp130 and calcineurin mediated signaling pathways also appear to play important regulatory roles in myocyte hypertrophy (83,86,95,96) (Fig. 7.4). As hypertrophy continues, there is an increase in the number of mitochondria in localized areas of the cell with demonstrable additional contractile elements. Cells subjected to longstanding hypertrophy show more obvious disruptions in cellular organization. The late stage of hypertrophy is characterized by a loss of contractile elements and severe disruption of the normal arrangement of sarcomeres (94).

The alterations in myocyte biology that accompany myocyte hypertrophy and eventually lead to the development of heart failure also include alterations in excitation–contraction coupling (97), sarcoplasmic reticulum protein structure and function (namely SERCA2A) (97), as well as a reduction in the mRNA expression of L-type calcium channels (97) and an increase in mRNA expression and activity of the Na$^+$/Ca$^+$ exchanger (98).

MYOCYTE NECROSIS AND APOPTOSIS

Hypertrophy of noninfarcted portions of the myocardium, seen early after infarction, serves as an adaptive mechanism initially resulting in compensated function. However, at some critical stage that is not yet well understood, these pro-hypertrophic signaling mechanisms may be downregulated or even exhausted, shifting the signaling balance from myocyte hypertrophy to necrosis and apoptosis. This loss of contractile function eventually leads to the development of clinical heart failure.

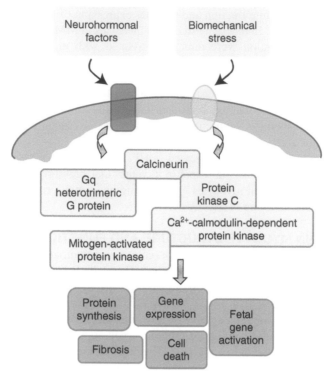

Figure 7.4 Extracellular signals triggering intracellular events in the cardiac myocyte. *Source*: Adapted from Ref. 195.

Myocyte necrosis and apoptosis have been increasingly recognized as playing an important role in the remodeling process (6,7,84,99). Necrotic myocyte death has been well described in ischemic heart disease. Neurohormonal activation, as seen in patients with heart failure, can also lead to necrotic cell death. For example, local (within myocardial tissue) as well as circulating concentrations of NE are sufficient to provoke myocyte necrosis in experimental model systems (94). Moreover, excessive stimulation with either angiotensin II or endothelin has been shown to provoke myocyte necrosis in experimental models. Myocyte necrosis was sevenfold greater than apoptosis in explanted hearts from male and female HF patients. Interestingly, necrotic cell death was twofold higher in men than in women (100).

Cardiac myocyte apoptosis has been shown to occur in failing human hearts (101). Indeed, many factors that have been implicated in the pathogenesis of HF, including catecholamines acting through β_1-adrenergic receptors, angiotensin II, reactive oxygen species, nitric oxide, inflammatory cytokines, and mechanical strain have been shown to trigger apoptosis in vitro. Moreover, activation of either the extrinsic (102) or intrinsic (103) cell death pathways provokes progressive LV dilation and decompensation in transgenic mice. Caspases, a family of serine proteases, are the intracellular mediators of apoptosis and execute cellular death by cleavage of cellular proteins. Caspases are activated in the cardiac myocyte by two main signaling pathways: (*i*) activation of death receptors on the cell surface, and (*ii*) apoptotic mediators released by mitochondria (84,104–107). Interestingly, the rate of apoptosis is noted to be increased in noninfarcted myocardium, although it remains at a relatively low overall rate (84). In addition, the rate of apoptosis appears to correlate

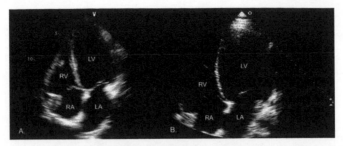

Figure 7.5 Demonstration of left ventricular sphericity by echocardiography. A normal ellipsoid left ventricle is shown in panel A. Panel B depicts a patients with multiple myocardial infarcts whose ventricle has lost its normal elliptical shape and has become more spherical. *Abbreviations*: LV, left ventricle; LA, left atrium; RV, right ventricle; RA, right atrium.

with degree of ventricular thinning and dilation and the development of heart failure (108), suggesting that apoptosis plays an important role in the remodeling process and its prevention may be an important therapeutic intervention.

REMODELING CHANGES ON A MACROSCOPIC LEVEL

Changes in the extracellular matrix and myocyte architecture, lead to changes at the macroscopic level, which involve ventricular dilatation, ventricular hypertrophy, and changes in ventricular shape, such as the development of a less elliptical and more spherical ventricle (Fig. 7.5), and LV scar and LV aneurysm formation. In postinfarct animal models and in humans, LV remodeling usually begins as early as within the first few hours postinfarct and progresses over time (24–26,109). The remote areas of well-perfused myocardium undergo a structural process of growth and remodeling that may be in part mediated by physical forces related to the nonfunctional segment of the cardiac chamber (110). As well, the structural changes may result from hormonal activation and gene reprogramming (111). Ultimately, these changes in LV geometry result in adverse ventricular mechanics and inefficiencies in ventricular contraction, further increasing myocardial oxygen demand and wall stress and resulting in contractile dysfunction and heart failure. With infarction, myocardial necrosis occurs, with eventual replacement of the necrotic region with scar (112), a process that is generally completed by six to eight weeks.

Continued expansion of infarcted tissue begins acutely after myocardial infarction. A more gradual remodeling process, however, also involves dilation of the noninfarcted regions (4,113), which while initially compensatory, ultimately becomes maladaptive, changing the normally ellipsoid shape of the LV to a larger, more spherical, and poorly contracting ventricle (26,114,115). A more spherical LV results in detrimental ventricular mechanics and is associated with an adverse prognosis (4,116–120). Changes in its mass and composition also accompany the changes in geometry of the LV; all of which may adversely affect contractile function (23,27,29,121). This remodeling process, while initially compensatory, ultimately becomes maladaptive (114,115). The change in the shape of the LV from an ellipse to a more spherical shape results in an increase in wall stress and myocardial oxygen demand, thereby placing further energy requirements on the failing heart. Shortly following MI, ventricular dilatation in the area of the noninfarcted myocardium occurs. Initially, this is considered an adaptive response aimed at maintaining an adequate cardiac output by utilizing the Frank–Starling mechanism (117). Ventricular dilation increases the end-diastolic dimension and allows the ventricle to maintain the same stroke volume despite loss of contractile function. At the same time, dilation of the ventricle results in increased wall stress according to Laplace's Law, which states that wall stress

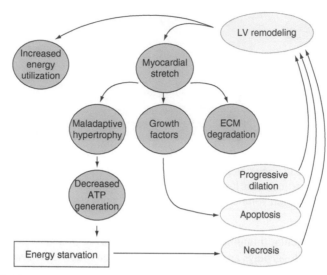

Figure 7.6 Self-amplifying nature of LV remodeling. LV remodeling results in increased afterload on the heart, which increases energy utilization and further stimulates cardiac growth through stretch-mediated activation of growth factors. The former contributes directly to a state of energy starvation, whereas the latter contributes to further cardiac remodeling including increased myocyte hypertrophy and further matrix remodeling. The sustained activation of growth stimuli also promotes apoptosis and myocardial fibrosis, which contribute to LV dysfunction and LV remodeling. *Abbreviations*: ATP, adenosine triphosphate; LV, left ventricular. *Source*: Adapted from Ref. 94.

is directly proportional to the pressure and radius of a sphere. Increased wall stress leads to an increase in myocardial oxygen demand, which reduces the efficiency of contraction. In response to ventricular dilation and increased wall stress, cardiac myocytes hypertrophy leading to an increase in wall thickness, and thereby reducing wall stress back toward normal. As ventricular dilation progresses, however, this adaptive mechanism is eventually overwhelmed resulting in wall thinning and, along with the increase in afterload created by LV dilation, leads to a functional "afterload mismatch" that may further cause decreased contractile function and heart failure (Fig. 7.6). Increased LV wall stress can also lead to sustained expression of stretch-activated genes (angiotensin II, endothelin, and tumor necrosis factor (TNF)) and/or stretch activation of hypertrophic signaling pathways. Moreover, the high end-diastolic wall stress might lead to episodic hypoperfusion of the subendocardium with consequent worsening of LV function and increased oxidative stress. The resultant free radical generation activated families of genes coding for inflammatory mediators, such as TNF and interleukin-1β (5).

In addition to global changes in ventricular shape, more segmental deformation, such as aneurysm formation also contributes to the decline in LV function. An LV aneurysm is defined as a focal area of thinned and scarred myocardium (Fig. 7.7). The development of LV aneurysm is a serious complication of MI and is associated with increased mortality. The incidence of LV aneurysm postmyocardial infarction is approximately 10–30% (120–122), although this seems to be decreasing in the era of more rapid and complete reperfusion with thrombolytics and primary coronary intervention (123). Pathologically, this area has no contractile elements and is composed entirely of scar tissue. The LV aneurysm, due to its noncontractile properties, leads to stagnation of blood within it and inefficient LV contraction. The development of an LV aneurysm is not only influenced by the

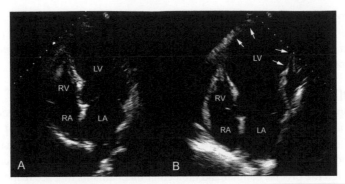

Figure 7.7   Echocardiographic image of a left ventricular aneurysm. These echocardiographic images show the development of an apical aneurysm in a patient following an anterior myocardial infarction. Panel (**A**) shows mild dilation of the left ventricular apex two weeks following myocardial infarction. Six weeks following infarction, there has been interval focal thinning and dilation of the apex (**B**), (arrows). *Abbreviations*: LV, left ventricle; LA, left atrium; RV, right ventricle; RA, right atrium.

molecular and cellular changes initiated by myocardial injury but also by hemodynamic variables such as heart rate and loading conditions of the ventricle (116). In addition to loss of contractile function and decrease in ventricular mechanics with the formation of an LV aneurysm, studies have demonstrated decreased function at the border zone of an LV aneurysm. This may occur because of an increase in wall stress at the border zone of the aneurysm, resulting in increased myocardial oxygen consumption, further reducing the efficiency of left ventricular function (118,119). In addition to reduction in mechanical function, LV aneurysms predispose to the formation of thrombus and can serve as foci for ventricular arrhythmias.

FUNCTIONAL CHANGES

The initial remodeling phase after an MI results in repair of the necrotic area and scar formation that may, to some extent, be considered beneficial because there is an improvement in or maintenance of LV function and cardiac output (13,124). However, once the threshold for afterload mismatch is reached, the ventricle starts to dilate and fail.

The time, course, and extent of remodeling are influenced by a variety of factors including the severity of the underlying disease, secondary events, such as recurrent ischemia, neuroendocrine activation, genotype, and treatment (24,32,113). In postinfarct animal models and humans, following MI the extent of remodeling changes is roughly related to infarct size (27,113). In a human study, left ventricular end-diastolic and end-systolic volumes increased progressively from hospital discharge to one year after an initial, moderately large anterior wall Q-wave infarction, but remained stable in patients with an initial small inferior wall infarction (113). In patients with progressive postinfarct left ventricular dilation, the end-systolic volume index increases progressively and LVEF declines due in part to the chamber enlargement itself and in part to loss of function in initially normally contracting myocardium (23,29). These changes are important predictors of all-cause mortality (125).

Diastolic dysfunction and changes in the passive elastic properties of the ventricular walls have been well documented in a rat postinfarct heart failure model. The pressure–volume relationship is displaced rightward with a profound increase in operating end-diastolic volume (1). Antecedent hypertension is found to be associated with adverse ventricular remodeling and increased the risk of developing HF requiring hospitalization within a time period of two years after a MI (126). This was demonstrated in a series of 1093 post-MI patients, where hypertensive patients were found to have significantly higher plasma levels of neurohormones and significantly greater increase in LV volumes (i.e., remodeling) at five months post-MI.

REVERSIBILITY OF LEFT VENTRICULAR REMODELING

Currently approved medical and device therapies for HF have favorable effects on cardiac remodeling, and studies have demonstrated a stabilization and/or reversal of LV chamber mass and LV chamber dilation. This process of myocardial recovery has been referred to as "reverse remodeling" and involves changes at the molecular, cellular, tissue, and organ levels. Although the precise cellular and molecular mechanisms that are responsible for the "normalization" of LV size and shape have not been fully elucidated, most studies have reported consistent results with respect to the parameters that return toward baseline following pharmacologic or device therapy (Table 7.1). Some studies in patients who have been treated with β-blockers showed that patients who had an improvement in ejection fraction also had an increase in SERC2A mRNA and α-myosin heavy chain mRNA and a decrease in β-myosin heavy chain mRNA, thus demonstrating that the improvement in ventricular function following treatment with β-blockers is associated with favorable changes in myocardial gene expression (127). Similar findings have been seen when evaluating myocardial recovery following therapy with ACE inhibitors and left ventricular assist devices (LVAD), suggesting that there may be specific gene programs that accompany myocardial recovery. In patients with dilated cardiomyopathy who were supported with an LVAD, treatment with an ACE inhibitor, an angiotensin receptor blocker, an aldosterone antagonist, and a β-blocker, followed by treatment with a β$_2$-agonist (clenbuterol), resulted in sufficient myocardial recovery to allow for explantation of the LVAD with a subsequent

Table 7.1 Cellular and Molecular Determinants of Myocardial Recovery

	ACE Inhibitor	β-Blocker	LVAD	CSD
Myocyte defects				
Hypertrophy	↓	↓	↓	↓
Myocytolysis	–	↓	↓	–
Excitation–contraction coupling	↑	↑	↑	↑
Fetal gene expression	↓	↓	↓	↓
Beta-adrenergic desensitization	↓	↓	↓	↓
Cytoskeletal proteins	–	–	↑	–
Myocyte contractility	–	↑	↑	↑
Myocardial defects				
Myocyte necrosis	↓	↓	↓	–
Myocyte apoptosis	↓	↓	↓	↓
MMP activation	↓	↓	↓	↓
Fibrosis	↓	↓	↓	↓
LV chamber size				
Dilation	Stabilized	↓	↓	↓

Abbreviations: ACE, angiotensin-converting enzyme; CSD, cardiac support device; LVAD, left ventricular assist device; MMP, matrix metalloproteinase; –, not done.
Source: From Ref. 94.

reported improvement in quality of life (128). Despite many encouraging studies, it is still not clear how the decrease in LV chamber mass and LV chamber dilation are coordinated during the process of myocardial recovery. Furthermore, clinical studies have so far shown that there are limits to the amount of myocardial recovery that can occur with currently available pharmacologic and device support.

ASSESSMENT OF LEFT VENTRICULAR REMODELING USING MULTIMODALITY IMAGING TECHNIQUES

Imaging techniques such as echocardiography, computed tomography (CT), and magnetic resonance imaging (MRI) have been applied to quantify the manifestations of LV remodeling, such as chamber volumes, mass, and function. For sequential monitoring of the remodeling process and the response to therapeutic strategies, the chosen imaging technique has to be highly accurate and reproducible.

Echocardiography is extremely useful in the assessment of global and regional cardiac dysfunction. Assessment of ventricular function is widely available and feasible in the vast majority of patients and the safety of ultrasound makes it ideal for serial assessment. Stress echocardiography with dobutamine has also been used to identify viable, yet chronically dysfunctional myocardium. Despite its widespread use, there are many limitations to the use of echocardiography in this setting. These range from interobserver variability, the necessity for an adequate acoustic window to accurate endocardial border definition.

The advancements in CT have allowed analysis of left ventricular size and function from the data set collected during noninvasive coronary angiography without additional radiation or contrast. Multidetector CT (MDCT) is able to accurately measure LVEF and LV volumes. The assessment of LV structure and function by CT compares favorably with MRI (129) and three-dimensional echocardiography (130), with low intraobserver variability. Rapidly improving temporal resolution, decreased radiation, widespread availability, and ease of use suggest that MDCT eventually may play a role in assessing ventricular remodeling, but further research and development are needed.

Published MRI studies have shown that serial and repeated quantification of LV dimensions and function can be achieved with high reproducibility and low interstudy variability, making MRI ideally suited for monitoring LV remodeling (131–134). Contrast-enhanced MRI with nonspecific extracellular agents, such as gadolinium-diethylenetriamine-pentaacetic acid (Gd-DTPA) have been applied to measure infarct size in acute (135,136) and chronic phases (137), to determine the transmural extent of MI (138), to determine residual viability (139), and to predict later LV remodeling (140). In a mouse model of reperfused MI, MRI has been shown to accurately and noninvasively determine infarct size, LV mass, and volumes as well as reveal that contractile dysfunction occurs not only in the infarcted and adjacent zones but also in areas remote from the infarcted zone (141).

SECONDARY VALVULAR DYSFUNCTION

The LV remodeling process eventually leads to LV dilation and secondary valvular dysfunction, primarily mitral regurgitation (MR). MR in this setting, in which the mitral leaflets are morphologically normal, is often referred to as functional or ischemic MR and is characterized by valve leaflets that coapt apically within the left ventricle restricting leaflet closure in a pattern known as incomplete mitral leaflet closure (Fig. 7.8) (142). Functional MR develops in up to 20% of patients following MI (143,144) and is present in up to 50% of patients with dilated cardiomyopathy (145–147). Functional MR is associated with an adverse prognosis; the development of MR following MI nearly doubling mortality (148,149). This relationship seems to be associated in a quantitative manner, as a greater

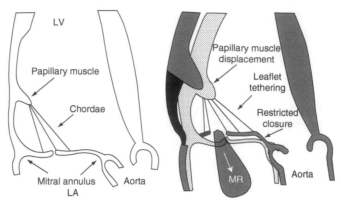

Figure 7.8 Schematic depicting the balance of forces applied to the mitral valve (left). Demonstration of the potential effect of a posterior and lateral shift of the posterolateral papillary muscle, combined with annular dilatation, restraining the mitral leaflets from meeting each other and causing mitral regurgitation (*right*). *Source*: Adapted from Ref. 152.

degree of MR correlates with higher mortality (148). It is important to emphasize that mitral valve function should be understood in terms of its relationship to its ventricular support structures and not as freestanding leaflets attached at the annulus. The mitral valve apparatus includes anterior and posterior mitral leaflets, the mitral annulus, papillary muscles, and associated chordae tendineae. The mitral leaflets are attached to the mitral annulus and tethered to the ventricle by the papillary muscles via the chordae tendineae. The posteromedial and anterolateral papillary muscles, located along the inferior and posterolateral surfaces of the left ventricle, respectively, give off chordae to each mitral leaflet. The papillary muscles and chordae tendineae serve to anchor the leaflets at the annular level during coaptation. The mechanism underlying functional MR relates to an altered mitral valve geometry resulting from the underlying LV remodeling process. Although a spectrum of morphologic abnormalities of the LV and papillary muscles exists, considerable evidence points to the central and predominant role of tethering as the final common pathway in inducing functional MR (150–154).

With infarction, the papillary muscles and surrounding left ventricle remodel, becoming thinned and dilated, and resulting in posterolateral displacement of the papillary muscles. Posterolateral displacement of the papillary muscles leads to stretching of the chordae tendineae and increased tethering forces on the mitral valve leaflets. In turn, an increase in mitral leaflet tethering leads to more apical leaflet coaptation and restricted leaflet closure, with resultant regurgitation (Fig. 7.8). Because of the posterolateral location of the papillary muscles, infarctions in this coronary territory have a greater incidence of associated MR compared with anterior infarctions (155). In patients who develop diffuse LV dysfunction, and global LV dilation, either from a nonischemic myopathic process or from multiple infarctions, similar papillary muscle displacement occurs. Dilation of the mitral annulus also plays a role in the development of functional MR (156). Annular dilation results in stretching of the mitral leaflets causing incomplete closure of the mitral leaflets.

MR can itself initiate and worsen LV remodeling. MR alters left ventricular loading (157) and increases wall stress, both of which can induce eccentric LV hypertrophy and dilation (158). This can result in further distortion of the mitral valve apparatus and worsening of the MR leading to a vicious cycle in which MR begets MR (159,160). In addition, MR induces neurohumoral and cytokine promoters of remodeling (161–163).

REMODELING OF THE RIGHT VENTRICLE AND ASSOCIATED VALVULAR DYSFUNCTION

Most of what is known about the remodeling process has been described or demonstrated in the left ventricle. Less is known about the right ventricular remodeling process, although there is evidence that right ventricular dilation and hypertrophy with decreased contractility occur following LV MI (164,165). Tricuspid regurgitation resulting from right ventricular remodeling is present in approximately 30% of patients with cardiomyopathy and is associated with an adverse prognosis (146,166).

THERAPEUTIC TARGETS

Ventricular remodeling is an important aspect of disease progression in heart failure, and hence it is emerging as an important therapeutic target. LV remodeling involves a number of molecular and cellular processes, which are initiated in response to myocardial injury. These processes provide a useful framework for targeting therapy to prevent or limit the deleterious effects of LV remodeling on myocardial function. ACE inhibitors, which antagonize the effects of angiotensin II, have well-known beneficial effects on LV remodeling and survival. They also restrict the breakdown of a novel peptide that lessens TGF-β expression (167). As well, atorvastatin inhibits TGF-β-mediated collagen production by cardiac fibroblasts (168). Data exist for the successful improvement of remodeling after therapy to block the RAAS (57,169,170). Spironolactone added to ACE-inhibitor therapy lessened remodeling, improved the ejection fraction, and reduced markers of myocardial fibrosis (171). New data showing that adrenergic activation promotes central activation of angiotensinogen, suggests an additional mode of action of β-blockade. Furthermore, β-blockade inhibits the activation of MMP-2 associated with increased circulating norepinephrine in human studies (172).

Endothelin-A antagonism has added little to existing methods of RAAS blockade, which already inhibit endothelin synthesis. Other measures of attenuating LV remodeling include stimulation of adaptive prosurvival pathways (Fig. 7.9) (173). Overexpression of IGF-I in mice restricts apoptotic and necrotic cell death in viable myocardium, decreasing left ventricular dilation and cardiac hypertrophy (174). Prosurvival signaling is probably achieved via the AKT pathway (175), which is stimulated by IGF-I, insulin, and statins and reduces experimental reperfusion-induced apoptosis (176). Novel therapeutic techniques have focused on targeting nitroso-oxidative stress (177,178) or alterations in myocyte energetics (179). Activation of physiologic growth by means of exercise, activation of PI3K–Akt signaling (180), or treatment with growth hormone may be beneficial in patients with heart failure (181). Some studies point to microRNAs (small, noncoding RNAs that form base pairs with specific mRNAs and inhibit translation or promote mRNA degradation) as both sufficient and necessary for stress-dependent cardiac growth (182).

Restoration of function in advanced heart failure can occur in response to various experimental mechanical interventions, such as a new left ventricular external pocket constraining device that improves left ventricular dimensions and peri-infarct collagen accumulation (183), biventricular pacing (184,185), and LVAD (186,187). Tissue sampling before and after implantation of such an assist device provides evidence to demonstrate myocardial recovery. Anatomically, there is regression of cell thickening and elongation (188). Improved myocyte contractile activity can be attributed to the recovery of function of the sarcoplasmic reticulum (187) and increased L-calcium-channel density (189)

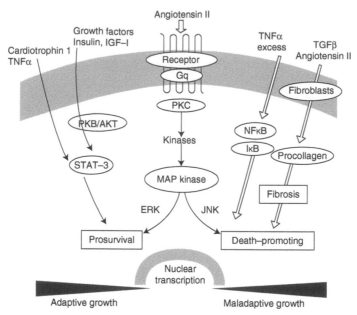

Figure 7.9 Consequences of physiological versus pathological signaling for mechanical function.

including reverse molecular remodeling of the genes controlling calcium cycling (190). Calcium content of the myocytes has been shown to increase (191), and MMPs are subsequently downregulated resulting in reduced collagen damage (192). β-adrenergic-receptor density and response to stimulation is increased (186), with reduced hyperphosphorylation of the sarcoplasmic reticulum (193), which is thought to promote calcium leakage from the sarcoplasmic reticulum. Similar reverse remodeling of the sarcoplasmic reticulum can result from β-blockade (194).

SUMMARY

Left ventricular remodeling is directly related to future deterioration in LV performance and a less favorable clinical course in patients with heart failure. The process of LV remodeling, while initially adaptive, has an important effect on the biology of the cardiac myocyte, on changes in the volume of myocyte and nonmyocyte components of the myocardium, and on the geometry and architecture of the LV chamber. The changes eventually result in deleterious effects on ventricular shape and function and secondarily on valvular function.

Numerous efforts have been aimed at identifying new therapeutic targets to prevent LV remodeling and halt the, sometimes inevitable, progression toward end-stage heart failure. Advances in pharmacology, myocardial biology, and stem cell research as well as in mechanical devices hold promise for future treatments.

REFERENCES

1. Smith WM. Epidemiology of congestive heart failure. Am J Cardiol 1985; 55: 3A–8A.
2. Rosamond W, Flegal K, Furie K, et al. Heart disease and stroke statistics–2008 update: a report from the American Heart Association Statistics Committee and Stroke Statistics Subcommittee. Circulation 2008; 117: e25–146.
3. Bristow M. New approaches to therapy for congestive heart failure. In: American Heart Association Twenty-First Science Writers Forum. Clearwater, FL: 1994.

4. Cohn JN, Ferrari R, Sharpe N. Cardiac remodeling–concepts and clinical implications: a consensus paper from an international forum on cardiac remodeling. Behalf of an International Forum on Cardiac Remodeling. J Am Coll Cardiol 2000; 35: 569–82.
5. Cohn JN, Anand IS. Overview: cardiac remodeling and its relationship to the development of heart failure, in cardiac remodeling: mechanisms and Treatment. Greenberg BH, ed. Informa Healthcare. 2005.
6. Sharov VG, Sabbah HN, Shimoyama H, et al. Evidence of cardiocyte apoptosis in myocardium of dogs with chronic heart failure. Am J Pathol 1996; 148: 141–9.
7. Teiger E, Than VD, Richard L, et al. Apoptosis in pressure overload-induced heart hypertrophy in the rat. J Clin Invest 1996; 97: 2891–7.
8. Olivetti G, Abbi R, Quaini F, et al. Apoptosis in the failing human heart. N Engl J Med 1997; 336: 1131–41.
9. Tan LB, Jalil JE, Pick R, et al. Cardiac myocyte necrosis induced by angiotensin II. Circ Res 1991; 69: 1185–95.
10. Villarreal FJ, Kim NN, Ungab GD, et al. Identification of functional angiotensin II receptors on rat cardiac fibroblasts. Circulation 1993; 88: 2849–61.
11. Anderson KR, Sutton MG, Lie JT. Histopathological types of cardiac fibrosis in myocardial disease. J Pathol 1979; 128: 79–85.
12. Weber KT, Pick R, Silver MA, et al. Fibrillar collagen and remodeling of dilated canine left ventricle. Circulation 1990; 82: 1387–401.
13. Ning XH, Zhang J, Liu J, et al. Signaling and expression for mitochondrial membrane proteins during left ventricular remodeling and contractile failure after myocardial infarction. J Am Coll Cardiol 2000; 36: 282–7.
14. Reiss K, et al. ANG II receptors, c-myc, and c-jun in myocytes after myocardial infarction and ventricular failure. Am J Physiol 1993; 264: H760–9.
15. Sadoshima J, Izumo S. Molecular characterization of angiotensin II–induced hypertrophy of cardiac myocytes and hyperplasia of cardiac fibroblasts. critical role of the AT1 receptor subtype. Circ Res 1993; 73: 413–23.
16. Everett AD, Tufro-McReddie A, Fisher A, et al. Angiotensin receptor regulates cardiac hypertrophy and transforming growth factor-beta 1 expression. Hypertension 1994; 23: 587–92.
17. Scherrer-Crosbie M, Ullrich R, Bloch KD, et al. Endothelial nitric oxide synthase limits left ventricular remodeling after myocardial infarction in mice. Circulation 2001; 104: 1286–91.
18. Hutchins GM, Bulkley BH. Infarct expansion versus extension: two different complications of acute myocardial infarction. Am J Cardiol 1978; 41: 1127–32.
19. Opie LH, Commerford PJ, Gersh BJ, et al. Controversies in ventricular remodelling. Lancet 2006; 367: 356–67.
20. Anversa P, et al. Left ventricular failure induced by myocardial infarction. I. Myocyte hypertrophy. Am J Physiol 1985; 248: H876–82.
21. Mitchell GF, Lamas GA, Vaughan DE, et al. Left ventricular remodeling in the year after first anterior myocardial infarction: a quantitative analysis of contractile segment lengths and ventricular shape. J Am Coll Cardiol 1992; 19: 1136–44.
22. Pfeffer JM, Pfeffer MA, Braunwald E. Influence of chronic captopril therapy on the infarcted left ventricle of the rat. Circ Res 1985; 57: 84–95.
23. McKay RG, Pfeffer MA, Pasternak RC, et al. Left ventricular remodeling after myocardial infarction: a corollary to infarct expansion. Circulation 1986; 74: 93–702.
24. Weisman HF, Bush DE, Mannisi JA, et al. Global cardiac remodeling after acute myocardial infarction: a study in the rat model. J Am Coll Cardiol 1985; 5: 1355–62.
25. Korup E, Dalsgaard D, Nyvad O, et al. Comparison of degrees of left ventricular dilation within three hours and up to six days after onset of first acute myocardial infarction. Am J Cardiol 1997; 80: 449–53.
26. Giannuzzi P, Temporelli PL, Bosimini E, et al. Heterogeneity of left ventricular remodeling after acute myocardial infarction: results of the Gruppo Italiano per lo Studio della Sopravvivenza nell'Infarto Miocardico-3 Echo Substudy. Am Heart J 2001; 141: 131–8.
27. Anversa P, Olivetti G, Capasso JM. Cellular basis of ventricular remodeling after myocardial infarction. Am J Cardiol 1991; 68: 7D–16D.
28. Olivetti G, Capasso JM, Sonnenblick EH, et al. Side-to-side slippage of myocytes participates in ventricular wall remodeling acutely after myocardial infarction in rats. Circ Res 1990; 67: 23–34.
29. Gaudron P, Eilles C, Kugler I, et al. Progressive left ventricular dysfunction and remodeling after myocardial infarction. Potential mechanisms and early predictors. Circulation 1993; 87: 755–63.
30. Weber KT, Brilla CG. Pathological hypertrophy and cardiac interstitium. Fibrosis and renin-angiotensin-aldosterone system. Circulation 1991; 83: 1849–65.

31. Mann DL, Bristow MR. Mechanisms and models in heart failure: the biomechanical model and beyond. Circulation 2005; 111: 2837–49.
32. Jugdutt BI. Effect of captopril and enalapril on left ventricular geometry, function and collagen during healing after anterior and inferior myocardial infarction in a dog model. J Am Coll Cardiol 1995; 25: 1718–25.
33. Cohn JN, Levine TB, Olivari MT, et al. Plasma norepinephrine as a guide to prognosis in patients with chronic congestive heart failure. N Engl J Med 1984; 311: 819–23.
34. Chidsey CA, Braunwald E, Morrow AG, et al. Myocardial Norepinephrine concentration in man. effects of reserpine and of congestive heart failure. N Engl J Med 1963; 269: 653–8.
35. Francis GS, Benedict C, Johnstone DE, et al. Comparison of neuroendocrine activation in patients with left ventricular dysfunction with and without congestive heart failure: a substudy of the studies of left ventricular dysfunction (SOLVD). Circulation 1990; 82: 1724–9.
36. Torre-Amione G, Kapadia S, Benedict C, et al. Proinflammatory cytokine levels in patients with depressed left ventricular ejection fraction: a report from the studies of left ventricular dysfunction (SOLVD). J Am Coll Cardiol 1996; 27: 1201–6.
37. Vaughan DE, Rouleau JL, Ridker PM, et al. Effects of ramipril on plasma fibrinolytic balance in patients with acute anterior myocardial infarction. Heart Study Investigators. Circulation 1997; 96: 442–7.
38. Packer M. The neurohormonal hypothesis: a theory to explain the mechanism of disease progression in heart failure. J Am Coll Cardiol 1992; 20: 248–54.
39. Vantrimpont P, Rouleau JL, Ciampi A, et al. Two-year time course and significance of neurohumoral activation in the survival and ventricular enlargement (SAVE) study. Eur Heart J 1998; 19: 1552–63.
40. Maeda K, Tsutamoto T, Wada A, et al. High levels of plasma brain natriuretic peptide and interleukin-6 after optimized treatment for heart failure are independent risk factors for morbidity and mortality in patients with congestive heart failure. J Am Coll Cardiol 2000; 36: 1587–93.
41. Tamura N, Ogawa Y, Chusho H, et al. Cardiac fibrosis in mice lacking brain natriuretic peptide. Proc Natl Acad Sci USA 2000; 97: 4239–44.
42. Gonzalez A, Lopez B, Ravassa S, et al. Stimulation of cardiac apoptosis in essential hypertension: potential role of angiotensin II. Hypertension 2002; 39: 75–80.
43. Konstam MA, Rousseau MF, Kronenberg MW, et al. Effects of the angiotensin converting enzyme inhibitor enalapril on the long-term progression of left ventricular dysfunction in patients with heart failure. SOLVD investigators. Circulation 1992; 86: 431–8.
44. Konstam MA, et al. Effects of the angiotensin converting enzyme inhibitor enalapril on the long-term progression of left ventricular dilatation in patients with asymptomatic systolic dysfunction. SOLVD (studies of left ventricular dysfunction) investigators. Circulation 1993; 88: 2277–83.
45. Greenberg B, Quinones MA, Koilpillai C, et al. Effects of long-term enalapril therapy on cardiac structure and function in patients with left ventricular dysfunction. Results of the SOLVD echocardiography substudy. Circulation 1995; 91: 2573–81.
46. Sadoshima J, Xu Y, Slayter HS, et al. Autocrine release of angiotensin II mediates stretch-induced hypertrophy of cardiac myocytes in vitro. Cell 1993; 75: 977–84.
47. Hokimoto S, Yasue H, Fujimoto K, et al. Expression of angiotensin-converting enzyme in remaining viable myocytes of human ventricles after myocardial infarction. Circulation 1996; 94: 1513–18.
48. Harada K, Sugaya T, Murakami K, et al. Angiotensin II type 1A receptor knockout mice display less left ventricular remodeling and improved survival after myocardial infarction. Circulation 1999; 100: 2093–9.
49. Hafizi S, Wharton J, Morgan K, et al. Expression of functional angiotensin-converting enzyme and AT1 receptors in cultured human cardiac fibroblasts. Circulation 1998; 98: 2553–9.
50. McEwan PE, Gray GA, Sherry L, et al. Differential effects of angiotensin II on cardiac cell proliferation and intramyocardial perivascular fibrosis in vivo. Circulation 1998; 98: 2765–73.
51. Kawano H, Do YS, Kawano Y, et al. Angiotensin II has multiple profibrotic effects in human cardiac fibroblasts. Circulation 2000; 101: 1130–7.
52. Paradis P, Dali-Youcef N, Paradis FW, et al. Overexpression of angiotensin II type I receptor in cardiomyocytes induces cardiac hypertrophy and remodeling. Proc Natl Acad Sci USA 2000; 97: 931–6.
53. van Kats JP, Duncker DJ, Haitsma DB, et al. Angiotensin-converting enzyme inhibition and angiotensin II type 1 receptor blockade prevent cardiac remodeling in pigs after myocardial infarction: role of tissue angiotensin II. Circulation 2000; 102: 1556–63.
54. Tamura T, Said S, Harris J, et al. Reverse remodeling of cardiac myocyte hypertrophy in hypertension and failure by targeting of the renin-angiotensin system. Circulation 2000; 102: 253–9.
55. Pfeffer MA, McMurray JJ, Velazquez EJ, et al. Valsartan, captopril, or both in myocardial infarction complicated by heart failure, left ventricular dysfunction, or both. N Engl J Med 2003; 349: 1893–906.

56. Hayashi M, Tsutamoto T, Wada A, et al. Relationship between transcardiac extraction of aldosterone and left ventricular remodeling in patients with first acute myocardial infarction: extracting aldosterone through the heart promotes ventricular remodeling after acute myocardial infarction. J Am Coll Cardiol 2001; 38: 1375–82.

57. Lal A, Veinot JP, Ganten D, et al. Prevention of cardiac remodeling after myocardial infarction in transgenic rats deficient in brain angiotensinogen. J Mol Cell Cardiol 2005; 39: 521–9.

58. Lijnen P, Petrov V. Induction of cardiac fibrosis by aldosterone. J Mol Cell Cardiol 2000; 32: 865–79.

59. Fullerton MJ, Funder JW. Aldosterone and cardiac fibrosis: in vitro studies. Cardiovasc Res 1994; 28: 1863–7.

60. Enomoto S, Yoshiyama M, Omura T, et al. Effects of eplerenone on transcriptional factors and mRNA expression related to cardiac remodelling after myocardial infarction. Heart 2005; 91: 1595–600.

61. Zannad F, Alla F, Dousset B, et al. Limitation of excessive extracellular matrix turnover may contribute to survival benefit of spironolactone therapy in patients with congestive heart failure: insights from the randomized aldactone evaluation study (RALES). rales investigators. Circulation 2000; 102: 2700–6.

62. Hwang MW, Matsumori A, Furukawa Y, et al. Neutralization of interleukin-1beta in the acute phase of myocardial infarction promotes the progression of left ventricular remodeling. J Am Coll Cardiol 2001; 38: 1546–53.

63. Maekawa Y, Anzai T, Yoshikawa T, et al. Prognostic significance of peripheral monocytosis after reperfused acute myocardial infarction: a possible role for left ventricular remodeling. J Am Coll Cardiol 2002; 39: 241–6.

64. Sakai S, Miyauchi T, Kobayashi M, et al. Inhibition of myocardial endothelin pathway improves long-term survival in heart failure. Nature 1996; 384: 353–5.

65. Mishima T, Tanimura M, Suzuki G, et al. Effects of long-term therapy with bosentan on the progression of left ventricular dysfunction and remodeling in dogs with heart failure. J Am Coll Cardiol 2000; 35: 222–9.

66. Levine B, Kalman J, Mayer L, et al. Elevated circulating levels of tumor necrosis factor in severe chronic heart failure. N Engl J Med 1990; 323: 236–41.

67. Bozkurt B, Kribbs SB, Clubb FJ, et al. Pathophysiologically relevant concentrations of tumor necrosis factor-alpha promote progressive left ventricular dysfunction and remodeling in rats. Circulation 1998; 97: 1382–91.

68. Miyamoto S, Nagaya N, Ikemoto M, et al. Elevation of matrix metalloproteinase-2 level in pericardial fluid is closely associated with left ventricular remodeling. Am J Cardiol 2002; 89: 102–5.

69. Fedak PW, Moravec CS, McCarthy PM, et al. Altered expression of disintegrin metalloproteinases and their inhibitor in human dilated cardiomyopathy. Circulation 2006; 113: 238–45.

70. Chancey AL, Brower GL, Peterson JT, et al. Effects of matrix metalloproteinase inhibition on ventricular remodeling due to volume overload. Circulation 2002; 105: 1983–8.

71. Peterson JT, et al. Matrix metalloproteinase inhibition attenuates left ventricular remodeling and dysfunction in a rat model of progressive heart failure. Circulation 2001; 103: 2303–9.

72. Rohde LE, Ducharme A, Arroyo LH, et al. Matrix metalloproteinase inhibition attenuates early left ventricular enlargement after experimental myocardial infarction in mice. Circulation 1999; 99: 3063–70.

73. Akhter SA, Luttrell LM, Rockman HA, et al. Targeting the receptor-Gq interface to inhibit in vivo pressure overload myocardial hypertrophy. Science 1998; 280: 574–7.

74. Force T, Michael A, Kilter H, et al. Stretch-activated pathways and left ventricular remodeling. J Card Fail 2002; 8: S351–8.

75. Gudi SR, et al. Equibiaxial strain and strain rate stimulate early activation of G proteins in cardiac fibroblasts. Am J Physiol 1998; 274: C1424–8.

76. Hu H, Sachs F. Stretch-activated ion channels in the heart. J Mol Cell Cardiol 1997; 29: 1511–23.

77. Ingber D. Integrins as mechanochemical transducers. Curr Opin Cell Biol 1991; 3: 841–8.

78. Dostal DE, Hunt RA, Kule CE, et al. Molecular mechanisms of angiotensin II in modulating cardiac function: intracardiac effects and signal transduction pathways. J Mol Cell Cardiol 1997; 29: 2893–902.

79. Ross RS, Borg TK. Integrins and the myocardium. Circ Res 2001; 88: 1112–19.

80. Mann DL, Spinale FG. Activation of matrix metalloproteinases in the failing human heart: breaking the tie that binds. Circulation 1998; 98: 1699–702.

81. Spinale FG, Coker ML, Thomas CV, et al. Time-dependent changes in matrix metalloproteinase activity and expression during the progression of congestive heart failure: relation to ventricular and myocyte function. Circ Res 1998; 82: 482–95.

82. Rude MK, Duhaney TA, Kuster GM, et al. Aldosterone stimulates matrix metalloproteinases and reactive oxygen species in adult rat ventricular cardiomyocytes. Hypertension 2005; 46: 555–61.

83. Dorn GW II, Mann DL. Signaling pathways involved in left ventricular remodeling: summation. J Card Fail 2002; 8: S387–8.

84. Mani K, Kitsis RN. Myocyte apoptosis: programming ventricular remodeling. J Am Coll Cardiol 2003; 41: 761–4.

85. Rubin SA, Fishbein MC, Swan HJ. Compensatory hypertrophy in the heart after myocardial infarction in the rat. J Am Coll Cardiol 1983; 1: 1435–41.

86. Sutton MG, Sharpe N. Left ventricular remodeling after myocardial infarction: pathophysiology and therapy. Circulation 2000; 101: 2981–8.

87. Weisman HF, Bush DE, Mannisi JA, et al. Cellular mechanisms of myocardial infarct expansion. Circulation 1988; 78: 186–201.

88. van Krimpen C, Smits JF, Cleutjens JP, et al. DNA synthesis in the non-infarcted cardiac interstitium after left coronary artery ligation in the rat: effects of captopril. J Mol Cell Cardiol 1991; 23: 1245–53.

89. Volders PG, Willems IE, Cleutjens JP, et al. Interstitial collagen is increased in the non-infarcted human myocardium after myocardial infarction. J Mol Cell Cardiol 1993; 25: 1317–23.

90. Cleutjens JP, Kandala JC, Guarda E, et al. Regulation of collagen degradation in the rat myocardium after infarction. J Mol Cell Cardiol 1995; 27: 1281–92.

91. Iwanaga Y, Aoyama T, Kihara Y, et al. Excessive activation of matrix metalloproteinases coincides with left ventricular remodeling during transition from hypertrophy to heart failure in hypertensive rats. J Am Coll Cardiol 2002; 39: 1384–91.

92. Lopez B, Gonzalez A, Querejeta R, et al. Alterations in the pattern of collagen deposition may contribute to the deterioration of systolic function in hypertensive patients with heart failure. J Am Coll Cardiol 2006; 48: 89–96.

93. Ducharme A, Frantz S, Aikawa M, et al. Targeted deletion of matrix metalloproteinase-9 attenuates left ventricular enlargement and collagen accumulation after experimental myocardial infarction. J Clin Invest 2000; 106: 55–62.

94. Mann DL. Pathophysiology of heart failure. In: Libby P, ed. Braunwald's Heart Disease: A Textbook of Cardiovascular Medicine, 8th edn. Saunders, 2007.

95. Bueno OF, Molkentin JD. Involvement of extracellular signal-regulated kinases 1/2 in cardiac hypertrophy and cell death. Circ Res 2002; 91: 776–81.

96. Wilkins BJ, Molkentin JD. Calcineurin and cardiac hypertrophy: where have we been? Where are we going? J Physiol 2002; 541: 1–8.

97. Houser SR, Margulies KB. Is depressed myocyte contractility centrally involved in heart failure? Circ Res 2003; 92: 350–8.

98. Margulies KB, Houser SR. Myocyte abnormalities in human heart failure. In: Mann DL, ed. Heart Failure: A Companion to Braunwald's Heart Disease. Philadelphia: Saunders, 2003: 41–56.

99. Palojoki E, Saraste A, Eriksson A, et al. Cardiomyocyte apoptosis and ventricular remodeling after myocardial infarction in rats. Am J Physiol Heart Circ Physiol 2001; 280:H2726–31.

100. Guerra S, Leri A, Wang X, et al. Myocyte death in the failing human heart is gender dependent. Circ Res 1999; 85: 856–66.

101. Garg S, Narula J, Chandrashekhar Y. Apoptosis and heart failure: clinical relevance and therapeutic target. J Mol Cell Cardiol 2005; 38: 73–9.

102. Wencker D, Chandra M, Nguyen K, et al. A mechanistic role for cardiac myocyte apoptosis in heart failure. J Clin Invest 2003; 111: 1497–504.

103. Yussman MG, Toyokawa T, Odley A, et al. Mitochondrial death protein Nix is induced in cardiac hypertrophy and triggers apoptotic cardiomyopathy. Nat Med 2002; 8: 725–30.

104. Ashkenazi A, Dixit VM. Death receptors: signaling and modulation. Science 1998; 281: 1305–8.

105. Bialik S, Geenen DL, Sasson IE, et al. Myocyte apoptosis during acute myocardial infarction in the mouse localizes to hypoxic regions but occurs independently of p53. J Clin Invest 1997; 100: 1363–72.

106. Green DR, Reed JC. Mitochondria and apoptosis. Science 1998; 281: 1309–12.

107. Jeremias I, Kupatt C, Martin-Villalba A, et al. Involvement of CD95/Apo1/Fas in cell death after myocardial ischemia. Circulation 2000; 102: 915–20.

108. Abbate A, Biondi-Zoccai GG, Bussani R, et al. Increased myocardial apoptosis in patients with unfavorable left ventricular remodeling and early symptomatic post-infarction heart failure. J Am Coll Cardiol 2003; 41: 753–60.

109. Hochman JS, Bulkley BH. Expansion of acute myocardial infarction: an experimental study. Circulation 1982; 65: 1446–50.

110. Weisman HF, Healy B. Myocardial infarct expansion, infarct extension, and reinfarction: pathophysiologic concepts. Prog Cardiovasc Dis 1987; 30: 73–110.

111. Swynghedauw B. Molecular mechanisms of myocardial remodeling. Physiol Rev 1999; 79: 215–62.

112. Reimer KA, Jennings RB. The changing anatomic reference base of evolving myocardial infarction. underestimation of myocardial collateral blood flow and overestimation of experimental anatomic infarct size due to tissue edema, hemorrhage and acute inflammation. Circulation 1979; 60: 866–76.

113. Rumberger JA, Behrenbeck T, Breen JR, et al. Nonparallel changes in global left ventricular chamber volume and muscle mass during the first year after transmural myocardial infarction in humans. J Am Coll Cardiol 1993; 21: 673–82.

114. Pfeffer MA. Left ventricular remodeling after acute myocardial infarction. Annu Rev Med 1995; 46: 455–66.

115. Picard MH, Wilkins GT, Ray PA, et al. Progressive changes in ventricular structure and function during the year after acute myocardial infarction. Am Heart J 1992; 124: 24–31.

116. Bartel T, Vanheiden H, Schaar J, et al. Biomechanical modeling of hemodynamic factors determining bulging of ventricular aneurysms. Ann Thorac Surg 2002; 74: 1581–7.

117. Frank O. On the dynamics of cardiac muscle. (Translated by C.B. Chapman and E. Wasserman). Am Heart J 1959; 58: 282–317.

118. Jackson BM, Gorman JH, Moainie SL, et al. Extension of borderzone myocardium in postinfarction dilated cardiomyopathy. J Am Coll Cardiol 2002; 40: 1160–7.

119. Moustakidis P, Maniar HS, Cupps BP, et al. Altered left ventricular geometry changes the border zone temporal distribution of stress in an experimental model of left ventricular aneurysm: a finite element model study. Circulation 2002; 106: I168–75.

120. Visser CA, Kan G, Meltzer RS, et al. Incidence, timing and prognostic value of left ventricular aneurysm formation after myocardial infarction: a prospective, serial echocardiographic study of 158 patients. Am J Cardiol 1986; 57: 729–32.

121. Arvan S, Badillo P. Contractile properties of the left ventricle with aneurysm. Am J Cardiol 1985; 55: 338–41.

122. Kirklin J, Barratt-Boyes B. Left ventricular aneurysm chapter 8. In: Cardiac Surgery. New York: Churchill Livingstone Inc, 1993: 383–401.

123. Tikiz H, et al. The effect of thrombolytic therapy on left ventricular aneurysm formation in acute myocardial infarction: relationship to successful reperfusion and vessel patency. Clin Cardiol 2001; 24: 656–62.

124. Cohen MV, Yang XM, Neumann T, et al. Favorable remodeling enhances recovery of regional myocardial function in the weeks after infarction in ischemically preconditioned hearts. Circulation 2000; 102: 579–83.

125. White HD, Norris RM, Brown MA, et al. Left ventricular end-systolic volume as the major determinant of survival after recovery from myocardial infarction. Circulation 1987; 76: 44–51.

126. Richards AM, Nicholls MG, Troughton RW, et al. Antecedent hypertension and heart failure after myocardial infarction. J Am Coll Cardiol 2002; 39: 1182–8.

127. Lowes BD, Gilbert EM, Abraham WT, et al. Myocardial gene expression in dilated cardiomyopathy treated with beta-blocking agents. N Engl J Med 2002; 346: 1357–65.

128. Birks EJ, Tansley PD, Hardy J, et al. Left ventricular assist device and drug therapy for the reversal of heart failure. N Engl J Med 2006; 355: 1873–84.

129. Dewey M, Muller M, Eddicks S, et al. Evaluation of global and regional left ventricular function with 16-slice computed tomography, biplane cineventriculography, and two-dimensional transthoracic echocardiography: comparison with magnetic resonance imaging. J Am Coll Cardiol 2006; 48: 2034–44.

130. Sugeng L, Mor-Avi V, Weinert L, et al. Quantitative assessment of left ventricular size and function: side-by-side comparison of real-time three-dimensional echocardiography and computed tomography with magnetic resonance reference. Circulation 2006; 114: 654–61.

131. Buser PT. MR studies of left ventricular remodeling. Magma 1998; 6: 150–1.

132. Kramer CM, Lima JA, Reichek N, et al. Regional differences in function within noninfarcted myocardium during left ventricular remodeling. Circulation 1993; 88: 1279–88.

133. Nahrendorf M, Wiesmann F, Hiller KH, et al. Serial cine-magnetic resonance imaging of left ventricular remodeling after myocardial infarction in rats. J Magn Reson Imaging 2001; 14: 547–55.

134. Semelka RC, Tomei E, Wagner S, et al. Interstudy reproducibility of dimensional and functional measurements between cine magnetic resonance studies in the morphologically abnormal left ventricle. Am Heart J 1990; 119: 1367–73.

135. de Roos A, Matheijssen NA, Doornbos J, et al. Myocardial infarct size after reperfusion therapy: assessment with Gd-DTPA-enhanced MR imaging. Radiology 1990; 176: 517–21.

136. Lima JA, Judd RM, Bazille A, et al. Regional heterogeneity of human myocardial infarcts demonstrated by contrast-enhanced MRI. Potential mechanisms. Circulation 1995; 92: 1117–25.

137. Kim RJ, Fieno DS, Parrish TB, et al. Relationship of MRI delayed contrast enhancement to irreversible injury, infarct age, and contractile function. Circulation 1999; 100: 1992–2002.
138. Choi KM, Kim RJ, Gubernikoff G, et al. Transmural extent of acute myocardial infarction predicts long-term improvement in contractile function. Circulation 2001; 104: 1101–7.
139. Kramer CM, Rogers WJ, Mankad S, et al. Contractile reserve and contrast uptake pattern by magnetic resonance imaging and functional recovery after reperfused myocardial infarction. J Am Coll Cardiol 2000; 36: 1835–40.
140. Watzinger N, et al. The potential of contrast-enhanced magnetic resonance imaging for predicting left ventricular remodeling. J Magn Reson Imaging 2002; 16: 633–40.
141. Yang Z, Berr SS, Gilson WD, et al. Simultaneous evaluation of infarct size and cardiac function in intact mice by contrast-enhanced cardiac magnetic resonance imaging reveals contractile dysfunction in noninfarcted regions early after myocardial infarction. Circulation 2004; 109: 1161–7.
142. Godley RW, Wann LS, Rogers EW, et al. Incomplete mitral leaflet closure in patients with papillary muscle dysfunction. Circulation 1981; 63: 565–71.
143. Barzilai B, Gessler C, Perez JE, et al. Significance of Doppler-detected mitral regurgitation in acute myocardial infarction. Am J Cardiol 1988; 61: 220–3.
144. Lehmann KG, Francis CK, Dodge HT. Mitral regurgitation in early myocardial infarction. incidence, clinical detection, and prognostic implications. TIMI Study Group. Ann Intern Med 1992; 117: 10–17.
145. Junker A, et al. The hemodynamic and prognostic significance of echo-Doppler-proven mitral regurgitation in patients with dilated cardiomyopathy. Cardiology 1993; 83: 14–20.
146. Koelling TM, Aaronson KD, Cody RJ, et al. Prognostic significance of mitral regurgitation and tricuspid regurgitation in patients with left ventricular systolic dysfunction. Am Heart J 2002; 144: 524–9.
147. Stevenson LW, Bellil D, Grover-McKay M, et al. Effects of afterload reduction (diuretics and vasodilators) on left ventricular volume and mitral regurgitation in severe congestive heart failure secondary to ischemic or idiopathic dilated cardiomyopathy. Am J Cardiol 1987; 60: 654–8.
148. Grigioni F, Enriquez-Sarano M, Zehr KJ, et al. Ischemic mitral regurgitation: long-term outcome and prognostic implications with quantitative Doppler assessment. Circulation 2001; 103: 1759–64.
149. Lamas GA, Mitchell GF, Flaker GC, et al. Clinical significance of mitral regurgitation after acute myocardial infarction. Survival and Ventricular Enlargement Investigators. Circulation 1997; 96: 827–33.
150. He S, Fontaine AA, Schwammenthal E, et al. Integrated mechanism for functional mitral regurgitation: leaflet restriction versus coapting force: in vitro studies. Circulation 1997; 96: 1826–34.
151. Otsuji Y, Handschumacher MD, Liel-Cohen N, et al. Mechanism of ischemic mitral regurgitation with segmental left ventricular dysfunction: three-dimensional echocardiographic studies in models of acute and chronic progressive regurgitation. J Am Coll Cardiol 2001; 37: 641–8.
152. Otsuji Y, Handschumacher MD, Schwammenthal E, et al. Insights from three-dimensional echocardiography into the mechanism of functional mitral regurgitation: direct in vivo demonstration of altered leaflet tethering geometry. Circulation 1997; 96: 1999–2008.
153. Rankin JS, et al. Ischemic mitral regurgitation. Circulation 1989; 79: I116–21.
154. Yiu SF, Enriquez-Sarano M, Tribouilloy C, et al. Determinants of the degree of functional mitral regurgitation in patients with systolic left ventricular dysfunction: a quantitative clinical study. Circulation 2000; 102: 1400–6.
155. Kumanohoso T, Otsuji Y, Yoshifuku S, et al. Mechanism of higher incidence of ischemic mitral regurgitation in patients with inferior myocardial infarction: quantitative analysis of left ventricular and mitral valve geometry in 103 patients with prior myocardial infarction. J Thorac Cardiovasc Surg 2003; 125: 135–43.
156. Boltwood CM, Tei C, Wong M, et al. Quantitative echocardiography of the mitral complex in dilated cardiomyopathy: the mechanism of functional mitral regurgitation. Circulation 1983; 68: 498–508.
157. Carabello BA. Mitral valve regurgitation. Curr Probl Cardiol 1998; 23: 202–41.
158. Spinale FG, Ishihra K, Zile M, et al. Structural basis for changes in left ventricular function and geometry because of chronic mitral regurgitation and after correction of volume overload. J Thorac Cardiovasc Surg 1993; 106: 1147–57.
159. Corin WJ, Monrad ES, Murakami T, et al. The relationship of afterload to ejection performance in chronic mitral regurgitation. Circulation 1987; 76: 59–67.
160. Zile MR, Gaasch WH, Levine HJ. Left ventricular stress-dimension-shortening relations before and after correction of chronic aortic and mitral regurgitation. Am J Cardiol 1985; 56: 99–105.
161. Dell'Italia LJ, et al. Increased ACE and chymase-like activity in cardiac tissue of dogs with chronic mitral regurgitation. Am J Physiol 1995; 269: H2065–73.
162. Kapadia SR, Yakoob K, Nader S, et al. Elevated circulating levels of serum tumor necrosis factor-alpha in patients with hemodynamically significant pressure and volume overload. J Am Coll Cardiol 2000; 36: 208–12.

163. Talwar S, Squire IB, Davies JE, et al. The effect of valvular regurgitation on plasma Cardiotrophin-1 in patients with normal left ventricular systolic function. Eur J Heart Fail 2000; 2: 387–91.

164. Hirose K, Shu NH, Reed JE, et al. Right ventricular dilatation and remodeling the first year after an initial transmural wall left ventricular myocardial infarction. Am J Cardiol 1993; 72: 1126–30.

165. Nahrendorf M, Hu K, Fraccarollo D, et al. Time course of right ventricular remodeling in rats with experimental myocardial infarction. Am J Physiol Heart Circ Physiol 2003; 284:H241–8.

166. Hung J, Koelling T, Semigran MJ, et al. Usefulness of echocardiographic determined tricuspid regurgitation in predicting event-free survival in severe heart failure secondary to idiopathic-dilated cardiomyopathy or to ischemic cardiomyopathy. Am J Cardiol 1998; 82: 1301–3, A10.

167. Borlaug BA, Melenovsky V, Marhin T, et al. Sildenafil inhibits beta-adrenergic-stimulated cardiac contractility in humans. Circulation 2005; 112: 2642–9.

168. Martin J, Denver R, Bailey M, et al. In vitro inhibitory effects of atorvastatin on cardiac fibroblasts: implications for ventricular remodelling. Clin Exp Pharmacol Physiol 2005; 32: 697–701.

169. Kuster GM, Kotlyar E, Rude MK, et al. Mineralocorticoid receptor inhibition ameliorates the transition to myocardial failure and decreases oxidative stress and inflammation in mice with chronic pressure overload. Circulation 2005; 111: 420–7.

170. Katada J, Meguro T, Saito H, et al. Persistent cardiac aldosterone synthesis in angiotensin II type 1A receptor-knockout mice after myocardial infarction. Circulation 2005; 111: 2157–64.

171. Hayashi M, Tsutamoto T, Wada A, et al. Immediate administration of mineralocorticoid receptor antagonist spironolactone prevents post-infarct left ventricular remodeling associated with suppression of a marker of myocardial collagen synthesis in patients with first anterior acute myocardial infarction. Circulation 2003; 107: 2559–65.

172. Banfi C, Cavalca V, Veglia F, et al. Neurohormonal activation is associated with increased levels of plasma matrix metalloproteinase-2 in human heart failure. Eur Heart J 2005; 26: 481–8.

173. Opie LH. Heart Physiology. Philadelphia: Lippincott Williams and Wilkins, 2004.

174. Li Q, Li B, Wang X, et al. Overexpression of insulin-like growth factor-1 in mice protects from myocyte death after infarction, attenuating ventricular dilation, wall stress, and cardiac hypertrophy. J Clin Invest 1997; 100: 1991–9.

175. Howes AL, Arthur JF, Zhang T, et al. Akt-mediated cardiomyocyte survival pathways are compromised by G alpha q-induced phosphoinositide 4,5-bisphosphate depletion. J Biol Chem 2003; 278: 40343–51.

176. Vinten-Johansen J, Yellon DM, Opie LH. Postconditioning: a simple, clinically applicable procedure to improve revascularization in acute myocardial infarction. Circulation 2005; 112: 2085–8.

177. Moens AL, Kass DA. Tetrahydrobiopterin and cardiovascular disease. Arterioscler Thromb Vasc Biol 2006; 26: 2439–44.

178. Takimoto E, Kass DA. Role of oxidative stress in cardiac hypertrophy and remodeling. Hypertension 2007; 49: 241–8.

179. Neubauer S. The failing heart: an engine out of fuel. N Engl J Med 2007; 356: 1140–51.

180. McMullen JR, Amirahmadi F, Woodcock EA, et al. Protective effects of exercise and phosphoinositide 3-kinase(p110alpha) signaling in dilated and hypertrophic cardiomyopathy. Proc Natl Acad Sci USA 2007; 104: 612–17.

181. Fazio S, Palmieri EA, Affuso F, et al. Effects of growth hormone on exercise capacity and cardiopulmonary performance in patients with chronic heart failure. J Clin Endocrinol Metab 2007; 92: 4218–23.

182. van Rooij E, Sutherland LB, Qi X, et al. Control of stress-dependent cardiac growth and gene expression by a microRNA. Science 2007; 316: 575–9.

183. Blom AS, Mukherjee R, Pilla JJ, et al. Cardiac support device modifies left ventricular geometry and myocardial structure after myocardial infarction. Circulation 2005; 112: 1274–83.

184. Yu CM, Fung WH, Lin H, et al. Predictors of left ventricular reverse remodeling after cardiac resynchronization therapy for heart failure secondary to idiopathic dilated or ischemic cardiomyopathy. Am J Cardiol 2003; 91: 684–8.

185. Yu CM, Lin H, Yang H, et al. Progression of systolic abnormalities in patients with "isolated" diastolic heart failure and diastolic dysfunction. Circulation 2002; 105: 1195–201.

186. Dipla K, Mattiello JA, Jeevanandam V, et al. Myocyte recovery after mechanical circulatory support in humans with end-stage heart failure. Circulation 1998; 97: 2316–22.

187. Terracciano CM, Hardy J, Birks EJ, et al. Clinical recovery from end-stage heart failure using left-ventricular assist device and pharmacological therapy correlates with increased sarcoplasmic reticulum calcium content but not with regression of cellular hypertrophy. Circulation 2004; 109: 2263–5.

188. Katz AM. Regression of left ventricular hypertrophy: new hope for dying hearts. Circulation 1998; 98: 623–4.

189. Chen X, Piacentino V, Furukawa S, et al. L-type Ca2+ channel density and regulation are altered in failing human ventricular myocytes and recover after support with mechanical assist devices. Circ Res 2002; 91: 517–24.
190. Heerdt PM, Holmes JW, Cai B, et al. Chronic unloading by left ventricular assist device reverses contractile dysfunction and alters gene expression in end-stage heart failure. Circulation 2000; 102: 2713–19.
191. Terracciano CM, Harding SE, Adamson D, et al. Changes in sarcolemmal Ca entry and sarcoplasmic reticulum Ca content in ventricular myocytes from patients with end-stage heart failure following myocardial recovery after combined pharmacological and ventricular assist device therapy. Eur Heart J 2003; 24: 1329–39.
192. Li YY, Feng Y, McTiernan CF, et al. Downregulation of matrix metalloproteinases and reduction in collagen damage in the failing human heart after support with left ventricular assist devices. Circulation 2001; 104: 1147–52.
193. Klotz S, Barbone A, Reiken S, et al. Left ventricular assist device support normalizes left and right ventricular beta-adrenergic pathway properties. J Am Coll Cardiol 2005; 45: 668–76.
194. Reiken S, Wehrens XH, Vest JA, et al. Beta-blockers restore calcium release channel function and improve cardiac muscle performance in human heart failure. Circulation 2003; 107: 2459–66.
195. Hill JA, Olson EN. Cardiac Plasticity. N Engl J Med 2008; 358: 1370–80.

8

Neurohormonal and cytokine activation in heart failure

Dennis M. McNamara

Dropsy is usually produced when the patient remains for a long time with impurities of the body...the flesh is consumed and becomes water...the abdomen fills..., the legs and feet swell, the shoulders, clavicles, chest and thighs melt away.

—*Affections XXII*, Hippocrates. (410–470, BC)

INTRODUCTION

Whether ischemic, viral, or inflammatory in etiology, the clinical syndrome of heart failure begins with myocardial injury. The hemodynamic consequences of the initial injury elicit a complex humoral response involving the central nervous system, the kidney, and the vascular endothelium. Progression to the syndrome of heart failure is determined by the degree of myocardial injury and the nature and magnitude of the resultant humoral activation. Pharmacologic interventions targeted to improve cardiac contractility have not improved clinical outcomes (2,3). In contrast, all therapies that improve heart failure survival inhibit aspects of the systemic response (4–6).

The systemic response has two major components: the sympathetic nervous system and the renin–angiotensin–aldosterone pathway (7), collectively referred to as neurohormonal activation (8). Circulating mediators such as natriuretic peptides, vascular regulators such as endothelin and nitric oxide (NO) (9) also play a significant role in the circulatory adaptations to the heart failure state. Myocardial injury and the heart failure syndrome stimulate the production of cytokines, circulating peptide mediators of inflammation such as tumor necrosis factor (TNF) and interleukin-6 (IL-6) (10). These cytokines help regulate the balance between programmed cell death (apoptosis) and myocardial recovery (11,12). Neurohormonal and cytokine activation are systemic reflexes designed for acute injury, which have maladaptive consequences in chronic disease states. Understanding their impact on myocardial dysfunction and vascular adaptation is critical to deciphering the systemic nature of the syndrome and essential for the optimal application of clinical therapeutics. While neurohormonal inhibition consistently improves survival in populations with heart failure (13), optimization of therapeutic blockade for the individual patient is complex (14). The variability among patients in heart failure progression likely reflects genetic differences in the neurohormonal response, and the delineation of the genomic basis for this heterogeneity would allow tailoring of therapy for individual patients.

RENIN–ANGIOTENSIN–ALDOSTERONE SYSTEM

The renin–angiotensin–aldosterone system (RAAS) is a compensatory pathway primarily designed for preservation of renal blood flow (15,16). A decrease in renal perfusion pressure results in the secretion of renin by juxtaglomerular cells lining the afferent renal arterioles. This release is also under the control of the autonomic nervous system through beta$_1$-adrenergic receptors in the kidney. Renin, an aspartyl protease, cleaves a propeptide produced by the liver, angiotensinogen, to form the decapeptide angiotensin-1. The angiotensin-converting enzyme (ACE), a dipeptidyl carboxypeptidase bound to the plasma membrane of endothelial cells, cleaves the two C-terminal amino acids to form the vasoactive octapeptide angiotensin-2, the primary effector of the system (Fig. 8.1). Receptors for angiotensin-2 are divided into subtypes, AT-1 and AT-2, based on antagonist binding affinity (17). AT-1 is the predominant subtype in the vascular endothelium, and the primary target for pharmacologic blockade (18). Binding of angiotensin-2 to AT-1 receptors results in increased release of intracellular calcium from the sarcoplasmic reticulum through activation of protein kinase C. Binding of angiotensin-2 in the vasculature results in vasoconstriction, an increase in systemic vascular resistance and restoration of blood pressure.

While during acute declines in renal perfusion, such as from blood loss or dehydration, this compensatory pathway has salutary effects on renal perfusion, in chronic heart failure the increase in systemic vascular resistance increases myocardial work, decreases cardiac output, and results in compensatory left ventricular (LV) hypertrophy (7,19). In addition, angiotensin-2 has direct effects on the myocardium that increases remodeling of the extracellular matrix (20), induces myocyte hypertrophy, and initiates apoptosis and interstitial fibrosis (21–24). This worsens myocardial relaxation and contributes to diastolic

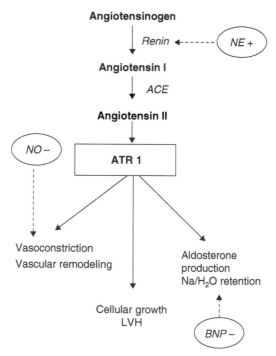

Figure 8.1   Renin–angiotensin pathway. Physiologic effects of angiotensin II and interactions with other neurohormones. *Abbreviations*: ACE, angiotensin-converting enzyme; NE, norepinephri1ne; NO, nitric oxide; ATR1, angiotensin receptor type 1; BNP, brain natriuretic peptide.

dysfunction (25). The impact of angiotensin-2 on the myocardium and the peripheral vasculature decreases cardiac output and renal blood flow, and thus leads to further increases in renin–angiotensin activation and a progressive decline in cardiac function.

The potential benefit of renin–angiotensin inhibition was first demonstrated in postinfarction animal models, in which ACE inhibitors decreased LV remodeling after myocardial infarction. These preclinical models provided the rationale for landmark clinical investigations, which demonstrated that the ACE inhibitor captopril limited LV remodeling (26,27) and improved clinical outcomes in patients after significant myocardial infarction. The improvement of heart failure survival with ACE inhibitors has been consistently demonstrated in clinical trials (4,28) supporting the central role renin–angiotensin activation plays in progression of heart failure. However, the impact of ACE inhibitors in heart failure reflects more than simple reductions in circulating angiotensin-2, as the therapeutic effects persist, whereas the decline in angiotensin-2 is transient (29,30) and incomplete, even at high doses (31).

In addition to the effects on the vasculature and the myocardium, angiotensin-2 increases plasma volume by initiating production of the mineralocorticoid aldosterone by the adrenal cortex (32). Aldosterone acts on the distal tubules of the renal nephron and activates a sodium potassium exchange pump. This results in the retention of sodium and water at the expense of increased kaluresis. As with the other compensatory action of RAAS, with acute volume loss the elevations in aldosterone result in a restoration of plasma volume, however, in chronic heart failure this increase exacerbates fluid overload and peripheral edema. In addition aldosterone, similar to angiotensin-2 (33), has a direct effect on vascular and ventricular remodeling, and chronic excess leads to an increase in fibrosis in the atria, ventricles, kidneys, and the perivasculature. Both angiotensin-2 and aldosterone contribute to adverse ventricular remodeling and progressive heart failure (34). The addition of aldosterone receptor antagonists to a background of ACE inhibitor therapy improves survival in patients with severe chronic heart failure (35) and in subjects with LV dysfunction post-myocardial infarction (36). In contrast, attempts to improve survival with the addition of angiotensin receptor blockers to ACE inhibitors have not been successful (37).

Through control of vascular tone and plasma volume, the two primary effectors of the RAAS play a central role in regulating blood pressure. A homologue of the angiotensin-converting enzyme, *ACE2*, has been cloned and mapped to a position on the X chromosome (38,39). It has significant cardiac expression (40), primarily in the endocardium and cleaves the C terminal amino acid from the vasoconstrictive octapeptide angiotensin-2 to form a seven-amino acid peptide with vasodilatory properties. Overexpression in transgenic models produces a hypotensive phenotype, and decreased expression has been demonstrated in hypertensive rat models. While it is clear that *ACE2* plays a counter regulatory role to *ACE* in terms of blood pressure control, the role of this second ACE enzyme in the inhibition and modulation of neurohormonal activation in heart failure remains uncertain.

SYMPATHETIC ACTIVATION

Increased sympathetic nerve activity plays a central role in the physiologic maladaptations of chronic heart failure (41). The decline in cardiac output and stroke volume is sensed by vascular baroreceptors and results in an increase in sympathetic nerve activity and release of norepinephrine. Sympathetic activation, the "fight or flight response" of the autonomic nervous system, improves cardiac output through increased heart rate, myocardial contractility, and stroke volume. In the peripheral vasculature, sympathetic activation increases systemic resistance and blood pressure. Stimulation of beta$_1$-adrenergic receptors in the kidney increases renin release and angiotensin-2 production, further increasing vascular resistance and afterload.

The direct augmentation of myocardial contractility by sympathetic activation is primarily mediated through beta-adrenergic receptors (42). The predominant receptor subtypes in the myocardium are beta$_1$ and beta$_2$. Agonist binding of both subtypes results in increased cyclic adenosine monophosphate (cAMP) and the activation of several cAMP-dependent protein kinases and phosphorylation of intracellular proteins (43). Beta$_1$-receptors are the predominant subtype in the nonfailing heart, comprising roughly 80% of the beta-adrenergic receptors (44). However, chronic sympathetic stimulation results in significantly more downregulation of beta$_1$-receptors than beta$_2$ and therefore in the failing heart the relative percentage of beta$_2$-receptors increases to approximately 40%. Although beta$_2$-receptors are less downregulated, they are inactivated by repetitive agonist stimulation and as a result become less responsive to adrenergic agonists in heart failure.

In addition to the effects on cardiac beta-receptors, chronic adrenergic stimulation has significant deleterious effects on cardiac function. The increase in cardiac contractility and heart rate increases myocardial metabolic demands, worsen ischemia, and has proarrhythmic effects. In addition, catecholamine stimulation of myocardial cells has direct cytotoxic effects and results in cell damage and cell death (45,46). Therefore, although norepinephrine acutely increases myocardial contractility, chronic stimulation of beta-adrenergic receptors worsens cardiac function and results in progression of the clinical syndrome of LV dysfunction, worsening pulmonary edema, and death.

In clinical heart failure, increasing severity of functional limitations and NYHA class is associated with increasing levels of plasma norepinephrine. Higher levels of circulating norepinephrine are associated with poorer survival in subjects with heart failure (47). The importance of sympathetic activation in the progression of LV dysfunction is best evidenced by clinical studies of beta-adrenergic blockade, which consistently demonstrate an improvement of left ventricular ejection fraction (LVEF) of 6–10 EF units after several months of therapy (48). This degree of improvement in LVEF far exceeds that achieved with any other pharmacologic therapeutics.

INTERACTION OF RENIN–ANGIOTENSIN AND SYMPATHETIC ACTIVATION

The complex interaction of renin–angiotensin and sympathetic activation in the pathophysiology of congestive heart failure suggests they act as two aspects of a single common pathway. The release of renin is regulated by the sympathetic nervous system through beta$_1$-receptors in the kidney and therapy with beta-adrenergic receptor antagonists reduces plasma renin and circulating angiotensin-2. The effect of beta-blockers on plasma renin is central to their antihypertensive mechanism, and their therapeutic impact in heart failure may also reflect their actions as "renin inhibitors" (49). In a similar fashion, treatment with ACE inhibitors reduces circulating plasma norepinephrine, and leads to increases in the myocardium cardiac beta-receptor density (50). Studies of pharmacologic perturbation of both the renin–angiotensin pathway and sympathetic activation demonstrate that it is impossible to inhibit either system without having significant impact on the other, and suggest they represent interdependent aspects of a single compensatory pathway of neurohormonal activation.

While treatment with ACE inhibitors and beta-blockers improves heart failure survival, determining the optimal degree of neurohormonal inhibition remains complex. The addition of angiotensin receptor antagonists to ACE inhibitors does not improve heart failure survival (37). In the ATLAS trial, high-dose ACE inhibition failed to improve survival when compared with low-dose therapy (51). In ValHeFT investigation of the angiotensin receptor blocker valsartan, subjects on a combination of beta-blockers, ACE inhibitors, and angiotensin receptor blockers (ARBs) appeared to have poorer outcomes than those on less therapy suggesting excessive neurohormonal inhibition may actually harm heart failure survival.

GENETIC DIVERSITY: PHARMACOGENETICS INTERACTIONS

Much of the clinical heterogeneity in response to heart failure therapy reflects genetic differences in the degree of neurohormonal activation. The common deletion/insertion polymorphism of the ACE has been extensively studied (52). The ACE D-allele, named for a 287 base pair deletion in intron-16, is associated with higher levels of ACE activity and circulating angiotensin-2 compared with the ACE-I (or insertion) polymorphism (53,54). Prospective studies have demonstrated that subjects homozygous for the D-allele have the poorest heart failure survival (55,56). This genetic risk can be modified by drug therapy, and the impact of the deletion allele is eliminated by treatment with beta-blockers (Fig. 8.2) (57,58). This ability of beta-blockers to eliminate the impact of the ACE D-allele reflects their roles as renin inhibitors (59) and is mediated by $beta_1$-adrenergic receptors (60). The genetic tendency toward poorer survival with the ACE D-allele and higher ACE activity also be diminished by treatment with high-dose ACE inhibitors (Fig. 8.3) (58). Genotyping at the ACE locus has significant utility in "tailoring" therapy and will allow clinicians to determine which subjects benefit from maximal neurohormonal inhibition.

Genomic heterogeneity of beta-adrenergic receptors also appears to affect heart failure outcomes and influences the response to beta-blockade. Three polymorphisms exist for the $beta_2$-receptor, two in the extracellular portion at codons 16 and 27, and one in the

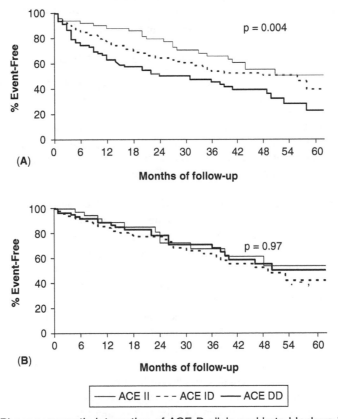

Figure 8.2 Pharmacogenetic interaction of ACE D-allele and beta-blockers in a cohort in subjects from the GRACE study. **(A)** Transplant-free survival by ACE genotype for subjects with systolic heart failure not treated with beta-blockers (*n* = 277). ACE D-allele associated with poor outcome (*P* = 0.004). **(B)** Transplant-free survival by ACE genotype for subjects treated with beta-blocker (*n* = 202) demonstrates the impact of the ACE D-allele is no longer evident (*P* = 0.97). *Abbreviation*: ACE, angiotensin-converting enzyme. *Source*: From Ref. 58.

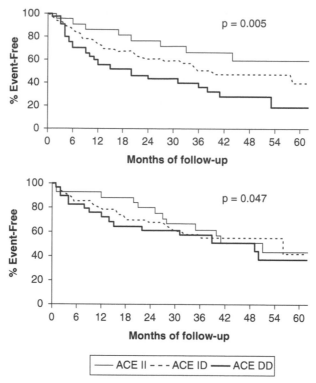

Figure 8.3 Pharmacogenetic interaction of ACE D-allele and ACE inhibitor dose in a cohort in *GRACE*. **(A)** Transplant-free survival by ACE genotype for subjects with systolic heart failure on low-dose ACE inhibitors and no beta-blockers (*n* = 130). ACE D-allele associated with markedly poor outcome (*P* = 0.005). **(B)** Transplant-free survival by ACE genotype for subjects treated with high-dose ACE inhibitors and no beta-blockers (*n* = 117) demonstrates the impact of the ACE D-allele is diminished (*P* = 0.47). Abbreviation: ACE, angiotensin-converting enzyme. *Source*: From Ref. 58.

transmembrane core at position 164 (Fig. 8.4B) (61). An isoleucine residue at codon 164 (Ile164) results in a receptor less responsive to agonist stimulation (62), and this less active Ile164 variant is associated with significantly poor outcomes in subjects with heart failure (63,64). The Ile164 variant is found in less than 5% of the population and pharmacogenetic interactions appear to be more powerful for the more common beta$_1$-receptor polymorphisms (Fig. 8.4A), particularly for the Arg389Gly polymorphism on the intracellular portion of the receptor. The Arg389 variant is more responsive to agonist stimulation, and in the NHLBI sponsored Beta-blocker Evaluation and Survival Trial (BEST) (65) therapy was most effective in the 50% of heart failure subjects homozygous for Arg389 receptor (66).

Ultimately genetic predictions of heart failure outcomes will have to incorporate many genetic variants which influence neurohormonal variation. An alpha-adrenergic receptor variant (67) impairs reuptake of catecholamines at the presynaptic level (68) and magnifies the impact of the beta$_1$-adrenergic receptor Arg389 variant. Co-inheritance of Arg389 and the alpha2C deletion increases the risk of heart failure in African Americans (69) and may target a subset of patients who receive the greatest benefit from beta-blockade (70). A promoter polymorphism of aldosterone synthase (-344C allele) (71) enhances the production of aldosterone (72), increases the risk of hypertension (73) and worsens heart failure outcomes (74). The frequency of many of these variants differs between white and black cohorts with heart failure, and may help explain the genomic basis for the racial differences in the impact of heart failure therapeutics (75).

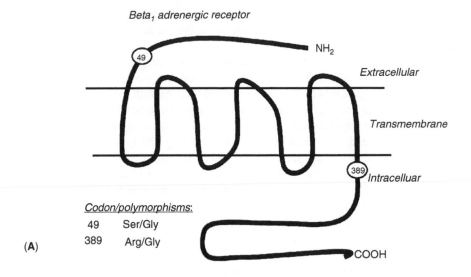

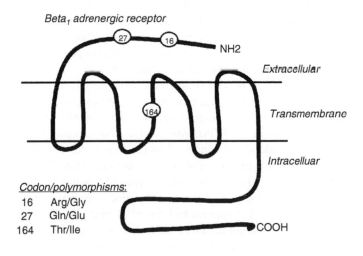

Figure 8.4 **(A)** Structure of the beta$_1$-adrenergic receptor: common polymorphisms. Arg389 variant more responsive to agonist stimulation and is predictive of enhanced benefit from beta-blockade. **(B)** Structure of the beta$_2$-adrenergic receptor: common polymorphisms. *Abbreviations*: Arg, arginine; Gly, glycine; Gln, glutamine; Glu, glutamate; Ser, serine; Thr, threonine; Ile, isoleucine; NH$_2$, amino terminus; COOH, carboxyl terminus. Ile164 variant in the transmembrane region (3–5% of the general population) causes a loss of function and is associated with poor survival in chronic heart failure. *Source*: From Ref. (61).

CYTOKINE ACTIVATION

Cardiac inflammation plays a significant role in the initiation of myocardial injury, ventricular remodeling, and the progression of LV dysfunction (76). Cytokines, circulating peptides initially isolated from cells of the immune system, are important mediators of systemic inflammation. Tumor necrosis factor-α (TNFα) is a 17-kDa polypeptide that activates endothelial cells, recruits inflammatory cells, and enhances the production of other proinflammatory cytokines. Initially called "cachectin" (77), it promotes weight loss and

muscle wasting in end-stage malignancy. The similar wasting phenotype in end-stage cardiac cachexia led to the investigation of TNFα in severe chronic heart failure where it was
found to be markedly elevated (78).

The cytokine hypothesis proposes that heart failure progression is an inflammatory
process and that elaboration of proinflammatory cytokines worsens LV dysfunction and
facilitates the development of the clinical syndrome (10). As with the neurohormonal mediators norepinephrine and angiotensin, clinical trial data demonstrate that increasing levels
of circulating TNFα correlate with increasing levels of functional limitations in heart failure (79). Early in the disease process, much of circulating TNFα is derived from immune
cell lines such as activated macrophages. However, late in disease progression the heart
itself becomes a secretory organ and much of the TNFα is produced by the cardiac myocytes themselves (Fig. 8.5A) (80). An examination of myocardial TNF expression in
recent-onset cardiomyopathy and in end-stage disease suggests a strong correlation of
myocardial TNF levels with levels in the peripheral circulation (Fig. 8.5B) (80). TNF
appears to be particularly important in the transition from compensated to decompensated
heart failure.

The effects of TNFα on myocardial function have been evaluated extensively in animal models. Transgenic mice with cardiac-specific overexpression of TNFα developed an
inflammatory myocarditis early on which later progresses to myocyte hypertrophy, LV
dilatation, and progressive LV dysfunction (81). In the transgenic model, TNFα activates
expression of matrix metalloproteinases (82), which contribute to LV remodeling and dilatation. Exogenously administered TNFα in animal models produces significant declines in
myocardial contractility, increasing pulmonary edema (83), and progressive LV enlargement accompanied by degradation of the extracellular matrix (84).

The negative inotropic effects of TNFα are mediated through the expression of
inducible nitric oxide synthase (NOS_2) and the production of NO (85,86). Chronic adrenergic stimulation induces myocardial TNFα expression (87), which in turn attenuates beta-
adrenergic responsiveness. Blockade of TNFα with soluble TNF receptor limits cardiac
inflammation (88) in animal models, and hence led to the hypothesis that inhibition of
TNFα activation would improve LV function and clinical outcomes (89). However, while
initial small clinical studies suggested soluble receptor improved function in chronic heart
failure (90,91), two larger randomized multicenter studies failed to prove benefit (92).

In models of myocarditis, TNFα appears to limit viral injury as TNFα knockout
mice have less cardiac inflammation but also less viral clearing and more myocyte cell
death (93). Myocardial expression of TNFα is elevated in human myocarditis, and in
clinical investigations of recent-onset cardiomyopathy, higher levels of circulating TNFα
at presentation predicted a higher probability of subsequent recovery of LV function
(94). These studies suggest a cardioprotective role for TNFα in early heart failure pathogenesis that appears quite distinct from the deleterious impact evident in end-stage disease (95).

IL-6 is also significantly elevated in heart failure, particularly in end-stage disease
(96). Initially thought to be a proinflammatory signal, such as TNFα, some evidence suggests more of an immune modulatory role (97). IL-6 knockout mice stimulated with lipo-
polysaccharide produce more TNFα than wild time litter mates, suggesting IL-6 limits
TNFα production. Murine transgenic models with chronic IL-6 overexpression are at a
greater risk for viral injury (98). In contrast, animals treated with short-term exogenous
IL-6 appear protected from viral injury. In addition to potential immune modulatory interactions with TNFα, IL-6 has direct effects on the myocardium and decreases contractility,
induces myocyte hypertrophy, activates matrix metalloproteinases, and contributes to LV
remodeling (99).

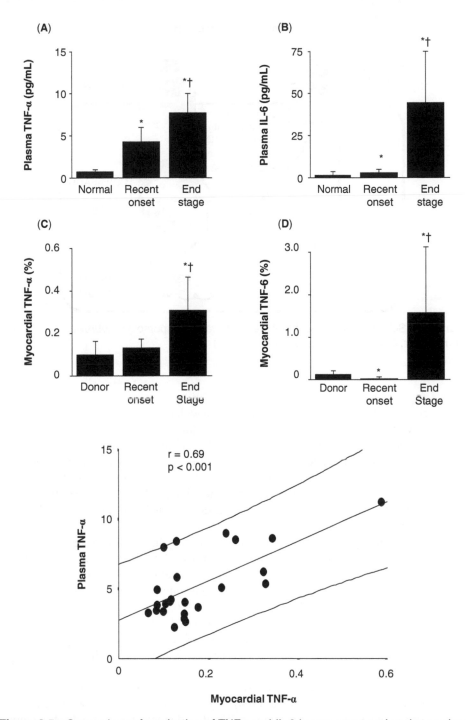

Figure 8.5 Comparison of production of TNFα and IL-6 in new-onset and end-stage heart failure. **(A)** Plasma and myocardial TNFα (A,C) and IL-6 (B,D) levels in recent-onset cardio-myopathy and end-stage patients [plasma levels: protein (pg/mL), myocardial levels: mRNA expressed as percent of GAPDH mRNA level]. *Significantly different ($P < 0.05$) from normal or donor group. †Significantly different ($P < 0.05$) from recent-onset group. **(B)** Correlation of plasma TNFα (pg/mL) with myocardial mRNA levels (percent of GAPDH mRNA level); $r = 0.69$, $P < 0.001$. *Abbreviations*: GAPDH, Glyceraldehyde 3-phosphate dehydrogenase; TNFα, tumor necrosis factor-alpha. *Source*: From Ref. 80.

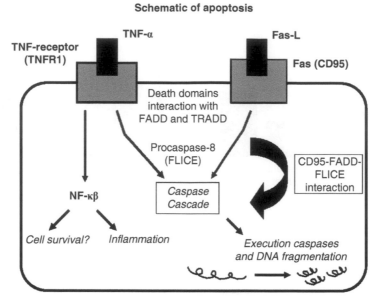

Figure 8.6 Schematic of receptor-initiated pathways for apoptosis. *Abbreviations*: TNFR1, TNF receptor; CD95, Fas (receptor for Fas ligand).

In clinical investigations, IL-6 levels correlate with measures of myocardial function, including LVEF, NYHA class, and cardiac hemodynamics (89,95). Myocardial expression of IL-6 is evident in severe end-stage heart failure but not in mild-to-moderate disease suggesting that cardiac IL-6 production occurs later in the disease process than TNFα (80). Higher circulating levels of IL-6 are associated with a poorer prognosis (100,101). IL-6 plays a central role in the acute phase response, inducing production of C-reactive protein (CRP) and fibrinogen. CRP levels are also markedly elevated in heart failure and predict poor outcomes.

Proinflammatory cytokines, in particular TNFα, may have cardioprotective effects in myocarditis and recent-onset cardiomyopathy. However, in end-stage disease increased production of inflammatory cytokines by the myocardium facilitates progression from compensated to decompensated heart failure. Through stimulation of the myocardial receptors, particularly Fas, TNF can initiate apoptosis (Fig. 8.6), resulting in the irreversible loss of myocytes. For subjects with new-onset cardiomyopathy, myocardial expression of the "cell death" cytokine receptor Fas was predictive of less recovery of LVEF at 6- and 12-month follow-up (102) (Fig. 8.7). There has been increasing interest in the utilization of left ventricular device (LVAD) support to facilitate myocardial recovery (103). For subjects with end-stage heart failure requiring LVAD support, myocardial expression of TNF was tightly correlated with expression of Fas (104), and this relationship was not affected by the hemodynamic unloading of LVAD support. Whether therapy directed against apoptosis could facilitate recovery remains to be determined.

REGULATION OF PLASMA VOLUME

Natriuretic peptides represent an additional hormonal response designed to control plasma volume and are activated in heart failure by excess fluid retention (105). Increased atrial and ventricular filling pressures, dilatation, and wall stress result in the secretion of

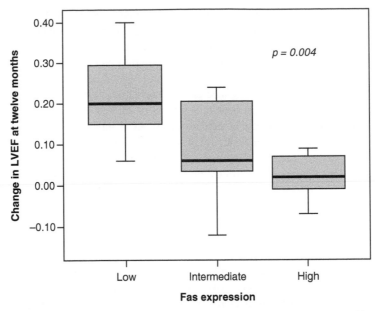

Figure 8.7 Box plot of distribution change in LVEF at 12 months by tertiles of baseline Fas expression. Solid black line = median, rectangle = quartile range, bars = total range. Higher Fas expression associated with less improvement in LVEF at six months, $P = 0.004$. Abbreviation: LVEF, left ventricular ejection fraction. *Source*: From Ref. 102.

peptides that act on the kidney to increase natriuresis and decrease plasma volume (106). Brain natriuretic peptide (BNP) is a 32-amino acid peptide synthesized by the ventricle. BNP is markedly elevated in congestive heart failure and correlates with cardiac filling pressures. Higher levels of BNP in subjects with heart failure predict a poor prognosis (107,108). In addition to natriuresis, BNP induces vasodilatation, decreases renin–angiotensin and sympathetic activation (109). Therefore, as neurohormonal activation drives the heart failure pathway forward, the increase in secretion of BNP driven by fluid overload diminishes their impact and serves as an important counter regulatory mechanism. The natriuretic peptides are cleaved into their active form by a converting enzyme, corin, a serine protease (110). Less active genetic variants of corin have been linked to hypertension (111) and LV hypertrophy (112), presumably due to a loss of the protective effect of the active natriuretic peptides.

VASCULAR REACTIVITY

Heart failure leads to endothelial dysfunction (113,114) and changes in the peripheral vasculature. Elevations in angiotensin-2 increase peripheral vascular resistance initially to preserve perfusion pressure. Over time vascular remodeling becomes evident with smooth muscle cell hypertrophy, cellular proliferation, and interstitial fibrosis that results ultimately in the loss of capillary vascular volume. Similar vascular changes occur in the pulmonary vasculature, driven by chronic elevations in pulmonary capillary wedge pressure, and leads to pulmonary hypertension. In addition to angiotensin-2, several important mediators are released by the endothelium that help regulate vascular tone: the endothelins and the nitric oxide (NO) pathway.

The primary mediator of endothelium-dependent vasodilatation, initially functionally described as endothelium-derived relaxation factor, is now known to be NO and its derivatives. NO, a freely diffusible gas with a short half-life, is produced from arginine from a family of enzymes, the three isoforms of nitric oxide synthase (NOS) (9). Endothelial nitric oxide synthase (NOS_3) is the primary source of vascular NO production and is a constitutively active enzyme. However, in heart failure inducible nitric oxide synthase (NOS_2) is upregulated and may be an important source of circulating NO (115).

The primary effect of NO on vascular function is vasodilatation. In heart failure, this results in decreased peripheral resistance and reduced after load, and the effects of NO improve cardiac performance. The beneficial effects of ACE inhibitors in heart failure are mediated through NO-dependent mechanisms (116). ACE inhibitors limit post -infarction LV remodeling in wild-type animals but not in NOS_3 knockout mice suggesting that the protective effects of therapy require the presence of NOS_3 (117,118). The impact of ACE inhibitors on endothelial function can be limited by pretreatment with L-N^G-Monomethylarginine (L-NMMA), an inhibitor of NO production (119). Although ACE inhibitors improve endothelial function by increasing NO production, circulating TNFα impairs the action of NOS_3 (120), and may tip the balance toward vasoconstriction and endothelial dysfunction.

Expression of NOS_3 in the myocardium is increased in heart failure and affects myocardial function as well as vascular reactivity (121,122). NO is an important mediator of the impact of both cytokine and neurohormonal activation on myocyte function. TNFα induces the expression of NOS_2 in cardiac myocytes, and the negative inotropic effect of this cytokine is mediated through increased NO. NO also improves myocyte relaxation (123) and calcium homeostasis. In addition, NO reduces beta-receptor responsiveness to catecholamine stimulation, and therefore may diminish the effects of sympathetic activation on myocyte function (124,125).

The African American Heart Failure Trial (AHeFT) demonstrated that isosorbide dinitrate and hydralazine in fixed combination improved survival in a cohort of self-designated African Americans with systolic heart failure (126). NO clearly plays a protected mechanism in heart failure, although balance between its cardioprotective effects and potential deleterious superoxide formation remains important (127). Genomic variation at the NOS_3 locus affects heart failure outcomes (128), and racial differences in NOS_3 genomics may explain the enhanced efficacy of isosorbide dinitrate and hydralazine in black heart failure (129).

Endothelin-1 is a 21-amino acid peptide released by the endothelium (130). Endothelin-1 is upregulated in circulating plasma but not in cardiac tissues in heart failure suggesting local production of endothelin-1 is responsible for heart failure elevations. Endothelin causes potent vasoconstriction mediated by type A endothelin receptors (131). Endothelin is promitogenic and promotes cell division and hypertrophy among smooth muscle cells and increased matrix production, leading to the permanent vascular changes of chronic heart failure. Activation of a separate class of endothelin receptors, type B, acts in a counter regulatory manner and stimulates NO production and vascular relaxation (132). Endothelin receptor antagonists are important therapeutic agents for pulmonary arterial hypertension, however, they have not been proved to be effective in heart failure (133). Some investigations have focused on the protective effects of a peptide hormone relaxin (134), which promotes vasodilatation and serve an important counter regulatory mechanism to angiotensin-2 and endothelin.

SUMMARY

Heart failure begins with myocardial injury but progresses as a systemic illness. The compensatory pathways (Table 8.1) designed to respond to acute injury lead to maladaptive consequences in the chronic heart failure state, including progressive myocardial dysfunction and regression of the vascular bed. This pathologic progression is driven by circulating mediators, in particular angiotensin-2 and norepinephrine. Natriuretic peptides play a significant role in the regulation of plasma volume and the downregulation of neurohormonal activation. In the

Table 8.1   Neurohormones: Initiation, Impact, and Interaction

	Initiation	Impact in Heart Failure	Interactions
RAAS			
Angiotensin II	Low cardiac output (renal perfusion) Beta-receptor stimulation	Increased vascular resistance (afterload) Cardiac myocyte hypertrophy Plasma expansion (aldosterone)	Sympathetic activation increases renin release BNP reduces RAAS activation
Sympathetic activation			
Norepinephrine	Baroreceptors (decreased stroke volume)	Increased myocardial work, cardiotoxicity, ischemia, arrhythmias	Increases renin release. Nitric oxide modulates beta receptor activation
Cytokine activation			
TNF-alpha	Myocardial injury	Decrease contractility chronic: worsen LV remodeling acute: facilitate viral clearing	Induce expression of NOS_2 in cardiac myocytes
Natriuretic peptides			
BNP	Ventricular pressure and wall stretch, increased volume	Sodium excretion, vasodilation	Inhibits RAAS activation
Nitric oxide pathway			
Nitric oxide	Constitutively active if endothelium intact (NOS_3) Cytokine induction of NOS_2	Vasodilation Decrease contractility Improve myocardial relaxation	TNF induces NOS_2 NO decreases adrenergic responsiveness

Abbreviations: BNP, brain natriuretic peptide; LV, left ventricular; NOS, nitric oxide synthase; RAAS, renin–angiotensin–aldosterone system; TNF, tumor necrosis factor.

vasculature, NO, relaxin, endothelin-1, and angiotensin-2 are important mediators of vascular tone. Beginning with the initial myocardial injury, cardiac inflammation is mediated by cytokines that can worsen both cardiac and endothelial dysfunction as the heart failure state progresses. While these pathways have been described separately, they are critically interdependent in the systemic response to heart failure. All medical interventions in heart failure that improve survival directly inhibit neurohormonal activation. Further investigation of the interactions of these pathways should lead to improved therapeutics. Given the importance of genetic diversity in the neurohormonal response, targeting of medical therapeutics to genetic background should be an important addition to the treatment of heart failure in the near future.

REFERENCES
1. Thomas C. The Aphorisims of Hippocrates. London: Longman and Co, 1822.
2. Cohn JN, Goldstein SO, Greenberg BH, et al. A dose-dependent increase in mortality with vesnarinone among patients with severe heart failure. Vesnarinone Trial Investigators. N Engl J Med 1998; 339: 1810–16.

3. Thackray S, Easthaugh J, Freemantle N, Cleland JG. The effectiveness and relative effectiveness of intravenous inotropic drugs acting through the adrenergic pathway in patients with heart failure-a meta-regression analysis. Eur J Heart Fail 2002; 4: 515–29.

4. Pfeffer MA, Braunwald E, Moye LA, et al. Effect of captopril on mortality and morbidity in patients with left ventricular dysfunction after myocardial infarction. Results of the survival and ventricular enlargement trial. The SAVE Investigators. New Engl J Med 1992; 327: 669–77.

5. The SOLVD Investigators. Effect of enalapril on survival in patients with reduced left ventricular ejection fractions and congestive heart failure. New Engl J Med 1991; 325: 293–302.

6. Hjalmarson A, Goldstein S, Fagerberg B, et al. The MERIT-HF Study Group. Effects of controlled-release metoprolol on total mortality, hospitalizations, and well-being in patients with heart failure: the Metoprolol CR/XL Randomized Intervention Trial in congestive heart failure (MERIT-HF). JAMA 2000; 283: 1295-302.

7. Dzau VJ. Tissue renin-angiotensin system in myocardial hypertrophy and failure. Arch Int Med 1993; 153: 937–42.

8. Packer M. The neurohormonal hypothesis: a theory to explain the mechanism of disease progression in heart failure. J Am Coll Cardiol 1992; 20: 248–54.

9. Kelly RA, Balligand J-L, Smith TW. Nitric oxide and cardiac function. Circulation 1996; 79: 363–80.

10. Mann DL. Inflammatory mediators and the failing heart. Circ Res 2002; 91: 988–98.

11. Chen D, Assad-Kottner C, Orrego C, Torre-Amione G. Cytokines and acute heart failure. Crit Care Med 2008; 36: S9–S16.

12. Lee Y, Gustafsson AB. Role of apoptosis in cardiovascular disease. Apoptosis. 2009 Apr; 14: 536–48.

13. Massie BM. Neurohormonal blockade in chronic heart failure. J Am Coll Cardiol 2002; 39: 79–82.

14. Mehra MR, Uber PA, Francis GS. Heart failure therapy at a crossroad: are there limits to the neuro-hormonal model? J Am Coll Cardiol 2003; 41: 1606–10.

15. Lavoie JL, Sigmund CD. Minireview: overview of the renin-angiotensin system – an endocrine and paracrine system. Endocrinology 2003; 144: 2179–83.

16. Volpe M, Savoia C, DePaolis P, et al. The renin-angiotensin system as a risk factor and therapeutic target for cardiovascular and renal disease. J Am Soc Nephrol 2002; 13: S173–8.

17. Opie LH, Sack MN. Enhanced angiotensin II activity in heart failure. Reevaluation of the counter-regulatory hypothesis of receptor subtypes. Circ Res 2001; 88: 654–8.

18. Manohar P, Pina IL. Therapeutic role of angiotensin II receptor blockers in the treatment of heart failure. Mayo Clin Proc 2003; 78: 334–8.

19. Shah M, Ali V, Lamba S, et al. Pathophysiology and clinical spectrum of acute congestive heart failure. Rev Cardiovasc Med 2001; 2: S2–6.

20. Weber KT. Extracellular matrix remodeling in heart failure. A role for denovo angiotensin II generation. Circulation 1997; 96: 4065–82.

21. Valgimigli M, Curello S, Ceconi C, et al. Neurohormones, cytokines and programmed cell death in heart failure: a new paradigm for the remodeling heart. Cardiovasc Drugs and Ther 2001; 15: 529–37.

22. Ichihara S, Senbonmatsu T, Price E, et al. Angiotensin II type 2 receptor is essential for left ventricular hypertrophy and cardiac fibrosis in chronic angiotensin II-induces hypertension. Circulation 2001; 104: 346–51.

23. Sadoshima J, Izumo S. Molecular characterization of angiotensin II-induced hypertrophy of cardiac myocytes and hyperplasia of cardiac fibroblasts. Critical role of the AT1 receptor subtype. Circ Res 1993; 73: 413–23.

24. Sackner-Bernstein JD. Activation and release of degradative proteinases within the myocardium are the trigger for ventricular remodeling in chronic heart failure. Med Hypotheses 2002; 58: 18–23.

25. Pouleur H. Rousseau MF, vanEyll C, et al. Effects of long-term enelapril therapy on left ventricular diastolic properties in patients with depressed ejection fraction. Circulation 1993; 88: 481–91.

26. Pfeffer MA, Lamas GA, Vaughan DE, et al. Effect of captopril on progressive ventricular dilatation after anterior myocardial infarction. N Engl J Med 1988; 319: 80–6.

27. Pfeffer MA, Pfeffer JM, Lamas GA. Development and prevention of congestive heart failure following myocardial infarction. Circulation 1993; 87: IV120–5.

28. The CONSENSUS Trial Study Group. Effects of enalapril on mortality in severe congestive heart failure. N Engl J Med 1987; 316: 1429–35.

29. Roig E, Perez-Villa F, Morales M, et al. Clinical implications of increased plasma angiotensin II despite ACE inhibitor therapy in patients with congestive heart failure. Eur Heart J 2000; 21: 53–7.

30. Farquharson CAJ, Struthers AD. Gradual reactivation over time of vascular tissue angiotensin I to angiotensin II conversion during chronic lisinopril therapy in chronic heart failure. J Am Coll Cardiol 2002; 39: 767–75.

31. Tang WH, Vagelos RH, Yee Y-G, et al. Neurohormonal and clinical responses to high- versus low-dose enalapril therapy in chronic heart failure. J Am Coll Cardiol 2002; 39: 69–78.
32. Weber KT. Aldosterone in congestive heart failure. N Engl J Med 2001; 345: 1689–97.
33. Brasier AR, Recinos III A, Eledrisi M. Vascular inflammation and the renin-angiotensin system. Arterioscler Thromb Vasc Biol 2002; 22: 1257–66.
34. Mehra MR, Uber PA, Potluri S. Renin angiotensin aldosterone and adrenergic modulation in chronic heart failure: contemporary concepts. Am J Med Sci 2002; 324: 267–75.
35. Pitt B, Zannad F, Remme WJ, et al. The effect of spironolactone on morbidity and mortality in patients with severe heart failure. N Engl J Med 1999; 341: 709–17.
36. Pitt B, Remme W, Zannad F, et al. Eplerenone a selective aldosterone blocker, in patients with left ventricular dysfunction after myocardial infarction. N Engl J Med 2003; 348: 1309–21.
37. Cohn JN, Tognoni G. The Valsartan Heart Failure Investigators. A randomized trial of the angiotensin-receptor blocker valsartan in chronic heart failure. N Engl J Med 2001; 345: 1667–75.
38. Tipnis SR, Hooper NM, Hyde R, et al. A human homolog of angiotensin-converting enzyme. Cloning and functional expression as a captopril-insensitive carboxypeptidase. J Biol Chem 2000; 275: 33238–43.
39. Donoghue M, Hsieh F, Baronas E, et al. A novel angiotensin-converting enzyme-related carboxypeptidase (ACE2) converts angiotensin I to angiotensin 1-9. Circ Res 2000; 87: E1–9.
40. Crackower MA, Sarao R, Oudit GY, et al. Angiotensin-converting enzyme 2 is an essential regulator of heart function. Nature 2002; 417: 822–8.
41. Felder RB, Francis J, Zhang Z-H, et al. Heart failure and the brain: new perspectives. Am J Physiol Regul Integr Comp Physiol 2004; 284: R259–76.
42. Steinberg SF. The molecular basis for distinct β-adrenergic receptor subtype actions in cardiomyocytes. Circ Res 1999; 85: 1101–11.
43. Feldman AM, McTiernan C. New insight into the role of enhanced adrenergic receptor-effector coupling in the heart. Circulation 1999; 100: 579–82.
44. Bristow MR. β-Adrenergic receptor blockade in chronic heart failure. Circulation. 2000; 101: 558–69.
45. Zaugg M, Xu W, Lucchinetti E, et al. β-Adrenergic receptor subtypes differentially affect apoptosis in adult rat ventricular myocytes. Circulation 2000; 102: 344–50.
46. Lefkowitz RJ, Rockman HA, Koch WJ. Catecholamines, cardiac β-adrenergic receptors, and heart failure. Circulation 2000; 101: 1634–7.
47. Cohn JN, Levine TB, Olivari MT, et al. Plasma norepinephrine as a guide to prognosis in patients with chronic heart failure. NEJM 1984; 311: 819–23.
48. Bristow MR, Gilbert EM, Abraham WT; MOCHA Investigators, et al. Carvedilol produces dose-related improvements in left ventricular function and survival in subjects with chronic heart failure. Circulation 1996; 94: 2807–16.
49. Roden DM, Brown NJ. Preprescription genotyping: not yet ready for prime time, but getting there. Circulation 2001; 103: 1608–10.
50. Gilbert EM, Sandoval A, Larrabee P, et al. Lisinopril lowers cardiac adrenergic drive and increases beta-receptor density in the failing human heart. Circulation 1993; 88: 472–80.
51. Packer M, Poole-Wilson PA, Armstrong PW, et al. Comparative effects of low and high doses of the angiotensin-converting enzyme inhibitor, lisinopril, on morbidity and mortality in chronic heart failure. Circulation 1999; 100: 2312–18.
52. Rigat B, Hubert C, Corvol P, Soubrier F. PCR detection of the insertion/deletion polymorphism of the human angiotensin converting enzyme gene (DCP) (dipeptidyl carboxypeptidase 1). Nucleic Acids Res 1992; 20: 1433.
53. Tiret L, Rigat B, Visvikis S, et al. Evidence, from combined segregation and linkage analysis, that a variant of the angiotensin I-converting enzyme (ACE) gene controls plasma ACE levels. Am J Hum Genet 1992; 51: 197–205.
54. Danser AH, Derkx FH, Hense HW, et al. Angiotensinogen (M235T) and angiotensin-converting enzyme (I/D) polymorphisms in association with plasma renin and prorenin levels. J Hypertens 1998; 16: 1879–83.
55. Andersson B, Sylven C. The DD genotype of the angiotensin-converting enzyme gene is associated with increased mortality in idiopathic heart failure. J Am Coll Cardiol 1996; 28: 162–7.
56. Palmer BR, Pilbrow AP, Yandle TG, et al. Angiotensin-converting enzyme gene polymorphism interacts with left ventricular ejection fraction and brain natriuretic peptide levels to predict mortality after myocardial infarction. J Am Coll Cardiol 2003; 41: 729–36.
57. McNamara DM, Holubkov R, Janosko K, et al. Pharmacogenetic Interactions Between Beta Blocker Therapy and the Angiotensin Converting Enzyme Deletion Polymorphism in Patients with Congestive Heart Failure. Circulation 2001; 103: 1644–8.

58. McNamara DM, Holubkov R, Postava L, et al. Pharmacogenetic interactions between ACE inhibitor therapy and the angiotensin-converting enzyme deletion polymorphism in patients with congestive heart failure. J Am Coll Cardiol 2004; 44: 2019–26.

59. Oates HF, Stoker LM, Monaghan JC, Stokes GS. The beta-adrenergic receptor controlling renin release. Arch Int Pharmacodyn 1978; 234: 205–13.

60. Ishizawar D, Teuteberg JJ, Cadaret LM, Mathier MA, McNamara DM. Impact of B selectivity on the pharmacogenetic Interaction of the ACE D/I Polymorphisms and B Blockers. Clinical Translational Science 2008; 1: 151–4.

61. McNamara DM, MacGowan GA, London B. Clinical importance of β-adrenoceptor polymorphisms in cardiovascular disease. Am J Pharmacogenomics 2002; 2: 73–8.

62. Brodde OE, Buscher R, Tellkamp R, et al. Blunted cardiac responses to receptor activation in subjects with Thr164Ile β2-adrenoceptors. Circulation 2001; 103: 1048–50.

63. Wagoner LE, Craft LL, Singh B, et al. Polymorphisms of the [beta]$_2$-adrenergic receptor determine exercise capacity in patients with heart failure. Circ Res 2000; 86: 834–40.

64. Liggett SB, Wagoner LE, Craft LL, et al. The Ile164 β2-adrenergic receptor polymorphism adversely affects the outcome of congestive heart failure. J Clin Invest 1998; 102: 1534–9.

65. The BEST Investigators. A trial of the beta blocker bucindolol in patients with advanced chronic heart failure. New Engl J Med 2001; 344: 1659–67.

66. Liggett SB, Mialet-Perez J, Thaneemit-Chen S, et al. A polymorphism within a conserved β1-adrenergic receptor motif alters cardiac function and β-blocker response in human heart failure. PNAS 2006; 103: 11288–93.

67. Small KM, Forbes SL, Rahman FF, et al. A four amino acid deletion polymorphism in the third intracellular loop of the human α2C-adrenergic receptor confers impaired coupling to multiple effectors. J Biol Chem 2000; 275: 23059–64.

68. Gerson MC, Wagoner LE, McGuire N, Liggett SB. Activity of the uptake-1 norepinephrine transporter as measured by I-123 MIBG in heart failure patients with a loss-of-function polymorphism of the presynaptic α2C-adrenergic receptor. J Nucl Cardiol 2003; 10: 583–9.

69. Small KM, Wagoner LE, Levin AM, et al. Synergistic polymorphisms of beta1- and alpha2C-adrenergic receptors and the risk of congestive heart failure. N Engl J Med 2002; 347: 1135–42.

70. Lobmeyer MT, Gong Y, Terra SG, et al. Synergistic polymorphisms of β1 and α2c-adrenergic receptors and the influence on left ventricular ejection fraction response to β-blocker therapy in heart failure. Pharma and Geno 2007; 17: 277–82.

71. White PC, Hautanen A, Kupari M. Aldosterone synthase (CYP11B2) polymorphisms and cardiovascular function. J Steroid Biochem Mol Biol 1999; 69: 409–12.

72. Pojoga L, Gautier S, Blanc H, et al. Genetic determination of plasma aldosterone levels in essential hypertension. Am J Hypertens 1998; 11: 856–60.

73. Davies E, Holloway CD, Ingram MC, et al. Aldosterone excretion rate and blood pressure in essential hypertension are related to polymorphic differences in the aldosterone synthase gene CYP11B2. Hypertension 1999; 33: 703–7.

74. McNamara DM, Tam SW, Sabolinski ML, et al. Aldosterone synthase promoter polymorphism predicts outcome in African Americans with heart failure. J Am Coll Cardiol 2006; 48: 1277–82.

75. Cooper RS, Kaufman JS, Ward R. Race and genomics. N Eng J Med 2003; 348: 1166–75.

76. Ferrari R. The role of TNF in cardiovascular disease. Pharmacol Res 1999; 40: 97–105.

77. Sharma R, Anker SD. Cytokines, apoptosis and cachexia: the potential for TNF antagonism. International J Cardol 2002; 85: 161–71.

78. Levine B, Kalman J, Mayer L, Fillit HM, Packer M. Elevated circulating levels of tumor necrosis factor in severe chronic heart failure. N Engl J Med 1990; 323: 236–41.

79. Koller-Strametz J, Pacher R, Frey B, et al. Circulating tumor necrosis factor-α levels in chronic heart failure: relation to its soluble receptor II, interleukin-6, and neurohumoral variables. J Heart Lung Transplant 1998; 17: 356–62.

80. Kubota T, Miyagishima M, Alvarez R, et al. Expression of proinflammatory cytokines in the failing human heart: comparison of recent-onset and end-stage congestive heart failure. J Heart and Lung Transplantation 2000; 19: 819–24.

81. Kubota T, McTiernan CF, Frye CS, et al. Dilated cardiomyopathy in transgenic mice with cardiac-specific overexpression of tumor necrosis factor-alpha. Circ Res 1997; 81: 627–35.

82. Sivasubramanian N, Coker ML, Kurrelmeyer KM, et al. Left ventricular remodeling in transgenic mice with cardiac restricted overexpression of tumor necrosis factor. Circulation 2001; 104: 826–31.

83. Bozkurt B, Kribbs SB, Clubb FJ Jr, et al. Pathophysiologically relevant concentrations of tumor necrosis factor-alpha promote progressive left ventricular dysfunction and remodeling in rats. Circulation 1998; 97: 1382–91.

84. Bradham WS, Bozkurt B, Gunasinghe H, et al. Tumor necrosis factor-alpha and myocardial remodeling in progression of heart failure: a current perspective. Cardiovasc Res 2002; 53: 822–30.
85. Funakoshi H, Kubota T, Machida Y, et al. Involvement of inducible nitric oxide synthase in cardiac dysfunction with tumor necrosis factor-α. Am J Physiol Heart Circ Physiol 2002; 282: H2159–66.
86. Ferdinandy P, Danial H, Ambrus I, et al. Peroxynitrite is a major contributor to cytokine-induced myocardial contractile failure. Circ Res 2000; 87: 241–7.
87. Murray DR, Prabhu SD, Chandrasekar B. Chronic β-adrenergic stimulation induces myocardial pro-inflammatory cytokine expression. Circulation 2000; 101: 2338–41.
88. Kubota T, Bounoutas GS, Miyagishima M, et al. Soluble tumor necrosis factor receptor abrogates myocardial inflammation but not hypertrophy in cytokine-induced cardiomyopathy. Circulation 2000; 101: 2518–25.
89. Francis GS. TNF-α and heart failure. The difference between proof of principle and hypothesis testing. Circulation 1999; 99: 3213–14.
90. Bozkurt B, Torre-Amione G, Warren MS, et al. Results of targeted anti-tumor necrosis factor therapy with etanercept (ENBREL) in patients with advanced heart failure. Circulation 2001; 103: 1044–7.
91. Deswal A, Bozkurt B, Seta Y, et al. Safety and efficacy of a soluble P75 tumor necrosis factor receptor (Enbrel, etanercept) in patients with advanced heart failure. Circulation 1999; 99: 3224–6; 15.
92. Mann DL, McMurray JJ, Packer M, et al. Targeted anticytokine therapy in patients with chronic heart failure: results of the Randomized Etanercept Worldwide Evaluation (RENEWAL). Circulation 2004; 109: 1594–602.
93. Wada H, Saito K, Kanda T, et al. Tumor necrosis factor-α (TNF-α) plays a protective role in acute viral myocarditis in mice. A study using mice lacking TNF-α. Circulation 2001; 103: 743–9.
94. McNamara DM, Starling R, Dec GW, et al. Plasma cytokines in acute cardiomyopathy: evolution over time, correlations with functional studies, and potential role in recovery. Circulation [abstr] 2000; 102: 2020.
95. Mann D. Tumor necrosis factor and viral myocarditis. The fine line between innate and inappropriate immune responses in the heart. Circulation 2001; 103: 626–9.
96. MacGowan GA, Mann DL, Kormos RL, et al. Circulating interleukin-6 in severe heart failure. Am J Cardiol 1997; 79: 1128–31.
97. Mann DL. Interleukin-6 and viral myocarditis: the yin-yang of cardiac innate immune responses. J Mol Cell Cardiol 2001; 33: 1551–3.
98. Tanaka T, Kanda T, McManus BM, et al. Overexpression of interleukin-6 aggravates viral myocarditis: impaired increase in tumor necrosis factor-α. J Mol Cell Cardiol 2001; 33: 1627–35.
99. Wollert KC, Drexler H. The role of interleukin-6 in the failing heart. Heart Failure Reviews 2001; 95–103.
100. Vasan RS, Sullivan LM, Roubenoff R, et al. Inflammatory markers and risk of heart failure in elderly subjects without prior myocardial infarction. The Framingham Heart Study. Circulation 2003; 107: 1486–91.
101. Roig E, Orus J, Pare C, et al. Serum interleukin-6 congestive heart failure secondary to idiopathic dilated cardiomyopathy. Am J Cardiol 1998; 82: 688–90.
102. Sheppard R, Bedi M, Kubota K, et al. Myocardial expression of Fas and recovery of left ventricular function in patients with recent-onset cardiomyopathy. J Am Coll Cardiol 2005; 46: 1036–42.
103. Simon MA, Kormos RL, Murali S, et al. Myocardial recovery using ventricular assist devices: prevalence, clinical characteristics, and outcomes. 2005; Circulation 112: I32–6.
104. Bedi MS, Alvarez RJ, Kubota T, et al. Myocardial Fas expression in end-stage heart failure: impact of LVAD support. Clinical Translational Science 2008; 1: 245–8.
105. Kalra PR, Bolger AP, Coats AJ, et al. The regulation and measurement of plasma volume in heart failure. J Am Coll Cardiol 2002; 39: 1901–8.
106. Braunwald E, Bristow MR. Congestive heart failure: fifty years of progress. Circulation 2000; 102: IV14–23.
107. Lemos JA, Morrow D, Bentley JH, et al. The prognostic value of B-type natriuretic peptide in patients with acute coronary syndromes. N Engl J Med 2001; 345: 1014–21.
108. Latini R, Masson S, deAngelis N, et al. Role of brain natriuretic peptide in the diagnosis and management of heart failure: current concepts. J Card Fail 2002; 8: 288–99.
109. Shi SJ, Ngyuyen HT, Sharma GD, et al. Genetic disruption of atrial natriuretic peptide receptor-A alters renin and angiotensin II levels. Am J Physiol Renal Physiol 2001; 281: F665–73.
110. Wang W, Liao X, Fukuda K, et al. Corin variant associated with hypertension and cardiac hypertrophy exhibits impaired zymogen activation and natriuretic peptide processing activity. Circ Res 2008; 103: 502–8; Epub 2008.

111. Dries DL, Victor RG, Rame JE, et al. Corin gene minor allele defined by 2 missense mutations is common in blacks and associated with high blood pressure and hypertension. Circulation 2005; 112: 2403–10; Epub 2005 Oct 10.

112. Rame JE, Drazner MH, Post W, et al. Corin I555(P568) allele is associated with enhanced cardiac hypertrophic response to increased systemic afterload. Hypertension 2007; 49: 857–64.

113. Fang ZY, Marwick TH. Vascular dysfunction and heart failure: epiphenomenon or etiologic agent? Am Heart J 2002; 143: 383–90.

114. Mathier MA, Rose GA, Fifer MA, et al. Coronary endothelial dysfunction in patients with acute-onset idiopathic dilated Cardiomyopathy. J Am Coll Cardiol 1998; 32: 216–24.

115. Drexler H. Nitric oxide synthases in the failing human heart. A doubled-edged sword? Circulation 1999; 99: 2972–5.

116. Nikolaidis LA, Doverspike A, Huerbin R, et al. Angiotensin-converting enzyme inhibitors improve coronary flow reserve in dilated Cardiomyopathy by a bradykinin-mediated, nitric oxide-dependent mechanism. Circulation 2002; 105: 2785–90.

117. Yang X-P, Liu Y-H, Shesely EG, et al. Endothelial nitric oxide gene knockout mice. Cardiac phenotypes and the effect of angiotensin-converting enzyme inhibitor on myocardial ischemia/reperfusion injury. Hypertension 1999; 34: 24–30.

118. Liu YH, Xu J, Yang XP, et al. Effect of ACE inhibitors and angiotensin II type 1 receptor antagonists on endothelial NO synthase knockout mice with heart failure. Hypertension 1992; 39: 375–81.

119. Wittstein IS, Kass DA, Pak PH, et al. Cardiac nitric oxide production due to angiotensin-converting enzyme inhibition decreases beta-adrenergic myocardial contractility in patients with dilated cardiomyopathy. J Am Coll Cardiol 2001; 38: 429–35.

120. Agnoletti L, Curello S, Bachetti T, et al. Serum from patients with severe heart failure down regulates eNOS and is proapoptotic: role of tumor necrosis factor-α. Circulation 1999; 100: 1983–91.

121. Kojda G, Kottenberg K. Regulation of basal myocardial function by NO. Cardiovasc Res 1999; 41: 514–23.

122. Paulus WJ, Frantz S. Kelly RA. Nitric oxide and cardiac contractility in human heart failure. Time for reappraisal. Circulation 2001; 104: 2260–2.

123. Heymes C, Vanderheyden M, Bronzwaer JGF, et al. Endomyocardial nitric oxide synthase and left ventricular preload reserve in dilated cardiomyopathy. Circulation 1999; 99: 3009–16.

124. Hare JM, Givertz MM, Creager MA, et al. Increased sensitivity to nitric oxide synthase inhibition in patients with heart failure. Potentiation of β-adrenergic inotropic responsiveness. Circulation 1998; 97: 161–6.

125. Ashley EU, Sears CE, Bryant SM, et al. Cardiac nitric oxide synthase 1 regulates basal and adrenergic contractility in murine ventricular myocytes. Circulation 2002; 105: 3011–16.

126. Taylor AL, Ziesche S, Yancy C, Carson P et al. Combination of Isosorbide Dinitrate and Hydralazine in Blacks with Heart Failure. N Engl J Med 2004; 351: 2049–57.

127. Hare JM. Nitroso-redox balance in the cardiovascular system. N Engl J Med 2004; 351: 2112–14.

128. McNamara DM, Holubkov R, Postava L, et al. The Asp298 variant of endothelial nitric oxide synthase: effect on Survival for patients with congestive heart failure. Circulation 2004; 107: 1598–602; 129.

129. McNamara DM, Tam SW, Sabolinski ML, et al. Endothelial nitric oxide synthase (NOS3) polymorphisms in African Americans with heart failure: results from the A-HeFT trial. J Card Fail 2009; in press.

130. Teerlink JR. The role of endothelin in the pathogenesis of heart failure. Curr Cardiol Rep 2002; 4: 206–12.

131. Greenberg B. Endothelin and endothelin receptor antagonists in heart failure. Congest Heart Fail 2002; 8: 257–61.

132. Alonso D, Radomski MW. The nitric oxide-endothelin 1 connection. Heart Fail Rev 2003; 8: 107–15.

133. Kirkby NS, Hadoke PW, Bagnall AJ, Webb DJ. The endothelin system as a therapeutic target in cardiovascular disease: great expectations or bleak house? Br J Pharmacol 2008; 153: 1105–19.

134. Teichman SL, Unemori E, Dschietzig T, et al. Relaxin, a pleiotropic vasodilator for the treatment of heart failure. Heart Fail Rev. 2009 Dec; 14: 321–9.

9
Cardiomyopathies in the adult

Richard Rodeheffer

CLASSIFICATION

The traditional cardiomyopathy classification, based on gross morphology and the principal form of functional cardiac impairment, is to divide the cardiomyopathies into the dilated, hypertrophic, and restrictive phenotypes (Fig. 9.1). The cardinal features of the dilated forms are multichamber dilation with marked impairment of systolic function, as well as reduced diastolic function. The features of the hypertrophic forms are atrial dilatation, marked left ventricular (LV) muscle hypertrophy with vigorous systolic function, impaired ventricular diastolic relaxation and compliance, and a small LV volume (1,2). Restrictive cardiomyopathy is characterized by normal ventricular size, relatively preserved systolic function, marked biatrial enlargement, and severe diastolic dysfunction. While descriptively useful, this grouping has been revised in the light of advances in clinical genetics.

A new classification has been proposed based on the following definition: "Cardiomyopathies are a heterogeneous group of diseases of the myocardium associated with mechanical and/or electrical dysfunction that usually (but not invariably) exhibit inappropriate ventricular hypertrophy or dilatation and are due to a variety of causes that frequently are genetic. Cardiomyopathies either are confined to the heart or are part of generalized systemic disorders, often leading to cardiovascular death or progressive heart failure-related disability" (2). Of note, this definition includes primary myocardial pump failure or arrhythmia, and includes genetic etiology as a prominent feature. According to this scheme cardiomyopathies are divided into two large groups: (*i*) primary cardiomyopathies are confined to heart muscle or the electrical system and may be genetic or acquired, (*ii*) secondary cardiomyopathies manifest myocardial dysfunction as part of a systemic multiorgan disorder, and may also be genetic or acquired (Tables 9.1 and 9.2). This review will be structured according to the new classification.

PRIMARY CARDIOMYOPATHIES
Genetic Primary Cardiomyopathy
Hypertrophic Cardiomyopathy

Morphology and Pathology

Hypertrophic cardiomyopathy (HCM) is a hereditary condition characterized by regional LV hypertrophy, normal or hyperdynamic systolic function, markedly impaired diastolic relaxation and compliance, left atrial enlargement, and a small LV chamber volume (3–5). A minority of patients have a detectable intraventricular pressure gradient across the outflow tract, and the degree of increase in LV mass is out of proportion to the increase in wall

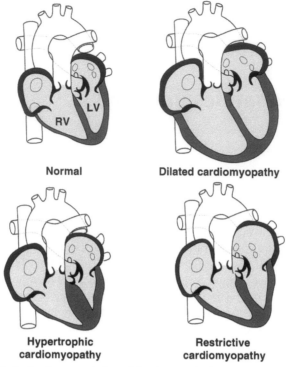

Figure 9.1   Morphologic characteristics of the three principal cardiomyopathy phenotypes.

Table 9.1   Primary Cardiomyopathies

A. Genetic
   HCM
   ARVC
   LVNC
   Conduction detects (Lenegre disease, sick sinus syndrome)
   Mitochondrial myopathies
   Ion channel disorders (Brugada, LQTS, SQTS, Asian SUNDS, CPUT)

B. Mixed Genetic & Acquired
   DCM
   Restrictive (nonhypertrophied nondilated)

C. Acquired
   Myocarditis
   Stress-provoked (apical ballooning)
   Peripartum
   Tachycardia induced

Abreviations: HCM, hypertrophic cardiomyopathy; ARVC, arrhythmic right ventricular cardiomyopathy/dysplasia; LVNC, left ventricular noncompaction; DCM, dilated cardiomyopathy.
Source: From Ref. 2.

Table 9.2 Secondary Cardiomyopathies

Infiltrative[a]
  Amyloidosis (primary, familial autosomal dominant[b], senile secondary forms)
  Gaucher disease[b]
  Hurler's disease[b]
  Hunter's disease[b]
Storage[c]
  Hemochromatosis
  Fabry's disease[b]
  Glycogen storage disease[b] (type II, Pompe)
  Niemann–Pick disease[b]
Toxicity
  Drugs, heavy metals, chemical agents
Endomyocardial
  Endomyocardial fibrosis
  Hypereosinophilic syndrome (Loeffler's endocarditis)
Inflammatory (granulomatous)
  Sarcoidosis
Endocrine
  Diabetes mellitus[b]
  Hyperthyroidism
  Hypothyroidism
  Hyperparathyroidism
  Pheochromocytoma
  Acromegaly
Cardiofacial
  Noonan syndrome[b]
  Lentiginosis[b]
Neuromuscular/neurologic
  Friedreich's ataxia
  Duchenne–Becker muscular dystrophy[b]
  Emery–Dreifuss muscular dystrophy[b]
  Myotonic dystrophy[b]
  Neurofibromatosis[b]
  Tuberous sclerosis[b]
Nutritional deficiencies
  Beriberi (thiamine), pallagra, scurvy, selenium, carnitine, kwashiorkor
Autoimmune/collagen
  Systemic lupus erythematosis
  Dermatomyositis
  Rheumatoid arthritis
  Scleroderma
  Polyarteritis nodosa
Electrolyte imbalance
Consequence of cancer therapy
  Anthracyclines: doxorubicin (adriamycin), daunorubicin
  Cyclophosphamide
  Trastuzumab
  Radiation

[a]Accumulation of abnormal substances between myocytes (i.e., extracellular).
[b]Genetic (familial) origin.
[c]Accumulation of abnormal substances within myocytes (i.e., intracellular).
Source: Adapted from Ref. 2.

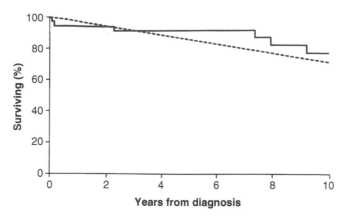

Figure 9.2 Survival in a population-based community cohort of 37 hypertrophic cardio-myopathy patients compared with age-and gender-matched population controls. *Source*: From Ref. 13.

stress associated with the pressure gradient. The distribution of LV hypertrophy is variable, and often includes especially prominent thickening of the intraventricular septum and anterolateral wall or, less commonly, the apex. A global LV hypertrophy pattern is occasionally seen. The histology is notable for widespread myocyte hypertrophy and disarray, scattered fibrosis, and reduced intramuscular coronary artery lumen size (6,7).

Epidemiology and Natural History
In population-based studies the prevalence of HCM has been estimated at 0.1–0.2%, approximately half the frequency of dilated cardiomyopathy (DCM) (8). Among children HCM also presents less commonly than DCM (9,10).

The natural history of HCM is not uniform, and may depend significantly on the specific underlying genetic defect responsible for the condition in an individual patient. Early reports from tertiary HCM referral centers described patients with advanced symptoms, severe hypertrophy, and high annual mortality rates (11,12). The high mortality reported from these specialty clinics represents is likely the effect of referral bias. In population-based community studies many patients are found to be asymptomatic and have mortality similar to age-matched controls (Fig. 9.2) (13). If they develop, symptoms are usually mild for many years. A few patients, progress to a "burned out" HCM characterized by LV dilatation, and reduced LV ejection fraction (14). The most common mode of death is sudden, particularly in younger patients in whom the disease is not suspected (15–18). Indeed, HCM is the most common cause of sudden death in young athletes (15–17). A history of syncope has predictive value for sudden cardiac death (18,19). Severe dyspnea, chest pain, or a very high intraventricular gradient are also predictors of poor prognosis (Table 9.3) (19–21). Finally, patients whose HCM is associated with eight of the most common myofilament or sarcomeric gene mutations have been shown to have a fourfold greater risk of progressing to NYHA Class III or IV symptoms (22).

Etiology
The etiology of HCM has been an area of considerable research over the last two decades (4,5,11,12). Although abnormalities in sarcomeric protein function, intracellular calcium handling, and Z-disc structure have been associated with HCM, the common physiologic consequence is impaired diastolic dysfunction. Subendocardial ischemia, a consequence of high intramural wall stress and reduced coronary lumen diameter, may play a secondary role.

Table 9.3 Factors Associated with Increase Risk of Sudden Cardiac Death in Hypertrophic Cardiomyopathy

---

Genetic

  Family history of sudden death

  Specific mutations of sarcomeric proteins (i.e., Arg403Gln mutation of ß-myosin heavy chain or Arg92Gln mutation of troponin T)

Clinical

  Prior cardiac arrest

  Recurrent syncope

  Ventricular tachycardia on monitoring

Morphologic

  Extreme left ventricular hypertrophy (>30 mm)

Hemodynamic

  Left ventricular outflow pressure gradient >30 mmHg

  Decline in blood pressure during exercise testing

  Limited myocardial coronary blood flow reserve

Source: Adapted from Ref. 19.

Great advances have been made in understanding the genetic basis of HCM (23,25). An estimated 60–80% of cases are familial and 20–40% are sporadic new mutations (24). Mendelian autosomal dominant patterns of inheritance are characteristic, but there is considerable genetic heterogeneity, that is, HCM can be caused by mutations at scores of different loci. At this time well over a hundred mutations have been shown to be associated with HCM. Mutations in the eight most common myofilament and sarcomeric genes account for approximately 60% of HCM cases (22,25). More recently a number of mutations affecting Z-disc function have also been associated with HCM (23). Intracellular calcium flux is a central factor controlling excitation–contraction coupling and mutations in genes coding for phospholamban and the cardiac ryanodine receptor have been found to cause HCM (11,12,23,25).

In addition to genotypic heterogeneity, HCM manifests phenotypic heterogeneity. A recent phenotypic characterization of 283 genotyped HCM patients showed that 47% of the cohort had a massively thickened septum resulting in a "reverse" septal curve configuration and 35% manifested basal septal hypertrophy resulting in a "sigmoidal septal curvature" (Fig. 9.3) (26). Myofilament mutations were strongly associated with the reverse septal phenotype, whereas Z-disc mutations were strongly associated with the sigmoidal septal curvature phenotype.

In some patients the hypertrophic walls, hypercontractile state, and the small LV chamber size combine to produce systolic intracavitary pressure gradients and small stroke volume. However, diastolic dysfunction, caused by a reduced rate of diastolic relaxation and increased chamber stiffness, is a more universal characteristic of HCM than are systolic intracavitary LV pressure gradients. Prolonged relaxation, likely related to altered intracellular calcium flux and subendocardial ischemia, combines with decreased distensibility due to hypertrophy and fibrosis to produce high diastolic filling pressures and atrial enlargement. Mitral regurgitation, usually proportional to the intracavitary pressure gradient, is often a feature (3). Finally, in addition to these hemodynamic abnormalities there is a significant impairment of coronary microvascular dilatation (21).

Some mutations in the B-myosin heavy chain and troponin T appear to be characterized by a higher risk of sudden death, but referral bias may contribute to these observations

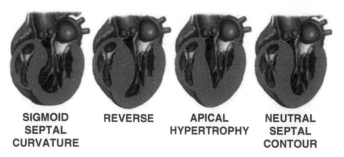

SIGMOID   REVERSE   APICAL   NEUTRAL
SEPTAL   HYPERTROPHY   SEPTAL
CURVATURE   CONTOUR

Figure 9.3 Configurations of the major phenotypes of hypertrophic cardiomyopathy: sigmoid septal curvature, reverse septal curvature, apical hypertrophy, neutral septal curvature.

(11,17–19,27). The frequency with which these "malignant" mutations are found in large referral clinics may be low, on the order of 1% of patients (28). Although some families do appear to manifest an unusually high frequency of sudden death, it is clear that all patients with the same mutation may not be at equally high risk. Confounding factors may influence the phenotypic expression of the mutation, such as variable penetrance within families, modifier genes, and the role of other nongenetic factors (28,29).

Finally, a small percentage of HCM patients present with restrictive hemodynamics but little or no gross hypertrophy despite having characteristic myofiber disarray. In this group, mutations in beta-myosin heavy chain and troponin have been reported (30,31).

Clinical Presentation

The age of presentation is variable and may depend in part on the specific underlying mutation. Many patients are asymptomatic when discovered by screening the relatives of an index HCM patient. Symptomatic patients present most commonly with effort dyspnea, but may also have angina, palpitations, syncope, or fatigue (32). Unfortunately, an initial manifestation may be sudden cardiac death, as observed in young athletes (15–17).

Physical examination usually features a sustained LV impulse. It may include a ventricular gallop, and patients with intracavitary pressure gradients usually have a prominent murmur and may have a bifid carotid upstroke. The murmur is typically midsystolic and harsh along the left sternal border, suggestive of aortic outflow tract obstruction, and more holosystolic at the apex due to mitral regurgitation. Maneuvers that increase peripheral resistance (e.g., squatting) tend to reduce murmur intensity and, conversely, maneuvers that reduce afterload (standing from the squatting position) augment murmur intensity.

Evaluation

The evaluation aims to establish the diagnosis and, if possible, prognosis. The electrocardiogram (ECG) usually demonstrates LV hypertrophy. Echocardiography is the fundamental diagnostic tool, providing information on the distribution of ventricular hypertrophy (septal, reverse curvature, septal sigmoid curvature, apical, or concentric), the presence and magnitude of an intraventricular pressure gradient, the severity of mitral regurgitation, systolic anterior motion of the mitral valve, the size of the LV chamber, the degree of diastolic dysfunction, and atrial size.

Most patients can be effectively diagnosed with echocardiography, and routine cardiac catheterization is not indicated. However, in older patients with chest pain coronary angiography is necessary to exclude concomitant coronary disease. In patients who do undergo catheterization, a number of hemodynamic abnormalities are observed: An intraventricular pressure gradient that varies with afterload and displays postextrasystolic potentiation (increased intracavitary gradient during the postextrasystolic beat), increased LVEDP and atrial a-wave, diminished aortic pressure during beats with increased intraventricular pressure gradient, and a bifid aortic peak systolic pressure form.

Management

Treatment has been offered primarily to patients who have symptoms associated with LV outflow tract obstruction (i.e., approximately 30–40% of patients) and is directed toward reduction of symptoms and prevention of sudden death. Drugs that increase myocardial contractility and intraventricular pressure gradient should be avoided. Diuretics should be used with caution since excessively decreased ventricular preload may result in orthostatic hypotension.

Beta-blockers are the first-line pharmacologic agents, their benefits being related to preventing tachycardia, reducing LV intracavitary gradient, prolonging diastolic filling, and reducing myocardial oxygen consumption (4). Approximately half of patients report improvement in angina or dyspnea with beta-blockade (32–34). A reasonable therapeutic goal is to keep the heart rate at 60–80 bpm at rest, and this may require relatively high doses.

In patients who do not respond to or tolerate beta-blockers, the calcium channel blockers verapamil or diltiazem may be employed. Since these agents have afterload-reducing vasodilatory effects that could exacerbate an intracavitary pressure gradient, they should be started at low dose and titrated upward slowly. Patients who do not respond well to beta-blockers or calcium channel blockers may improve with the addition of disopyramide.

Atrial fibrillation may result in an abrupt increase in heart rate, dyspnea, and may cause serious hypotension. Prompt electrical cardioversion is sometimes needed, and amiodarone added to help maintain sinus rhythm.

Implantation of DDD pacemaker devices in patients with high intracavitary gradients has been employed to optimize AV conduction and the atrial contribution to LV filling. DDD pacing results in a modest LV gradient reduction in most patients but improved exercise capacity in only about 15% of cases (35,36). DDD pacing should not be considered a primary form of HCM therapy. However, for patients who also need pacing for symptomatic bradyarrhythmias, or in those who are not candidates for surgical myectomy, DDD pacing should be considered.

In patients felt to be at high risk for ventricular arrhythmias and sudden death ICD implantation is warranted (37). Risk factors for sudden death are younger age, previous sustained ventricular tachycardia, massive LV hypertrophy, or a family history of HCM with sudden death (18,19). Registry data in such high-risk persons suggest that appropriate primary prevention defibrillator discharges occur in 3.6% of patients per year, and secondary prevention discharges in 10.6% of patients per year (38). As noted previously, early data suggested that some mutations may predispose especially to sudden death (11,12,17–19,23,28,29,39). Antiarrhythmic drugs such as amiodarone have not been well studied for the prevention of ventricular arrhythmias in HCM. Patients should be advised to avoid vigorous physical activity, such as that implicated in precipitating sudden death in apparently healthy athletes with HCM (15–18).

Surgical septal myectomy has traditionally been offered to patients whose symptoms cannot be controlled medically, with the goal of reducing intracavitary outflow tract gradient (40–42). Effective surgery also eliminates or reduces the mitral regurgitation and relieves symptoms. In experienced centers the procedural mortality is <1.0% and the 10-year survival is not different than that of the general population matched for age and gender (42). Symptomatic improvement occurs in 80–90% of patients and is long-lasting (41).

Percutaneous alcohol ablation of the septum has recently been employed as a catheter-based alternative to surgical myectomy (43,44). Injection of alcohol into the first septal perforator produces focal myocardial infarction in the basal septum, and thereby reduces the outflow tract obstruction. The most common complication of the procedure is complete heart block resulting from conduction system damage, occurring in about 10% of patients. Nonrandomized patient series suggest that alcohol septal ablation and surgical septal myectomy both have beneficial effects, but that surgical myectomy results in lower postintervention LV outflow gradients, NYHA symptom class, and long-term mortality (45).

Family Screening

Because HCM has a genetic basis, echocardiographic screening of first-degree relative every 3–5 years is recommended.

ARRHYTHMIC RIGHT VENTRICULAR CARDIOMYOPATHY/DYSPLASIA
Morphology, Pathology, and Clinical Features

Arrhythmic right ventricular cardiomyopathy/dysplasia (ARVC) is a genetic cardiomyopathy principally affecting the right ventricle, characterized by ventricular tachycardia (VT), sudden death, and right heart failure (46). Symptoms typically manifest in the fourth or fifth decade. The pathology is that of fibrofatty infiltration in the right (occasionally also left) ventricle associated with right ventricular dysfunction, histologic signs of inflammation, and myocyte apoptosis.

Natural History

Mortality rates among ARVC patients referred to tertiary centers are about 3% per year, whereas family kindred studies that include earlier asymptomatic cases report a lower mortality rate of <1% per year (46). Risk stratification is still imprecise, but poorer outcomes are observed in patients who are young, have a history of syncope or cardiac arrest, have a family history of juvenile sudden death, or who have severe right ventricular dysfunction (46).

Diagnostic criteria continue to evolve. Magnetic resonance imaging (MRI) may disclose focal right ventricular hypokinesis associated with signs of fatty infiltration (47). Endocardial biopsy may disclose characteristic histology.

At this point multiple causative mutations have been identified that affect desmosomal structure and function, and approximately 40% of patients can be successfully genotyped (48,49). Mutations in desmosome proteins and the ryanodine receptor have been particularly implicated (25). The clinical value of genotyping resides primarily in identifying preclinical disease in relatives of known ARVC patients, since sudden death is the presenting symptom in about half of index cases (48). Variable age-related penetrance, however, make the timing of antiarrhythmic interventions uncertain.

Management

Although controlled trial data are lacking, patient series suggest that sotalol may reduce inducible ventricular tachycardia (VT) (46). Catheter ablation also reduces VT events, but only 50% of patients have VT recurrence-free survival at five years (50). The lack of more long-lasting benefits from VT ablation may be due to the progressive and diffuse nature of the disease. The incomplete efficacy of drugs and ablation has made ICD implantation an important part of effective management.

LEFT VENTRICULAR NONCOMPACTION

LV noncompaction (LVNC) is characterized by normal compaction of the epicardial myocardium and noncompaction of the endocardium. Prominent endocardial trabeculations are thought to represent persistence of hypertrabeculated embryonic myocardium (51). Unambiguous diagnostic criteria have not yet emerged, and the finding of LVNC in kindreds of HCM and DCM raises the question of whether LVNC is part of a cardiomyopathy spectrum rather than a unique disease (51). LVNC has been linked to mutations in sarcomeric, Z-line, cytoskeletal, and mitochondrial proteins (51,52).

LVNC is probably asymptomatic for many years. Tertiary referral patients typically present in the fourth and fifth decade with heart failure or sudden death (53). Population-based studies are not available. In a clinical series of 34 patients followed for 3.5 years, 53% developed heart failure, 24% had thromboembolic events, and 41% manifested ventricular tachycardia (53). Survival free of death or heart transplantation was 58% at five years.

GLYCOGEN STORAGE

Glycogen storage is critical for meeting energy supply demands during sudden increases in muscle activity. Genetic defects in regulators of cardiac metabolism may result in excessive intracellular glycogen storage and may present with a hypertrophic cardiomyopathy phenotype in childhood and has been associated with poor prognosis (25,54).

CONDUCTION DEFECTS

The heritable conduction defects overlap with the ion channel disorders and the heritable DCMs (below). Mutations in genes coding for ion channels, gap junctions, energy metabolism, and transcription factors may cause combinations of conduction system disease, arrhythmia, and multichamber dilatation (25,55). Mutations in the sodium channel genes (SCN5A) have been of particular interest (56). As more such mutations are identified, further studies of environmental factors and modifier genes that influence phenotypic penetrance will be important (57).

Mitochondrial Cardiomyopathies

Mitochondrial DNA mutations cause a heterogeneous group of cardiomyopathies. Defects in respiratory chain enzyme activity or in mitochondrial structural proteins may produce a DCM phenotype, usually presenting early in life (25,58). Occasional cases are associated with skeletal myopathy and present in adulthood (59).

Ion Channel Disorders

Ion channel disorders are included in the new cardiomyopathy classification. These constitute a large and growing array of mutations primarily affecting Na+, Ca++, and K+ channels (60–62). Since these disorders present most often as arrhythmias rather than as a structural cardiomyopathy they are not considered in detail in this chapter. The reader is referred to some earlier reviews (60,61).

MIXED GENETIC AND ACQUIRED CARDIOMYOPATHY
Nonischemic Dilated Cardiomyopathy

Morphology and Pathology

In nonischemic DCM there is relatively widespread involvement of all the myocardium. In its fully evolved form, therefore, DCM manifests impressive cardiomegaly (Fig. 9.1). Although there is impairment of muscle function during both diastole and systole, the dominant feature is that of decreased systolic ejection. A small minority of patients present with globally reduced contractile function and only mild chamber dilatation. The atrioventricular valve rings are dilated, atria are enlarged, and there is LV hypertrophy. Histologic evaluation reveals myocyte hypertrophy, variable degrees of diffuse fibrosis (particularly in the subendocardium), occasional lymphocytes and, rarely, focal myocyte necrosis.

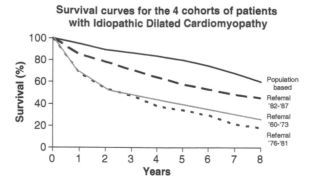

Figure 9.4 Survival in nonischemic dilated cardiomyopathy: comparison of referral and population-based community patients. The three lower curves represent cohorts of referral patients from 1976 to 81; 1960 to 1973; 1982 to 1987.

Epidemiology and Natural History

The incidence of DCM is based on autopsy series and population-based studies. Data from Sweden and Minnesota indicate 5–8 cases/100,000 persons/year (8,63). Pediatric surveillance registries report an annual incidence of 0.6–0.7 cases/100,000 children/year, with most children presenting in the first year of life (9,10). Although the incidence has been reported to be increasing, some of this apparent increase could be related to ascertainment bias consequent to widespread application of noninvasive diagnostic tools such as echocardiography (8). The age- and sex-adjusted prevalence rate is estimated at 36.5/100,000 population (8). Among adults, blacks have a two- to threefold greater prevalence than whites (64).

Prognosis has been assessed in both population-based and referral cohorts. DCM patients identified in the community appear to have better survival than those referred to tertiary hospitals, likely as a result of the referral bias that results from tertiary hospital clinic patients being at a more advanced stage of their disease (Fig. 9.4) (65). Even among referral cohorts, however, there is evidence of improved survival beginning in the 1980s (65). Factors associated with poor survival in DCM are similar to those associated with early death in heart failure in general: severe hemodynamic derangement, advanced neurohumoral activation, NYHA Class III–IV symptom severity, and marked cardiomegaly.

Etiology

Four chamber dilatation with depressed systolic contractile function is a final common phenotype that may result from a range of myocardial stresses or injuries (66). The source of injury may be known, as in the secondary DCMs (e.g., inflammatory injury, metabolic deficiency states, excessive stimulation by hyperactive endogenous endocrine systems or exogenous toxins). There is a growing body of evidence that viral myocarditis may cause some cases (see Myocarditis section). When the nature of the injury cannot be determined, the disease is idiopathic DCM.

Familial DCM was once believed to be rare but studies in the 1990s, involving systematic echocardiographic and electrocardiographic screening of the first-degree relatives of idiopathic DCM patients, revealed that at least 25% of presumably sporadic idiopathic DCM cases were actually familial (67–70). Importantly, 83% of these familial DCM cases would not have been identified on the basis of the family history alone, that is, other affected family members were only identified by echocardiographic screening (67). Gene mutations leading to DCM now number in the dozens, and they involve contractile proteins, ion channel proteins, and transcription binding proteins (Fig. 9.5) (25,62). Interestingly, mutations

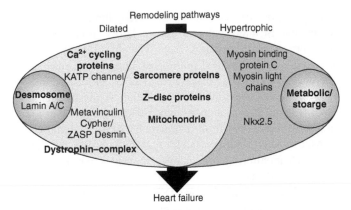

Figure 9.5   Human gene mutations causing cardiac hypertrophy (right), dilatation (left), or both (center). A hypertrophic phenotype can also result from gene mutations causing glycogen accumulation (metabolic/storage). A dilated phenotype with fibrofatty myocardial degeneration can occur with mutations (desmosome). *Source*: Adapted from Ref. 25.

resulting in a DCM phenotype may occur in the same proteins as mutations that give rise to an HCM phenotype (25). To date, great heterogeneity has been observed in these mutations, with no single mutation accounting for a substantial portion of familial cases.

Clinical Presentation

DCM can present at any age, although it is most common to present in infancy or during the fourth to sixth decades. There may be an asymptomatic phase, lasting months to years, during which the disease is occasionally discovered by chance if cardiomegaly is noted on a chest radiograph, left bundle branch block, or ST-T changes are noted on an ECG, or ectopic beats are found on a routine physical examination. Although the presenting symptoms may seem to evolve over only a few weeks, it is often difficult to determine when the onset of ventricular dysfunction actually occurred. Some patients appear to develop symptoms after a viral infection syndrome but proof of a viral inflammatory injury to the heart is difficult to establish. In patients who present in atrial fibrillation and DCM it may be difficult to determine if the atrial fibrillation is secondary to a previously established but undiagnosed cardiomyopathy, or whether the ventricular systolic dysfunction and dilatation are due to prolonged tachycardia (71,72).

Typical symptoms include exertional or supine dyspnea, effort fatigue, and edema. Physical findings depend on the stage of disease, and include cardiac enlargement, S4 and S3 gallop, mitral and tricuspid regurgitation murmurs, jugular venous distention, pulmonary rales, liver enlargement, and edema. Prominent right ventricular failure signs are evidence of end-stage deterioration. In addition to physical findings indicative of circulatory decompensation one should be alert to noncardiac findings that may provide clues to etiology: signs of thyroid dysfunction, hemochromatosis, sarcoidosis, pheochromocytoma, or alcoholism. Many patients are initially misdiagnosed as having asthma or recurrent episodes of pneumonitis.

Evaluation

The goals of clinical assessment are to establish etiology and estimate prognosis. In screening for secondary causes of DCM measuring thyroid stimulating hormone, creatinine, phosphorous, calcium, potassium, ferritin, complete blood count, and HIV serology may provide valuable clues. The ECG may disclose left bundle branch block, sometimes an early precursor of DCM, or clinically silent tachyarrhythmias. Nonsustained ventricular tachycardia is detectable in many patients if ambulatory monitoring is performed, and tends to be more severe as the disease progresses. The chest radiograph, in addition to providing information on cardiac size and pulmonary congestion, may also show signs of pulmonary infection or other thoracic disease, such as sarcoidosis.

Measurement of ventricular function is essential. While this may be performed by echocardiographic, radionuclide, or angiographic means, the echocardiogram has merit in that it provides a wealth of corollary information on LV mass, regional wall and valve function, chamber sizes, estimated right ventricular systolic pressure and the presence of pericardial effusion. When monitoring for changes in ventricular function it is helpful to perform serial measurements using the same methodology.

Since coronary disease can present as a DCM without a history of documented myocardial infarction, it is important to exclude occult ischemic disease. In DCM stress echocardiography or thallium scintigraphy may show regional abnormalities even in the absence of significant coronary occlusions. Therefore, a low threshold for performing coronary angiography in persons over 35 years of age is appropriate.

The use of endocardial biopsy should be selective. Knowledge of histology may point toward a specific etiology in approximately 15% of DCM cases seen in referral centers, but in only a few of these is an effective etiology-specific therapy available (66). Examples of potentially treatable conditions include sarcoidosis, eosinophilic hypersensitivity myocarditis and giant cell myocarditis.

Right heart catheterization provides prognostic information when it is performed after a comprehensive medical treatment program is established and a stable hemodynamic state is achieved. If ventricular filling pressures remain high despite optimal medical therapy, the prognosis is particularly worrisome.

Treatment

The approach to management of DCM is similar to that of systolic heart failure in general: neurohormonal blockade with angiotensin-converting enzyme inhibitors or angiotensin II blockers, beta-blockers, and aldosterone blockade; digoxin, diuretics, biventricular pacing, ventricular assist devices, and cardiac transplantation. Patients having sustained ventricular arrhythmias and/or an ejection fraction below 35% are candidates for implantable defibrillators.

Patients with treatable underlying etiologic conditions, such as myocardial ischemia, hypertension, sustained atrial tachyarrhythmias, or others, should have optimal therapy for those conditions. Concomitant anemia or obstructive sleep apnea needs to be aggressively managed. Avoidance of cardiotoxins such as alcohol is advised and moderate conditioning exercise is recommended. Coumadin anticoagulation is important for preventing emboli in those with atrial fibrillation; for patients in sinus rhythm with severely depressed systolic function the value of anticoagulation is being evaluated in controlled clinical trials at this time.

Patients with idiopathic DCM need genetic counseling to alert them to the 25% or greater probability that they have a heritable condition. Although longitudinal data are not yet available, it is prudent to offer periodic screening with ECG and echocardiography to adult first-degree relatives of the DCM patient, perhaps repeated every five years.

RESTRICTIVE CARDIOMYOPATHY
Morphology and Pathology

Restrictive cardiomyopathy (RCM) is characterized by severe diastolic dysfunction, relatively preserved systolic function, and LV cavity size, biatrial enlargement, and extensive

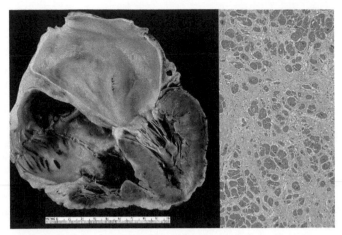

Figure 9.6 Configuration of ventricles and atria in idiopathic restrictive cardiomyopathy. Photomicrograph shows extensive myocardial fibrosis. *Source*: Courtesy of Dr. William D. Edwards, Department of Laboratory Medicine and Pathology, Mayo Clinic.

myocardial fibrosis (Fig. 9.6) (73). Its physiology is very similar to that constrictive pericarditis (74). Several different processes may produce severely impaired ventricular filling and restrictive cardiomyopathy. Infiltrative conditions (such as amyloidosis) and endocardial fibrosis typically present with diastolic dysfunction and are considered below under Secondary Cardiomyopathies section. After known secondary causes have been excluded there remain a small number of patients with idiopathic progressive myocardial fibrosis, and these are considered to have a primary cardiomyopathy. Patients with this phenotype have been evaluated and mutations in troponin and actin genes have been reported (75). The relationship between such patients and similar patients considered to have HCM remains to be clarified (30).

Epidemiology, Natural History, and Etiology
Since different etiologic events can lead to the final common pathway of RCM, the epidemiology and natural history of RCM depend on the particular etiology (30,75–77). Patients with a primary idiopathic RCM, for whom no cause can be identified, have a five-year survival rate of approximately 65% (Fig. 9.7) (77).

Clinical Presentation
The clinical features of restrictive cardiomyopathy may be difficult to distinguish from those of constrictive pericarditis: ascites, dependent edema, exercise intolerance, low systemic blood pressure, anorexia, and hepatic congestion. Since cardiac restriction may affect right-sided filling as much as left-sided filling, pulmonary congestion symptoms, such as paroxysmal nocturnal dyspnea, are not prominent symptoms.

The physical examination is dominated by signs of right-sided heart failure: jugular venous distention, which increases on inspiration, hepatic enlargement, icterus, ascites, and anasarca. The right ventricle may be palpable, the P_2 augmented, and S_3 or S_4 gallops are common.

Evaluation
The workup centers on determining the etiology and distinguishing restrictive cardiomyopathy from constrictive pericarditis, the latter requiring surgical pericardiectomy. To

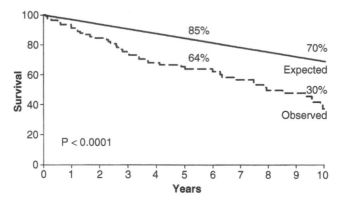

Figure 9.7 Survival in a cohort of 94 referral patients with idiopathic restrictive cardiomyopathy.

distinguish constrictive from restrictive disease thorough noninvasive imaging assessment and invasive hemodynamic evaluation are indicated. Echocardiography is valuable to assess systolic and diastolic function and to look for evidence of amyloidosis. MRI or CT scanning may provide important information on pericardial thickness and calcification. An optimal catheterization study should include simultaneous high fidelity right and LV pressure measurements and respirometry recordings. In restrictive disease respiratory maneuvers produces concordant changes in RV and LV systolic pressures, whereas constriction usually results in discordant respiratory variation in ventricular systolic pressures (i.e., greater ventricular interdependence) (74). The measurement of ventricular interdependence appears to be more sensitive and specific for identification of constrictive pericarditis than does measurement of more traditional hemodynamic parameters (74). Finally, endocardial biopsy may provide useful diagnostic information, such as the extent of myocardial fibrosis, amyloid infiltration, or evidence of sarcoidosis or storage disease; in constrictive pericarditis the myocardium is usually normal.

Management
Management is challenging. General measures include employing only as much diuretic as needed to control fluid retention without producing clinically significant orthostatic hypotension. If tachycardia is contributing to impaired diastolic filling beta-blockade may be beneficial. The onset of atrial fibrillation can produce an abrupt increase in symptoms, and urgent efforts to restore sinus rhythm may need to be undertaken. Inotropic agents are of little benefit.

ACQUIRED CARDIOMYOPATHY
Myocarditis
Myocarditis describes a group of inflammatory diseases of the myocardium characterized by a cellular infiltrate, usually lymphocytic but sometimes predominantly eosinophilic or giant cell. Myocyte necrosis and myocardial fibrosis may also be present.

Lymphocytic myocarditis may present as fulminant heart failure, requiring inotropic or even mechanical circulatory support, and often resolves within days to weeks without residual chronic heart failure (78). This stands in contrast to cases that have a less dramatic onset but which more often result in significant chronic heart failure and a poor prognosis (78).

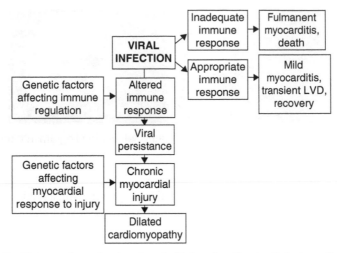

Figure 9.8   Proposed mechanism for viral injury leading to dilated cardiomyopathy.

It is widely suspected that a lymphocytic myocarditis can lead to widespread myocyte injury, and that this can lead ultimately to DCM (79–81). The cause of the initial inflammation is commonly unknown, although it has long been speculated that many cases are due to infection by a cardiotropic virus (certain strains of coxsackie, adenovirus, parvovirus). There are epidemiologic data and rodent viral myocarditis models to support this hypothesis (79–81). Proposed mechanisms of viral injury involve persistence of virus, a sustained and inappropriately modulated host immunologic response to the virus, and the development of a low-grade chronic active myocarditis leading to progressive myocyte destruction (Fig. 9.8). Current human studies have focused on the chronic presence of viral DNA in the myocardium, the development of cross-reactive antibodies to myocyte proteins, and the roles of T-cell regulation, cytokine release, and myocyte apoptosis (82–87). Why the majority of persons infected with cardiotropic viruses do not develop myocarditis may be related to individual genetic susceptibility, appropriate immunomodulation in response to viral infection or other environmental factors. Viral myocarditis should be distinguished from other infectious myocarditides, from lymphocytic myocarditis that may be associated with other systemic inflammatory diseases, and from other forms of local inflammatory injury, such as grant cell and eosinophilic myocarditis.

The diagnosis of lymphocytic myocarditis has traditionally depended on endocardial biopsy, a technique limited by significant sampling error. Although recent reports suggest a role for MRI in the diagnosis it is clear that the lack of a sensitive and specific diagnostic test is an ongoing problem in myocarditis research and treatment (88).

Management of fulminant myocarditis consists of pharmacologic and/or mechanical hemodynamic support as a bridge to recovery. For acute or chronic lymphocytic myocarditis controlled trial data have not supported the use of immunosuppression (89). Future trials, employing better diagnostic and therapeutic strategies, may further clarify the role of immunosuppression.

Giant cell myocarditis, a rarer disease, characteristically presents with heart failure, chest pain, ventricular arrhythmias, and heart block, often mimicking an acute coronary syndrome (90,91). Diagnosis depends on histology and a biopsy should be obtained if the clinical findings are suggestive. The prognosis is poor and the use of immunosuppression, although unproven in controlled trials, may be of value. Cardiac transplantation is an option for refractory patients.

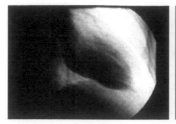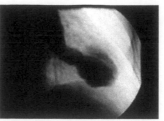

Figure 9.9 Stress-induced acute cardiomyopathy: left ventriculogram in diastole and systole showing "apical ballooning."

Drug-induced hypersensitivity myocarditis may present with a predominantly eosinophilic infiltrate on biopsy. It usually responds to removal of the offending substance and corticosteroid anti-inflammatory therapy.

Stress-Induced Cardiomyopathy (Apical Ballooning)
Apical ballooning or "takotsubo" cardiomyopathy is a form of acute stress-induced DCM (92,93). Typically affecting women aged 50–75 years, patients present with chest pain, dyspnea, and sometimes hypotension. Because these symptoms are usually accompanied by mild ST elevation evolving into diffuse T-wave inversion patients are often believed to have an acute coronary syndrome. Coronary angiography, however, shows little or no obstructive disease. In most patients the history reveals an antecedent severe emotional or physiologic stress (e.g., death of a family member, sudden medical illness).

During the acute phase ejection fraction may decrease to the 15–30% range accompanied by a brief cardiac enzyme rise and markedly elevated plasma catecholamine levels (94). The characteristic ventricular configuration is that of apical and midventricular akinesis–dyskinesis with preserved basal function (Fig. 9.9). Treatment focuses on pharmacologic and/or mechanical support. In almost all patients ejection fraction returns to normal within several weeks.

Peripartum Cardiomyopathy
Peripartum cardiomyopathy (PPCM) is defined as heart failure and decreased ejection fraction developing in the last gestational month or the first five postpartum months, absent prior heart disease or other identifiable cause of heart failure (91–98). The time frame is specified in an attempt to distinguish PPCM from preexisting DCM unmasked by the stress of pregnancy. The incidence of PPCM varies in different regions of the world and in the United States occurs in from 1 in 3000 and 1 in 4000 births (96–99). PPCM incidence appears to be higher among African Americans than whites, Hispanics, or Asians (99). Risk factors include age > 30 years, race, multiparity, and hypertension.

The PPCM heart is morphologically like the idiopathic DCM heart and PPCM presents with symptoms and signs typical of systolic heart failure. The etiology is unknown but biopsy evidence for inflammation in some cases suggests the possibility of an autoimmune or virally induced chronic inflammatory state (95,100). Elevations of circulating TNFα, C-reactive protein, and markers of apoptosis also support the presence of an inflammatory mechanism (95).

Treatment of PPCM is similar to other forms of systolic heart failure. During pregnancy diuretics, digoxin, and beta-blockers may be used, whereas hydralazine and ACE inhibitors are to be avoided (96).

The natural history among tertiary referral patients is notable for recovery of ejection fraction in about 50% of persons in the 6–12 months after delivery (97,98). While referral centers have reported high mortality rates among PPCM, population-based studies suggest a five-year mortality of about 5% (98). Although information is limited, follow-up survey data on PPCM women whose ejection fraction has returned to normal show that a subsequent pregnancy is associated with an average ejection fraction decrease from 56% to 49% and a 20% incidence heart failure symptoms (101). In contrast, among women whose ejection fraction had not recovered after the first pregnancy the subsequent pregnancy was associated with an ejection fraction decline from 36% to 32%, heart failure symptoms in about 45% of cases, and 20% mortality (101).

Tachycardia-Induced Cardiomyopathy

Unrelieved tachycardia can produce reversible LV systolic dysfunction. Indeed, the canine pacing tachycardia model produces systolic heart failure so reliably that it is widely used in heart failure research (72,102). Reduced ejection fraction may be caused by rapid atrial fibrillation, accessory pathway, and AV nodal reentrant tachycardias, and incessant atrial or ventricular tachycardia (71,103,104). With rhythm or rate control and conventional heart failure therapy most patients recover normal systolic function within several months. A similar reversible tachycardia has been reported in persons with very frequent premature ventricular contractions (>20,000 per 24 hours) (109).

SECONDARY CARDIOMYOPATHIES

As listed in Table 9.2, the secondary cardiomyopathies encompass a wide range of systemic diseases that include myocardial involvement and result in systolic or diastolic heart failure. These multisystem disorders may be genetic or acquired. Because a complete discussion of each of these entities is beyond the scope of this review only selected diseases will be considered.

Infiltrative Cardiomyopathies

Cardiac amyloidosis may be considered a paradigm for infiltrative cardiomyopathy leading to restrictive physiology. Amyloidosis occurs as a consequence of the widespread multiorgan deposition of amyloid protein, most commonly caused by a plasma cell dyscrasia that results in excessive production of an immunoglobulin fragment (AL amyloid). Cardiac involvement is common in primary AL amyloidosis and contributes significantly to the overall morbidity and mortality of the disease. Early manifestations include thickening of the LV walls and biatrial enlargement. Initially ejection fraction is maintained, but with progressive amyloid infiltration it begins to decrease and the prognosis for survival is then usually less than a year.

Cardiac amyloidosis often presents as right heart failure, with ascites, increased central venous pressure, edema, pleural effusions, and exercise intolerance. Concomitant renal involvement may include significant proteinuria, which aggravates the symptoms of fluid retention. The diagnosis is based on the typical echocardiographic features described above, as well as Doppler evidence of impaired diastolic function. While endocardial biopsy can confirm the diagnosis, an amyloid positive tissue biopsy from elsewhere (e.g., fat aspirate), combined with identification of an amyloid protein in serum or urine, are usually sufficient to explain the echocardiographic findings. Treatment, in highly selected cases, may involve autologous bone marrow stem cell transplantation, or cardiac transplantation (105).

Storage Diseases

Hemochromatosis presents with a clinical picture typical of the DCM (106,107). Patients with liver dysfunction, diabetes, and dilated ventricles should be evaluated with serum iron, iron-binding capacity, and ferritin levels.

Endomyocardial Fibrotic Conditions

Eosinophilic heart disease includes disorders in which hypereosinophilia and/or eosino-philic myocarditis are associated with endocardial and/or myocardial fibrosis. Hypereo-sinophilic syndrome with cardiac involvement is known as Löffler endocarditis (108–110). The disorder is characterized by thromboembolic events, widespread arteritis, and eosino-philic myocarditis. Both ventricles are subject to mural thrombosis and dense fibrotic thickening. Damage to valvular support may produce significant mitral regurgitation, and biatrial enlargement predisposes to atrial fibrillation.

In equatorial Africa a similar disease, known as endomyocardial fibrosis, is not asso-ciated with peripheral eosinophilia (111–113). There are significant regional variations in prevalence. A random sample of persons in a rural area of Mozambique revealed a 20% prevalence of endomyocardial fibrosis, and frequent family clustering was observed (114). Endomyocardial fibrosis may involve either or both ventricles and sometimes responds favorably to surgical resection of fibrotic endocardium (112–114).

Toxicity

Alcoholic cardiomyopathy deserves special comment. Alcohol depresses myocardial contractility, and the risk of developing DCM is related to the volume and duration of alcohol consumption (111–118). Women appear to be susceptible at a lower level of alcohol exposure than men (117). Abstinence from alcohol has been observed to allow recovery of ventricular function if achieved early in the course of alcoholic cardiomy-opathy. Avoidance of significant alcohol consumption is recommended in all DCM patients, whether or not alcohol toxicity is believed to be the primary underlying etiology.

Cardiotoxic Cancer Chemotherapy

In addition to radiation, which can cause coronary artery disease and restrictive myocardial fibrosis, several chemotherapeutic agents can cause DCM (119). Anthracycline toxicity is dose dependent and risk increases at doses above 400 mg/m^2. Most cases present in the first year after chemotherapy exposure. In addition to dose, risk factors include mediastinal radiation, hypertension, age, and prior cardiac disease. Patients with risk factors should have ventricular function monitored at baseline and periodically during treatment. Patients without risk factors should have ventricular function at baseline and after the cumulative dose reaches 350 mg/m^2 (119). Ventricular dysfunction should be treated with conventional heart failure agents.

Cyclophosphamide-related depression of ventricular function may occur after doses of 120–170 mg/kg and may resolve after several weeks of conventional heart failure man-agement. In combination with an anthracycline about 5% of patients have significant decreases in ejection fraction (120).

Recombinant humanized monoclonal antibodies that bind the HER2 protein (present in 25% of breast cancer patients), such as trastuzumab, are now widely employed. In recent trials trastuzumab caused decreased ejection fraction in about 9% of patients during treat-ment and about 6% after treatment (120). Half of these decreases were transient. Clinical heart failure occurred in approximately 3% of patients.

Patients treated with cardiotoxic chemotherapy should be monitored at baseline and serially as exposure increases. This is especially important in persons receiving more than one cardiotoxic agent, in elderly patients, and in those with prior hyper-tension or cardiac disease. Medical management for heart failure should be instituted promptly.

SUMMARY

The cardiomyopathies constitute a diverse group of diseases, but can be usefully categorized into three clinical phenotypes: dilated, hypertrophic, and restrictive. Within each class a variety of etiologies give rise to a similar morphologic phenotype and pathophysiology. The current classification is based on whether the cardiomyopathy is primary or secondary (associated with an identifiable systemic multiorgan disorder). Within each category disease may be genetic or acquired. As more etiologies and genetic associations are elucidated, it is anticipated that classification systems will change to account for new findings.

REFERENCES

1. Richardson P, McKenna W, Bristow M, et al. Report of the 1995 world health organization/international society and federation of cardiology task force on the definition and classification of cardiomyopathies. Circulation 1996; 93: 841.
2. Maron BJ, Towbin JA, Theine G, et al. Contemporary definitions and classification of the cardiomyopathies. Circulation 2006; 113: 1807–16.
3. Wigle ED, Rakowski H, Kimball BP, et al. Hypertrophic cardiomyopathy. Clinical Spectrum and Treatment. Circulation 1995; 92: 1680–92.
4. Braunwald E, Seidman CE, Sigwart U. Contemporary evaluation and management of hypertrophic cardiomyopathy. Circulation 2002; 106: 1312–16.
5. Maron BJ. Hypertrophic cardiomyopathy. A systematic review. JAMA 2002; 287: 1308–20.
6. Maron BJ, Wolfson JK, Epstein SE, et al. Intramural ("small vessel") coronary artery disease in hypertrophic cardiomyopathy. J Am Coll Cardiol 1986; 8: 545–57.
7. Maron BJ, Anan TJ, Roberts WC. Quantitative analysis of the distribution of cardiac muscle cell disorganization in the left ventricular wall of patients with hypertrophic cardiomyopathy. Circulation 1981; 63: 882–94.
8. Codd MB, Sugrue DD, Gersh BJ, et al. Epidemiology of idiopathic dilated and hypertrophic cardiomyopathy: a population-based study in Olmsted County, Minnesota, 1975–1984. Circulation 1989; 80: 564–72.
9. Nugent AW, Piers BS, Daubeney EF, et al. The epidemiology of childhood cardiomyopathy in Australia. N Engl J Med 2003; 348: 1639–46.
10. Lipschultz SE, Sleeper LA, Towbin JA, et al. The incidence of pediatric cardiomyopathy in two regions of the United States. N Engl J Med 2003; 348: 1647–55.
11. Roberts R, Sigwart U. New concepts in hypertrophic cardiomyopathies, part I. Circulation 2001; 104: 2113–16.
12. Roberts R, Sigwart U. New concepts in hypertrophic cardiomyopathies, part II. Circulation 2001; 104: 2249–52.
13. Cannan CR, Reeder GS, Bailey KR, et al. Natural history of hypertrophic cardiomyopathy. A population-based study, 1976 through 1990. Circulation 1995; 92: 2488–95.
14. Spirito P, Maron BJ, Bonow RO, et al. Occurrence and significance of progressive left ventricular wall thinning and relative cavity dilatation in hypertrophic cardiomyopathy. Am J Cardiol 1987; 60: 123–9.
15. Maron BJ, Shirani J, Poliac LC, et al. Sudden death in young competitive athletes. Clinical, demographic, and pathological profiles. JAMA 1996; 276: 199–204.
16. Spirito P, Seidman CE, McKenna WJ, et al. The management of hypertrophic cardiomyopathy. N Engl J Med 1997; 336: 775–85.
17. Maron BJ. Sudden death in young athletes. N Engl J Med 2003; 349: 1064–75.
18. Watkins H. Sudden death in hypertrophic cardiomyopathy. N Engl J Med 2000; 342: 422–4.
19. Cannon RO III. Assesing risk in hypertrophic cardiomyopathy. N Engl J Med 2003; 349: 11.
20. Maron MS, Olivotto I, Betocchi S, et al. Effect of left ventricular outflow tract obstruction in clinical outcome in hypertrophic cardiomyopathy. N Engl J Med 2003; 348: 295–303.
21. Cecchi F, Olivotto I, Gistri R, et al. Coronary microvascular dysfunction and prognosis in hypertrophic cardiomyopathy. N Engl J Med 2003; 349: 1027–35.
22. Olivotto I, Girolami F, Ackerman MJ, et al. Myofilament protein gene mutation screening and outcome of patients with hypertrophic cardiomyopathy. Mayo Clin Proc 2008; 83: 630–8.
23. Bos JM, Ommen SR, Ackerman MJ. Genetics of hypertrophic cardiomyopathy: one, two, or more diseases? Curr Opin Cardiol 2007; 22: 193–9.
24. Dandona A, Roberts R. Identification of myofilament mutations: its role in the diagnosis and management of hypertrophic cardiomyopathy. Mayo Clin Proc 2008; 83: 523–5.

25. Morita H, Seidman J, Seidman C. Genetic causes of human heart failure. J Clin Invest 2005; 115: 518–26.
26. Binder J, Ommen SR, Gersh BJ, et al. Echocardiography-guided genetic testing in hypertrophic cardiomyopathy: septal morphological features predict the presence of myofilament mutations. Mayo Clin Proc 2006; 81: 459–67.
27. Anan R, Greve G, Thierfelder L, et al. Prognostic implications of novel beta cardiac myosin heavy chain gene mutations that cause familial hypertrophic cardiomyopathy. J Clin Invest 1994; 93: 280–5.
28. Ackerman MJ, VanDriest SL, Ommen SR, et al. Prevalence and age-dependence of malignant mutations in the beta-myosin heavy chain and troponin T genes in hypertrophic cardiomyopathy: a comprehensive outpatient perspective. J Am Coll Cardiol 2002; 39: 2042–8.
29. Van Driest SL, Ackerman MJ, Ommen SR, et al. Prevalence and severity of "benign" mutations in the β-myosin heavy chain, cardiac troponin T, and α-tropomyosin genes in hypertrophic cardiomyopathy. Circulation 2002; 106: 3085–90.
30. Kubo T, Gimeno JR, Bahl A, et al. Prevalence, clinical significance, and genetic basis of hypertrophic cardiomyopathy with restrictive phenotype. J Am Coll Cardiol 2007; 49: 2419–26.
31. Niimura H, Patton KK, McKenna WJ, et al. Sarcomere protein gene mutations in hypertrophic cardiomyopathy of the elderly. Circulation 2002; 105: 446–51.
32. Maron BJ, Bonow RO. Cannon RO 3rd, et al. Hypertrophic cardiomyopathy. Interrelations of clinical manifestations, pathophysiology and therapy. N Engl J Med 1987; 316: 780–9.
33. Maron BJ, Bonow RO. Cannon RO 3rd, et al. Hypertrophic cardiomyopathy. Interrelations of clinical manifestations, pathophysiology and therapy. N Engl J Med 1987; 316: 844–52.
34. Louie EK, Edwards LC 3rd. Hypertrophic cardiomyopathy. Prog Cardiovasc Dis 1994; 36: 275.
35. Maron BJ, Nishimura RA, McKenna WJ, et al. Assessment of permanent dual-chamber pacing as a treatment for drug-refractory symptomatic patients with obstructive hypertrophic cardiomyopathy. A randomized, double-blind, crossover study (M-PATHY). Circulation 1999; 99: 2927–33.
36. Ommen SR, Nishimura RA, Squires RW, et al. Comparison of dual-chamber pacing versus septal myectomy for the treatment of patients with hypertrophic obstructive cardiomyopathy: a comparison of objective hemodynamic and exercise end points. J Am Coll Cardiol 1999; 34: 191–6.
37. Maron BJ, Shen WK, Link MS, et al. Efficacy of implantable cardioverter-defibrillators for the prevention of sudden death in patients with hypertrophic cardiomyopathy. N Engl J Med 2000; 342: 365–673.
38. Maron BJ, Spirito P, Shen W-K, et al. Implantable cardioverter-defibrillators and prevention of sudden cardiac death in hypertrophic cardiomyopathy. JAMA 2007; 298: 405–12.
39. Van Driest SL, Maron BJ, Ackerman MJ. From malignant mutations to malignant domains: the continuing search for prognostic significance in the mutant genes causing hypertrophic cardiomyopathy. Heart 2004; 90: 7–8.
40. Schulte HD, Borisov K, Gams E, et al. Management of symptomatic hypertrophic obstructive cardiomyopathy-long-term results after surgical therapy. Thorac Cardiovasc Surg 1999; 47: 213–18.
41. Merrill WH, Friesinger GC, Graham TP Jr, et al. Long-lasting improvement after septal myectomy for hypertrophic obstructive cardiomyopathy. Ann Thorac Surg 2000; 69: 1732–5; discussion 1735-6.
42. Ommen SR, Maron BJ, Olivotto I, et al. Long-term effects of surgical septal myectomy on survival in patients with obstructive hypertrophic cardiomyopathy. J Am Coll Cardiol 2005; 46: 470–6.
43. Braunwald E. Induced septal infarction: a new therapeutic strategy for hypertrophic obstructive cardiomyopathy. Circulation 1997; 95: 1981–2.
44. Braunwald E. Hypertrophic cardiomyopathy – the benefits of a multidisciplinary approach. N Engl J Med 2002; 347: 1306–7.
45. Ralph-Edwards A, Woo A, McCrindle BW, et al. Hypertrophic obstructive cardiomyopathy: comparison of outcomes after myectomy or alcohol ablation adjusted by propensity score. J Thorac Cardiovasc Surg 2005; 129: 351–8.
46. Buja G, Estes M III, Wichter T, et al. Arrhythmogenic right ventricular cardiomyopathy/dysplasia: risk stratification and therapy. Prog Cardiovasc Dis 2008; 50: 282–93.
47. Tandri H, Macedo R, Calkins H, et al. Role of magnetic resonance imaging in arrhythmogenic right ventricular dysplasia: insights from the North American arrhythmogenic right ventricular dysplasia (ARVD/C) study. Am Heart J 2008; 155: 147–53.
48. Sen-Chowdhry S, Syrris P, McKenna WJ. Role of genetic analysis in the management of patients with arrhythmogenic right ventricular dysplasia/cardiomyopathy. J Am Coll Cardiol 2007; 50: 1813–21.
49. Merner ND, Hodgkinson KA, Haywood AFM, et al. Arrhythmogenic right ventricular cardiomyopathy type 5 is a fully penetrant, lethal arrhythmic disorder caused by a missense mutation in the TMEM43 gene. Am J Hum Genet 2008; 82: 809–21.

50. Dalal D, Jain R, Tandri H, et al. Long-term efficacy of catheter ablation of ventricular tachycardia in patients with arrhythmogenic right ventricular dysplasia/cardiomyopathy. J Am Coll Cardiol 2007; 50: 432–40.

51. Sen-Chowdhry S, McKenna WJ. Left ventricular noncompaction and cardiomyopathy: cause, contributor, or epiphenomenon? Curr Opin Cardiol 2008; 23: 171–5.

52. Klaassen S, Probst S, Oechslin E, et al. Mutations in sarcomere protein genes in left ventricular noncompaction. Circulation 2008; 117: 2893–901.

53. Oechslin EN, Attenhofer CH, Jost A, et al. Long-term follow-up of 34 adults with isolated left ventricular noncompaction: a distinct cardiomyopathy with poor prognosis. J Am Coll Cardiol 2000; 36: 493–500.

54. Kollberg G, Tulinius M, Gilljam T, et al. Cardiomyopathy and exercise intolerance in muscle glycogen storage disease. N Engl J Med 2007; 357: 1507–14.

55. Wolf CM, Berul CI. Inherited conduction system abnormalities: one group of diseases, many genes. J Cardiovasc Electrophysiol 2006; 17: 446–55.

56. Tan HL, Bink-Boelkens MTE, Bezzina CR, et al. A sodium-channel mutation causes isolated cardiac conduction disease. Nature 2001; 49: 1043–7.

57. Niu DM, Hwang B, Hwang HW, et al. A common SCN5A polymorphism attenuates a severe cardiac phenotype caused by a nonsense SCN5A mutation in a Chinese family with an inherited cardiac conduction defect. J Med Genet 2006; 43: 817–21.

58. Sebastiani M, Giordano C, Nediani C, et al. Induction of mitochondrial biogenesis is a maladaptive mechanism in mitochondrial cardiomyopathies. J Am Coll Cardiol 2007; 50: 1362–9.

59. van der Kooi AJ, van Langen IM, Aronica E, et al. Extension of the clinical spectrum of Danon disease. Neurology 2008; 70 :1358–63.

60. Morita H, Wu J, Zipes DP. The QT syndromes: long and short. The Lancet 2008; 372: 750–63.

61. Ellinor PT, Yi BA, MacRae CA. Genetics of atrial fibrillation. Med Clin N Am 2008; 92: 41–51.

62. Olson TM, Michael VV, Ballew JD, et al. Sodium channel mutations and susceptibility to heart failure and atrial fibrillation. JAMA 2005; 293: 447–54.

63. Torp A. Incidence of congestive cardiomyopathy. Postgrad Med J 1978; 54: 435–7.

64. Coughlin SS, Szklo M, Baughman K, et al. The epidemiology of idiopathic dilated cardiomyopathy in a biracial community. Am J Epidemiol 1990; 131: 48–56.

65. Redfield MM, Gersh BJ, Bailey KR, et al. Natural history of idiopathic dilated cardiomyopathy: effect of referral bias and secular trend. J Am Coll Cardiol 1993; 22: 1921–6.

66. Kasper EK, Agema WRP, Hutchins GM, et al. The causes of dilated cardiomyopathy: A clinicopathologic review of 673 consecutive patients. J Am Coll Cardiol 1994; 23: 586–90.

67. Michels VV, Moll PP, Miller FA, et al. The frequency of familial dilated cardiomyopathy in a series of patients with idiopathic dilated cardiomyopathy. N Engl J Med 1992; 326: 77–82.

68. Keeling PJ, Gang Y, Smith G, et al. Familial dilated cardiomyopathy in the United Kingdom. Br Heart J 1995; 73: 417–21.

69. Grunig E, Tasman JA, Kucherer H, et al. Frequency and phenotypes of familial dilated cardiomyopathy. J Am Coll Cardiol 1998; 31: 186–94.

70. Baig MK, Goldman JH, Caforio ALP, et al. Familial dilated cardiomyopathy: cardiac abnormalities are common in asymptomatic relatives and may represent early disease. J Am Coll Cardiol 1998; 31: 195–201.

71. Grogan M, Smith HC, Gersh BJ, et al. Left ventricular dysfunction due to atrial fibrillation in patients initially believed to have idiopathic dilated cardiomyopathy. Am J Cardiol 1992; 69: 1570–3.

72. Kajstura J, Zhang X, Liu Y, et al. The cellular basis of pacing-induced dilated cardiomyopathy. Myocyte cell loss and myocyte cellular reactive hypertrophy. Circulation 1995; 92: 2306–17.

73. Kushwaha SS, Fallon JT, Fuster V. Restrictive cardiomyopathy. N Engl J Med 1997; 336: 267–76.

74. Hurrell DG, Nishimura RA, Higano ST, et al. Value of dynamic respiratory changes in left and right ventricular pressures for the diagnosis of constrictive pericarditis. Circulation 1996; 93: 2007–13.

75. Kaski JP, Syrris P, Burch M, et al. Idiopathic restrictive cardiomyopathy in children is caused by mutations in cardiac sarcomere protein genes. Heart 2008; 94: 1478–84.

76. Hirota Y, Shimizu G, Kita Y, et al. Spectrum of restrictive cardiomyopathy: Report of the national survey in Japan. Am Heart J 1990; 120: 188.

77. Ammash MA, Seward JB, Bailey KR, et al. Clinical profile and outcomes of idiopathic restrictive cardiomyopathy. Circulation 2000; 101: 2490–6.

78. McCarthy RE, III, Boehmer JP, Hruban RH, et al. Long-term outcome of fulminant myocarditis as compared with acute (nonfulminant) myocarditis. N Engl J Med 2000; 342: 690–5.

79. Feldman AM, McNamara D. Myocarditis. N Engl J Med 2000; 373: 1388–98.

80. Liu P, Martino T, Opavsky MA, et al. Viral myocarditis: balance between viral infection and immune response. Can J Cardiol 1996; 12: 935–43.
81. Kawai C. From myocarditis to cardiomyopathy: mechanisms of inflammation and cell death. Circulation 1999; 99: 1091–100.
82. Why HJR, Meany BT, Richardson PJ, et al. Clinical and prognostic significance of detection of enteroviral RNA in the myocardium of patients with myocarditis or dilated cardiomyopathy. Circulation 1994; 89: 2582–9.
83. Li Y, Bourlet T, Andreoletti L, et al. Enteroviral capsid protein VP1 is present in myocardial tissues from some patients with myocarditis or dilated cardiomyopathy. Circulation 101: 231–4.
84. Archard LC, Bowles NE, Cunningham L, et al. Molecular probes for detection of persisting enterovirus infection of human heart and their prognostic value. Eur Heart J 1991; 12: 56–9.
85. Cooper LT. Myocarditis. N Engl J Med 2008; in press.
86. Kuhl U, Pauschinger M, Seeberg B, et al. Viral persistence in the myocardium is associated with progressive cardiac function. Circulation 2005; 112: 1965–70.
87. Kuhl U, Lassner D, Pauschinger M, et al. Prevalence of erythrovirus genotypes in the myocardium of patients with dilated cardiomyopathy. J Med Virol 2008; 80: 1243–51.
88. Mahrholdt H, Goedecke C, Wagner A, et al. Cardiovascular magnetic resonance assessment of human myocarditis: a comparison to histology and molecular pathology. Circulation 2004; 109: 1250–8.
89. Mason JW, O'Connell JB, Herskowitz A, et al. A clinical trial of immunosuppressive therapy for myocarditis. N Engl J Med 1995; 333: 269–75.
90. Cooper LT, Berry GJ. Shabetai, R. Idiopathic giant-cell myocarditis; natural history and treatment. N Engl J Med 1997; 336: 1860–6.
91. Davidoff R, Palacios I, Southern J, et al. Giant cell versus lymphocytic myocarditis. A comparison of their clinical features and long-term outcomes. Circulation 1991; 83: 953–61.
92. Prasad A. Apical ballooning syndrome: An important differential diagnosis of acute myocardial infarction. Circulation 2007; 115: e56–9.
93. Bybee KA, Kara T, Prasad A, et al. Systematic review: transient left ventricular apical ballooning: a syndrome that mimics ST-segment elevation myocardial infarction. Ann Intern Med 2004; 141: 858–65.
94. Wittstein IS, Thiemann DR, Lima JAC, et al. Neurohumoral features of myocardial stunning due to sudden emotional stress. N Engl J Med 2005; 352: 539–48.
95. Pearson GD, Veille JC, Rahimtoola S, et al. Peripartum cardiomyopathy. JAMA 2000; 283: 1183–8.
96. Sliwa K, Fett J, Elkayam U. Peripartum cardiomyopathy. Lancet 2006; 368: 687–93.
97. Abboud J, Murad Y, Chen-Scarabelli C, et al. Peripartum cardiomyopathy: a comprehensive review. Int J Cardiol 2007; 118: 295–303.
98. Elkayam U, Akhter MW, Singh H, et al. Pregnancy-associated cardiomyopathy: clinical characteristics and a comparison between early and late presentation. Circulation 2005; 111: 2050–5.
99. Brar SS, Khan SS, Sandhu GK, et al. Incidence, mortality and racial differences in peripartum cardiomyopathy. Am J Cardiol 2007; 100: 302–4.
100. Lamparter S, Pankuweit S, Maisch B. Clinical and immunologic characteristics in peripartum cardiomyopathy. Int J Cardiol 2007; 118: 14–20.
101. Elkayam U, Tummala PP, Rao K, et al. Maternal and fetal outcomes of subsequent pregnancies in women with peripartum cardiomyopathy. N Engl J Med 2001; 344: 1567–71.
102. Shinbane JS, Wood MA, Jensen DN, et al. Tachycardia-induced cardiomyopathy: a review of animal models and clinical studies. J Am Coll Cardiol 1997; 29: 709–15.
103. Nerheim P, Birger-Botkin S, Piracha L, et al. Heart failure and sudden death in patients with tachycardia-induced cardiomyopathy and recurrent tachycardia. Circulation 2004; 110: 247–52.
104. Duffee DF, Shen WK, Smith HC. Suppression of frequent premature ventricular contractions and improvement of left ventricular function in patients with presumed idiopathic dilated cardiomyopathy. Mayo Clin Proc 1998; 73: 430–3.
105. McGregor CGA, Rodeheffer RJ, Daly RC, et al. Heart transplantation for AL amyloidosis. J Heart Lung Transplant 2000; 19: 51.
106. Olson LJ, Edwards WD, McCall JT, et al. Cardiac iron deposition in idiopathic hemochromatosis: histologic and analytic assessment of 14 hearts from autopsy. J Am Coll Cardiol 1987; 10: 1239–43.
107. Olson LJ, Baldus WP, Tajik AJ. Echocardiographic features of idiopathic hemochromatosis. Am J Cardiol 1987; 60: 885–9.
108. Parrillo JE. Heart disease and the eosinophil. N Engl J Med 1990; 323: 1560–1.
109. deMello DE, Liapis H, Jureidini S, et al. Cardiac localization of eosinophil-granule major basic protein in acute necrotizing myocarditis. N Engl J Med 1990; 323: 1542–5.

110. Weller PF, Bubley GJ. The idiopathic hypereosinophilic syndrome. Blood 1994; 83: 2759–79.
111. Gupta PN, Valiathan MS, Balakrishnan KG, et al. Clinical course of endomyocardial fibrosis. Br Heart J 1989; 62: 450–4.
112. Shaper AG. What's new in endomyocardial fibrosis? Lancet 1993; 342: 255–6.
113. Barretto AC, Lemos da Luz P, de Oliveira SA, et al. Determinants of survival in endomyocardial fibrosis. Circulation 1989; 80(Suppl I): I-177–I-182.
114. Mocumbi AO, Ferreira MB, Sidi D, et al. A population study of endomyocardial fibrosis in a rural area of Mozambique. N Engl J Med 2008; 359: 43–9.
115. Regan TJ. Alcohol and the cardiovascular system. JAMA 1990; 264: 377–81.
116. Urbano-Marquez A, Estruch R, Navarro-Lopez F, et al. The effects of alcoholism on skeletal and cardiac muscle. N Engl J Med 1989; 320: 409–15.
117. Urbano-Marquez A, Estruch R, Fernandez-Sola J, et al. The greater risk of alcoholic cardiomyopathy and myopathy in women compared with men. JAMA 1995; 274: 149–54.
118. Kupari M, Koskinen P. Relation of left ventricular function to habitual alcohol consumption. Am J Cardiol 1993; 72: 1418–24.
119. Floyd JD, Nguyen DT, Lobins RL, et al. Cardiotoxicity of cancer therapy. J Clin Oncol 2005; 23: 7685–96.
120. Perez EA, Suman VJ, Davidson NE, et al. Cardiac safety analysis of doxorubicin and cyclophosphamide followed by paclitaxel with or without trastuzumab in the N9831 Adjuvant Breast Cancer Trial. J Clin Oncol 2008; 26: 1231–8.

10

Water and salt: The cardiorenal syndrome

Maria Rosa Costanzo

INTRODUCTION

The term "cardiorenal syndrome" often refers to a condition in which renal impairment occurs as a result of cardiac dysfunction (1). This view has been supported by the observation that a previously impaired renal function normalizes after a cardiac assist device is implanted in a patient with end-stage heart failure (HF) (2). The expression "cardiorenal syndrome" has also been used to describe the negative effects of renal disorders on heart structure and function (3). Thus, although the term "cardiorenal syndrome" is loosely applied to many pathologic interactions between the heart and the kidney, a comprehensive definition is lacking. To be inclusive of the damage/dysfunction produced in either the heart or the kidney by an acute or chronic disease of the other organ, the cardiorenal syndrome should be classified according to whether the impairment of each organ is primary, secondary or whether abnormal heart and kidney functions occur simultaneously as a result of a systemic disease (4). For example, acute HF decompensation can cause both acute renal injury and chronic kidney disease: a decreased cardiac output is associated with renal arterial underfilling and increased venous pressure which, in turn, result in a reduced glomerular filtration rate (GFR) (3). Activation of the renin–angiotensin–aldosterone system (RAAS), initially aimed at restoring GFR, eventually leads to increased renal expression of endothelin-1 (ET-1), a potent proinflammatory and profibrotic vasoconstrictor peptide known to mediate acute and chronic kidney injury (4).

In chronic HF, increased sympathetic nervous system (SNS) and RAAS activity augment oxidative stress to the kidneys, and impair action of nitric oxide (NO) on the vascular endothelium (5). Activation of the RAAS, which increases the production of angiotensin II (A II) and aldosterone within the kidney, is a key factor in the development of end-organ damage in the heart, vasculature, and kidneys (6). Chronic HF is often complicated by anemia, known to independently worsen hemodynamic and clinical outcomes, and by the release of inflammatory cytokines, including tumor necrosis factor-alpha (TNF-α), interleukin-1 (IL-1), and interleukin-6 (IL-6). This inflammation leads to gradual toxic injury to renal cells and eventually to chronic kidney damage and functional loss (4).

Conversely, acute kidney injury can provoke cardiac failure. Models of postischemic renal injury have demonstrated the intrarenal accumulation of neutrophils, macrophages/monocytes, and lymphocytes and increased circulating levels of inflammatory cytokines, which can impair contractility and trigger myocyte apoptosis (4).

Chronic kidney disease independently increases the risk of cardiovascular disease by promoting myocardial hypertrophy, coronary atherosclerosis and fluid overload. Anemia, advanced glycation end-products (AGEs), abnormal calcium–phosphate metabolism, nutritional factors, extracellular fluid accumulation, inflammation, insulin resistance, hyperhomocysteinemia, oxidative stress, and dyslipidemia have all been implicated in the amplification of cardiovascular morbidity by chronic kidney disease (5). In addition, by inhibiting Na–potassium–adenosine triphosphatase (Na–K–ATPase), uremic toxins may increase contractile force and impair relaxation of cardiac myocytes, thus contributing to the diastolic dysfunction commonly encountered in patients with chronic kidney disease (4).

Finally, highly prevalent conditions, such as diabetes and hypertension, and less common ones, including autoimmune diseases, amyloidosis, pulmonary arterial hypertension, and sepsis can simultaneously damage heart and kidneys (4,5).

This chapter examines the epidemiology of the cardiorenal syndrome, reviews the mechanisms of renal handling of sodium (Na) and water, describes how these mechanisms are altered in the setting of acute and chronic HF and kidney disease, and describes the therapeutic challenges posed by the cardiorenal syndrome.

EPIDEMIOLOGY

Renal impairment in HF patients is common and independently associated with increased morbidity and mortality (7–11). In the Candesartan in Heart Failure Assessment of Reduction in Mortality and Morbidity (CHARM) study, the level of renal dysfunction was a powerful independent predictor of death or hospitalization for HF (12). The Acute Decompensated Heart Failure National Registry (ADHERE), a large U.S. database of 105,388 hospitalized HF patients, reported that 30% had chronic kidney disease (13). Approximately 20% of the patients had serum creatinine (Cr) > 2.0 mg/dL, 9% had Cr > 3.0 mg/dL, and 5% were treated with dialysis (13). A meta-analysis of 16 studies spanning 60 years and including 80,098 HF patients with variably defined renal impairment showed that 63% of patients had any renal impairment, and 29% had moderate to severe impairment. Adjusted all-cause mortality was significantly increased in patients with any renal impairment. Mortality worsened incrementally across the range of renal dysfunction, with 15% increased risk for every 0.5 mg/dL increase in Cr and 7% increased risk for every 10 mL/min decrease in estimated GFR (eGFR) (14). Among 6440 HF patients hospitalized between 1987 and 2002, age and admission Cr increased, eGFR and hemoglobin decreased over the 16-year period analyzed (15). The Evaluation Study of Congestive Heart Failure and Pulmonary Artery Catheterization Effectiveness (ESCAPE) trial showed that, compared with historical data, episodes of HF decompensation were more commonly associated with renal dysfunction and the requirement of higher diuretic doses at discharge (16). Thus cardiorenal failure in patients hospitalized for HF is becoming more frequent and severe and equally frequent in patients with preserved or decreased left ventricular ejection fraction (LVEF) (14,15,17). Several studies have documented that, during hospitalization for HF, >70% of patients will experience some increase in Cr, with approximately 20–30% having increments >0.3 mg/dL (15,17–22). Worsening renal function (WRF) occurs early in the course of hospitalization and is independently associated with longer hospitalizations, greater costs, and higher short- and long-term mortality (15,17–23). Nonetheless, it remains unclear whether the WRF itself contributes to the increased mortality or whether it represents more advanced disease. Rates of WRF during hospitalization are similar in patients with decreased or preserved LVEF (14,15,17). The ADHERE documented that almost 90% of hospitalized HF patients are treated with intravenous (IV) diuretics. With this approach the average weight loss is only 2.5 lb and 20% of patients actually gain weight during hospitalization (13). Furthermore, more than 40% of these patients are discharged with unresolved congestion (13). These disappointing outcomes have been attributed to diuretic resistance, defined as persistent pulmonary and peripheral congestion with or without worsening renal function despite attempts at diuresis (24). Patients with under-lying renal disease are at especially high risk for developing diuretic-induced WRF before euvolemia can be achieved (24).

The common risk factors of hypertension, diabetes mellitus, and atherosclerosis explain the high prevalence of coexistent cardiac and renal dysfunction (23). Successful reduction in mortality from HF, acute myocardial infarction (MI), stroke, and extracar-diac disease may result in protracted exposure to risk factors for renal dysfunction. Importantly, because Cr is secreted by the kidney, Cr clearance or eGFR, as calculated with the simplified Modification of Diet in Renal Disease (MDRD) or Cockcroft–Gault equations, provide a more accurate appraisal of renal function than Cr (25,26). On aver-age, persons developing WRF are older and more often have prior HF, renal dysfunction, diabetes, and hypertension. Cox regression analysis in 1004 diverse HF patients permit-ted the development of a risk score for predicting which patients with acutely decompen-sated HF would develop WRF. With the allocation of 1 point each to HF history, diabetes, and systolic blood pressure >160 mmHg at admission; 2 points to Cr 1.5–2.4 mg/dL; and 3 points to Cr ≥ 2.5 mg/dL, 35% of the patients had a score of ≥3 and a 43% likelihood of WRF (17).

The data summarized above illustrate that renal dysfunction is common in HF patients, portends a poor prognosis and poses complex therapeutic challenges.

BASIC PRINCIPLES FOR RENAL SODIUM AND WATER HANDLING
Salt and Water Transport Across the Nephron

The body content of Na, chloride (Cl), and water is regulated by control of their renal excre-tion (27). The normal kidney can vary NaCl excretion over daily ingestion amounts ranging from 0.05 to 25 g and daily urinary water excretion from approximately 0.4 to 25 L. Water, Na, and Cl are freely filtered by the renal gomeruli and undergo more than 99% tubular reabsorption and no secretion (28). While Na reabsorption is mainly an active, transcellular process driven by Na–K–ATPase, that of Cl is both by passive paracellular diffusion and by active transcellular transport coupled with Na. Water is reabsorbed by osmosis secondary to NaCl reabsorption (Fig. 10.1) (29).

Of the filtered Na, 65% is reabsorbed at the proximal tubule (PT), 25% at the loop of Henle, and most of the remaining 10% at the distal convoluted tubule (DCT) and collecting duct system, so that the final urine contains <1% of the filtered Na (Table 10.1). Reabsorption of Na throughout the nephron is under neural, hormonal, and paracrine control (30–32). Due to the large quantity of filtered Na, small changes in reabsorption can result in large differences in excretion. Throughout the nephron, the key event is the active transfer of Na from cell to interstitial fluid by the Na–K–ATPase pumps in the basolateral cell membrane. Because these pumps keep the intra-cellular Na concentration below that of the interstitium and the intracellular compartment is negatively charged compared with the tubular lumen, Na ions enter the cell passively, down their electrochemical gradient. The entry processes for Na at the luminal mem-brane of the PT include various symporters, Na–hydrogen (H) antiporters and Na chan-nels (Fig. 10.1) (33).

Because of the restriction of electroneutrality, 1 L of normal filtrate containing 140 mEq of Na, must contain about 140 mEq of anions, mainly Cl (110 mEq) and bicarbonate (24 mEq). If 91 mEq (65%) of filtered Na is reabsorbed in the PT, approximately 91 mEq of Cl and bicarbonate must also be reabsorbed to accompany Na. A sufficiently high intra-cellular Cl concentration must be achieved to cause Cl movement out of the cell across the basolateral membrane. The luminal membrane Cl transporters function similarly to the Na–K–ATPase pumps located in the basolateral cell membrane (34). The movement of Cl

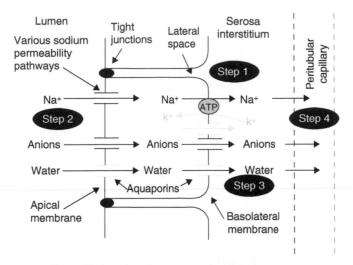

Figure 10.1 Steps involved in solute and water transport from the tubular lumen to the peritubular capillary. Events depend on and follow logically from Step 1, which is the active extrusion of sodium into the interstitium. This induces a parallel transport of anions (Step 2). The movement of sodium and anions generates an osmotic drive that causes reabsorption of water (Step 3). Finally, the increased volume in the interstitium alters peritubular Starling forces and induces the bulk flow of water and solute from interstitium into the peritubular capillary (Step 4). *Source*: From Ref. 364.

Table 10.1 Sodium and Water Reabsorption along the Tubule

	Percentage of Filtered Load Reabsorbed (%)	
Tubular segment	Sodium	Water
Proximal tubule	65	65
Descending thin limb of loop of Henle	—	10
Ascending thin limb and thick Ascending limb of loop of Henle	25	—
Distal convoluted tubule	5	—
Collecting duct system	4–5	5 (with water loading) >24 (with dehydration)

across this membrane is also facilitated by the negative intracellular potential. The major routes of Cl movement are paracellular absorption and Na–H and Cl–base antiporters. Thus, transmembrane Cl movements are linked to those of Na (34).

Water constitutes approximately 55–65% of body weight. Of total body water (TBW) 55–65% resides in the intracellular fluid (ICF) and 35–45% in the extracellular fluid (ECF), three-fourths of which is interstitial- and one-fourth intravascular fluid (plasma) (35) (Table 10.2). Membrane-bound Na/K pumps maintain Na in a primarily extracellular- and K in a primarily intracellular location. Osmotic pressure, a function of the concentrations of all the solutes in a fluid compartment, is always equivalent in the ICF and ECF because most biologic membranes are freely permeable to water but not to aqueous solutes (semipermeable). Thus, water will flow across membranes into a compartment with a higher solute concentration until a steady state is reached where the osmotic pressures have equalized on both sides of the cell membrane (36). Osmolality is defined as the

Table 10.2 Body Fluid Compartments in Man

Compartment	Amount	Volume (L) in a 70 kg Male
Total body fluid	60% of body weight	42
Intracellular fluid	40% of body weight	28
Extracellular fluid	20% of body weight	14
Interstitial fluid	2/3 of extracellular fluid	9.4
Intravascular fluid (plasma)	1/3 of extracellular fluid	4.6
Venous fluid	85% of plasma	3.9
Arterial fluid	15% of plasma	0.7

concentration of all of the solutes in a given weight of water. Plasma osmolality can be estimated as:

$$P_{osm} \text{(mOsm/kg } H_2O) = 2 \times \text{serum [Na](mmol/L + glucose (mmol/L) + blood urea nitrogen (mmol/L)}$$

Serum [Na] ([.] means concentration) is doubled because of its accompanying anions. Solutes that are impermeable to cell membranes (mannitol) are restricted to the ECF compartment and are effective in creating osmotic pressure gradients across cell membranes favoring the movement of water from ICF to ECF. Solutes permeable to cell membranes (urea, ethanol, and methanol) are not associated with such water shifts. Only the effective solutes in plasma determine whether there is clinically significant hyperosmolality or hypo-osmolality. Thus, elevation of serum [Na], does not cause cellular dehydration, and consequently does not activate mechanisms that increase body water stores (37).

The kidney can produce large quantities of hypotonic urine in response to a water load, and low volume, hypertonic urine during dehydration. To alter urine osmolality, the kidney must be able to *independently* control excretion of salt and water. Diluted urine reflects solute reabsorption in excess of water, whereas urine is concentrated when water is reabsorbed in excess of solute (38).

The two sources of body water are oxidation of carbohydrates and ingestion. Of the filtered water 65% is reabsorbed in PT, 10% in the descending thin limb of Henle's loop, and a variable amount in the collecting duct system. In the PT Na and water are reabsorbed to the same extent. In Henle's loop, the fraction of Na reabsorbed always exceeds that of water. Sodium, but not water reabsorption, occurs in the DCT. Both Na and water are reabsorbed in the collecting duct system in highly variable amounts (Table 10.1) (39).

Permeability of luminal membranes to water is high in the PT and descending thin limb of Henle's loop, low in the ascending limbs of Henle's loop and DCT, intrinsically low, but highly regulated in the collecting duct system. The ability of the kidneys to produce hyperosmotic urine up to 1400 mOsm/kg, or five times the osmolality of plasma, is a major defense from dehydration. Because the daily sum of the urea, sulfate, phosphate, and other ions averages approximately 600 mOsm/day, the smallest volume of water in which this mass of solute can be dissolved is roughly 600 mmol/1400 mOsm/L, or 0.43 L/day.

In the PT, a large fraction of the filtered Na enters the cell across the luminal membrane via antiport with carbon dioxide- and water-derived protons, which cause the secondary active reabsorption of filtered bicarbonate. Early in the PT Cl reabsorption occurs primarily via paracellular diffusion, because the reabsorption of water, driven by that of Na and its cotransported solutes and bicarbonate, causes [Cl] in the tubular lumen to exceed that of peritubular capillaries. Furthermore, in the PT Cl is also actively transported from lumen to cell by parallel Na–H and Cl–base antiporters. Transport of Cl into the cell is powered by the downhill antiport of organic bases continuously generated in the cell by dissociation of their respective acids into proton and base (34). Simultaneously, these protons are actively transported into the lumen by Na–H antiporters. In the lumen, the protons and organic bases recombine to form the neutral form of the acid, which then diffuses across the luminal membrane back into the cell, where the entire process is repeated. All these processes depend on the ability of the basolateral membrane Na–K–ATPases to establish the gradient for Na that powers the luminal Na–H antiporter (33). Due to the PT's high water permeability, very small differences in osmolality created by solute reabsorption (1–2 mOsm/L) suffice to drive the reabsorption of approximately 65% of the filtered water. Early in the PT, intraluminal fluid osmolality is nearly equal to that of plasma and interstitial fluid. Solute reabsorption from the lumen lowers luminal osmolality below that of interstitial fluid. The resulting osmotic gradient causes osmosis of water from the lumen across the plasma membranes or tight junctions into the interstitial fluid (40). Because the Starling forces across the peritubular capillaries in the interstitium favor reabsorption, water and solutes then move into the peritubular capillaries and are returned to the general circulation. This iso-osmotic volume reabsorption in the PT can be disrupted by *osmotic diuresis*, a process in which unreabsorbed solute (such as glucose exceeding its tubular maximum) prevents water from following Na, causing [Na] in the PT lumen to fall slightly below that in the interstitial fluid, driving a net passive diffusion of Na across the epithelium back into the lumen and increasing the amount of Na reaching the loop of Henle (41). This segment reabsorbs proportionally more Na and Cl (≈25% of the filtered loads) than water (≈10% of the filtered water). The *descending* limb reabsorbs predominantly water, whereas the *ascending* limbs reabsorb Na and Cl but little water (42). Sodium and Cl are reabsorbed passively in the thin- and actively in the thick ascending limb. Water reabsorption in the descending limb concentrates luminal Na and creates a favorable gradient for passive paracellular Na reabsorption. In the ascending limb the luminal entry steps for Na and Cl include the Na–K–2Cl symporter, which is the target of loop diuretics and, to a lesser extent, an Na-H antiporter similar to that present in the PT. In addition to active transcellular reabsorption, as much as 50% of total Na reabsorption in this segment occurs by paracellular diffusion, made possible by the continuous operation of the Na–K–ATPase. Because the ascending limb reabsorbs NaCl but not water, the DCT is hypo-osmotic compared with plasma (43).

In the DCT Na and Cl are actively reabsorbed by the Na–Cl symporter, the target of thiazide diuretics. In the collecting ducts reabsorption of Na and water occurs in the principal cells, which also play a major role in potassium homeostasis. Reabsorption of Cl is partially passive, via paracellular pathways, and active in the intercalated cells of the collecting ducts (34). The principal cells reabsorb Na via epithelial Na channels whose regulation is critical for overall body fluid homeostasis. Some NaCl reabsorption continues in the medullary collecting ducts through epithelial Na channels.

Water permeability of the DCT is always very low, rendering tubular fluid more hypo-osmotic than in the thick ascending limb of Henle's. The water permeability of the collecting duct system is controlled by the hormone arginine–vasopressin (AVP), also known as antidiuretic hormone (44). When water permeability is very low, the fluid entering the collecting duct system remains hypo-osmotic. When this fluid reaches the medullary collecting ducts, the large osmotic gradient favors some water reabsorption. However, because of the high tubular volume not reabsorbed in the cortex, most of the water entering the medullary collecting duct reaches the ureter (water diuresis) (45). In these tubular segments the intraluminal Na concentration can be lowered almost to zero and osmolality can be as low as 50 mOsm/kg because the "tight epithelia" minimize back-leak of Na (46). When water permeability of the collecting ducts is high, as the hypo-osmotic fluid entering the collecting duct system from the DCT flows through the cortical collecting ducts, water is rapidly reabsorbed due to the large difference in osmolality between the hypo-osmotic luminal fluid and the iso-osmotic (285 mOsm/kg) cortical interstitial fluid. Once luminal fluid and interstitial fluids are nearly iso-smotic, the cortical collecting duct reabsorbs similar amounts of NaCl and water. As a result, the tubular fluid leaving the cortical collecting duct to enter the medullary collecting duct is iso-osmotic with cortical plasma, and its volume is greatly reduced compared with the amount arriving from the distal tubule. In the medullary collecting duct solute reabsorption continues but water reabsorption is proportionally even greater, rendering tubular fluid increasingly more hyperosmotic and contracted in its passage through the medullary collecting ducts because the interstitial fluid of the medulla is very hyperosmotic (46). Without AVP the water permeability of the cortical and outer medullary collecting duct is very low, and water diuresis occurs. As plasma AVP concentrations increase, water permeability of the collecting ducts gradually increases resulting in progressively more hyperosmotic urine (Fig. 10.2). Binding of AVP to its type 2 (V2) receptors in the basolateral membrane of the principal cells activates adenylate cyclase, the catalyst of intracellular production of cyclic adenosine monophosphate (cAMP), which induces the migration to, and fusion with the luminal membrane of intracellular vesicles containing an isoform of the water channel protein, aquaporin 2, through which water is reabsorbed (46). In the absence of AVP, the aquaporins are withdrawn from the luminal membrane by endocytosis (47).

The osmolality of the medullary interstitium increases from a nearly iso-osmotic value at the corticomedullary border, to >1000 mOsm/kg at the papilla (48). This osmotic gradient is produced by active NaCl transport from lumen to interstitium in the thick ascending limb; the vascular configuration of the medulla with closely located descending and ascending blood vessels; and the recycling of urea between medullary collecting ducts and deep portions of the loops of Henle. At the junction of inner and outer medulla, the thick ascending limbs of all loops of Henle simultaneously dilute the luminal fluid and concentrate the interstitium by removing water-free solute. This is the process inhibited by loop diuretics that block the Na–K–2Cl symporter. As a result, the urine becomes iso-osmotic. In the cortex, the solute reabsorbed by the ascending thick limb mixes with that reabsorbed by the nearby PT and, because of the abundant peritubular capillaries, moves into the vasculature and returns to the general circulation. In contrast, the low blood flow of the medulla and the parallel arrangement of the vasa recta, throughout which the solute and water move freely, allow the solute to accumulate in the medullary interstitium and produce an osmolality much greater than that of the entering blood. Because the vasa recta return to the corticomedullary junction, as the hyperosmotic plasma flows upward, it again tends to equilibrate with the surrounding interstitium, which is now decreasing in osmolality (48). The flow of blood in opposite directions in parallel vessels and the ability of the vessels to at least partially equilibrate with the surrounding interstitium constitute the *countercurrent exchange system*, which is critically important in maintaining the medullary osmotic gradient (49). Of the freely filtered urea (plasma concentration 5 mmol/L), 50% is reabsorbed in the PT and 50% is secreted in the thin portion of the loop of Henle, thus restoring the amount of tubular urea back to the filtered load, which remains unchanged up to the origin of the inner medullary collecting ducts (49). Because by this point the vast majority of water has been reabsorbed, the luminal urea concentration is 50 times higher than its plasma value (≥500 mmol/L). In the inner medullary collecting ducts, some urea is reabsorbed via specialized uniporters. Because blood flow in this region is low, the reabsorbed urea raises the interstitial concentration close to that in the lumen. Thus by moving back into the interstitium, urea contributes greatly to the hyperosmolality of the medulla, allowing the kidneys to excrete hyperosmotic urine. In fact, when metabolic urea production is reduced by low protein intake, the ability of kidneys to produce highly concentrated urine is compromised (37).

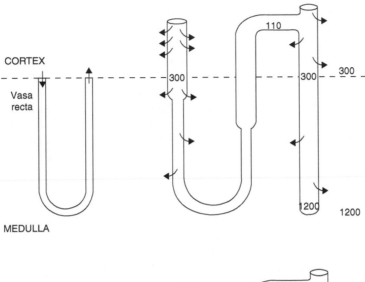

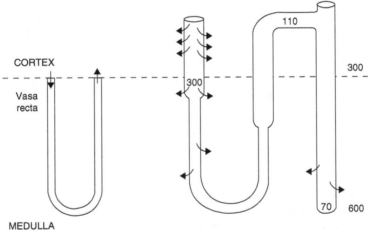

Figure 10.2 Renal water handling in states of maximum antidiuresis (**A**) and maximum diuresis (**B**). Numbers to the right indicate interstitial osmolarity, whereas those in the tubules indicate luminal osmolarity. Arrows indicate sites of water reabsorption. In both antidiuresis and diuresis, 65% of the filtered water is reabsorbed in the proximal tubule and another 10% in the descending loop of Henle. The relatively greater reabsorption of solute by the loop as a whole results in luminal fluid that is quite dilute in the distal tubule (110 mOsm). During antidiuresis, the actions of AVP permit further water reabsorption in the cortical and medullary collecting tubules, resulting in a final fluid that is very hyperosmotic (1200 mOsm). During diuresis, no water reabsorption occurs in the cortical collecting tubule, but some occurs in the inner medullary collecting tubule. Continued solute reabsorption reduces solute content even more than water content, and the final urine is very dilute (70 mOsm). In the parallel vasa recta, there is considerable exchange of both solute and water, so that plasma osmolarity and solute concentration equilibrate with the surrounding interstitium. The vasa recta remove solute and water reabsorbed in the medulla. Because there is always some net volume reabsorption in the medulla even in states of diuresis, the vasa recta plasma flow out of the medulla always exceeds plasma inflow. *Source*: From Ref. 364.

Importantly, AVP raises urea permeability by stimulating a specific AVP-sensitive isoform of the urea uniporters in the inner medullary collecting ducts. Dehydration decreases GFR and AVP levels rise (48). Because AVP-induced water extraction in the cortical collecting duct removes most of the water from the lumen, a greatly reduced luminal volume flows through the hyperosmolar medulla, where further concentration occurs. With overhydration GFR increases and AVP levels decline. Because only a small amount of tubular fluid is reabsorbed in the cortical collecting ducts, a high volume of very dilute fluid with a modest urea concentration is delivered to the inner medullary collecting ducts, which have poor water permeability without AVP. Because the local osmotic driving force is great, some water, but little urea is reabsorbed. In fact, urea may initially be secreted due to a lower concentration in the lumen than in the medullary interstitium. Thus during maximum dehydration the osmolality of the medullary interstitium falls to about half of its value (500–600 mOsm/kg) (50).

RENAL REGULATION OF PLASMA VOLUME, PLASMA OSMOLALITY, AND SYSTEMIC BLOOD PRESSURE

Blood pressure is crucial in salt and water balance because it plays a key role in generating the signals that alter renal handling of Na and water. Blood pressure is regulated around a value controlled by a group of brainstem nuclei (the *vasomotor center*). The two major types of detectors for the short-term control blood pressure are nerve cells with sensory endings in the carotid arteries and aortic arch (high-pressure baroreceptors), which through sensory neural pathways report arterial blood pressure to the vasomotor center and nerve cells with sensory endings in the atria and parts of the pulmonary vasculature (low-pressure baroreceptors) (51). These cardiopulmonary baroreceptors function as blood volume detectors, because atrial and pulmonary vascular pressures rise and fall, respectively, when blood volume increases and decreases. High- and low-pressure baroreceptors send afferent neural information to the brainstem vasomotor center, which, in response to the information from these baroreceptors, sends regulatory autonomic signals to effector systems, such as the heart, blood vessels, and kidneys (51). The activity of the vasomotor center mediates SNS signals that directly alter vascular tone, with consequent changes in peripheral vascular resistance and central venous pressure (CVP). A decrease in blood pressure increases SNS activity, which raises peripheral vascular resistance, CVP, heart rate, and cardiac contractility to produce a rapid restoration of normal blood pressure. These rapid mechanisms are activated for blood pressure alterations due to muscular activity or postural changes and stabilize arterial pressure at a mean arterial pressure, which is typically slightly below 100 mmHg. Mean arterial pressure, which has diurnal fluctuations related to activity, emotions, and sleep, is determined, in the long term, by the kidney through salt and water handling (52). If renal excretion is inappropriate for several days, mean arterial pressure is reset to a new value.

In addition to initiating rapid blood pressure responses (few seconds), changes in SNS signals also have effects on intrarenal baroreceptors that contribute to the intermediate-term (> few tens of seconds) regulation of blood pressure. These baroreceptors are the afferent arteriole's pressure-sensitive granular cells that detect renal afferent arteriolar pressure and form part of the *juxtaglomerular apparatus* (53). Neural signals generated by the vasomotor center in response to inputs from vascular baroreceptors reach the granular cells via the renal sympathetic nerve. In response to changes in afferent arteriolar pressure *or* signals from the renal sympathetic nerves, the granular cells release the peptide hormone *renin*, a proteolytic enzyme that cleaves angiotensinogen of hepatic origin to form angiotensin I (Fig. 10.3) (54). The angiotensin-converting enzyme (ACE) in endothelial cells of pulmonary and renal capillaries further cleaves angiotensin I to produce A II, a potent

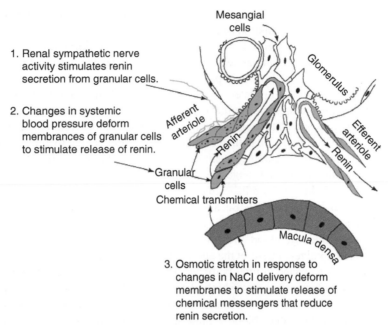

1. Renal sympathetic nerve activity stimulates renin secretion from granular cells.

2. Changes in systemic blood pressure deform membrances of granular cells to stimulate release of renin.

3. Osmotic stretch in response to changes in NaCl delivery deform membranes to stimulate release of chemical messengers that reduce renin secretion.

Figure 10.3 There are three primary mechanisms regulating renin secretion. First, when blood pressure falls, renal sympathetic nerve activity increases and activates β_1-adrenergic receptors on granular cells of the afferent arteriole to stimulate renin secretion. Second, the granular cells also act as "intrarenal baroreceptors." They respond to changes in pressure within the afferent arteriole, which, except in cases of renal artery stenosis, is a reflection of changes in systemic blood pressure. Deformation of the membranes of the granular cells alters renin secretion: When pressure falls, renin production increases. Third, macula densa cells in the thick ascending limb sense sodium chloride delivery by changing the uptake of salt, with subsequent osmotic swelling. Changes in cell volume lead to the release of chemical transmitters that alter renin secretion from the granular cells: When sodium chloride delivery increases, renin production decreases. *Source*: From Ref. 364.

vasoconstrictor, which increases total peripheral resistance and blood pressure (55). Vascular changes mediated by A II occur at a slower pace and last longer (tens of seconds or minutes). Activation of β_1-adrenergic receptors on the granular cells by renal sympathetic nerves stimulates renin secretion via a cAMP and protein kinase A-dependent process and decreases renal blood flow (RBF) by afferent arteriolar constriction (56). Intrarenal baroreceptors on granular cells are deformed by changes in afferent arteriolar pressure, and therefore function both as detectors of renal arteriolar pressure and effectors, through renin release. Communication between the vasomotor system and the renin-producing granular cells ensures tight coordination between the rapid baroreceptor reflexes and the slower-acting RAAS. Importantly, intrareneal mechanisms regulate renin release not by direct blood pressure detection but by sensing the amount of NaCl that leaves the thick ascending limb, bathes *macula densa* cells and is delivered to the DCT. Such NaCl amount depends on Na filtration and reabsorption rates in all nephron segments proximal to the macula densa (57). Because filtration rate is partially regulated by SNS-mediated afferent arteriolar vasoconstriction, the macula densa NaCl load detector integrates blood pressure and SNS activity with the reabsorptive capacity of the PT and loop of Henle to regulate renin release (58). When [NaCl] and flow rate increase, the enhanced uptake of NaCl by the macula densa cells causes their osmotic swelling which, in turn, mediates inhibition of renin release (54). Thus the salt load detector in the macula densa couples the short-term SNS activity and A II-mediated regulation of blood pressure with the long-term blood pressure regulation achieved by the control of NaCl and water excretion. Furthermore, the binding of A II to AT1 receptors on granular cells acts as a negative feedback to increase intracellular [Ca], which, in turn, inhibits renin production. Thus the mean blood pressure around which the baroreceptor reflex operates, is ultimately established by the kidneys (59). The intravascular pressure required for optimal organ perfusion can be generated only when the cardiac chambers and vasculature are filled by an adequate blood volume which, in turn, depends on total ECF volume. Sustained changes in ECF volume due to altered renal handling of Na and water, will eventually overcome the ability of baroreceptor reflexes to keep blood pressure within the normal range. Because ECF volume is the ratio of total osmoles and osmolarity, the kidney accomplishes the task of regulating ECF volume by regulating the total osmotic content of the ECF. Because Na and its anions account for more than 90% of the ECF osmotic content, by controlling plasma osmolality the kidney regulates ECF volume and, consequently, blood pressure (60). According to the physiologic events described above, the kidneys interpret the alterations in blood pressure detected by vascular and renal sensors as a change in total body Na. Thus an increased renal artery pressure is interpreted by the kidney as excess of both plasma Na and volume, which then promotes Na and water excretion (pressure natriuresis and diuresis) (45). In other words the kidney produces isotonic urine to reduce blood volume and, consequently, pressure. This is largely achieved by reduction in Na reabsorption in the PT and increased Na delivery to the loop of Henle, made possible by a reduction in apical membrane Na–H antiporters and in the activity of basolateral Na–K–ATPase. Because proximal Na transport mechanisms are primarily modulated by A II and SNS signals, failure of peritubular A II levels to decrease despite an increased systemic blood pressure, blunts or even eliminates pressure natriuresis and diuresis (61). The body volume status acts as a "gain control" mechanism on pressure natriuresis and diuresis because for similar elevations in renal artery pressure, the degree of salt and water excretion is high when ECF volume is normal or high, and low when ECF volume is contracted.

Because Na excretion represents the difference between filtration and reabsorption, regulation of GFR obviously plays a role in the regulation of Na excretion (Table 10.3). The reflex control of GFR occurs through changes in afferent and efferent arteriolar resistance due to changes in renal SNS activity and circulating A II levels. Because a change in the amount of Na filtered due to a change in GFR is also accompanied by a change in the amount of filtered water, and any modification of GFR represents a mechanism for altering ECF volume rather than for the independent regulating of salt and water (62–66).

Changes in afferent arteriolar resistance also alter RBF and glomerular capillary pressure (Fig. 10.4). Glomerular damage can result from substantial reductions in RBF and marked increases in glomerular capillary pressures (62–66). In addition, the kidney's ability to preserve electrolyte and water homeostasis hinges on maintaining tubular flow (i.e., GFR) within a narrow range. Therefore, the kidney has specific mechanisms for blunting responses that would otherwise lead to large changes in GFR (*autoregulation*) or RBF (*tubuloglomerular feedback*) (62–67). Autoregulation of GFR depends on intrarenal synthesis of prostaglandins (which oppose the renal effects of A II), arteriolar vasodilation, and mesangial cells relaxation (62). Increased intrarenal A II concentrations resulting from renin release and increased SNS activity stimulate the production of prostaglandins, which protect RBF and GFR despite systemic vasoconstriction (67). Tubuloglomerular feedback is centered on the macula densa NaCl load detector (Fig. 10.5) (68). When GFR (i.e., NaCl delivery) is high, the macula densa cells swell due to avid NaCl and K uptake through Na–K–2Cl symporters (69). Increased luminal NaCl, by stimulating the Na–H antiporter,

Table 10.3 Summary of Direct Determinants of GFR

Direct Determinants of GFR = GFR = K_f $(P_{cg} - P_{bc} - \Pi_{gc})$			Factors which Increase the Magnitude of the Direct Determinants
Filtration coefficient (K_f)	1. ↑		Glomerular surface area (because of relaxation of glomerular mesangial cells) Result: ↑ GFR
Glomerular capillary hydrostatic pressure (P_{cg})	1. 2. 3.	↑ ↓ ↑	Renal artery pressure Afferent arteriolar resistance (afferent dilatation) Efferent arteriolar resistance (efferent constriction) Result: ↑ GFR
Bowman's capsule hydrostatic pressure (P_{bc})	1. ↑		Intratubular pressure due to tubule or extrarenal urinary system obstruction Result: ↓ GFR
Glomerular capillary oncotic pressure (Π_{gc})	1. 2.	↑ ↓	Systemic plasma oncotic pressure (sets Π_{gc} at the onset of glomerular capillaries) Renal plasma flow (causes increase of Π_{gc} along glomerular capillaries) Result: ↓ GFR

Abbreviation: GFR, glomerular filtration rate.

enables intracellular movement of Ca, which mediates the release of ATP from the basolateral surface of the cells in close proximity to the glomerular mesangial cells. The ATP stimulation of purinergic P2 and adenosine receptors on mesangial- and afferent arteriolar smooth muscle cells increases intracellular Ca and promotes contraction. Increased Ca in the afferent arteriolar cells also reduces renin secretion (66). Mesangial cells contraction decreases the effective filtration area, which decreases GFR. Afferent arteriolar smooth muscle cells contraction decreases RBF and GFR (62–69). As a relatively minor contribution, the increase in intracellular Ca of the granular cells inhibits their renin production, thus reducing local production of A II and of prostaglandins, which would normally counteract the vasoconstrictive effects of the purinergic agonists (64). Nitric oxide plays a secondary role in sustaining tubuloglomerular feedback whose net effect is to blunt pressure natriuresis and diuresis, and thus preserve other aspects of renal tubular function (70). A rise in interstitial pressure causes back-leak of reabsorbed fluid from the interstitial space across the tight junctions into the tubule, thus reducing net Na and water reabsorption. An increase in peritubular–capillary hydrostatic pressure (P_{PC}) reduces movement of fluid from the interstitium into the capillaries, causing fluid to accumulate in the interstitium and raise interstitial pressure. A decrease in peritubular–capillary oncotic pressure (Π_{PC}) has similar effects. The P_{PC} is set by arterial pressure and the combined afferent and efferent arteriolar resistances, which determine the extent of attenuation of the arterial pressure reaching the peritubular capillaries. The Π_{PC} depends on arterial oncotic pressure and filtration fraction (GFR/RPF), which determine the magnitude of oncotic pressure rise during passage through the glomeruli.

Fluid loss lowers GFR through neurohormonally mediated afferent and efferent arterioles constriction, decreased arterial hydrostatic pressure, and increased arterial oncotic

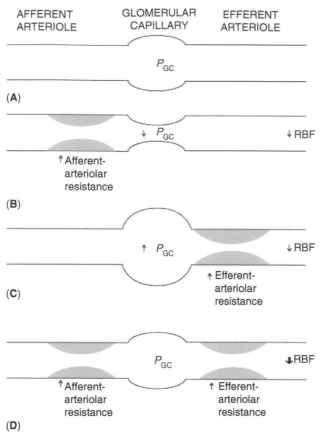

Figure 10.4 Effects of afferent- and/or efferent-arteriolar constriction on glomerular capillary pressure (P_{GC}) and renal blood flow (RBF). The RBF changes reflect changes in total renal arteriolar resistance, the location of the change being irrelevant. In contrast, the changes in P_{GC} on the specific site of altered arteriolar resistance. Pure afferent constriction lowers both P_{GC} and RBF, whereas pure efferent constriction raises P_{GC} and lowers RBF. Simultaneous constriction of both afferent and efferent arterioles has counteracting effects on P_{GC} but additive effects on RBF; the effect on P_{GC} may be a small increase, small decrease, or no change. Vasodilation of only one set of arterioles would have effects on P_{GC} and RBF opposite those shown in B and C. Vasodilation of both sets would cause little or no change in P_{GC}, the same result as constriction of both sets but would cause a large increase in RBF. Constriction of one set of arterioles and dilation of the other would have maximal effects on P_{GC} but little effect on RBF. *Source*: From Ref. 364.

pressure. Together these events decrease renal interstitial hydrostatic pressure and thus increase Na reabsorption. For example, expansion of the ECF volume due to a high salt intake, results in decreased plasma oncotic pressure from dilution of plasma proteins, increased arterial pressure, and renal vasodilation due to attenuation of neurohormonal activity. As a result of these events GFR and interstitial pressure increase and fluid reabsorption is reduced.

For the regulation of Na excretion, control of tubular Na *reabsorption* is more important than control of GFR, because a change in GFR automatically produces a proportional change in Na reabsorption by the PT, so that the *fraction*, but not the total amount, reabsorbed (65%) remains relatively constant (70). Therefore, a change in GFR produces a change in the Na and water presented to the loop of Henle. Reabsorbed fraction is changed by mechanisms distinct from alterations of GFR. The mechanisms responsible for matching

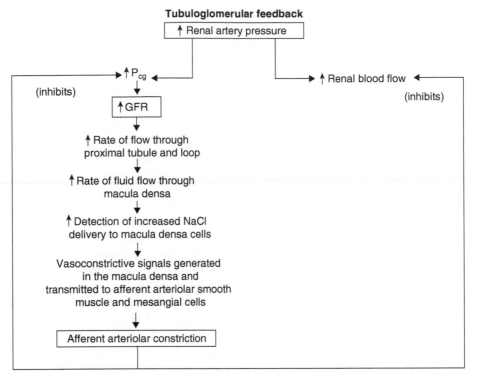

Figure 10.5 Tubuloglomerular feedback acts to prevent changes in renal artery pressure from causing extreme changes in sodium delivery to the macula densa. This mechanism acts in the opposite direction to the other reflexes and thus partially reduces or blunts their effectiveness. However, the overall effect of an increase in renal artery pressure is still a net increase in sodium excretion. *Abbreviations*: GFR, glomerular filtration rate; P_{GC}, hydrostatic pressure in glomerular capillaries.

changes in tubular reabsorption to those in GFR (glomerulotubular balance) constitute a second line of defense to prevent renal hemodynamic alterations from causing large changes in Na excretion (68). Autoregulation of GFR prevents it from changing excessively in response to changes in blood pressure, whereas glomerulotubular balance blunts the Na-excretion response to specific changes in GFR. Thus, tubuloglomerular feedback and glomerulotubular balance mediated by GFR autoregulation consign homeostatic control of Na excretion to the mechanisms, which influence tubular Na reabsorption independently of GFR changes (67–70). Most of these processes occur in the *distal* nephron, where Na reabsorption is modulated by aldosterone, whose blood levels are controlled by circulating A II levels (69). Thus, a decrease in blood pressure produces a rapid short-term baroreceptor-mediated vascular response followed by the intermediate-term renally mediated renin release and A II production, which reinforces the initial short-term vascular response. Despite blood pressure normalization, circulating A II stimulates adrenal aldosterone production, which acts on the principal cells of the DCT and collecting ducts to increase Na reabsorption (71). Retention of Na in these segments of the nephron will increase total body Na and blood volume to produce long-term correction of total body Na content and mean blood pressure.

Aldosterone controls reabsorption of 2% of the total filtered Na. This is a large amount because of the enormous volume of glomerular filtrate:

Total filtered Na/day = GFR × PNa = 180 L/day × 145 mmol/L = 26,100 mmol/day

Thus, aldosterone controls the reabsorption of 0.02 × 26,100 mmol/day = 522 mmol/day, which is approximately 30 g NaCl/day, a quantity far greater than that consumed by the average person (49,72). Therefore, with control of plasma aldosterone concentration, Na excretion can be finely adjusted to the intake to ensure homeostasis of total-body Na and ECF volume. After freely crossing principal cell membranes, aldosterone binds to cytoplasmic mineralocorticoid receptors in the cytoplasm. Aldosterone-bound receptors undergo conformational changes, which expose a nuclear localization molecule. In the nucleus, the receptor acts as a transcription factor that promotes gene expression and synthesis of messenger RNA for proteins that increase the activity or number of luminal membrane Na channels and basolateral membrane Na–K–ATPase pumps, which, in turn, mediate increased Na reabsorption (71). The two major signals stimulating aldosterone secretion from the adrenal gland are increased plasma [K] and A II, the latter mainly determined by plasma renin activity, which, in turn, depends on intrarenal baroreceptors, macula densa, and renal sympathetic nerves (Fig. 10.3) (72).

Secretion of aldosterone is attenuated by natriuretic peptides (NP), including atrial natriuretic peptide (ANP) and B-type natriuretic peptide (BNP) produced, respectively, by atrial and ventricular myocardium (73,74). The NP have both vascular and tubular actions, including afferent arteriolar relaxation, which increases filtration; inhibition of renin release; and Na reabsorption mediated by A II in the PT and by aldosterone in the medullary collecting duct (73–75). The major stimulus for increased secretion of NPs is cardiac chambers distention secondary to plasma volume expansion (75). Although the major function of AVP is to decrease water excretion by increasing the water permeability of the cortical and medullary collecting ducts, AVP also increases Na reabsorption by the same segment of the cortical collecting duct controlled by aldosterone (76).

Control of Water Excretion

Water excretion has two major components: a PT component, in which water is absorbed along with Na as an isotonic fluid, and a distal nephron component, in which water can be reabsorbed independent of Na (77,78). The PT component is primarily a mechanism to regulate ECF volume in response to changes in blood pressure (pressure diuresis) (77). Water reabsorption in the *distal* nephron is predominantly controlled by AVP. Thus total-body water is regulated mainly by reflexes that alter AVP secretion (Table 10.1) (77).

The groups of hypothalamic neurons that produce AVP have cell bodies in the supra-optic and paraventricular nuclei and axons terminating in the posterior pituitary gland, from which AVP is secreted into the blood. The key signals to these neurons arise from cardiovascular baroreceptors and hypothalamic osmoreceptors (78).

Decreased cardiovascular pressures due to ECF volume contraction reduce baroreceptor firing and, through afferent pathways to the hypothalamus, stimulate AVP secretion. Conversely, enhanced baroreceptors stimulation by increased cardiovascular pressures inhibits AVP secretion. Therefore, these baroreceptor reflexes help restore ECF volume and, hence, blood pressure (78).

With marked reductions in plasma volume AVP concentrations rise above those needed to produce maximal antidiuresis and produce arteriolar smooth muscle contraction. The resulting increase in peripheral vascular resistance raises arterial blood pressure independently of the slower restoration of body fluid volume. Renal arterioles and mesangial cells also participate in this constrictor response, so that high plasma AVP concentrations promote Na and water retention by lowering GFR, independently from AVP effects on water permeability (77,78).

Water gains or losses without corresponding changes in Na alter body fluids osmolality. An increase in plasma osmolality stimulates hypothalamic osmoreceptors which, through neural signals, increase hypothalamic AVP production (79). Water permeability of the collecting ducts is increased, water reabsorption is maximal and a very small volume of hyperosmotic urine is excreted. The smaller excretion of water relative to that of solute restores plasma osmolality toward normal. Conversely, a decrease in body fluid osmolality produced by excess water intake inhibits AVP secretion via the hypothalamic osmoreceptors (57). As a result, water permeability of the collecting ducts sharply declines, little or no water is reabsorbed, and a large volume of hypo-osmotic urine is excreted, thus eliminating excess water (77–79). The activity of hypothalamic baroreceptors and osmoreceptors is determined by the total synaptic input they receive. Thus, a simultaneous increase in plasma volume and decrease in body fluid osmolality cause strong inhibition of AVP secretion. Conversely, a simultaneous decrease in plasma volume and increase in osmolality produce very marked stimulation of AVP secretion. However, when both plasma volume and osmolality are decreased to a mild or moderate extent, the more sensitive osmoreceptors prevail over baroreceptors. In contrast, if a large change in plasma volume occurs, baroreceptors prevail over osmoreceptors in influencing AVP secretion; water is retained in excess of solute, and body fluids become hypo-osmotic and hyponatremic. In other words, maintenance of an adequate cardiac output through intravascular volume preservation takes precedence over maintenance of normal osmolality (35).

Large deficits of salt and water can be only partially compensated by renal conservation of these substances, and ingestion is the ultimate compensatory mechanism. Thirst centers reside in the hypothalamus near AVP-secreting areas. Interestingly, thirst is stimulated both by reduced plasma volume and increased body fluid osmolality, the same factors that stimulate AVP secretion (35). Moreover, osmoreceptors and nerve cells responding to cardiovascular baroreceptors, which initiate AVP-controlling reflexes are near those that stimulate thirst. The thirst response, however, is significantly less sensitive than the AVP response. Thirst is also stimulated by the direct action of A II on the brain in response to a decreased ECF volume (80,81). Salt appetite, a critically important determinant of Na homeostasis in most mammals, has a hedonistic component leading to ingestion of salt independent of salt deficit and a regulatory component driving intake when salt is lacking. In the United States there is a strong hedonistic appetite for salt, as illustrated by the fact that while a daily salt intake of <0.5 g is adequate for survival, the average daily salt intake in the United States is 10–15 g/day (82). In susceptible individuals this large salt intake may contribute to the pathogenesis of hypertension, which is a strong risk factor for the development of HF.

RENAL SODIUM AND WATER HANDLING IN HEART FAILURE

Knowledge of renal regulation of Na and water homeostasis is *indispensible* to understanding why patients with HF have expanded total plasma and blood volumes and yet their otherwise normal kidneys continue to retain Na and water (6,27).

The observation that renal Na and water retention occur in edematous disorders associated with *either* a low cardiac output *or* decreased peripheral vascular resistances points to underfilling of the arterial circulation as the event, which initiates Na and water retention by kidneys free of intrinsic disease. Importantly, the arterial circulation, which perfuses the body's vital organs and tissues, is the smallest body fluid compartment (<2% of TBW), thus providing the system regulating Na and water homeostasis with high sensitivity to detect small changes in total body volume (Table 10.2).

The function of the high- and low-pressure receptors, which control body fluid volume in mammals have been described earlier in this chapter (28,51–53). Maneuvers that decrease central venous return, including positive pressure breathing, lower extremities tourniquets, and prolonged standing are associated with decreased renal Na excretion. In contrast, maneuvers that increase thoracic venous return, such as negative pressure breathing, recumbency, and head-out water immersion result in significant increase in renal salt and water excretion without significant changes in either GFR or RBF (83–85). The role for atrial receptors in volume regulation is also supported by the finding in a canine model that renal Na excretion and left atrial pressure are directly correlated (85). Left atrial receptors contribute to ECF volume regulation also by exerting nonosmotic control over AVP (85). In addition, changes in atrial volume and pressure form the principal determinant of plasma ANP concentrations (86,87). An increase in left atrial pressure normally decreases renal sympathetic tone. These atrial–renal reflexes are impaired in both animal HF models and HF patients in whom a volume load fails to increase plasma ANP levels and natriuresis (88,89). Evidence identifying the fullness of the arterial circulation as a sensor for the regulation of renal Na excretion emerged from the observation that closure of an A–V fistula, which increases diastolic arterial pressure and decreases cardiac output, produces an immediate increase in renal Na excretion without changes in either GFR or RBF (90). Furthermore, pharmacologic or surgical interruption of sympathetic afferent neural pathways originating from high-pressure baroreceptors inhibited the natriuretic response to volume expansion (91–96). In addition, a pressure drop or stretch at the carotid sinus results in SNS activation and increased renal Na and water excretion. High-pressure baroreceptors play an important role in regulating nonosmotic AVP release which, in turn, modulates renal water excretion (91–96).

Both vagal and sympathetic afferent nerve endings in the heart and lungs also respond to various exogenous and endogenous compounds, including capsaicin, phenylguanidine, bradykinin, substance P, and prostaglandins. In particular prostaglandin I_2 (PGI_2), whose plasma concentration is increased in HF, attenuates the baroreflex control of renal nerve activity via a cardiac afferent vagal mechanism (97).

The GFR, which is usually preserved in mild HF, decreases with increasing severity of cardiac dysfunction. Renal vascular resistance is increased with a concomitant reduction in RBF, which is proportional to the degree of cardiac impairment. Therefore, in HF patients filtration fraction (GFR/RBF) is usually increased due to constriction of the efferent arterioles in the kidney. These renal hemodynamic changes alter hydrostatic and oncotic forces in the peritubular capillaries in a manner that increases Na and water reabsorption in the PT (Fig. 10.4). Renal hemodynamic changes in HF patients result from neurohormonal activation, which also directly enhances Na and water reabsorption in both the proximal and distal nephron (28,32,54–56).

Arterial underfilling, due to a decrease in either cardiac output or peripheral vascular resistance, activates SNS, RAAS, and nonosmotic AVP release to maintain the integrity of the arterial circulation with both peripheral vasoconstriction and ECF expansion through renal Na and water retention. Baroreceptor activation of the SNS appears to be the primary integrator of these neurohormonal responses, as indicated by the fact that nonosmotic AVP release requires stimulation of hypothalamic supraoptic and paraventricualr nuclei and RAAS activation requires renal adrenergic stimulation (27,28,30,32,46,47). Unloading of arterial baroreceptors in the carotid sinus and aortic arch decreases the tonic inhibitory effect of afferent vagal and glossopharyngeal pathways on the central nervous system and increases efferent sympathetic tone which, in turn, activates the RAAS and AVP release.

Counterregulatory vasodilatory and natriuretic hormones are also activated in HF, including the NPs and renal prostaglandins (73–75).

Activation of SNS is suggested by the finding of elevated norepinephrine (NE) levels in mild HF. Studies of NE kinetics using tritiated NE in advanced HF have shown both increased NE secretion and decreased NE clearance (98–100). The SOLVD has documented the presence of SNS activation, as determined by increased plasma NE concentrations in patients with asymptomatic LV dysfunction (101). Importantly, SNS activation occurs at both the cardiac and renal levels. In one study of whole body and organ-specific NE kinetics in HF patients, cardiac and renal NE spillover rates were increased, respectively, five- and twofold (102). The adverse effects of systemic and cardiac neurohormonal activation are described in detail in another chapter.

The renal effects of the SNS, which elicit avid Na and water reabsorption in HF patients, include renal vasoconstriction, RAAS stimulation, and direct PT effects. In both experimental animals and human HF, intrarenal adrenergic blockade increases natriuresis (103–105). Conversely, in rodent models renal nerves stimulation produces a 25% reduction in Na excretion and urine volume through efferent arteriolar vasoconstriction, which alters hemodynamic forces in peritubular capillaries in favor of increased tubular Na reabsorption (56,106,107). The occurrence of this phenomenon is also supported by the common finding in HF of an increased filtration fraction in the presence of a normal or only slightly decreased GFR. Whole kidney and single nephron studies in rats have shown that renal sympathetic nerves activation directly enhances PT Na reabsorption (103–106,108). The finding in these animals models that renal nerve stimulation increases the tubular fluid/plasma inulin concentration ratio in the late PT as a result of increased fractional Na and water reabsorption, provide evidence that increased renal nerve activity may promote Na retention independently form hemodynamic changes (56,107). However the fact that Na retention persists in dogs with denervated transplanted kidneys and chronic vena caval constriction suggests that in HF renal nerves contribute, but do not fully account for Na and water retention (109,110).

In HF A II promotes Na and water retention both through direct and indirect effects on Na reabsorption in the PT and by stimulation of adrenal aldosterone release. Similarly, to renal nerves stimulation, A II-induced renal efferent arteriolar vasoconstriction results in a decreased RBF and an increased filtration fraction. These hemodynamic changes increase peritubular capillary oncotic pressure and reduce peritubular capillary hydrostatic pressure, thus favoring Na and water reabsorption in the PT (108,111). In addition, A II directly activates the basolateral Na–bicarbonate cotransporter and the apical Na–H exchanger, an effect which is inhibited by A II receptor blockade (112,113). Finally, A II increases adrenal aldosterone secretion, which promotes Na reabsorption in the DCT and collecting duct, as described earlier in this chapter. Indeed, in HF patients urinary Na excretion inversely correlates with plasma renin activity and urinary aldosterone excretion. The observation that ACE inhibition inconsistently increases urinary Na excretion, despite a consistent decrease in plasma aldosterone concentration, suggests that the decrease in blood pressure associated with decreased circulating A II levels may activate hemodynamic and neurohormonal mechanisms, which attenuate the natriuresis expected to occur when A II and aldosterone levels are decreased (114).

Aldosterone antagonism can reverse HF's Na retention despite activation of renin–angiotensin and SNS. In fact in a group of patients with mild-to-moderate HF, all of whom retained Na after withdrawal of their medications, spironolactone administration increased daily urinary Na excretion despite being associated with increased plasma renin activity (PRA) and NE (115).

Plasma AVP levels are elevated in HF patients and correlate with HF severity and serum Na levels (116–120). Furthermore, in HF plasma AVP levels are elevated despite hypo-osmolality and are not normally suppressed by acute water loading (117,121). These data indicate that the principal cause of elevated AVP levels in HF is the nonosmotic release of the hormone driven by SNS baroreceptor activation.

Stimulation of renal (V_2) receptors by AVP enhances water reabsorption in the cortical and medullary collecting ducts. Three lines of evidence implicate nonosmotic AVP release in the abnormal water retention of HF (122–127). Selective V_2 receptors antagonists reverse the defect in water excretion in animal and humans with HF (125,126). Tolvaptan, an orally available nonpeptide AVP antagonist, has been shown to reverse impaired urinary diluting capacity, increase solute-free water excretion and correct hyponatremia (125–127). In a rodent HF model a nonpeptide V_2-receptor antagonist reversed upregulation of AVP-sensitive water channels in the cortex and papilla (128). Interestingly, in one study, both the ACE inhibitor captopril and the α_1-adrenergic blocker prazosin, despite having opposite effects on the RAAS, were shown to similarly improve water excretion and restore AVP suppression by an acute water load. Notably in this study, the average 5 mmHg decrease in mean arterial pressure was less than the 7–10% necessary to trigger nonosmotic AVP release (129). The observation that afterload reduction improved cardiac output and water excretion supports the belief that ventricular receptors and/or baroreceptors sensing arterial pressure and stroke volume contribute to the regulation of AVP release (129).

In HF increased concentrations of endothelin, a powerful vasoconstrictor, portend a poor prognosis (130–132). In the kidney, mesangial cells, endothelial cells, epithelial glomerular cells, and inner medullary collecting duct cells all synthesize endothelin. As an autocrine/paracrine hormone, endothelin influences Na and water regulation by mediating vasoconstriction (130,131).

The NPs are the subject of chapter 14. Briefly plasma concentrations of ANP and BNP are increased in HF patients (133–136). These peptide hormones possess natriuretic, vasorelaxant, and anti-neurohormonal actions aimed at attenuating the detrimental hemodynamic and tissue effects of the SNS and RAAS (115,131,137–143).

Micropuncture studies in the rat have shown that ANP causes afferent arteriolar dilatation and efferent arteriolar constriction. These findings explain why administration of NPs in normal human subjects increases GFR with no change or only a modest decrease in RBF. NP infusions appear to be associated with diminished Na reabsorption in the PT (143–145). However, enzymatic and binding studies of ANP in rat glomeruli and nephrons show that the glomerulus and distal nephron, rather than the PT are the renal sites where NPs inhibit Na reabsorption (146–148). In a dog model of low output HF caused by thoracic vena cava constriction, avid Na retention was associated with elevated PRA and plasma aldosterone concentration and normal plasma ANP levels. In these dogs exogenous administration of ANP prevented Na retention, renal vasoconstriction, and activation of the RAAS (149). These results suggest that the high plasma ANP, and probably BNP, levels in human HF are important in attenuating the renal Na retention. However, the intravenous infusion of synthetic NPs in patients with low-output HF results in only a modest increase in renal Na excretion and alteration of renal hemodynamics (149,150). These results suggest that resistance to the natriuretic effects of NPs is present in human HF (Fig. 10.6). Possible causes of NP resistance include downregulation of renal NP receptors, secretion of inactive immunoreactive NP, enhanced renal neutral endopeptidase activity limiting delivery of NPs to the collecting duct receptor sites, hyperaldosteronism caused by increased Na reabsorption in the distal renal tubule, increased intracellular phosphodiesterase activity diminishing second messenger cyclic guanosine monophosphate (cGMP) concentrations, and diminished Na delivery to the distal renal site of NP action. Several lines of evidence suggest that reduced distal Na delivery to the collecting ducts secondary to decreased GFR or increased PT Na reabsorption are the most likely causes of NP resistance in HF. A linear correlation between plasma ANP and urinary cGMP excretion is present in HF patients. In addition, ANP resistance in cirrhotic patients is reversed by increasing distal Na delivery to the collecting duct with mannitol infusion of (150,151). Finally, in HF distal tubular Na delivery is the best correlate of the natriuretic response to infused BNP (151). Reduced Na delivery to the DCT may be due to neurohormonally mediated renal vasoconstriction and may cause the impaired aldosterone escape occurring in HF.

Mechanisms of sodium and water retention in heart failure

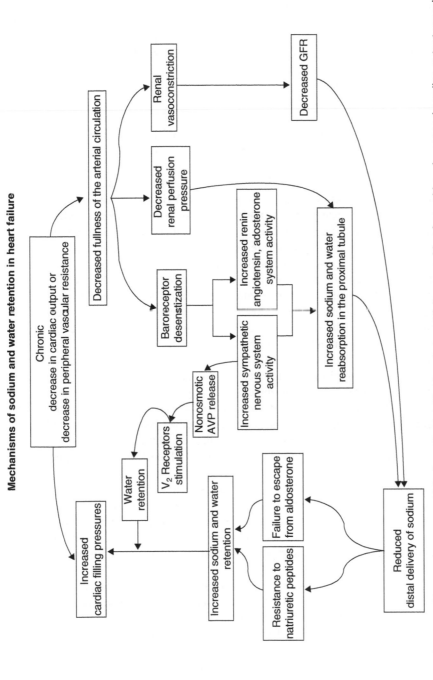

Figure 10.6   Decreased baroreceptor sensitivity in patients with chronic heart failure resulting from either decreased cardiac output or reduced peripheral vascule resistance can worsen cardiac function by increasing renin-angiotensin-aldosterone system and sympathetic activity, enhancing proximal fluid reabsorption, nonosmotic release of vasopressin, impairing aldosterone escape, and blunting the response to natriuretic peptides. *Source:* Adapted from Ref. 3.

Another attractive member of the NP family is urodilatin, a slightly extended form of ANP synthesized primarily in the distal nephron (141). Exogenous administration of urodilatin exerts vasodilating and natriuretic effects similar to those of ANP and BNP (141,152).

In normal subjects and in intact animals, renal prostaglandins have insignificant effects on renal Na excretion and hemodynamics (153,154). In HF patients, prostaglandin activity is increased and correlates with disease severity, as assessed by the degree of hyponatremia. Furthermore, reversible acute renal failure can occur in HF patients taking cyclooxygenase inhibitors (155). In fact in patients with moderate HF and a normal Na intake, administration of acetylsalicylic acid in doses that decrease the synthesis of renal PGE_2, significantly reduces urinary Na excretion (156).

DIMINISHED RENAL FUNCTION AND PROGRESSION OF HEART FAILURE

Death from cardiac causes is 10–20 times more common in patients with chronic renal failure (CRF) than in matched segments of the general population (157) and 43.6% of all deaths in patients with end-stage renal disease (ESRD) are due to cardiac causes (157). In ESRD, the prevalence of left ventricular hypertrophy (LVH) and coronary artery disease are, respectively, approximately 75% and 40% (158). As many as 50% of ESRD patients experience a myocardial infarction within two years of dialysis initiation and have high mortality rates (159). Even a slightly decreased kidney function independently correlates with higher cardiovascular disease risk and mortality (160–165). Both proteinuria and a decline in GFR are independent risk factors for the development of cardiovascular disease. Impaired renal function is also associated with adverse outcomes after acute coronary syndromes, percutaneous coronary intervention, coronary artery bypass surgery, or thrombolytic therapy (166–170). The incidence of HF as a cause of death is inversely related to GFR (171,172). Both the number of patients with moderate renal dysfunction and the prevalence of ESRD are increasing, along with the growing HF epidemic due to aging of the population and improved survival after cardiovascular events (173–177).

Intrinsic renal disease may contribute to HF progression because of its association with increased left ventricular volume, neurohormonal activation, decreased erythropoietin and resultant anemia, inflammation, and increased reactive oxygen species (ROS) (3–5). Each of these mechanisms may influence myocardial remodeling by increasing left ventricular dilatation, mitral regurgitation, left ventricular wall mass, myocardial fibrosis, and apoptosis.

Renal Na retention with ECF expansion causes increased cardiac preload, resulting in cardiac dilatation, which is closely correlated with both mortality and HF hospitalization (178). Cardiac dilatation increases myocardial wall stress, resulting in increased myocardial oxygen demand and mitral regurgitation, which leads to reduced forward cardiac output and increased pulmonary vascular pressures, thereby placing an additional burden on the right ventricle.

Increased wall stress results in increased LVH, which, in turn, increases diastolic dysfunction, wall stress, left ventricular filling pressures, and mortality. The anemia commonly present in patients with renal disease further increases LVH (179).

In the heart there appears to be a LVH disproportionate with the hemodynamic milieu and an accelerated type of coronary artery atherosclerosis (180–183). Intramyocardial arterioles wall thickening and reduced lumen diameter as a consequence of hypertrophy of smooth muscle cells have been described in patients with concomitant cardiac and renal dysfunction (184). Clinically, the narrowed lumen diameter further reduces coronary flow reserve. In fact uremic rats have been found to have a decreased intramyocardial capillary density, which increases the oxygen diffusion distance and may render the myocardium more vulnerable to hypoxia (185).

Uremic patients also have increased pulse wave velocity, a prognostically important measure of arterial stiffness, which is increased by A II, volume expansion, and vascular calcification (186–190).

When HF and renal dysfunction coexist, fluid retention, with the associated cardiac dilatation and mitral regurgitation, reduces cardiac output, resulting in diminished renal perfusion and further activation of the RAAS (191). Increased aldosterone levels may block myocardial NE reuptake, resulting in increased SNS activation and progressive myo-cardial dysfunction (192,193) Table 10.4. In HF A II generation in the cerebrospinal fluid, and decreased NO in the central nervous system, may be partially responsible for decreased baroreceptor sensitivity which, by reducing the tonic inhibition of renal sympathetic nerve activity, results in Na retention (193–195). Both A II and increased renal sympathetic activity activate PT epithelial receptors to enhance Na reabsorption (106,196). Decreased Na delivery to the distal nephron prevents escape from the Na-retaining effects of aldosterone. A II causes glomerular efferent arteriolar constriction resulting in enhanced Na and water retention due to increase in hydrostatic pressure in the peritubular capillaries (197). Thus in

Table 10.4 Effects of Neurohormonal Activation on the Kidney in Heart Failure

Vasoconstrictor Systems

  Renal Nerves
    Promote afferent and efferent arteriolar constriction
    Enhance sodium reabsorption in the proximal tubule
    Stimulate rennin release

  Renin–Angiotensin–Aldosterone System
    Promotes efferent greater than afferent arteriolar constriction
    Enhance sodium reabsorption in the proximal tubule
    Stimulates adrenal aldosterone synthesis and release
    Causes cardiac remodeling

  Aldosterone
    Enhances sodium reabsorption and potassium secretion in collecting duct
    Increases cardiac fibrosis

  Arginine vasopressin
    Increases water reabsorption in the cortical and medullary collecting duct
    Increases vasoconstriction predominantly of the efferent arteriole

  Endothelin
    Increases renal vasoconstriction
    Possible effects on tubular sodium handling

Vasodilator Systems

  Natriuretic Peptides
    Increase glomerular filtration rate
    Oppose sodium reabsorption in the collecting duct
    Suppress plasma rennin activity
    Inhibit aldosterone synthesis and release
    Possible inhibition of vasopressine release

  Renal Prostaglandins
    Promote renal vasodilatation
    Decrease sodium reabsorption in the ascending limb of the loop of Henle
    Inhibit vasopressin action in the collecting duct

the PT, enhanced Na reabsorption is due to the direct effects of A II, sympathetic stimulation and renal vasoconstriction. The decreased Na delivery to the macula densa caused by increased Na reabsorption in the PT, stimulates renin secretion and further activation of the RAAS (198,199).

It has been proposed that the combined abnormalities of the RAAS, the balance between NO and ROS, inflammation, and the SNS lead to a vicious circle, which results in acceleration and amplification of cardiorenal dysfunction and damage (Fig. 10.7) (5).

In addition to causing volume expansion and vasoconstriction, A II also activates NADPH-oxidase, which results in the formation of ROS in endothelial cells, vascular smooth muscle cells, renal tubular cells, and cardiomyocytes (200–204). Increased myocardial NADPH-oxidase activity in patients with end-stage HF and NADPH-oxidase-mediated ROS release in glomeruli of Dahl salt-sensitive rats with HF are both attenuated by ACE inhibition (205,206). Notably, ACE inhibition has also been shown to increase NO bioavailability in patients with coronary artery disease by reducing vascular oxidative stress or increasing extracellular superoxide dismutase (SOD) activity (207). By altering cellular redox state, A II may promote vascular inflammation via the nuclear factor kappa B (NF-κB) pathway, a transcription factor for chemotactic and adhesion molecules (208–215).

The inflammation associated with both HF and renal dysfunction, as documented by the high levels of circulating inflammatory cytokines, such as TNF-α and IL-6, may enhance the negative effects that the dysfunction of one organ has on the other (214,216). Indeed, TNF-α, which is increased in renal failure is also a myocardial depressant. Similar

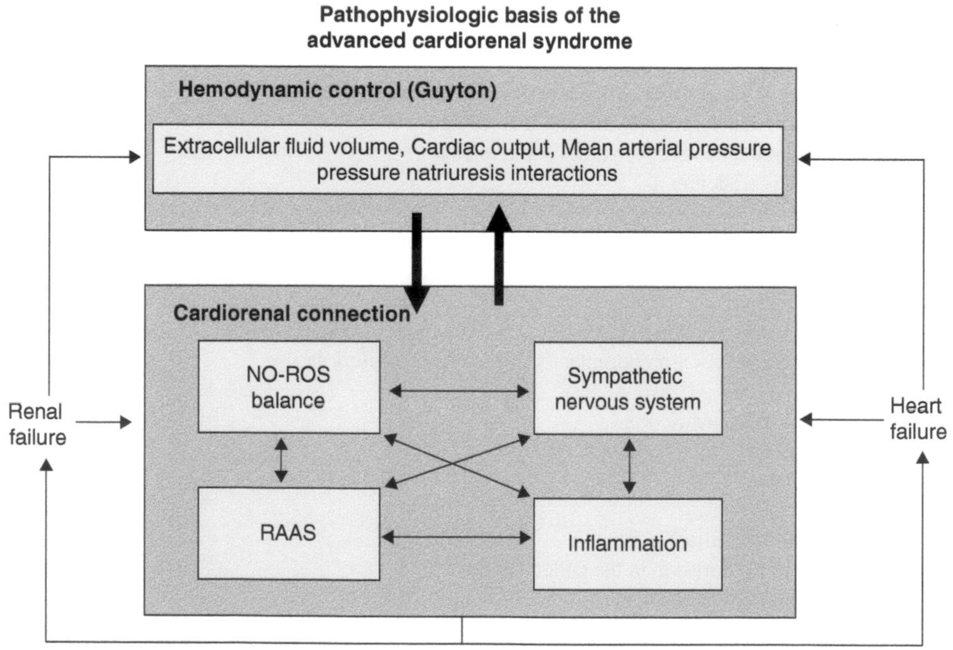

Figure 10.7   Pathophysiologic basis of the advanced cardiorenal syndrome. The model of Guyton explains heart/kidney interaction with respect to blood pressure and extracellular fluid volume. When one of the organs fails, a vicious cycle develops in which the renin–angiotensin system, the NO–ROS balance, the sympathetic nervous system and inflammation interact and synergize, forming additional cardiorenal connections. *Abbreviations*: NO, nitric oxide; ROS, reactive oxygen species. *Source*: Adapted from Ref. 232.

to neurohormonal activation, increased expression of cytokines has direct cardiac and renal toxicity (214,217,218). Both A II and TNF-α induce oxidative stress that results in myocytes hypertrophy (214). Thus, the enhanced inflammation occurring when renal dysfunction complicates HF is likely to exacerbate myocardial remodeling.

Nitric oxide is important in renal control of ECF volume and blood pressure because it mediates vasodilatation, natriuresis, and desensitization of tubuloglomerular feedback (219). Superoxide has opposite effects (220–223). When cardiac and renal disease coexist, the balance between NO and the ROS is shifted toward the latter by increased ROS production, low antioxidant state, and reduced NO availability. Increased levels of oxidative stress markers have been detected in ESRD patients (224–226). A relative NO deficiency in renal failure is caused by the reaction of NO with oxygen radicals, as well as by high circulatory concentrations of asymmetric di-methyl arginine (ADMA), an endogenous NOS inhibitor (227). Increased oxidative stress has also been demonstrated in HF (205,228). Interestingly, hemodynamic improvement by captopril and prazosin is associated with enhanced antioxidant status (229). In normotensive HF patients the relationship between reduced renal perfusion, impaired NO-mediated endothelial vasodilation, and high concentrations of ADMA is similar to that occurring in CRF patients (230,231). Oxidative stress by hydrogen peroxide (H_2O_2) has been shown to increase activity of preganglionic sympathetic neurons in vivo and in vitro in rats, raising mean arterial pressure and heart rate (232). In addition, renal sympathetic activity in spontaneously hypertensive rats was found to be regulated by vascular superoxide concentrations (233).

In renal failure, oxidative stress has damaging effects on DNA (8-oxo-OH-deoxyguanosine), proteins (carbonyl compounds, advanced oxidation protein products), carbohydrates (AGEs), and lipids (oxidized LDL). These substances mediate endothelial cells damage and inflammation, by attracting and activating leukocytes, with the resultant upregulation of cytokines, such as IL-1, IL-6, and TNFα (234–239).

Oxidative damage to the renal tubular or interstitial cells may interfere with feedback systems involved in renin secretion and A II formation. Chronic inhibition of NO synthesis causes upregulation of cardiac ACE and A II receptors, possibly mediating inflammatory changes (240).

Little data exist on therapies aimed at decreasing superoxide production (such as NADPH-oxidase inhibitors), scavenging ROS, or supporting the function of NO. In one relatively small trial, antioxidant therapy had a favorable effect on cardiovascular outcomes of patients with renal failure (241,242).

In addition to increased oxidative stress, inflammation is a hallmark of uremia (243). An elevated C-reactive protein in patients with CRF is associated with a more than additive effect on rates of MI and death (244). In CRF, circulating levels of C-reactive protein and several proinflammatory cytokines, such as IL-1β, IL-6, and TNFα, are predictors of atherosclerosis (245–247).

In HF patients, elevated levels of TNFα and IL-6 are present in both plasma and myocardium and correlate with disease progression (248,249). Although the exact role of inflammatory cells activation remains unclear, a state of chronic inflammation is present in both CRF and HF. This low-grade inflammation can cause ROS production by activating leukocytes to release their oxidative contents (250). In cultured rat vascular smooth muscle cells, IL-6 induced upregulation of the AT_1 receptor and A II-mediated production of ROS, providing evidence for a possible link between inflammation and RAAS activation (251). Cytokines may stimulate renin secretion as a component of the systemic stress response, and tubulointerstitial inflammation may affect adaptation of glomerular hemodynamics to impaired renal function (252). Production of IL-1β after a MI has been shown to stimulate NE release from sympathetic neurons (253–255).

As discussed earlier in this chapter, the SNS contributes to long-term regulation of ECF volume and blood pressure by stimulating renin release via renal sympathetic neurons. In fact, the increased peripheral sympathetic nerve activity documented in ESRD is corrected by removal of the diseased kidneys. In HF, SNS activation in response to arterial underfilling, ultimately results in cardiomyocyte apoptosis, hypertrophy, and focal myocardial necrosis (210,256–258). Interestingly, these effects appear to involve superoxide induction (257,258). Chronic SNS activation reduces β-adrenergic receptor sensitivity in both HF and renal failure, leading to altered baroreceptor reflexes, reduced heart rate variability, and increased susceptibility to arrhythmia. In addition, SNS activation has been shown to affect lipid metabolism and β-blockers appear to have antiatherosclerotic effects (259–263). The SNS also contributes to RAAS activation, production of ROS by SNS mediators, and activation of the immune system. Importantly, renin release is enhanced both directly by renal sympathetic nerves and indirectly because of intrarenal vascular hypertrophy due to the enhanced ROS production resulting from chronic SNS activation (264,265). In a renal ischemia/reperfusion model, H_2O_2 formation by monoamine oxidase enzymes initiated a proapoptotic cascade in proximal tubular cells (266). The finding that β-blockade after experimental myocardial infarction decreases myocardial cytokine gene expression, suggests that the SNS promotes inflammation by NE-mediated cytokine production in multiple organs (267–269). Furthermore, SNS activation results in the release of neuropeptide Y (NPY), a neurohormone that mediates prolonged vasoconstriction during stress, vascular intimal proliferation, and release of proinflammatory cytokines. High levels of NPY have been demonstrated after MI and in HF (270–274).

Anemia and relative resistance to erythropoietin are common in HF patients and contribute to both cardiac dysfunction and increased mortality (275). Renal dysfunction is one of the causes of the anemia occurring in HF (275). Anemia is associated with LVH even when kidney disease is mild (276). In addition, by causing peripheral vasodilation and thus relative arterial underfilling, anemia contributes to the reduction of renal perfusion pressure and exacerbation of Na and water retention. Since red blood cells contain antioxidants, anemia may also increase oxidative stress (277). The increase in erythropoietin levels commonly seen in HF may be inadequate for the severity of anemia (278–280). A possible cause of erythropoietin resistance in HF is the enhanced production of inflammatory cytokines (277,278,280). It should be noted that, in addition to stimulating hematopoiesis, erythropoietin binds to receptors on endothelial and smooth muscle cells and reduces both the production and release of proinflammatory cytokines and chemokines and the influx of inflammatory cells into injured myocardium with a potential decrease in myocardial remodeling (281–285). Thus resistance to the anti-inflammatory and antioxidant effects of erythropoietin may adversely affect myocardial remodeling in HF.

THERAPEUTIC STRATEGIES IN PATIENTS WITH THE CARDIORENAL SYNDROME
Role of Diuretics and Diuretic Resistance

In symptomatic HF patients diuretics are effective in treating the symptoms and signs of pulmonary and peripheral congestion. However, diuretic therapy in some HF patients may lead to deterioration of renal function. Therefore, the optimal management of volume overloaded HF patients requires in depth knowledge of the pharmacology of diuretics and of the factors responsible for the development of resistance to diuretic therapy (3).

In the relationship between dietary Na intake, urinary Na excretion, and mean arterial pressure, diuretics shift the renal function curve to the left, permitting Na excretion to increase at a constant mean arterial pressure (286). Currently available diuretics include the loop diuretics (furosemide, bumetanide, torsemide, and ethacrynic acid), the DCT diuretics (thiazides, metolazone, chlorthalidone), the Na channel-blocking drugs (amiloride and triamterene), and aldosterone antagonists (spironolactone and eplerenone) (Table 10.5).

A critically important initial step in controlling symptoms of ECF volume expansion is restriction of daily salt intake to 2 g or 86 mEq of Na. Dietary NaCl restriction is necessary to maximize the therapeutic benefit of diuretics. Loop diuretics, which are rapidly but incompletely absorbed in the gastrointestinal tract and have short half-lives, can increase Na excretion by as much as 25% of filtered Na. To produce natriuresis, a loop diuretic must achieve a critical renal tubular concentration. In edematous conditions, such as HF, this dose–response curve is shifted downward and to the right, indicating that achievement of natriuresis requires loop diuretic doses higher than those that effectively increase urinary NaCl excretion in normal individuals. A rightward shift of the dose–response curve also occurs with renal insufficiency, indicating that, compared with normal individuals, higher diuretic doses are needed to achieve the same fractional Na excretion (286). Considering that a furosemide dose >240 mg produces only a modest additional natriuresis, but is associated with considerable toxicity, it is currently recommended that such dose not be exceeded in HF patients (286). Importantly, most patients can correctly identify which diuretic dose produces a significant increase in urine output within 4 hours of ingestion. In the absence of increased diuresis, it is reasonable to double the diuretic dose. Although in HF loop diuretics' half-lives are lengthened, they remain ≤5–6 hours. Thus, after a period of natriuresis, the diuretic concentration in the renal tubular fluid declines below the diuretic threshold and renal Na reabsorption resumes (postdiuretic NaCl retention). Therefore, the net daily effect of a diuretic is the Na excretion occurring while NaCl reabsorption is inhibited minus the Na retention persisting until the next diuretic dose achieves sufficient tubular concentration to trigger the natriuresis. If dietary NaCl intake is excessive, postdiuretic NaCl retention can overcome initial natriuresis and a negative salt balance cannot be achieved. Thus dietary salt restriction is critically important to preserve the effectiveness of diuretics. To minimize postdiuretic Na retention, loop diuretics should be given at least twice daily (Figs. 10.8 and 10.9) (287,288).

Diuretics stimulate the RAAS via several mechanisms. Because NaCl uptake by the loop, diuretic-sensitive Na–K–2Cl cotransporter is the key mechanism for the macula densa-mediated renin secretion, by inhibiting NaCl uptake into macula densa cells, loop diuretics directly stimulate renin secretion, leading to a volume-independent increase in A II and aldosterone secretion (289). Loop diuretics also stimulate renal production of

Table 10.5 Pharmacokinetics of Loop Diuretics

| Loop Diuretic | Oral Bioavailability (%) | Elimination Half-Life (hr) | | |
		Normal Subjects	Patients with Renal Insufficiency	Patients with Heart Failure
Furosemide	10–100	1.5–2	2.8	2.7
Bumetanide	80–100	1	1.6	1.3
Torsemide	80–100	3–4	4–5	6

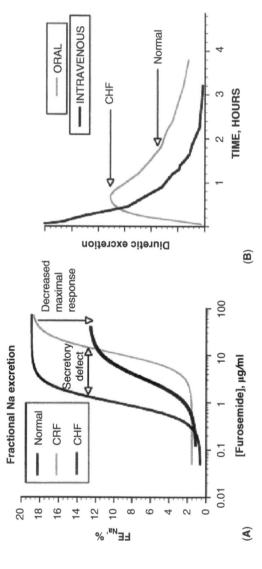

Figure 10.8 Dose–response curves for loop diuretics. (A) FENa as a function of loop diuretic concentration. Compared with normal patients, patients with CRF show a rightward shift in the curve, owing to impaired diuretic secretion. The maximal response is preserved when expressed as FENa, but not when expressed as absolute Na excretion. Patients with CHF demonstrate a rightward and downward shift, even when the response is expressed as FENa, and thus are relatively diuretic resistant. (B) Comparison of the response to intravenous and oral doses of loop diuretics. In a normal individual (Normal), an oral dose may be as effective as an intravenous dose because the time above the natriuretic threshold (indicated by the 'Normal' line) is approximately equal. If the natriuretic threshold increases [as indicated by the gray line, from a patient with CHF], then the oral dose may not provide a high enough serum level to elicit natriuresis. *Abbreviations*: CHF, congestive heart failure; CRF, chronic renal failure; FENa, fractional Na excretion. *Source*: From Ref. 286.

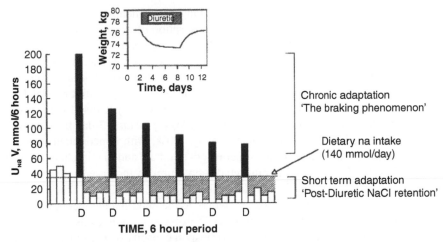

Figure 10.9 Effects of diuretics on urinary Na excretion and ECF volume. Inset: Effect of a diuretic on body weight, taken as an index of ECF volume. Note that steady state is reached within 6–8 days despite continued diuretic administration. Main graph: Effects of a loop diuretic on UNaV. Bars represent 6-hr periods before (in Na balance) and after doses of loop diuretic (D). The dotted line indicates dietary Na intake. The solid portion of the bars indicates the amount by which Na excretion exceeds intake during natriuresis. The hatched areas indicate the amount of positive Na balance after the diuretic effect has worn off. Net Na balance during 24 hr is the difference between the hatched area (postdiuretic NaCl retention) and the solid area (diuretic-induced natriuresis). Chronic adaptation is indicated by progressively smaller peak natriuretic effects (the braking phenomenon) and is mirrored by a return to neutral balance, as indicated in the inset, where the solid and hatched areas are equal. As discussed in the text, chronic adaptation requires ECF volume depletion. ECF, extracellular fluid; UNaV, urinary Na excretion. *Source*: From Ref. 286.

prostacyclin, which further enhances renin secretion (290). By contracting the ECF volume all types of diuretics can activate the vascular (volume-dependent) mechanism of renin release. However, only loop diuretics can stimulate renin secretion also by increasing its synthesis within the macula densa (291,292). When a loop diuretic is administered over a prolonged period, renal renin gene expression is strongly upregulated in a volume-independent manner (292). To attenuate RAAS activation, DCT diuretics, such as thiazides can be combined with low-dose loop diuretics. Furthermore, this approach may reduce the effects of the adaptive changes in the DCT, which limit diuretic effectiveness. In fact, combinations of low-dose loop and DCT diuretics are more effective than higher doses of a single diuretic type. When diuretics effectively decrease ECF volume, the NaCl balance gradually returns to neutral despite continued diuretic administration (293–295). Thus the magnitude of natriuresis decreases after each diuretic dose ("braking phenomenon"). The greater the contraction of the ECF volume, the greater is the decline in natriuresis with subsequent diuretic doses, because the amount of filtered NaCl is reduced and the amount of reabsorbed NaCl is increased (295). Rodent micropuncture studies have shown that when hydrochlorothiazide is administered for 7–10 days, ECF volume contraction *increases* PT solute reabsorption, limiting the delivery of NaCl to the distal tubule (296). Thus, during chronic treatment, inhibition of NaCl transport along the distal nephron (the predominant site of thiazide action) is counterbalanced by a reduction in distal NaCl delivery. Under these conditions, urinary NaCl equals dietary NaCl intake because enhanced proximal NaCl absorption equals inhibited distal NaCl absorption (296).

Various mechanisms contribute to the braking phenomenon: (*i*) *ECF volume contraction* increases filtration fraction proximal reabsorption of Na and water by decreasing renal interstitial pressure; (*ii*) *stimulation of efferent sympathetic nerves* reduces urinary NaCl excretion by reducing RBF, promoting renin release from the macula densa, enhancing NaCl reabsorption throughout the nephron and interacting with hormonal modulators of NaCl transport; (*iii*) loop diuretics *stimulate renin secretion* by inhibiting NaCl uptake into macula densa cells; and (*iv*) diuretics increase solute delivery to distal segments, causing *epithelial cells to undergo both hypertrophy and hyperplasia*. A 7-day furosemide infusion in rats increased DCT cell volume by nearly 100%, with concomitant increases in luminal- and basolateral membrane areas per length of tubule and in mitochondrial volume per cell (297–299). Chronically administered loop diuretics increase the Na–K–ATPase activity in the DCT and cortical collecting tubule and the number of thiazide-sensitive Na–Cl cotransporters, measured by Western blot or as the maximal number of binding sites for [3H]-metolazone (300–304). Cells of the DCT expressing high levels of transport proteins are hypertrophic and have a higher NaCl transport capacity than normal tubules (288). In normal human volunteers, one month loop diuretic therapy enhanced DCT ion transport capacity, measured as the requirement for larger thiazide diuretic doses to enhance Na excretion. The ECF volume-independent component of NaCl retention occurring after loop diuretic administration may also reflect changes in distal nephron structure and function (305,306).

An edematous patient may be deemed resistant to diuretic drugs when moderate doses of a loop diuretic do not achieve the desired ECF volume reduction. Before labeling the patient as "resistant" to diuretics potential reversible factors should be excluded. An inadequate reduction in ECF volume may reflect excessive NaCl intake rather than inadequate *natriuretic* response to loop diuretics. Understanding the mechanisms of diuretic action and adaptation, the causes of diuretic resistance and goals of diuretic treatment is key to identifying the optimal therapy for the diuretic-resistant patient (307). The addition of a proximal tubule- or a DCT (i.e., thiazides) diuretic to loop diuretics is often very effective (308–310). The combination of loop and DCT diuretics is synergistic (311,312). Because their half-life is longer than that of loop drugs, DCT diuretics may attenuate postdiuretic NaCl retention by continuing to inhibit NaCl reabsorption after the action of the loop diuretic ceases. By inhibiting carbonic anhydrase, DCT diuretics also inhibit salt transport in the PT, thereby increasing Na and fluid delivery to the loop of Henle, which, in turn, leads to enhanced NaCl delivery to the DCT (313). Because the loop diuretics inhibit loop solute reabsorption, the delivery of solute to the distal nephron will be magnified. The weak carbonic anhydrase inhibitors, such as acetazolamide, can be effective when added to loop diuretics (311). In addition, DCT diuretics inhibit distal NaCl reabsorption, thus attenuating the threefold increase in hypertrophy and hyperplasia of distal cells produced by chronic administration of loop diuretics (297). Because DCT diuretics can completely inhibit thiazide-sensitive Na–Cl cotransport even under these stimulated conditions, the effects of the thiazides will be greatly magnified in HF patients who have developed distal nephron hypertrophy loop diuretic as a result of protracted loop diuretic therapy (297,305,314). In general, when a second diuretic is added, the loop diuretic dose should not be modified, because the shape of the steep dose–response curve for loop diuretics is not altered by the addition of other diuretics. Metolazone is often the DCT diuretic of choice because it remains effective at low GFRs and has a longer half-life (315–317). Although DCT diuretics may be added in full doses (50–100 mg/day hydrochlorothiazide or 10 mg/day metolazone) when a rapid and robust response is needed, such an approach may lead to complications without close monitoring to prevent excessive fluid and electrolytes

Table 10.6 Maximal Intravenous Doses of Loop Diuretics in Patients with Diminished Responses to Oral Therapy

Maximal Intravenous Dose (mg)	Moderate Renal Insufficiency	Severe Renal Insufficiency	Heart Failure
Furosemide	80–160	160–200	40–80
Bumetanide	4–8	8–10	1–2
Torsemide	20–50	50–100	10–20

depletion, which can occur in up to two-thirds of the patients. One reasonable approach to combination therapy is to achieve control of ECF volume by initially adding full daily doses of DCT diuretics and then to maintain control by reducing DCT diuretic dosing to three times weekly. In fact, the finding in rats that thiazide diuretics down-regulate Na–K–ATPase activity and transport capacity along the DCT, suggests that addition of a DCT to a loop diuretic may decrease the structural and functional adaptation to loop diuretics (318,319).

In some reports a limited course of combination therapy was shown to be as effective as and perhaps safer than more prolonged courses (316). Thus, in the outpatient setting, either a small dose of DCT diuretic, such as 2.5 mg/day metolazone, or a limited course of a higher dose (three days of 10 mg/day metolazone) may be effective and safer. Because DCT diuretics are absorbed more slowly than loop diuretics, it may be reasonable to administer the DCT diuretic 0.5–1 hour prior to the loop diuretic. Although, at least acutely, their effects are less dramatic than those of DCT diuretics, collecting duct drugs, such as amiloride and spironolactone, can be added to loop diuretics. Aldosterone antagonists, while not synergistic with loop diuretics, have important roles in preventing hypokalemia and hypomagnesemia while maintaining renal Na excretion and they have been shown to prolong life (315).

In the hospital setting chlorothiazide (500–1,000 mg once or twice daily) and acetazolamide (250–375 mg up to four times daily) are available for intravenous administration to supplement loop diuretics (320). Chlorothiazide inhibits both carbonic anhydrase in the proximal tubule and the "thiazide-sensitive" Na–Cl cotransporter in the distal tubule and has a longer half-life than some other thiazides. Acutely, both chlorothiazide and acetazolamide are synergistic with loop diuretics. Acetazolamide is especially useful when the treatment of edema is complicated by hypokalemia and metabolic alkalosis, which renders both correction of hypokalemia and withdrawal of mechanical ventilatory support more difficult (319,321).

In diuretic-sensitive patients, the most common complications of loop diuretics stems from the hypokalemia, hyponatremia, and hypotension, which can occur because of excessive fluid and electrolyte losses. For diuretic-resistant patients, ototoxicity, more likely to occur with rapid high-dose administration, may limit intensity and duration of therapy, particularly in patients exposed to other ototoxic agents, such as the aminoglycosides (322–324). Myalgias may be more common after of bumetanide.

It has long been appreciated that many HF patients experience symptomatic relief after intravenous loop diuretics boluses before the occurrence of significant volume and NaCl losses (Table 10.6). The finding in one study that pretreatment of animals with indomethacin greatly attenuates furosemide-induced venodilation, suggests that loop diuretic-mediated acute reduction in pulmonary capillary wedge pressure is because of the stimulation of vasodilatory prostaglandins secretion. However, the hemodynamic response to intravenous loop diuretics may be more complex, as suggested by the findings in two series, that 1–1.5 mg/kg furosemide bolus administration in HF patients resulted in acute,

Table 10.7 Doses for Continuous Intravenous Infusion of Loop Diuretics

Diuretic	Intravenous Loading Dose (mg)	Creatinine Clearance <25 ml/min	Infusion Rate (mg/hr) Creatinine Clearance 25–75 mL/min	Creatinine Clearance >75 mL/min
Furosemide	40	20 then 40	10 then 20	10
Bumetanide	1	1 then 2	0.5 then 1	0.5
Torsemide	20	10 then 20	5 then 10	5

transient hemodynamic and symptomatic deterioration (325–327). These changes were related to activation of both the SNS and the RAAS by the diuretic drug (326,328). These data, however, do not negate the contribution of intravenous loop diuretics to symptomatic improvement once natriuresis begins within 15–20 min of administration.

Another possible complication of high-dose furosemide both in experimental animals and humans is the development of thiamine deficiency (329). In one study, in which HF patients receiving an 80 mg daily furosemide dose for at least three months were randomized to receive intravenous thiamine or placebo, thiamine supplementation was associated with improved hemodynamics, natriuresis, and erythropoiesis (330).

The intravenous administration of diuretics as continuous infusions has several potential advantages over bolus administration. By avoiding trough diuretic concentrations, continuous infusions prevent intermittent periods of positive Na–Cl balance (postdiuretic NaCl retention) (Table 10.7).

In fact comparison of the amount of NaCl excreted per mg of bumetamide in patients with chronic renal failure showed that continuous infusion was 32% more efficient than a bolus of the same dose (331). In a crossover study of nine patients with New York Health Association Class III–IV HF, 60–80 mg/day furosemide was more effective when given as a loading dose (30–40 mg) followed by continuous infusion than when given as three daily boluses (30–40 mg/dose) (332). Some patients refractory to large diuretic bolus doses respond to continuous infusion (322,333). Because continuous infusion of loop diuretics may reduce sympathetic discharge and RAAS activation and allow titration of the diuretic response it may be preferable for hemodynamically unstable patients in need of diuresis (334). Finally, adverse effects, such as ototoxicity and myopathy, appear to be less common when loop diuretics are administered as continuous infusions. Of note, although natriuretic efficacy may vary linearly with loop diuretic dose, high infusion rates (e.g., 2 g/day furosemide) might lead to toxic serum concentrations if continued for prolonged periods. In patients with renal failure, a drug such as torsemide that is partially cleared by hepatic metabolism may be preferred when high dose or prolonged therapy is needed.

Other Pharmacologic Therapies
Angiotensin-Converting Enzyme Inhibitors and Beta-Blockers
Prevention of renal dysfunction in patients with HF is likely to result in improved symptoms, fewer and shorter hospitalizations, and a lower mortality. However, currently available strategies to prevent renal dysfunction have limited success. While diuretics clearly improve symptoms in patients with HF, they have limited efficacy and may hasten HF progression. Conventional HF therapy, including dietary salt restriction, diuretics, and direct-acting vasodilators modestly improve survival in HF, but are limited by the

development of drug tolerance, partially attributable to their activation of vasoconstrictor mechanisms. In fact, Na depletion due to dietary salt restriction and the use of diuretics may itself activate the RAAS and SNS (191,326,335–337). Importantly, concomitant use of an ACE inhibitor prevents the development of nitrate tolerance, suggesting that the development of drug tolerance and expansion of body fluid volume associated with chronic nitrate therapy is mediated by activation of the RAAS (338–348). However, ACE inhibitors and angiotensin receptor blockers (ARBs) may worsen renal function by blocking A II-induced vasoconstriction of the efferent arteriole, which reduces glomerular hydrostatic pressure and thus GFR and perpetuates Na retention and volume overload (349). The HF patients most susceptible to this effect are those with an abnormal renal function who are treated with loop diuretics. In general, if vasodilation is not balanced by adequate improvement of cardiac output, there is elative worsening of arterial underfilling and reduced renal perfusion pressure, which, in turn, results in increased tubular Na reabsorption (119,350).

B-Type Natriuretic Peptide
The potential benefit of NPs on renal function in HF patients has been questioned (351,352). Although the reasons for this lack of benefit are uncertain, one might speculate that systemic vasodilatation with worsening arterial underfilling counteracts the potential benefits of BNP-induced reduction of cardiac filling pressures and neurohormonal activation.

Arginine Vasopressin Antagonists
Ongoing investigations of AVP receptor antagonists may broaden the application of such antihormonal therapy in HF. A trial with a vasopressin (V_2) antagonist in HF patients demonstrated weight loss accompanied by increased solute-free water excretion without changes in blood pressure, renal function, or neurohormones (127). Despite these encouraging results, it is important to understand that one-third of electrolyte-free water excretion comes from the ECF and two-thirds from the ICF compartment. Furthermore, vasopressin agonism of the unblocked V_1a receptors on cardiomyocytes and vascular smooth muscle may be detrimental. There are, however, nonpeptide orally active antagonists on both V_1a and V_2 AVP receptors under investigation.

Ultrafiltration
The use of ultrafiltration has been suggested when loop diuretics are associated with WRF. There are theoretic advantages to ultrafiltration in this setting. Diuretic resistance is often present when large doses of loop diuretics are used and, as previously discussed, these may have adverse effects (286). Ultrafiltration, however, may be associated with neurohormonal activation if the rate of fluid removal (and thus the transfer of fluid from the interstitium to vascular compartment) is too aggressive (353). The fluid removed by ultrafiltration is isotonic with plasma, whereas the fluid removed with diuretics is hypotonic to plasma. Thus, ultrafiltration is likely to remove more Na with fewer electrolyte disturbances than loop diuretics. Ultrafiltration is extensively discussed in another chapter (354,355).

Challenges in the Treatment of the Cardiorenal Syndrome in the Setting of Acutely Decompensated Heart Failure
It is clear from the foregoing discussion that renal dysfunction in HF patients is complex and multifactorial. Individualization of therapy is especially important in the setting of acutely decompensated HF and it requires careful determination of the patient's fluid status, cardiac output, and severity of intrinsic renal disease (Fig. 10.10).

Assessment of fluid status is critical, as volume status can be easily manipulated with the appropriate interventions. Patients can develop diuresis-induced hypovolemia during intensive treatment for HF or because of intercurrent illness. Although diuretics are an

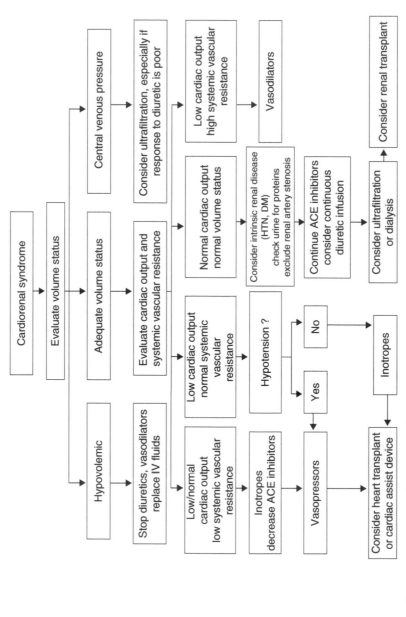

Figure 10.10 Therapeutic approaches to the Cardiorenal Syndrome in the setting of acutely decompensated heart failure. *Abbreviations:* ACE, angiotensin-converting enzyme; DM, diabetes mellitus; HTN, hypertension. *Source:* Adapted from Ref. 365.

integral part of HF therapy, overly aggressive use can decrease cardiac output because of an excessive reduction in preload. As described earlier in the chapter, diuretics also decrease GFR independently of their effect on cardiac output (356). Diuresis-induced hypotension must be reversed with fluids before irreversible renal damage occurs. Thus, when HF and renal insufficiency coexist, it is critically important to determine if the patient is hypovolemic. In this regard careful physical examination or echocardiographic estimation of right atrial pressure is especially helpful (357–359). In some cases invasive hemodynamic monitoring may be necessary to monitor cardiac filling pressures.

If the patient is euvolemic or hypervolemic, the adequacy of renal performance should be determined. If the patient is hypotensive, pressor therapy should be used to keep systolic blood pressure >80 mmHg, with a mean systolic blood pressure of 60 mmHg (360).

In the absence of hypotension, knowledge of cardiac output is helpful in directing therapy. The patient with cold extremities, low cardiac output, and increased systemic vascular resistance is excessively vasoconstricted and often responds very favorably to vasodilation (361). When such a patient has renal insufficiency, ACE inhibitors are often withdrawn in an attempt to improve renal function; however, such patients are the ones who truly benefit from vasodilator therapy, first acutely, with either nitroprusside or nesiritide, and later with ACE inhibitors. Renal function may actually improve as cardiac output and, consequently, renal perfusion increase. Systolic blood pressures of 80–90 mmHg should be tolerated as long as renal function does not worsen.

More problematic is the treatment of patients with hypotension, normal cardiac output, low systemic vascular resistance, and WRF. This hemodynamic picture, typically seen with sepsis, can also occur in patients with severe HF and is termed "vasodilatory shock" (362). In such cases either blood pressure is too low to support adequate renal perfusion, or blood is shunted away from the kidneys. Although the syndrome is far from being completely understood, a current hypothesis states that K channels on vascular smooth muscle cells remain abnormally open and allow K to leak extracellularly (362). The resulting hyperpolarization impairs normal depolarization by preventing Ca channels from opening, thus precluding movement of Ca intracellularly and activation of normal contraction. The resulting intense vasodilation is often refractory to NE and A II. The abnormal K channel activity may be due to acidosis, reduced levels of ATP, or inadequate AVP levels, the latter due to the depleted AVP stores in advanced HF. In a small randomized trial infusion of AVP increased blood pressure and allowed for a reduction in pressor medication dose in patients with hypotension and low system vascular resistance after implantation of a ventricular assist device (358). Early recognition and appropriate therapy for this form of cardiorenal syndrome is vital because it is associated with a high mortality. In patients who are eligible for cardiac transplantation, insertion of a ventricular assist device can reverse renal insufficiency and allow successful transplantation (363). Intrinsic renal disease is frequent in patients with the cardiorenal syndrome and should be suspected when hypovolemia has been excluded or corrected and cardiac output and systemic vascular resistance are normal (364–370). These patients are especially susceptible to the development of diuretic resistance.

SUMMARY

In depth knowledge of renal handling of sodium and water is critically important for the understanding of the hypervolemia, which increases morbidity and mortality of HF patients.

The control of Na excretion depends on the control of two variables of renal function: GFR and rate of Na reabsorption. The latter is controlled by the RAAS, renal sympathetic nerves, effects of arterial blood pressure on the kidneys (pressure natriuresis), and atrial natriuretic factors. The renal interstitial hydrostatic pressure and several renal paracrine agents play important roles in regulating Na reabsorption. The regulation of Na excretion depends on two distinct mechanisms: (*i*) proximal nephron processes (control of GFR, pressure natriuresis, and, to a lesser extent, changes in Starling forces) that lead to coupled changes in Na and water excretion; and (*ii*) distal nephron effects in which Na can be reabsorbed *independently* of water. Proximal mechanisms are primarily involved in excreting excess ECF volume, whereas the distal mechanisms alter Na excretion when ingestion of Na is not balanced by ingestion of water. Both types of mechanisms can alter blood pressure because of the intimate relationship between total body Na and water, blood volume, and pressure.

In HF normal kidneys retain abnormal amounts of Na and water due to the neurohormonal mechanisms activated by arterial underfilling. However, the bidirectional cardiorenal interactions go beyond purely hemodynamic effects and include the expanded effects of neurohormonal activation on inflammation and oxidative stress. Although neurohormonal blockade has some effectiveness in reducing oxidative stress and inflammation, currently there is no effective strategy that directly influences these factors.

Improved understanding of the complex relationship between cardiac and renal dysfunction may help to identify treatments aimed at reversing these complex cardiorenal interactions.

REFERENCES

1. Sica DA. Sodium and water retention in heart failure and diuretic therapy: basic mechanisms. Cleve Clin J Med 2006; 73: S2–7.
2. Farrar DJ, Hill JD. Recovery of major organ function in patients awaiting heart transplantation with Thoratec ventricular devices. Thoratec Ventricular Assist Device Principal Investigators. J Heart Lung Tansplant 1994; 13: 1125–32.
3. Schrier RW. Role of diminished renal function in cardiovascular mortality: marker or pathogenic factor? J Am Coll Cardiol 2006; 47: 1–8.
4. Ronco C, House AA, Haapio M. Cardiorenal syndrome: refining the definition of a complex symbiosis gone wrong. Intensive Care Med 2008; 34: 957–62.
5. Bongartz LG, Cramer MJ, Doevendans PA, et al. The severe cardiorenal syndrome. Guyton revisited. Eur Heart J 2005; 26: 11–17.
6. Schrier RW, Abraham WT. Hormones and hemodynamics in heart failure. N Engl J Med 1999; 341: 577–85.
7. Shlipak MG. Pharmacotherapy for heart failure in patients with renal insufficiency. Ann Intern Med 2003; 138: 917–24.
8. Bibbins-Domingo K, Lin F, Vittinghoff E, et al. Renal insufficiency as an independent predictor of mortality among women with heart failure. J Am Coll Cardiol 2004; 44: 1593–600.
9. Shlipak MG, Smith GL, Rathore SS, et al. Renal function, digoxin therapy, and heart failure outcomes: evidence from the digoxin intervention group trial. J Am Soc Nephrol 2004; 15: 2195–203.
10. Ezekowitz J, McAlister FA, Humphries KH, et al. The association among renal insufficiency, pharmacotherapy, and outcomes in 6,427 patients with heart failure and coronary artery disease. J Am Coll Cardiol 2004; 44: 1587–92.
11. Smith GL, Shlipak MG, Havranek EP, et al. Race and renal impairment in heart failure: mortality in blacks versus whites. Circulation 2005; 111: 1270–7.
12. Hillege HL, Nitsch D, Pfeffer MA, et al. Renal function as a predictor of outcome in a broad spectrum of patients with heart failure. Circulation 2006; 113: 671–8.
13. Adams KF Jr, Fonarow GC, Emerman CL, et al. Characteristics and outcomes of patients hospitalized for heart failure in the united states: rationale, design, and preliminary observations from the first 100,000 cases in the acute decompensated heart failure national registry (ADHERE). Am Heart J 2005; 149: 209–16.
14. Smith GL, Lichtman JH, Bracken MB, et al. Renal impairment and outcomes in heart failure: Systematic review and meta-analysis. J Am Coll Cardiol 2006; 47: 1987–96.
15. Owan TE, Hodge DO, Herges RM, et al. Secular trends in renal dysfunction and outcomes in hospitalized heart failure patients. J Card Fail 2006; 12: 257–62.
16. Binanay C, Califf RM, Hasselblad V, et al. Evaluation study of congestive heart failure and pulmonary artery catheterization effectiveness: the ESCAPE trial. JAMA 2005; 294: 1625–33.

17. Forman DE, Butler J, Wang Y, et al. Incidence, predictors at admission, and impact of worsening renal function among patients hospitalized with heart failure. J Am Coll Cardiol 2004; 43: 61–7.
18. Gottlieb SS, Abraham W, Butler J, et al. The prognostic importance of different definitions of worsening renal function in congestive heart failure. J Card Fail 2002; 8: 136–41.
19. Krumholz HM, Chen YT, Vaccarino V, et al. Correlates and impact on outcomes of worsening renal function in patients ≥ 65 years of age with heart failure. Am J Cardiol 2000; 85: 1110–13.
20. Weinfeld MS, Chertow GM, Stevenson LW. Aggravated renal dysfunction during intensive therapy for advanced chronic heart failure. Am Heart J 1999; 138: 285–90.
21. Nohria A, Lewis E, Stevenson LW. Medical management of advanced heart failure. JAMA 2002; 287: 628–40.
22. Smith GL, Vaccarino V, Kosiborod M, et al. Worsening renal function: what is a clinically meaningful change in creatinine during hospitalization with heart failure? J Card Fail 2003; 9: 13–25.
23. Mehrotra R, Kathuria P. Place of peritoneal dialysis in the management of treatment-resistant congestive heart failure. Kidney Int Suppl 2006; 103: S67– 71.
24. Costanzo MR. Management of volume overload in acute heart failure: diuretics and ultrafiltration. In: Mebaaza A, Gheorghiade M, Zannad FM, Parrillo JE, eds. Acute Heart Failure. London: Springer, 2008: 503–18.
25. Levey AS, Coresh J, Greene T, et al. Chronic kidney disease epidemiology collaboration using standardized serum creatinine values in the modification of diet in renal disease study equation for estimating glomerular filtration rate. Ann Intern Med 2006; 145: 247–54.
26. Cockroft DW, Gault MH. Prediction of creatinine clearance from serum creatinine. Nephron 1976; 16: 31–41.
27. Schrier RW. Body fluid volume regulation in health and disease: a unifying hypothesis. Ann Intern Med 1990; 113: 155–9.
28. Schreier RW, Gurevich AK, Abraham WT. Renal sodium excretion, edematous disorders and diuretic use. In: Schreier RW, ed. Renal and Electrolytes Disorders, 6th edn. Philadelphia: Lippincott Williams and Wilkins, 2002: 64–114.
29. Wesson LG Jr. Glomerular and tubular factors in the renal excretion of sodium chloride. Med Balt 1957; 36: 281–396.
30. McCormick SD, Bradshaw D. Hormonal control of salt and water balance in vertebrates. Gen Comp Endocrinol 2006; 147: 3–8.
31. Bard P. Anatomical organization of the central nervous system in relation to control of heart and blood vessels. Physiol Rev 1960; 40: S3–S26.
32. Di Bona GF. Neural control of renal function in health and disease. Clin Autom Res 1994; 4: 69–74.
33. Thomsen K. Lithium clearance a new method for determining proximal and distal tubular reabsorption of sodium and water. Nephron 1984; 37: 217–23.
34. Rector FC. Sodium, bicarbonate and chloride absorption by the proximal tubule. Am Physiol 1983; 13: F461–71.
35. Verbalis JG. Disorders of body water homeostasis. Best Pract Res Clin Endocrinol Metab 2003; 17: 471–503.
36. Nielsen S, Knepper M, Kwon T, et al. Regulation of water balance. In: Schrier RW, ed. Diseases of the Kidney and Urinary Tract, 7th edn. New York: Lippincott Williams and Wilkins, 2001: 109–34.
37. de Wardener HE, del Greco F. Influence of solute excretion on production of hypotonic urine in man. Clin Sci 1955; 14: 715–23.
38. Andreoli TE, Berliner RW, Kokko J, et al. Questions and replies: renal mechanisms of urinary concentration and diluting processes. Am J Physiol 1978; 235: F1–F11.
39. Knepper MA, Nielsen N, Chou Cl, et al. Mechanism of vasopressin action in the renal collecting duct. Semin Nephrol 1994; 14: 302–21.
40. Morgan T, Berliner RW. A study by continuous microperfusion of water and electrolytes movements in the loop of henle and distal tubule of the rat. Nephron 1969; 6: 388–405.
41. Molony DA, Reeves WB, Andreoli TE. Na+:K+: 2Cl-cotransport and the thick ascending limb. Kidney Int 1989; 36: 418–26.
42. Imai M, Taniguchi J, Yoshitomi K. Transition of permeability properties along the descending limb of long-loop nephron. Am Phisiol 1988; 254: F323–8.
43. Knepper MA. Urea permeability of mammalian inner medullary collecting ducts from rats. Am J Physiol 1983; 245: F634–9.
44. Verney EB. Renal excretion of water and salt. Lancet 1957; 273: 1295–8.
45. Borst JG, deVries LA. Three types of "natural diuresis". Lancet 1950; 2: 1–6.
46. Brown D, Nielsen S. Cell biology in vasopressin action. In: Brenner B, ed. The Kidney, 6th edn. Philadelphia: WB Saunders, 2000: 575–94.

47. Nielsen S, Chou CL, Marples D, et al. Vasopressin increases water permeability of kidney collecting duct by inducing translocation of aquaporin-CD water channels to plasma membrane. Proc Natl Acad Sci USA 1995; 92: 1013–17.

48. Anderson RJ, Schreier RW. Physiology of renal water excretion. Contrib Nephrol 1978; 14: 583–686.

49. Jamison RL, Maffly RH. The urinary concentrating mechanism. N Engl J Med 1976; 295: 1059–61.

50. Layton HE. Urea transport in a distributed loop model of the urine-concentrating mechanism. Am J Physiol 1990; 258: F1110–FF1124.

51. Gilmore JP. Contribution of baroreceptors to the control of renal function. Circ Res 1964; 14: 301–17.

52. Guyton AC. The surprising kidney-fluid mechanism for pressure control-its infinite gain! Hypertension. 1990; 16: 725–30.

53. Goetz KL, Bond GC, Bloxham DD. Atrial receptors and renal function. Physiol Rev 1975; 55: 157–205.

54. Brewster UC, Perazzella M. The renin angiotensin aldosterone system and the kidney: effects on kidney disease. Am J Med 2004; 116: 263–72.

55. Weir MR, Dzau VJ. The renin angiotensin aldosterone system: a specific target for hypertension management. Am J Hypertens 1999; 12(Suppl): 2053–135.

56. Bello-Reuss E, Trevino DL, Gottschalk CW. Effect of renal sympathetic nerve stimulation on proximal water and sodium reabsorption. J Clin Invest 1976; 57: 1104–7.

57. Rector FC. Sodium bicarbonate and chloride absorption by the proximal tubule. Am J Physiol 1983; 13: F46–F471.

58. Henrich WL, Berl T, MacDonald KM, et al. Angiotensin, renal nerves, and prostaglandins in renal hemodynamics during hemorrhage. Am J Physiol 1978; 235: F46–51.

59. Blaustein MP, Zhang J, Chen L, Hamilton BP. How does salt retention raise blood pressure? Am J Physiol Regul Integr Comp Physiol 2006; 290: R514–23.

60. Lev-Ran A, Porta M. Salt and hypertension: a phylogenetic prospective. Diab Metabol Res Rev 2005; 21: 118–31.

61. Guyton PC. Dominant role of the kidneys and accessory role of whole-body autoregulation in the pathogenesis of hypertension. Am J Hypertens 1989; 2: 575–85.

62. McDonough AA, Leong PKK, Yang LE. Mechanisms of pressure diuresis: how blood pressure regulates sodium transport. Ann NY Acad Sci 2003; 986: 669–77.

63. Cupples WA. Interactions contributing to kidney blood flow autoregulation. Curr Opin Nephrol Hypertens 2007; 16: 39–45.

64. Chou CL, Marsh DJ. Time course of proximal tubule response to acute arterial hypertension in the rat. Am J Physiol 1988; 254: F601–7.

65. Zhang Y, Mircheff AK, Hensley CB, et al. Rapid redistribution and inhibition of renal sodium transporters during acute pressure natriuresis. Am J Physiol 1996; 270: F1004–14.

66. Maygar CE, Zhang Y, Holstein-Rathlou NH, McDonough AA. Proximal tubule Na transporter responses are the same during acute and chronic hypertension. Am J Physiol 2000; 275: F358–69.

67. Cupples WA, Braam B. Assessment of renal autoregulation. Am J Physiol 2007; 292: F1105–23.

68. Braam B, Mitchell KD, Koomans HA, Navar LG. Relevance of the tubuloglomerular feedback mechanism and pathophysiology. J Am Soc Nephrol 1993; 4: 1257–74.

69. Vallon V. Tubuloglomerular feedback and the control of glomerular filtration rate. News Physiol Sci 2003; 18: 169–74.

70. Schnermann J, Traynor T, Yang T, et al. Tubuloglomerular feedback: new concept and developments. Kidney Int 1998; 54:S40–5.

71. Brewster UC, Setaro JF, Perazzella MA. The renin-angiotensin-aldosterone System: cardiorenal effects and implications for renal and cardiovascular disease states. Am J Med Sci 2003; 326: 15–24.

72. Goodfriend TL. Aldosterone: a hormone of cardiovascular adaptation and maladaptation. J Clin Hypertens 2006; 8: 133–9.

73. Molina CR, Fowler MB, McCrory S, et al. Hemodynamic, renal and endocrine effects of atrial natriuretic peptide in severe heart failure. J Am Coll Cardiol 1988; 12: 175–86.

74. Hosoda K, Nakao K, Mukoyama M, et al. Expression of brain natriuretic peptide gene in human heart: production in the ventricle. Hypertension 1991; 17: 1152–5.

75. Sato F, Kamoi K, Wakiya Y, et al. Relationship between plasma atrial natriuretic peptide levels and atrial pressure in man. J Clin Endocrinol Metab 1986; 63: 823–7.

76. Robertson GL. The regulation of vasopressin function in health and disease. Recent Prog Horm Res 1976; 33: 333–85.

77. Dunn FL, Brennan TJ, Nelson AE, et al. The role of blood osmolality and volume in regulating vasopressin secretion in the rat. J Clin Invest 1973; 52: 3212–19.

78. Schreier RW, Berl T, Anderson RJ, et al. Nonosmolar control of renal water excretion. In: Andreoli T, Grantham J, Rector F, eds. Disturbances in Body Fluid Osmolality. Bethesda, MD: American Physiological Society, 1977: 149.

79. Sklar AH, Schreier RW. Central nervous system mediators of vasopressin release. Physiol Rev 1983; 63: 1243.

80. Fitsimons JT. Physiology and pathophysiology of thirst and sodium appetite. In: Seldin DW, Glebisch G, eds. The Kidney, Physiology and Pathophysiology. New York: Raven Press, 1992: 1615–48.

81. deCastro J. A microregulatory analysis of spontaneous fluid intake in humans: evidence that amount of liquid ingested and its timing is mainly governed by feeding. Physiol Behav 1988; 3: 705–14.

82. Stricker EM, Verbalis JG. Water intake and body fluids. In: Zigmond MJ, et al., eds. Fundamental Neuroscience. San Diego: Academic Press, 1999: 1111–26.

83. Zucker IH, Earle AM, Gilmore JP. The mechanism of adaptation of left atrial stretch receptors in dogs with chronic congestive heart failure. J Clin Invest 1977; 60: 323–31.

84. Murdaugh HV Jr, Sieker HO, Manfredi F. Effect of altered intrathoracic pressure on renal hemodynamics, electrolyte excretion and water clearance. J Clin Invest 1959; 38: 834–42.

85. de Torrente A, Robertson GL, McDonald KM, et al. Mechanism of diuretic response to increased left atrial pressure in the ansthetized dog. Kidney Int 1975; 8: 355–61.

86. Nakaoka H, Imataka K, Amano M, et al. Plasma levels of atrial natriuretic factor in patients with congestive heart failure. N Engl J Med 1985; 313: 892–3.

87. Raine AE, Erne P, Burgisser E, et al. Atrial natriuretic peptide and atrial pressure in patients with congestive heart failure. N Engl J Med 1986; 315: 533–7.

88. Zucker IH, Gorman AJ, Cornish KG, et al. Impaired atrial receptor modulation or renal nerve activity in dogs with chronic volume overload. Cardiovasc Res 1985; 19: 411–18.

89. Volpe M, Tritto C, De Luca N, et al. Failure of atrial natriuretic factor to increase with saline load in patients with dilated cardiomyopathy and mild heart failure. J Clin Invest 1991; 88: 1481–9.

90. Epstein FH, Post RS, McDowell M. The effects of an arteriovenous fistula on renal hemodynamics and electrolyte excretion. J Clin Invest 1953; 32: 233–41.

91. Schrier RW, Humphreys MH. Factors involved in antinatriuretic effects of acute constriction of the thoracic and abdominal inferior vena cava. Circ Res 1971; 29: 479–89.

92. Schrier RW, Humphreys MH, Ufferman RC. Role of cardiac output and the autonomic nervous system in the antinatriretic response to acute constriction of the thoracic superior vena cava. Circ Res 1971; 29: 490–8.

93. Pearce JW, Sonnenberg H. Effects of spinal section and renal denervation on the renal response to blood volume expansion. Can J Physiol Pharmacol 1965; 43: 211–24.

94. Gilmore JP, Daggett WM. Response of the chronic cardiac denervated dog to acute volume expansion. Am J Physiol 1966; 210: 509–12.

95. Knox Fe, Davis BB, Berliner RW. Effect of chronic cardiac denervation on renal response to saline infusion. Am J Physiol 1967; 213: 174–8.

96. Schedl HP, Bartter FC. An explanation for and experimental correction of the abnormal water diuresis in cirrhosis. J Clin Invest 1967; 46: 1297–308.

97. Dzau VI, Packer M, Lilly LS, et al. Prostaglandins in severe congestive heart failure. Relation to activation of the renin angiotensin system and hyponatremia. N Engl J Med 1984; 310: 347–52.

98. Abraham WT, Hensen J, Schrier RW. Elevatedp lasma noradrenaline concentrations in patients with low-output cardiac failure: dependence on increased noradrenaline secretion rates. Clin Sci (Lond) 1990; 79: 429–35.

99. Cohn JN. Sympathetic nervous system in heart failure. Circulation 2002; 106: 2417–18.

100. Leimbach WN Jr, Wallin BG, Victor RG, et al. Direct evidence from intraneural recordings for increased central sympathetic outflow in patients with heart failure. Circulation 1986; 73: 913–19.

101. Francis GS, Benedict C, Johnstone DE, et al. Comparison of neuroendocrine activation in patients with left ventricular dysfunction with and without congestive heart failure: a substudy of the studies of left ventricular dysfunction (SOLVD). Circulation 1990; 82: 1724–9.

102. Hasking JG, Esler MD, Jennings GL, et al. Norepinephrine spillover to plasma in patients with congestive heart failure: evidence of increased overall and cardiorenal sympathetic nervous activity. Circulation 1986; 73: 615–21.

103. Brod J, Fejfar Z, Fejfarova MH. The role of neuro-humoral factors in the genesis of renal haemodynamic changes in heart failure. Acta Med Scand 1954; 148: 273–90.

104. Gill JR Jr, Mason DT, Bartter FC. Adrenergic nervous system in Na metabolism: effects of guanethidine and Na-retaining steroids in normal man. J Clin Invest 1964; 43: 177–84.

105. DiBona GF, Herman PJ, Sawin LL. Neural control of renal function in edema-forming states. Am J Physiol 1988; 254: RI017–24.

106. Bello-Reuss E. Effect of catecholamines on fluid reabsorption by the isolated proximal convoluted tubule. Am J Physiol 1980; 238: F347–52.
107. Meyers BD, Deen WM, Brenner BM. Effects of norepinephrine and angiotensin II on the determinants of glomerular ultrafiltration and proximal tubule fluid reabsorption in the rat. Circ Res 1975; 37: 101–10.
108. Ichikawa I, Pfeffer JM, Pfeffer MA, et al. Role of angiotensin II in the altered renal function of congestive heart failure. Circ Res 1984; 55: 669–75.
109. Carpenter CC, Davis JO, Holman JE, et al. Studies on the response of the transplanted kidney and the transplanted adrenal gland to thoracic inferior vena caval constriction. J Clin Invest 1961; 40: 196–204.
110. Lifschitz MD, Schrier RW. Alterations in cardiac output with chronic constriction of thoracic inferior vena cava. Am J Physiol 1973; 225: 1364–70.
111. Ichikawa I, Brenner BM. Importance of efferent arteriolar vascular tone in regulation of proximal tubule fluid reabsorption and glomerulotubular balance in the rat. J Clin Invest 1980; 65: 1192–201.
112. Liu FY, Cogan MG. Angiotensin II: a potent regulator of acidification in the rat early proximal convoluted tubule. J Clin Invest 1987; 80: 272–5.
113. Eiam-Ong S, Hilden SA, Johns CA, et al. Stimulation of basolateral Na(+)-HC03-cotransporter by angiotensin II in rabbit renal cortex. Am J Physiol 1993; 265: FI95–203.
114. Hensen J, Abraham WT, Durr JA, et al. Aldosterone in congestive heart failure: analysis of determinants and role in Na retention. Am J Nephrol 1991; 11: 441–6.
115. Hensen J, Abraham WT, Lesnefsky EJ, et al. Atrial natriuretic peptide kinetic studies in patients with cardiac dysfunction. Kidney Int 1992; 41: 1333–9.
116. Szatalowicz VL, Arnold PE, Chaimovitz C, et al. Radioimmune assay of plasma arginine vasopressin in hyponatremic patients with congestive heart failure. N Engl J Med 1981; 305: 263–6.
117. Riegger GA, Uebau G, Kochsiek K. Antidiuretic hormone in congestive heart failure. Am J Med 1982; 72: 49–52.
118. Pruszczynski W, Vahanian A, Ardaillou R, et al. Role of antidiuretic hormone in impaired water excretion of patients with congestive heart failure. J Clin Endocrinol Metab 1984; 58: 599–605.
119. Bichet DG, Kortas C, Mettauer B, et al. Modulation of plasma and platelet vasopressin by cardiac function in patients with heart failure. Kidney Int 1986; 29: 1188–96.
120. Goldsmith SR, Francis GS, Cowley AW Jr, et al. Hemodynamic effects of infused arginine vasopressin in congestive heart failure. J Am Coll Cardiol 1986; 8: 779–83.
121. Goldsmith SR, Francis GS, Cowley AW Jr. Arginine vasopressin and the renal response to water loading in congestive heart failure. Am J Cardiol 1986; 58: 295–9.
122. Anderson RJ, Cadnapaphornchai P, Harbottle JA, et al. Mechanism of effect of thoracic inferior vena cava constriction on renal water excretion. J Clin Invest 1974; 54: 1473–9.
123. Handelman W, Lum G, Schrier RW. Impaired water excretion in high output cardiac failure in the rat. Clin Res 1979; 27: 173A.
124. Abraham WT, Oren RM, Crisman TD. Effects of an oral, nonpeptide, selective V2 receptor vasopressin antagonist in patients with chronic heart failure. J Am Coll Cardiol 1997; 29: 169A.
125. Ishikawa S, Saito T, Okada K, et al. Effect of vasopressin antagonist on water excretion in inferior vena cava constriction. Kidney Int 1986; 30: 49–55.
126. Yared A, Kon V, Brenner BM, et al. Role for vasopressin with congestive heart failure. Kidney Int 1985; 27: 337.
127. Gheorghiade M, Gattis WA, O'Connor CM, et al. Effects of tolvaptan, a vasopressin antagonist, in patients hospitalized with worsening heart failure: a randomized controlled trial. JAMA 2004; 291: 1963–71.
128. Xu DL, Martin PY, Ohara M, et al. Upregulation of aquaporin-2 water channel expression in chronic heart failure rat. J Clin Invest 1997; 99: 1500–5.
129. Dunn FL, Brennan TJ, Nelson AE, et al. The role of blood osmolality and volume in regulating vasopressin secretion in the rat. J Clin Invest 1973; 52: 3212–19.
130. McMurray JJ, Ray SG, Abdullah I, et al. Plasma endothelin chronic heart failure. Circulation 1992; 85: 504–9.
131. Teerlink JR, Laffler BM, Hess P, et al. Role of ednothelin in the maintenance of blood pressure in conscious rats with chronic heart failure: acute effects of the endothelin receptor antagonist Ro 47-0203 (bosentan). Circulation 1994; 90: 2510–18.
132. Pacher R, Stanek B, Hulsmann M, et al. Prognostic impact of big endothelin-l plasma concentrations compared with invasive hemodynamic evaluation in severe heart failure. J Am Coll Cardiol 1996; 27: 633–41.
133. Burnett JC Jr, Kao PC, Hu DC, et al. Atrial natriuretic peptide elevation in congestive heart failure in the human. Science 1986; 231: 1145–7.

134. Hirata Y, Ishii M, Matsuoka H, et al. Plasma concentration of alpha-human atrial natriuretic polypeptide and cyclic GMP in patients with heart disease. Am Heart J 1987; 113: 1463–9.

135. Michel JB, Amal IE, Corvol P. Atrial natriuretic factor as a marker in congestive heart failure. Horm Res 1990; 34: 166–8

136. Mukoyama M, Nakao K, Saito Y, et al. Increased human natriuretic peptide in congestive heart failure. N Engl J Med 1990; 323: 757–8.

137. Molina CR, Fowler MB, McCrory S, et al. Hemodynamic, renal and endocrine effects of atrial natriuretic peptide infusion in heart failure. J Am Coll Cardiol 1988; 12: 175–86.

138. Cody RJ, Atlas SA, Laragh JH, et al. Atrial natriuretic factor in normal subjects and heart failure patients. Plasma levels and renal, hormonal, and hemodynamic responses to peptide infusion. J Clin Invest 1986; 78: 1362–74.

139. Saito Y, Nakao K, Arai H, et al. Atrial natriuretic polypeptide (ANP) in human ventricle. Increased gene expression of ANP in dilated cardiomyopathy. Biochem Biophys Res Commun 1987; 148: 211–17.

140. Drexler H, Hirth C, Stasch HP, et al. Vasodilatory action of endogenous atrial natriuretic factor in a rat model of chronic heart failure as determined by monoclonal ANP antibody. Circ Res 1990; 66: 1371–80.

141. Munagala VK, Burnett JC Jr, Redfield MM. The natriuretic peptides in cardiovascular medicine. Curr Probl Cardiol 2004; 9: 707–69.

142. Publication Committee for the VMAC Investigators. Intravenous nesiritide vs nitroglycerin for treatment of decompensated congestive heart failure: a randomized controlled trial. JAMA 2002; 287: 1531–40.

143. Biollaz J, Nussberger J, Porchet M, et al. Four-hour infusions of synthetic atrial natriuretic peptide in normal volunteers. Hypertension 1986; 8: II96–1I105

144. Borenstein HB, Cupples WA, Sonnenberg H, et al. The effect of natriuretic atrial extract on renal haemodynamics and urinary excretion in anaesthetized rats. J Physiol 1983; 334: 133–40.

145. Dunn BR, Ichikawa I, Pfeffer JM, et al. Renal and Systemic hemodynamic effects of synthetic atrial natriuretic peptide in the anesthetized rat. Circ Res 1986; 59: 237–46.

146. Kim JK, Summer SN, Durr JA, et al. Enzymatic and binding effects of atrial natriuretic factor in glomeruli and nephrons. Kidney Int 1989; 35: 799–805.

147. Koseki C, Hayashi Y, Torikai S, et al. Localization of binding sites for alpha-rat atrial natriuretic polypeptide in rat kidney. Am J Physiol 1986; 250: F210–16.

148. Healy DP, Fanestil DD. Localization of atrial natriuretic peptide binding sites within the rat kidney. Am J Physiol 1986; 250: F573–8.

149. Lee ME, Miller WL, Edwards BS, et al. Role of endogenous atrial natriuretic factor in acute congestive heart failure. J Clin Invest 1989; 84: 1962–6.

150. Abraham WT, Hensen J, Kim JK, et al. Atrial natriuretic peptide and urinary cyclic guanosine monophosphate in patients with chronic heart failure. J Am Soc Nephrol 1992; 2: 1697–703.

151. Abraham WT, Lauwaars ME, Kim JK, et al. Reversal of atrial natriuretic peptide resistance by increasing distal tubular Na delivery in patients with decompensated cirrhosis. Hepatology 1995; 22: 737–43.

152. Kistorp C, Raymond I, Pedersen F, et al. N-terminal pro-brain natriuretic peptide, C-reactive protein, and urinary albumin levels as predictors of mortality and cardiovascular events in older adults. JAMA 2005; 293: 1609–16.

153. Swain JA, Heyndrickx GR, Boettcher DH, et al. Prostaglandin control of renal circulation in the anesthetized dog and baboon. Am J Physiol 1975; 229: 826–30.

154. Walker RM, Massey TE, McElligott TF, et al. Acetaminophen-induced hypothermia, hepatic congestion, and modification by N-acetylcysteine in mice. Toxicol Appl Pharmacol 1981; 59: 500–7.

155. Walshe JJ, Venuto RC. Acute oliguric renal failure induced by indomethacin: possible mechanism. Ann Intern Med 1979; 91: 47–9.

156. Riegger GA, Kahles HW, Elsner D, et al. Effects of acetylsalicylic acid on renal function in patients with chronic heart failure. Am J Med 1991; 90: 571–5.

157. National Institutes of Health, National Institute of Diabetes and Digestive and Kidney Diseases. USRDS 1997 Annual Data Report. Bethesda, MD, USA: National Institutes of Health, National Institute of Diabetes and Digestive and Kidney Diseases, 1997. [Available from: http://www.usrds.org/adr_1997.htm] [11 November 2003].

158. Foley RN, Parfrey PS, Sarnak MJ. Epidemiology of cardiovascular disease in chronic renal disease. J Am Soc Nephrol 1998; 9: S16–23.

159. Herzog CA, Ma JZ, Collins AJ. Poor long-term survival after acute myocardial infarction among patients on long-term dialysis. N Engl J Med 1998; 339: 799–805.

160. Zoccali C. Cardiorenal risk as a new frontier of nephrology: research needs and areas for intervention. Nephrol Dial Transplant 2002; 17: 50–4.

161. Muntner P, He J, Hamm L, et al. Renal insufficiency and subsequent death resulting from cardiovascular disease in the united states. J Am Soc Nephrol 2002; 13: 745–53.

162. Henry RM, Kostense PJ, Bos G, et al. Mild renal insufficiency is associated with increased cardiovascular mortality: the hoorn study. Kidney Int 2002; 62: 1402–7.

163. Beddhu S, Allen-Brady K, Cheung AK, et al. Impact of renal failure on the risk of myocardial infarction and death. Kidney Int 2002; 62: 1776–83.

164. Fried LF, Shlipak MG, Crump C, et al. Renal insufficiency as a predictor of cardiovascular outcomes and mortality in elderly individuals. J Am Coll Cardiol 2003; 41: 1364–72.

165. Manjunath G, Tighiouart H, Ibrahim H, et al. Level of kidney function as a risk factor for atherosclerotic cardiovascular outcomes in the community. J Am Coll Cardiol 2003; 41: 47–55.

166. Sarnak MJ, Levey AS, Schoolwerth AC, et al. Kidney disease as a risk factor for development of cardiovascular disease: a statement from the american heart association councils on kidney in cardiovascular disease, high blood pressure research, clinical cardiology, and epidemiology and prevention. Circulation 2003; 108: 2154–69.

167. Al Suwaidi J, Reddan DN, Williams K, et al. Prognostic implications of abnormalities in renal function in patients with acute coronary syndromes. Circulation 2002; 106: 974–80.

168. Best PJ, Lennon R, Ting HH, et al. The impact of renal insufficiency on clinical outcomes in patients undergoing percutaneous coronary interventions. J Am Coll Cardiol 2002; 39: 1113–19.

169. Rao V, Weisel RD, Buth KJ, et al. Coronary artery bypass grafting in patients with non-dialysis-dependent renal insufficiency. Circulation 1997; 96(Suppl): II-38–43.

170. Gibson CM, Pinto DS, Murphy SA, et al. Association of creatinine and creatinine clearance on presentation in acute myocardial infarction with subsequent mortality. J Am Coll Cardiol 2003; 42: 1535–43.

171. Wright RS, Reeder GS, Herzog CA, et al. Acute myocardial infarction and renal dysfunction: a high-risk combination. Ann Intern Med 2002; 137: 563–70.

172. Hillege HL, van Gilst WH, van Veldhuisen DJ, et al. Accelerated decline and prognostic impact of renal function after myocardial infarction and the benefits of ACE inhibition: the CATS randomized trial. Eur Heart J 2003; 24: 412–20.

173. National Institutes of Health. National Institute of Diabetes and Digestive and Kidney Diseases. USRDS 1998 Annual Data Report. Bethesda, MD, USA: National Institutes of Health, National Institute of Diabetes and Digestive and Kidney Diseases, 1998. [Available from: http://www.usrds.org/adr_1998.htm] [20 January 2004].

174. National Kidney Foundation. K/DOQI clinical practice guidelines for chronic kidney disease: evaluation, classification and stratification. Am J Kidney Dis 2002; 39: S1–S266.

175. McCullough PA, Philbin EF, Spertus JA, et al. Confirmation of a heart failure epidemic: findings from the resource utilization among congestive heart failure (REACH) study. J Am Coll Cardiol 2002; 39: 60–9.

176. Dzau VJ. Renal and circulatory mechanisms in congestive heart failure. Kidney Int 1987; 31: 1402–15.

177. McAlister FA, Ezekowitz J, Tonelli M, Armstrong PW. Renal insufficiency and heart failure: prognostic and therapeutic implications from a prospective cohort study. Circulation 2004; 109: 1004–9.

178. Konstam MA, Udelson JE, Anand IS, et al. Ventricular remodeling in heart failure: a credible surrogate endpoint. J Card Fail 2003; 9: 350–3.

179. Levy D, Garrison RJ, Savage DD, et al. Prognostic implications of echocardiographically determined left ventricular mass in the framingham heart study. N Engl J Med 1990; 322: 1561–6.

180. Rambausek M, Ritz E, Mall G, et al. Myocardial hypertrophy in rats with renal insufficiency. Kidney Int 1985; 28: 775–82.

181. Stefanski A, Schmidt KG, Waldherr R, Ritz E. Early increase in blood pressure and diastolic left ventricular malfunction in patients with glomerulonephritis. Kidney Int 1996; 50: 1321–6.

182. Clyne N, Lins LE, Pehrsson SK. Occurrence and significance of heart disease in uraemia. An autopsy study. Scand J Urol Nephrol 1986; 20: 307–11.

183. Oh J, Wunsch R, Turzer M, et al. Advanced coronary and carotid arteriopathy in young adults with childhood-onset chronic renal failure. Circulation 2002; 106: 100–5.

184. Tornig J, Gross ML, Simonaviciene A, et al. Hypertrophy of intramyocardial arteriolar smooth muscle cells in experimental renal failure. J Am Soc Nephrol 1999; 10: 77–83.

185. Amann K, Breitbach M, Ritz E, Mall G. Myocyte/capillary mismatch in the heart of uremic patients. J Am Soc Nephrol 1998; 9: 1018–22.

186. Vuurmans TJ, Boer P, Koomans HA. Effects of endothelin-1 and endothelin-1 receptor blockade on cardiac output, aortic pressure, and pulse wave velocity in humans. Hypertension 2003; 41: 1253–8.

187. Safar ME, London GM, Plante GE. Arterial stiffness and kidney function. Hypertension 2004; 43: 163–8.
188. Schwarz U, Buzello M, Ritz E, et al. Morphology of coronary atherosclerotic lesions in patients with end-stage renal failure. Nephrol Dial Transplant 2000; 15: 218–23.
189. Goodman WG, Goldin J, Kuizon BD, et al. Coronary-artery calcification in young adults with end-stage renal disease who are undergoing dialysis. N Engl J Med 2000; 342: 1478–83.
190. Raggi P, Boulay A, Chasan-Taber S, et al. Cardiac calcification in adult hemodialysis patients: a link between end-stage renal disease and cardiovascular disease? J Am Coll Cardiol 2002; 39: 695–701.
191. Francis GS, Cohn JN, Johnson G, et al. Plasma norepinephrine, plasma renin activity, and congestive heart failure. Relations to survival and the effects of therapy in V-HeFT II: the V-HeFf VA cooperative studies group. Circulation 1993; 87: VI40–8.
192. Barr CS, Lang CC, Hanson J, et al. Effects of adding spironolactone to an angiotensin-converting enzyme inhibitor in chronic congestive heart failure secondary to coronary artery disease. Am J Cardiol 1995; 76: 1259–65.
193. Brooks VL. Interactions between angiotensin II and the sympathetic nervous system in the long-term control of arterial pressure. Clin Exp Pharmacol Physiol 1997; 24: 83–90.
194. Weber KT. Aldosterone in congestive heart failure. N Engl J Med 2001; 345: 1689–97.
195. Zucker IH, Schultz HD, Li YF, et al. The origin of sympathetic outflow in heart failure: the roles of angiotensin II and nitric oxide. Prog Biophys Mol Biol 2004; 84: 217–32.
196. Myers BD, Deen WM, Brenner BM. Effects of norepinephrine and angiotensin II on the determinants of glomerular ultrafiltration and proximal tubule fluid reabsorption in the rat. Circ Res 1975; 37: 101–10.
197. Schrier RW, De Wardener HE. Tubular reabsorption of Na ion: influence of factors other than aldosterone and glomerular filtration rate. N Engl J Med 1971; 285: 1292–303.
198. Castrop H, Schweda E, Mizel D, et al. Permissive role of nitric oxide in macula densa control of renin secretion. Am J Physiol Renal Physiol 2004; 286: F848–57.
199. He XR, Greenberg SG, Briggs IP, et al. Effects of furosemide and verapamil on the NaCI dependency of macula densa-mediated renin secretion. Hypertension 1995; 26: 137–42.
200. Warren DJ, Ferris TF. Renin secretion in renal hypertension. Lancet 1970; 1: 159–62.
201. Griendling KK, Minieri CA, Ollerenshaw JD, Alexander RW. Angiotensin II stimulates NADH and NADPH oxidase activity in cultured vascular smooth muscle cells. Circ Res 1994; 74: 1141–8.
202. Ushio-Fukai M, Zafari AM, Fukui T, et al. p22phox is a critical component of the superoxide-generating NADH/NADPH oxidase system and regulates angiotensin II-induced hypertrophy in vascular smooth muscle cells. J Biol Chem 1996; 271: 23317–21.
203. Chabrashvili T, Kitiyakara C, Blau J, et al. Effects of ANG II type 1 and 2 receptors on oxidative stress, renal NADPH oxidase, and SOD expression. Am J Physiol Regul Integr Comp Physiol 2003; 285: R117–24.
204. Nakagami H, Takemoto M, Liao JK. NADPH oxidase-derived superoxide anion mediates angiotensin II-induced cardiac hypertrophy. J Mol Cell Cardiol 2003; 35: 851–9.
205. Heymes C, Bendall JK, Ratajczak P, et al. Increased myocardial NADPH oxidase activity in human heart failure. J Am Coll Cardiol 2003; 41: 2164–71.
206. Tojo A, Onozato ML, Kobayashi N, et al. Angiotensin II and oxidative stress in dahl salt-sensitive rat with heart failure. Hypertension 2002; 40: 834–9.
207. Hornig B, Landmesser U, Kohler C, et al. Comparative effect of ace inhibition and angiotensin II type 1 receptor antagonism on bioavailability of nitric oxide in patients with coronary artery disease: role of superoxide dismutase. Circulation 2001; 103: 799–805.
208. Tojo A, Onozato ML, Kobayashi N, et al. Angiotensin II and oxidative stress in Dahl salt-sensitive rat with heart failure. Hypertension 2002; 40: 834–9.
209. Ruiz-Ortega M, Lorenzo O, Egido J. Angiotensin III increases MCP-1 and activates NF-kappa B and AP-1 in cultured mesangial and mononuclear cells. Kidney Int 2000; 57: 2285–98.
210. Reid IA. Interactions between ANG II, sympathetic nervous system, and baroreceptor reflexes in regulation of blood pressure. Am J Physiol 1992; 262: E763–78.
211. Converse RL Jr, Jacobsen TN, Toto RD, et al. Sympathetic overactivity in patients with chronic renal failure. N Engl J Med 1992; 327: 1912–18.
212. Ligtenberg G, Blankestijn PJ, Oey PL, et al. Reduction of sympathetic hyperactivity by enalapril in patients with chronic renal failure. N Engl J Med 1999; 340: 1321–8.
213. Klein IH, Ligtenberg G, Oey PL, et al. Enalapril and losartan reduce sympathetic hyperactivity in patients with chronic renal failure. J Am Soc Nephrol 2003; 14: 425–30.
214. Anker SD, Ponikowski PP, Clark AL, et al. Cytokines and neurohormones relating to body composition alterations in the wasting syndrome of chronic heart failure. Eur Heart J 1999; 20: 683–93.

215. Bryant D, Becker L, Richardson J, et al. Cardiac failure in transgenic mice with myocardial expression of tumor necrosis factor-alpha. Circulation 1998; 97: 1375–81.

216. Zhang W, Huang BS, Leenen FH. Brain renin-angiotensin system and sympathetic hyperactivity in rats after myocardial infarction. Am J Physiol 1999; 276: H1608–15.

217. Sekiguchi K, Li X, Coker M, et al. Cross-regulation between the renin-angiotensin system and inflammatory mediators in cardiac hypertrophy and failure. Cardiovasc Res 2004; 63: 433–42.

218. Knotek M, Rogachev B, Wang W, et al. Endotoxemic renal failure in mice: role of tumor necrosis factor independent of inducible nitric oxide synthase. Kidney Int 2001; 59: 2243–9.

219. Hernandez-Presa M, Bustos C, Ortego M, et al. Angiotensin converting enzyme inhibition prevents arterial nuclear factor-kappa B activation, monocyte chemoattractant protein-l expression, and macrophage infiltration in a rabbit model of early accelerated atherosclerosis. Circulation 1997; 95: 1532–41.

220. Braam B. Renal endothelial and macula densa NOS: integrated response to changes in extracellular fluid volume. Am J Physiol 1999; 276: R1551–61.

221. Zou AP, Li N, Cowley AW Jr. Production and actions of superoxide in the renal medulla. Hypertension 2001; 37: 547–53.

222. Welch WJ, Wilcox CS. AT1 receptor antagonist combats oxidative stress and restores nitric oxide signaling in the SHR. Kidney Int 2001; 59: 1257–63.

223. Ren Y, Carretero OA, Garvin JL. Mechanism by which superoxide potentiates tubuloglomerular feedback. Hypertension 2002; 39: 624–8.

224. Ortiz PA, Garvin JL. Interaction of O(2)(-) and NO in the thick ascending limb. Hypertension 2002; 39: 591–6.

225. Handelman GJ, Walter MF, Adhikarla R, et al. Elevated plasma F2-isoprostanes in patients on long-term hemodialysis. Kidney Int 2001; 59: 1960–6.

226. Maggi E, Bellazzi R, Gazo A, et al. Autoantibodies against oxidatively-modified LDL in uremic patients undergoing dialysis. Kidney Int 1994; 46: 869–76.

227. Ha TK, Sattar N, Talwar D, et al. Abnormal antioxidant vitamin and carotenoid status in chronic renal failure. Q J Med 1996; 89: 765–9.

228. Vallance P, Leone A, Calver A, et al. Accumulation of an endogenous inhibitor of nitric oxide synthesis in chronic renal failure. Lancet 1992; 339: 572–5.

229. Hill MF, Singal PK. Antioxidant and oxidative stress changes during heart failure subsequent to myocardial infarction in rats. Am J Pathol 1996; 148: 291–300.

230. Khaper N, Singal PK. Effects of afterload-reducing drugs on pathogenesis of antioxidant changes and congestive heart failure in rats. J Am Coll Cardiol 1997; 29: 856–61.

231. Kielstein JT, Bode-Boger SM, Klein G, et al. Endogenous nitric oxide synthase inhibitors and renal perfusion in patients with heart failure. Eur J Clin Invest 2003; 33: 370–5.

232. Bongartz LG, Cramer MJ, Braam B. The cardiorenal connection. Hypertension 2004; 43: e14.

233. Lin HH, Chen CH, Hsieh WK, et al. Hydrogen peroxide increases the activity of rat sympathetic preganglionic neurons in vivo and in vitro. Neuroscience 2003; 121: 641–7.

234. Shokoji T, Nishiyama A, Fujisawa Y, et al. Renal sympathetic nerve responses to tempol in spontaneously hypertensive rats. Hypertension 2003; 41: 266–73.

235. Miyata T, Sugiyama S, Saito A, Kurokawa K. Reactive carbonyl compounds related uremic toxicity ('carbonyl stress'). Kidney Int Suppl 2001; 78: S25–31.

236. Witko-Sarsat V, Friedlander M, Capeillere-Blandin C, et al. Advanced oxidation protein products as a novel marker of oxidative stress in uremia. Kidney Int 1996; 49: 1304–13.

237. Miyata T, Maeda K, Kurokawa K, van Ypersele de Strihou C. Oxidation conspires with glycation to generate noxious advanced glycation end products in renal failure. Nephrol Dial Transplant 1997; 12: 255–8.

238. Herbst U, Toborek M, Kaiser S, et al. 4-hydroxynonenal induces dysfunction and apoptosis of cultured endothelial cells. J Cell Physiol 1999; 181: 295–303.

239. Witko-Sarsat V, Friedlander M, Nguyen Khoa T, et al. Advanced oxidation protein products as novel mediators of inflammation and monocyte activation in chronic renal failure. J Immunol 1998; 161: 2524–32.

240. Nguyen-Khoa T, Massy ZA, Witko-Sarsat V, et al. Oxidized low-density lipoprotein induces macrophage respiratory burst via its protein moiety: a novel pathway in atherogenesis? Biochem Biophys Res Commun 1999; 263: 804–9.

241. Katoh M, Egashira K, Usui M, et al. Cardiac angiotensin II receptors are upregulated by long-term inhibition of nitric oxide synthesis in rats. Circ Res 1998; 83: 743–51.

242. Boaz M, Smetana S, Weinstein T, et al. Secondary prevention with antioxidants of cardiovascular disease in endstage renal disease (SPACE): randomised placebo-controlled trial. Lancet 2000; 356: 1213–18.

243. Himmelfarb J, Stenvinkel P, Ikizler TA, Hakim RM. The elephant in uremia: oxidant stress as a unifying concept of cardiovascular disease in uremia. Kidney Int 2002; 62: 1524–38.

244. Arici M, Walls J. End-stage renal disease, atherosclerosis, and cardiovascular mortality: is C-reactive protein the missing link? Kidney Int 2001; 59: 407–14.

245. Zebrack JS, Anderson JL, Beddhu S, et al. Do associations with C-reactive protein and extent of coronary artery disease account for the increased cardiovascular risk of renal insufficiency? J Am Coll Cardiol 2003; 42: 57–63.

246. Zoccali C, Benedetto FA, Mallamaci F, et al. Inflammation is associated with carotid atherosclerosis in dialysis patients. creed investigators. Cardiovascular risk extended evaluation in dialysis patients. J Hypertens 2000; 18: 1207–13.

247. Irish A. Cardiovascular disease, fibrinogen and the acute phase response: associations with lipids and blood pressure in patients with chronic renal disease. Atherosclerosis 1998; 137: 133–9.

248. Bologa RM, Levine DM, Parker TS, et al. Interleukin-6 predicts hypoalbuminemia, hypocholesterolemia, and mortality in hemodialysis patients. Am J Kidney Dis 1998; 32: 107–14.

249. Levine B, Kalman J, Mayer L, et al. Elevated circulating levels of tumor necrosis factor in severe chronic heart failure. N Engl J Med 1990; 323: 236–41.

250. Torre-Amione G, Kapadia S, Benedict C, et al. Proinflammatory cytokine levels in patients with depressed left ventricular ejection fraction: a report from the studies of left ventricular dysfunction (SOLVD). J Am Coll Cardiol 1996; 27: 1201–6.

251. Ward RA, McLeish KR. Polymorphonuclear leukocyte oxidative burst is enhanced in patients with chronic renal insufficiency. J Am Soc Nephrol 1995; 5: 1697–702.

252. Wassmann S, Stumpf M, Strehlow K, et al. Interleukin-6 induces oxidative stress and endothelial dysfunction by overexpression of the angiotensin II type 1 receptor. Circ Res 2004; 94: 534–41.

253. Sanchez-Lozada LG, Tapia E, Johnson RJ, et al. Glomerular hemodynamic changes associated with arteriolar lesions and tubulointerstitial inflammation. Kidney Int Suppl 2003; 64: S9–S14.

254. Deten A, Volz HC, Briest W, Zimmer HG. Cardiac cytokine expression is upregulated in the acute phase after myocardial infarction. Experimental studies in rats. Cardiovasc Res 2002; 55: 329–40.

255. Ono K, Matsumori A, Shioi T, et al. Cytokine gene expression after myocardial infarction in rat hearts: possible implication in left ventricular remodeling. Circulation 1998; 98: 149–56.

256. Niijima A, Hori T, Aou S, Oomura Y. The effects of interleukin-1 beta on the activity of adrenal, splenic and renal sympathetic nerves in the rat. J Auton Nerv Syst 1991; 36: 183–92.

257. Jackson G, Gibbs CR, Davies MK, Lip GY. ABC of heart failure. pathophysiology. Br Med J 2000; 320: 167–70.

258. Luo M, Hess MC, Fink GD, et al. Differential alterations in sympathetic neurotransmission in mesenteric arteries and veins in DOCA-salt hypertensive rats. Auton Neurosci 2003; 104: 47–57.

259. Amin JK, Xiao L, Pimental DR, et al. Reactive oxygen species mediate alpha-adrenergic receptor-stimulated hypertrophy in adult rat ventricular myocytes. J Mol Cell Cardiol 2001; 33: 131–9.

260. Leineweber K, Heinroth-Hoffmann I, Ponicke K, et al. Cardiac beta-adrenoceptor desensitization due to increased beta-adrenoceptor kinase activity in chronic uremia. J Am Soc Nephrol 2002; 13: 117–24.

261. Bristow MR, Ginsburg R, Minobe W, et al. Decreased catecholamine sensitivity and beta-adrenergic-receptor density in failing human hearts. N Engl J Med 1982; 307: 205–11.

262. Maurice JP, Shah AS, Kypson AP, et al. Molecular beta-adrenergic signaling abnormalities in failing rabbit hearts after infarction. Am J Physiol 1999; 276: H1853–60.

263. Ruffolo RR Jr, Feuerstein GZ. Pharmacology of carvedilol: rationale for use in hypertension, coronary artery disease, and congestive heart failure. Cardiovasc Drugs Ther 1997; 11: 247–56.

264. Wikstrand J, Berglund G, Hedblad B, Hulthe J. Antiatherosclerotic effects of beta-blockers. Am J Cardiol 2003; 91: 25H–9H.

265. Erami C, Zhang H, Ho JG, et al. Alpha(1)-adrenoceptor stimulation directly induces growth of vascular wall in vivo. Am J Physiol Heart Circ Physiol 2002; 283: H1577–87.

266. Bleeke T, Zhang H, Madamanchi N, et al. Catecholamine-induced vascular wall growth is dependent on generation of reactive oxygen species. Circ Res 2004; 94: 37–45.

267. Bianchi P, Seguelas MH, Parini A, Cambon C. Activation of pro-apoptotic cascade by dopamine in renal epithelial cells is fully dependent on hydrogen peroxide generation by monoamine oxidases. J Am Soc Nephrol 2003; 14: 855–62.

268. Prabhu SD, Chandrasekar B, Murray DR, Freeman GL. Beta-adrenergic blockade in developing heart failure: effects on myocardial inflammatory cytokines, nitric oxide, and remodeling. Circulation 2000; 101: 2103–9.

269. Liao J, Keiser JA, Scales WE, et al. Role of epinephrine in TNF and IL-6 production from isolated perfused rat liver. Am J Physiol 1995; 268: R896–901.

270. Oddis CV, Simmons RL, Hattler BG, Finkel MS. cAMP enhances inducible nitric oxide synthase mRNA stability in cardiac myocytes. Am J Physiol 1995; 269: H2044–50.

271. Li L, Lee EW, Ji H, Zukowska Z. Neuropeptide Y-induced acceleration of postangioplasty occlusion of rat carotid artery. Arterioscler Thromb Vasc Biol 2003; 23: 1204–10.

272. Schwarz H, Villiger PM, von Kempis J, Lotz M. Neuropeptide Y is an inducible gene in the human immune system. J Neuroimmunol 1994; 51: 53–61.

273. Zukowska-Grojec Z, Neuropeptide Y. A novel sympathetic stress hormone and more. Ann NY Acad Sci 1995; 771: 219–33.

274. Morris MJ, Cox HS, Lambert GW, et al. Region-specific neuropeptide Y overflows at rest and during sympathetic activation in humans. Hypertension 1997; 29: 137–4.

275. Lindenfeld J. Prevalence of anemia and effects on mortality in patients with heart failure. Am Heart J 2005; 149: 391–401.

276. McMurray JJ. What are the clinical consequences of anemia in patients with chronic heart failure? J Card Fail 2004; 10: S10–12.

277. Levin A, Thompson CR, Ethier I, et al. Left ventricular mass index increase in early renal disease: impact of decline in hemoglobin. Am J Kidney Dis 1999; 34: 125–34.

278. Silverberg DS, Wexler D, Iaina A. The role of anemia in the progression of congestive heart failure. Is there a place for erythropoietin and intravenous iron? J Nephrol 2004; 17: 749–61.

279. van der Meer P, Voors AA, Lipsic E, et al. Prognostic value of plasma erythropoietin on mortality in patients with chronic heart failure. J Am Coll Cardiol 2004; 44: 63–7.

280. Volpe M, Tritto C, Testa U, et al. Blood levels of erythropoietin in congestive heart failure and correlation with clinical, hemodynamic, and hormonal profiles. Am J Cardiol 1994; 74: 468–73.

281. Okonko DO, Anker SD. Anemia in chronic heart failure: pathogenetic mechanisms. J Card Fail 2004; 10: S5–9.

282. Maiese K, Li E, Chong ZZ. New avenues of exploration for erythropoietin. JAMA 2005; 293: 90–5.

283. Fisher JW. Erythropoietin: physiology and pharmacology update. Exp Biol Med (Maywood) 2003; 228: 1–14.

284. Smith KJ, Bleyer AJ, Little WC, et al. The cardiovascular effects of erythropoietin. Cardiovasc Res 2003; 59: 538–48.

285. Calvillo L, Latini R, Kajstura T. Recombinant human erythropoietin protects the myocardium from ischemia-reperfusion injury and promotes beneficial remodeling. Proc Natl Acad Sci USA 2003; 100: 2802–6.

286. Ellison DH. Diuretic therapy and resistance in congestive heart failure. Cardiology 2001; 96: 132–43.

287. Brater DC, Anderson SA, Brown-Cartright D. Response to furosemide in chronic renal insufficiency: rationale for limited doses. Clin Pharmacol Ther 1986; 40: 134–9.

288. Stroupe KT, Forthofer MM, Brater DC, Murray MD. Healthcare costs of patients with heart failure treated with torsemide or furosemide. Pharmacoeconomics 2000; 17: 429–40.

289. Ellison DH. Diuretic resistance: physiology and therapeutics. Semin Nephrol 1999; 19: 581–97.

290. Heird WC, Dell RB, Driscoll JM Jr, et al. Metabolic acidosis resulting from intravenous alimentation mixtures containing synthetic amino acids. N Engl J Med 1972; 287: 943–8.

291. Frölich JC, Hollifield JW, Dormois JC, et al. Suppression of plasma renin activity by indomethacin in man. Circ Res 1976; 39: 447–52.

292. Martinez-Maldonado M, Gely R, Tapia E, Benabe JE. Role of macula densa in diuretics induced renin release. Hypertension 1990; 16: 261–8.

293. Modena B, Holmer S, Eckardt KU, et al. Furosemide stimulates renin expression in the kidneys of salt-supplemented rats. Pflügers Arch 1993; 424: 403–9.

294. Knauf H, Mutschler E. Functional state of the nephron and diuretic dose-response – rationale for low-dose combination therapy. Cardiology 1994; 84: 18–26.

295. Grantham JJ, Chonko AM. The physiological basis and clinical use of diuretics. In: Brenner BM, Stein JH, eds. Sodium and Water Homeostasis. New York: Churchill Livingstone, 1978: 178–211.

296. Wilcox CS, Mitch WE, Kelly RA, et al. Response of the kidney to furosemide. 1. Effects of salt intake and renal compensation. J Lab Clin Med 1983; 102: 450–8.

297. Walter SJ, Shirley DG. The effect of chronic hydrochlorothiazide administration on renal function in the rat. Clin Sci (Lond) 1986; 70: 379–87.

298. Ellison DH, Velazquez H, Wright FS. Adaptation of the distal convoluted tubule of the rat: structural and functional effects of dietary salt intake and chronic diuretic infusion. J Clin Invest 1989; 83: 113–26.

299. Kaissling B, Bachmann S, Kriz W. Structural adaptation of the distal convoluted tubule to prolonged furosemide treatment. Am J Physiol 1985; 248: F374–81.

300. Kaissling B, Stanton BA. Adaptation of distal tubule and collecting duct to increased sodium delivery. 1. Ultrastructure. Am J Physiol 1988; 255: F1256–68.

301. Scherzer P, Wald H, Popovtzer MM. Enhanced glomerular filtration and Na+-K+-ATPase with furosemide administration. Am J Physiol 1987; 252: F910–15.

302. Wald H, Scherzer P, Popovtzer MM. Inhibition of thick ascending limb Na+-K+-ATPase activity in salt-loaded rats by furosemide. Am J Physiol 1989; 256: F549–55.

303. Chen ZF, Vaughn DA, Beaumont K, Fanestil DD. Effects of diuretic treatment and of dietary sodium on renal binding of 3H-metolazone. J Am Soc Nephrol 1990; 1: 91–8.

304. Obermüller N, Bernstein PL, Vela zquez H, et al. Expression of the thiazide-sensitive Na-Cl cotransporter in rat and human kidney. Am J Physiol 1995; 269: F900–10.

305. Abdallah JG, Schrier RW, Edelstein C, et al. Loop diuretic infusion increases thiazide-sensitive Na(+)/Cl(−)-cotransporter abundance: role of aldosterone. J Am Soc Nephrol 2001; 12: 1335–41.

306. Loon NR, Wilcox CS, Unwin RJ. Mechanism of impaired natriuretic response to furosemide during prolonged therapy. Kidney Int 1989; 36: 682–9.

307. Almeshari K, Ahlstrom NG, Capraro FE, Wilcox CS. A volume-independent component to postdiuretic sodium retention in humans. J Am Soc Nephrol 1993; 3: 1878–83.

308. Chemtob S, Doray J-L, Laudignon N, et al. Alternating sequential dosing with furosemide and ethacrynic acid in drug tolerance in the newborn. Am J Dis Child 1989; 143: 850–4.

309. Epstein M, Lepp BA, Hoffman DS, Levinson R. Potentiation of furosemide by metolazone in refractory edema. Curr Ther Res 1977; 21: 656–67.

310. Oster JR, Epstein M, Smoler S. Combined therapy with thiazide-type and loop diuretic agents for resistant sodium retention. Ann Intern Med 1983; 99: 405–6.

311. Oimomi M, Takase S, Saeki S. Combination diuretic therapy for severe refractory nephritic syndrome. Lancet 1990; 336: 1004–5.

312. Ellison DH. The physiologic basis of diuretic synergism: its role in treating diuretic resistance. Ann Intern Med 1991; 114: 886–94.

313. Marone C, Muggli F, Lahn W, Frey FJ. Pharmacokinetic and pharmacodynamic interaction between furosemide and metolazone in man. Eur J Clin Invest 1985; 15: 253–7.

314. Okusa MD, Persson AEG, Wright FS. Chlorothiazide effect on feedback-mediated control of glomerular filtration rate. Am J Physiol 1989; 257: F137–44.

315. Ellison DH, Velazquez H, Wright FS. Thiazide-sensitive sodium chloride cotransport in early distal tubule. Am J Physiol 1987; 253: F546–54.

316. Garin EH. A comparison of combinations of diuretics in nephrotic edema. Am J Dis Child 1987; 141: 769–71.

317. Channer KS, McLean KA, Lawson-Matthew P, Richardson M. Combination diuretic treatment in severe heart failure: a randomized controlled trial. Br Heart J 1994; 71: 146–50.

318. Fliser D, Schröter M, Neubeck M, Ritz E. Coadministration of thiazides increases the efficacy of loop diuretics even in patients with advanced renal failure. Kidney Int 1994; 46: 482–8.

319. Morsing P, Velazquez H, Wright FS, Ellison DH. Adaptation of distal convoluted tubule of rats. 2. effects of chronic thiazide infusion. Am J Physiol 1991; 261: F137–43.

320. Miller PD, Berns AS. Acute metabolic alkalosis perpetuating hypercarbia: a role for acetazolamide in chronic obstructive pulmonary disease. JAMA 1977; 238: 2400–1.

321. Vargo DL, Brater DC, Rudy DW, Swan SK. Dopamine does not enhance furosemide-induced natriuresis in patients with congestive heart failure. J Am Soc Nephrol 1996; 7: 1032–7.

322. Gerlag PGG, van Meijel JJM. High-dose furosemide in the treatment of refractory congestive heart failure. Arch Intern Med 1988; 148: 286–91.

323. Rybak LP. Ototoxicity of loop diuretics. Otolaryngol Clin North Am 1993; 26: 829–44.

324. Nierenberg DW. Furosemide and ethacrynic acid in acute tubular necrosis. West J Med 1980; 133: 163–70.

325. Dikshit K, Vyden JK, Forrester JS, et al. Renal and extrarenal hemodynamic effects of furosemide in congestive heart failure after acute myocardial infarction. N Engl J Med 1973; 288: 1087–90.

326. Francis GS, Siegel RM, Goldsmith SR, et al. Acute vasoconstrictor response to intravenous furosemide in patients with chronic congestive heart failure. Ann Intern Med 1985; 103: 1–6.

327. Curran KA, Hebert MJ, Cain BD, Wingo CS. Evidence for the presence of a K-dependent acidifying adenosine triphosphatase in the rabbit renal medulla. Kidney Int 1992; 42: 1093–8.

328. Goldsmith SR, Francis G, Cohn JN. Attenuation of the pressor response to intravenous furosemide by angiotensin converting enzyme inhibition in congestive heart failure. Am J Cardiol 1989; 64: 1382–5.

329. Leslie D, Gheorghiade M. Is there a role for thiamine supplementation in the management of heart failure? Am Heart J 1996; 131: 1248–50.

330. Shimon I, Almog S, Vered Z, et al. Improved left ventricular function after thiamine supplementation in patients with congestive heart failure receiving long-term furosemide therapy. Am J Med 1995; 98: 485–90.

331. Salvador DRK, Rey NR, Ramos GC, Punzalan FER. Continuous infusion versus bolus injection of loop diuretics in congestive heart failure. Cochrane Database Syst Rev 2005; 20: CD003178.pub3; doi: 10.1002/14651858.CD003178.pub3.

332. Lahav M, Regev A, Raanani P, Thodor E. Intermittent administration of furosemide vs continuous infusion preceded by a loading dose for congestive heart failure. Chest 1992; 102: 725–31.

333. Van Meyel JJM, Smits P, Dormans T, et al. Continuous infusion of furosemide in the treatment of patients with congestive heart failure and diuretic resistance. J Intern Med 1994; 235: 329–34.

334. Agostoni P, Marenzi G, Lauri G, et al. Sustained improvement in functional capacity after removal of body fluid with isolated ultrafiltration in chronic cardiac insufficiency: failure of furosemide to provide the same result. Am J Med 1994; 96: 191–9.

335. Cohn IN, Archibald DG, Ziesche S, et al. Effect of vasodilator therapy on mortality in chronic congestive heart failure: results of a veterans administration cooperative study. N Engl J Med 1986; 314: 1547–52.

336. Bayliss J, Norell M, Canepa-Anson R, et al. Untreated heart failure: clinical and neuroendocrine effects of introducing diuretics. Br Heart J 1987; 57: 17–22.

337. Packer M, Lee WH, Kessler PD, et al. Prevention and reversal of nitrate tolerance in patients with congestive heart failure. N Engl J Med 1987; 317: 799–804.

338. Katz RI, Levy WS, Buff L, et al. Prevention of nitrate tolerance with angiotensin converting enzyme inhibitors. Circulation 1991; 83: 1271–7.

339. The cardiac insufficiency bisoprolol study II (CIBIS-II): a randomized trial. Lancet 1999; 353: 9–13.

340. Hjalmarson A, Goldstein S, Fagerberg B, et al. Effects of controlled-release metoprolol on total mortality, hospitalizations, and well-being in patients with heart failure: the metoprolol CR/XL randomized intervention trial in congestive heart failure (MERIT-HF). MERIT-HF Study Group. JAMA 2000; 283: 1295–302.

341. Packer M, Bristow MR, Cohn JN, et al. The effect of carvedilol on morbidity and mortality in patients with chronic heart failure. U.S. carvedilol heart failure study group. N Engl J Med 1996; 334: 1349–55.

342. Taylor AL, Ziesche S, Yancy C, et al. Combination of isosorbide dinitrate and hydralazine in blacks with heart failure. N Engl J Med 2004; 351: 2049–57.

343. Waagstein F, Bristow MR, Swedberg K, et al. Beneficial effects of metoprolol in idiopathic dilated cardiomyopathy, metoprolol in dilated cardiomyopathy (MDC) trial study group. Lancet 1993; 342: 1441–6

344. Bristow MR, Gilbert EM, Abraham WT, et al. Carvedilol produces dose-related improvements in left ventricular function and survival in subjects with chronic heart failure. MOCHA investigators. Circulation 1996; 94: 2807–16.

345. Captopril Multicenter Research Group. A placebo-controlled trial of captopril in refractory chronic congestive heart failure. J Am Coll Cardiol 1983; 2: 755–63.

346. The CONSENSUS Trial Study Group. CONSENSUS Trial Study Group: effects of enalapril on mortality in severe congestive heart failure: results of the Cooperative North Scandinavian Enalapril Survival Study (CONSENSUS). N Engl J Med 1987; 316: 1429–35.

347. The SOLVD Investigators. SOLVD Investigators: effect of enalapril on survival in patients with reduced left ventricular ejection fractions and congestive heart failure. N Engl J Med 1991; 325: 293–302.

348. Cohn JN. Future directions in vasodilator therapy for heart failure. Am Heart J 1991; 121: 969–74.

349. Suki WN. Renal hemodynamic consequences of angiotensin converting enzyme inhibition in congestive heart failure. Arch Intern Med 1989; 149: 669–73.

350. Tobian I, Coffee K, Ferriera D, et al. The effect of renal pressure on net transport out of distal tubular urine as studied with stop-flow technique. J Clin Invest 1964; 43: 118–28.

351. Wang DJ, Dowling TC, Meadows D, et al. Nesiritide does not improve renal function in patients with chronic heart failure and worsening serum creatinine. Circulation 2004; 110: 1620–5.

352. Sackner-Bemstein JD, Skopicki HA, Aaronson KD. Risk of worsening renal function with nesiritide in patients with acutely decompensated heart failure. Circulation 2005; 111: 1487–91.

353. Fauchauld P. Effects of ultrafiltration of body fluid and transcapillary colloid osmotic gradient in hemodialysis patients: improvements in dialysis therapy. Contrib Nephrol 1989; 74: 170–5.

354. Costanzo MR, Saltzberg M, O'Sullivan J, Sobotka P. Early ultrafiltration in patients with decompensated heart failure and diuretic resistance. J Am Coll Cardiol 2005; 46: 2047–51.

355. Costanzo MR, Guglin M, Saltzberg M, et al. Ultrafiltration versus intravenous diuretics for patients hospitalized for acute decompensated heart failure. J Am Coll Cardiol 2007; 49: 675–83.

356. Gottlieb SS, Brater DC, Thomas I, et al. BG9719 (CVT-124), an Al adenosine receptor antagonist, protects against the decline in renal function observed with diuretic therapy. Circulation 2002; 105: 1348–53.

357. Butman SM, Ewy GA, Standen JR, et al. Bedside cardiovascular examination in patients with severe chronic heart failure: importance of rest or inducible jugular venous distension. J Am Coll Cardiol 1993; 22: 968–74.

358. Kircher BJ, Himelman RB, Schiller NB. Noninvasive estimation of right atrial pressure from the inspiratory collapse of the inferior vena cava. Am J Cardiol 1990; 66: 493–6.

359. Ommen SR, Nishimura RA, Appleton CP, et al. Clinical utility of doppler echocardiography and tissue doppler imaging in the estimation of left ventricular filling pressures: a comparative simultaneous doppler catheterization study. Circulation 2000; 102: 1788–94.

360. Stevenson LW. Clinical use of inotropic therapy for heart failure: looking backward or forward? Part I: inotropic infusions during hospitalization. Circulation 2003; 108: 367–72.

361. Chatterjee K, Parmley WW, Cohn JN, et al. A cooperative multicenter study of captopril in congestive heart failure: hemodynamic effects and long-term response. Am Heart J 1985; 110: 439–47.

362. Landry DW, Oliver JA. The pathogenesis of vasodilatory shock. N Engl J Med 2001; 345: 588–95.

363. Khot UN, Mishra M, Yamani MH, et al. Severe renal dysfunction complicating cardiogenic shock is not a contraindication to mechanical support as a bridge to cardiac transplantation. J Am Coll Cardiol 2003; 41: 381–5.

364. Renal blood flow and glomerular filtration. In: Eaton DC, Pooler JP, eds. Vander's Renal Physiology, 6th edn. New York: McGraw Hill, 2002.

365. Patel J, Heywood JT. Management of the cardiorenal syndrome in heart failure. Curr Cardiol Rep 2006; 8: 211–16.

366. Lee WH, Packer M. Prognostic importance of serum Na concentration and its modification by converting-enzyme inhibition in patients with severe chronic heart failure. Circulation 1986; 73: 257–67.

367. Pueyo ME, Gonzalez W, Nicoletti A, et al. Angiotensin II stimulates endothelial vascular cell adhesion molecule-1 via nuclear factor-kappa B activation induced by intracellular oxidative stress. Arterioscler Thromb Vasc Biol 2000; 20: 645–51.

368. Woldbaek PR, Tonnessen T, Henriksen UL, et al. Increased cardiac IL-18 mRNA, pro-IL-18 and plasma IL-18 after myocardial infarction in the mouse; a potential role in cardiac dysfunction. Cardiovasc Res 2003; 59: 122–31.

369. Garg LC, Narang N. Effects of hydrochlorothiazide on Na-K-ATPase activity along the rat nephron. Kidney Int 1987; 31: 918–22.

370. Argenziano M, Choudhri AF, Oz MC, et al. A prospective randomized trial of arginine vasopressin in the treatment of vasodilatory shock after left ventricular assist device placement. Circulation 1997; 96:11286–90.

11

The clinical syndrome of heart failure

Thomas DiSalvo and Jordan Shin

INTRODUCTION

Heart failure (HF) remains the only common cardiovascular syndrome increasing in preva-lence and incidence (1). Despite significant advances in pharmacologic and device thera-pies, morbidity, and mortality for those afflicted with HF remains high (2). Following a brief discussion of epidemiology and pathophysiology, this chapter focuses on the clinical syndrome of HF with particular emphasis on clinical presentation and diagnosis.

EPIDEMIOLOGY
Definition

Given the pathophysiologic and clinical heterogeneity, it is not surprising that there is not yet any firm consensus definition of the clinical syndrome of HF (Table 11.1) (3). Over the past several decades, basic and clinical research elucidating the complex and continuous interplay of adaptive and maladaptive myocyte, myocardial extracellular matrix, hemody-namic, biochemical, energetic, genetic, neurohormonal, renal, pulmonary, skeletal muscle, vascular endothelial alterations, and adaptations in HF has rendered consensus definition even more challenging (4). However, virtually all clinical instances of HF may be broadly conceptualized as a primary failure of the heart to render sufficient pressure–volume work over the range of physiologic resting and exercise pressure–volume conditions, and thereby maintain organ perfusion at ventricular filling pressures below the threshold for the precipi-tation of systemic or pulmonary venous congestion.

Classification

Heart failure may be classified as either predominantly systolic or diastolic (3). Almost all instances of systolic HF also exhibit diastolic abnormalities; most instances of diastolic HF also exhibit systolic abnormalities, usually inadequate systolic functional reserve (5,6). The cardiomyopathies have traditionally been classified as either dilated, restrictive, or hypertrophic (7). Neither classification schema necessarily provides sufficient insight into disease etiology, severity, or prognosis. It is important to distinguish HF from states of extreme or supraphysiologic circulatory pressure or volume overload (e.g., acute severe hypertension, severe anemia, arteriovenous fistula) or from the occasional metabolic (e.g., hypoxemia, acidosis), endocrinologic (e.g., hypo- or hyperthyroidism), and diverse medi-cal conditions (e.g., sepsis) associated with transient and reversible myocardial dysfunction (2,3). In such instances, transient signs and/or symptoms of HF may appear in the absence of true myocardial dysfunction or disease.

Table 11.1 Definitions of Heart Failure

- "A condition in which the heart fails to disrg its contents adequately"—*Thomas Lewis, 1933*
- "A state in which the heart fails to maintain n adequate circulation for the needs of the body despite
- a satisfactory filling pressure"—*Paul Wood, 1950*
- "A pathophysiological state in which an abnormality of cardiac function is responsible for the failure
- of the heart to pump blood at a rate commensurate with the requirements of the metabolizing
- tissues"—*Eugene Braunwald, 1980*
- "Heart failure is the state of any heart disease in which, despite adequate ventricular filling, the heart's
- output is decreased or in which the heart is unable to pump blood at a rate adequate for satisfying
- the requirements of the tissues with functional parameters remaining within normal limits"—*H.*
- *Denolin, H. Kuhn, H.P. Krayenbuehl, F. Loogen, A. Reale, 1983*
- "A clinical syndrome caused by an abnormality of the heart and recognized by a characteristic pattern
- of hemodynamic, renal, neural and hormonal responses"—*Philip A. Poole-Wilson, 1985*
- "...syndrome ... which arises when the heart if chronically unable to maintain an appropriate blood
- pressure without support"—*Peter Harris, 1987*
- "A syndrome in which cardiac dysfunction is associated with reduced exercise tolerance, a high
- incidence of ventricular arrhythmias and shortened life expectancy"—*Jay Cohn, 1988*
- "Symptoms of heart failure, objective evidence of cardiac dysfunction and response to treatment
- directed towards heart failure"—*Task Force of ESC, 1995*
- "Heart failure is a complex clinical syndrome that can result from any cardiac disorder that impairs
- the ability of the ventricle to eject blood"—*Consensus Recommendations for the Management of*
- *Chronic Heart Failure, 1999 Source*: From Ref. 11.
- "Heart failure is a complex clinical syndrome that can result from any structural of functional cardiac
- disorder that impairs the ability of the ventricle to fill with or eject blood"—*ACC/AHA Consensus*
- *Guidelines, 2001 Source*: From Ref. 2.

Source: Adapted from Ref. 60.

Incidence and Prevalence

Heart failure is the only common cardiovascular disease with rising incidence and prevalence (8,9). In the United States, HF afflicts approximately 6.6 million people (1) with approximately 400,000–700,000 new symptomatic cases, and 250,000 deaths annually (10). Between 1.5% and 2% of the U.S. population has symptomatic HF, with a prevalence of 6–10% in those older than 65 years (11). In the Framingham Heart Study, the lifetime HF risk for men and women free of HF at age 40 years was 21% for men and 20.3% for women (12). In the Framingham cohort, the incidence of HF declined for women but not for men between 1950 and 1999 (13). There is a marked age-dependence in HF prevalence and incidence with elderly patients being disproportionately afflicted (14). Given the continued successes in managing coronary artery disease, the incidence and prevalence of HF will probably only increase in the future (8).

The largest pool of patients with HF are, in fact, minimally symptomatic (15). Up to 3–6% of the general population may have asymptomatic left ventricular systolic dysfunction and be at high risk of developing symptomatic HF within five years (Fig. 11.1)

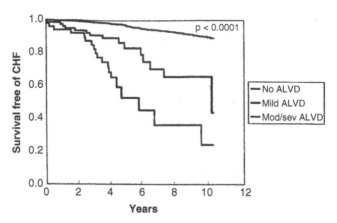

Figure 11.1   Kaplan–Meier curves for survival free of symptomatic heart failure. Referent group consists of subjects with normal left ventricular systolic function (LVEF > 50%). Mild ALVD indicates mild asymptomatic left ventricular systolic dysfunction (LVEF 40–50%). Mod/Sev ALVD indicates moderate to severe asymptomatic left ventricular systolic dysfunction (LVEF < 40%). *Abbreviations*: LVEF, left ventricular ejection fraction; ALVD, *Source*: From Ref. 16.

(10,15,16). Up to 20% of the asymptomatic general population may have evidence of dia-stolic dysfunction by screening echocardiography (16). The recognition and importance of these phenomena for public health and cardiovascular disease prevention inform the ratio-nale for the "redefinition" of HF by the American College of Cardiology/American Heart Association (ACC/AHA) consensus guidelines (2). The ACC/AHA reclassification seeks to emphasize the large number of "at-risk" future HF patients in the United States, and empowers physicians to deploy HF preventative strategies analogous to the life-long pre-vention and management strategies deployed in the management of patients with risk fac-tors for coronary artery disease and its sequelae. In the current ACC/AHA classification schema, patients in HF stage "A" (high risk for HF but without structural heart disease) and HF stage "B" (structural heart disease without symptoms of HF) are, in fact, without symptoms or signs of heart HF (2). Reducing the morbidity and mortality of HF in the future may well rest upon the success with which physicians extend the recommended life-long preventative strategies to at-risk patients long before the symptoms, signs, and overt echocardiographic features of HF supervene.

Economics

Heart failure poses an enormous societal financial burden with an estimated cost of between $20 and $40 billion dollars annually in the United States (10). Care of HF con-sumes approximately 11% of total expenditure for cardiovascular disease (17,18). The elderly bear a disproportionate economic burden given the rising prevalence of heart HF with age (14).

Risk Factors

Observational and epidemiologic studies have identified multiple risk factors for HF, including systemic hypertension, coronary artery disease, diabetes mellitus, cardiotoxic drug therapy, alcohol abuse, history of rheumatic fever, family history of cardiomyopathy, and obesity (2,12–14). Although these risk factors are well recognized, HF does not develop in all patients so exposed. For example, some instances of noncoronary disease-related HF

Table 11.2 Risk Factors for Heart Failure

- Coronary artery disease
- Hypertension
- Heavy alcohol use
- Familial or genetic cardiomyopathy
- Significant mitral of aortic valvular heart disease
- Myocarditis
- Toxin exposure (chemotherapy, cocaine)
- Underlying systemic disorders (e.g., thyroid
- disease, hemochromatosis, sarcoidosis, amyloidosis)
- Nutritional deficiencies
- Collagen vascular disease
- Peripartum disease
- Neuromuscular disorders
- Age
- Obesity

may well require more than a single genetic abnormality, epidemiologic or environmental exposure, or coexistent disease condition to evolve (19). A "multiple hit" hypothesis has been promoted to account for these epidemiologic observations in HF pathophysiology analogous to the "multiple hit" hypothesis advanced in cancer pathophysiology (20). According to this attractive paradigm, the population-attributable risk bequeathed by a single HF risk factor is modified by a unique constellation of individual genetic characteristics, other risk factors, concurrent cardiovascular and noncardiovascular diseases or conditions, environmental exposures, body habitus, physical condition, and medications. Known risk factors for the development of HF appear in Table 11.2. Of particular interest in clinical research at present are the single or multiple gene defects that may either precipitate HF directly (19,21–29) or enhance the predisposition to HF given a specific environmental exposure or exposures (30). The "customization" of both "prophylactic" and chronic pharmacologic therapy based on genotype is the long-term aim of much current HF clinical and translational research (chap. 7) (31–33).

PATHOPHYSIOLOGY
Normal Integrated Function of the Heart
As a pump, the normal heart is designed to apply circumferential compressive force to the blood pool resident within the heart following diastolic filling (34). Since blood is a relatively incompressible fluid, the pressure within the blood pool rises steeply as compressive force develops during isovolumic contraction. Eventually the pressure within the relatively noncompressible blood pool exceeds the pressure across the aortic valve, the aortic valve opens, and ventricular ejection ensues. In healthy circumstances, the anatomy and physiology of the heart are carefully construed and maintained so as to perform compressive mechanical work at near-maximal efficiency to deliver an adequate cardiac output over the normal range of rest and exertional pressure–volume conditions, commensurate with the demands of the body's metabolizing tissues.

Heart Failure
Heart failure, systolic or diastolic, may be conceived as a pathophysiologic state in which either the delivery of cardiac output is inadequate to meet the metabolic demands of tissues or an adequate cardiac output is delivered only under conditions of abnormally elevated

Table 11.3   Causes of Systolic Heart Failure

• Coronary artery disease
• Hypertension
• Alcohol
• Valvular heart disease
• Familial/genetic cardiomyopathy
• Myocarditis
• Toxins (chemotherapy, cocaine)
• Collagen vascular disease
• Metabolic disorders
• Endocrine disorders
• Electrolyte disorders
• Acidosis
• Sepsis
• Hypoxia
• Severe sleep apnea
• Peripartum

intracardiac pressures, which prematurely precipitate systemic or pulmonary venous congestion (35). In the latter instance, exertion is curtailed prematurely as the supranormal intracardiac pressures exceed the maximal capacitance of either the systemic or pulmonary venous and lymphatic circulations. An excessive volume of interstitial fluid accumulates in response constitutively elevating systemic or pulmonary hydraulic capillary pressure gradients and resulting in symptoms or signs and exertional limitation.

Although still debated, the primary "locus" of dysfunction in most instances of systolic HF appears to reside largely within the myocyte compartment of the heart. At least in the end-stage human heart, both in vivo and in vitro studies support a marked reduction in "contractility reserve" in response to increasing heart rate of sympathetic stimulation (36). Whether this reduction in myocardial "contractility reserve" results from intrinsic abnormalities of myocyte contractile function or myocyte response to alterations in the myocardial and extracellular matrix neurohormonally modulated "milieu," is still uncertain.

Normal integrated function of the heart depends on a host of factors that include normal ultrastructural and gross architecture of the heart, an adequate number of myocytes, normal myocyte contractile and relaxant function, normal structure and function of cardiacvalves, normal structure, composition, and metabolism of the myocardial extracellular matrix, adequate myocardial perfusion, and normal myocardial metabolism. Not surprisingly, abnormalities in any of these major anatomic and functional components may result in HF. Among the more common causes of HF are loss of myocytes (ischemic, inflammatory or toxic necrosis, apoptosis), acute or chronic contractile dysfunction of myocytes (inflammation, alcohol, chemotherapeutic agents, sepsis, hypoxia), excessive myofiber architectural disorganization or disarray (hypertrophic cardiomyopathy, infiltrative cardiomyopathy), extracellular matrix structural or functional abnormalities (excessive fibrosis leading to abnormal force transduction, myocyte linkage, and inadequate "compressive force" efficiency), distortion of the three-dimensional shape of the heart itself (aneurysm, infarction, chronic valvular disease), and intractable pressure or volume overload (hypertension, valvular heart disease) (Table 11.3).

Under the current "neurohormonal" hypothesis, the initial myocardial injury or overload results in a perceived diminution in the rate, pattern, or distribution of perfusion to the vital regulatory organs and centers of the circulation (37). Such alterations in perfusion invoke a complex cascade of initially "homeostatic" responses (positive inotropy and chronotropy, vasoconstriction, sodium retention) mediated largely by multiple interacting and amplifying neurohormonal axes (such as the renin–angiotensin–aldosterone systems and the sympathetic nervous system) that provide initial restoration of perfusion. Over time, however, the constitutive activation of these diverse neurohormonal systems, particularly the ongoing elaboration of high circulating, and tissue levels, of key effector molecules (e.g., angiotensin II, norepinephrine, epinephrine, aldosterone, and the endothelin family of peptides) proves progressively pathologic and promotes both: (*i*) deleterious alterations in circulatory dynamics, which impose greater myocardial load (e.g., volume expansion due to excessive salt and water retention, vasoconstriction); and (*ii*) deleterious changes in myocardial structure and function, which effect adverse ventricular remodeling (e.g., accelerated myocyte loss via apoptosis, increasing myocardial fibrosis). Many instances of adverse myocardial remodeling are accompanied, likely, by an ever-dwindling myocyte mass due to ongoing necrosis, apoptosis, or aging. Although there appears to be a small population of cardiac stem-like cells within myocardial tissue capable of terminal differentiation into functional myocytes, the majority of preexisting terminally differentiated myocytes cannot undergo hyperplasia at a rate sufficient to repopulate a dwindling myocyte mass (38).

Central to the progression of HF, once initiated and the target of current pharmacologic management of heart failure, is the process of adverse ventricular remodeling (chap. 6) (4). Once exposed to significant injury or unrelieved pressure and volume overload, the heart responds by remodeling itself with, at times, a remarkable degree of plasticity with respect to structure and function (39). Remodeling is largely mediated by exogenous and endogenous neurohormonal axes activated in response to altered systemic perfusion or chronic myocardial pressure and volume overload itself. The process of remodeling alters ventricular dimensions and shape as well as myocyte and extracellular matrix composition, integration, and function. In addition to the neurohormonal axes previously described, diverse autocrine, paracrine, and endocrine signaling systems are simultaneously activated and play important roles in modulating the pace and outcome of remodeling (40).

Underappreciated is the heterogeneity of the mechanisms, not only initiating HF but also influencing the course of remodeling once HF supervenes. For example, genetic defects underlie up to one-third of cases of idiopathic dilated cardiomyopathy and likely all instances of hypertrophic cardiomyopathy (19). Undoubtedly, other genetic factors impact the myocardial response to injury or overload and determine, in part, the course of remodeling. These diverse and intersecting pathophysiologic mechanisms are often paradoxically "hidden" in individuals by the stereotypical clinical symptoms and signs, and histopathologic features of established chronic systolic HF.

Systolic Heart Failure

In addition to the structural and functional considerations previously presented, normal systolic function also depends on a precise sequence of electrical activation of the myocardium (apex to base), a torsional translational motion of the ventricle (a "wringing" out), a precise anatomic array of myofibers that mechanically maximizes force generation (myofibers wrapped in orthogonal layers), an appropriate degree of hypertrophy of myocytes given load, and a suitably deformable and elastic extracellular matrix that maintains myocardial orientation and recoil. Systolic dysfunction, signifying inadequate "compressive force generation" requisite over the normal range of circulatory pressure and volume conditions, may, thus, also result or be exacerbated by diverse alterations in myocardial activation, contractile sequence, macro- or microanatomy, and abnormalities of the extracellular matrix.

Despite evidence for abnormal "contractile reserve" in end-stage human HF, in may instances it is not yet possible in clinical practice to adequately characterize the precise anatomic (submyocyte, myocyte, myofiber, matrix), physiologic, molecular, or metabolic "loci"

Table 11.4   Abnormalities Resulting in Systolic Dysfunction

Myocyte compartment

- Myocyte loss (necrosis, apoptosis, aging)
- Abnormal force transduction (e.g., dystrophin mutations)
- Abnormal force generation (calcium release, substrate deficiency)
- Abnormal relaxation (abnormal calcium reuptake)
- Excessive myocyte hypertrophy

Myocardial load

- Volume overload (mitral or aortic regurgitation, renal or hepatic failure)
- Pressure overload (hypertension, increased arterial stiffness)

Heart rate and conduction

- Excessive tachycardia (weeks)
- Discoordinate contraction (right ventricular pacing)

Extracellular matrix compartment

- Fibrosis
- Altered metabolism (cardiofibroblast function, protein synthesis and degradation, paracrine/ autocrine signaling)

Cardiac structure

- Abnormal myocardial fiber "wrapping" or alignment
- Focal infarction or aneurysm
- Advanced remodeling (increased sphericity)

---

of clinically encountered "failing" myocardial tissue (37,41). Some important myocardial characteristics are not easily quantifiable in the intact heart, such as the number of viable myocytes, myocyte and myofiber array, the degree of individual myocyte hypertrophy, the integrity, composition, and metabolic activity of the extracellular matrix. Undoubtedly, incomplete "phenotyping" of failing myocardial tissue has hampered not only a more intimate understanding of HF pathophysiology and ventricular remodeling, but also the customization of pharmacologic and device therapies to individual patients (42–45). Several of the most important abnormalities accounting for systolic dysfunction appear in Table 11.4.

Diastolic Heart Failure

The clinical syndrome of normal or near-normal left ventricular dimension and resting ejection fraction, coupled with the symptoms of dyspnea, exertional limitation, and episodic pulmonary congestion, accounts for up to 40–50% of HF diagnosed and treated in the community (chap. 9) (2,3). A cause of considerable morbidity, including a high rate of recurrent hospitalization, mortality from diastolic HF is lower than in systolic HF but is increased fourfold compared with age-adjusted baseline mortality (46).

Controversy abounds regarding the existence, definition, diagnosis, and therapy of heart failure with preserved EF (HFpEF) or "diastolic" HF (Table 11.5) (5,47–52). The incidence and prevalence of diastolic HF are steeply age-dependent due to the confluence of several age-dependent processes, including progressive loss of myocytes (by age 80 years, one-third of myocytes have been lost), myocardial fibrosis, arterial stiffening (attrition of elastic fibers, atherosclerosis, calcification and fibrosis, and loss of normal endothelial-dependent vasodilation), and the long-term sequelae of hypertension and atherosclerotic coronary artery and peripheral vascular disease (53). In the less common instances of diastolic HF in younger patients, myocardial tissue typically exhibits abnormally relaxant, non-compliant, nondistensible, or excessively stiffened characteristics under the normal range of

Table 11.5 Criteria for Diagnosis of Diastolic Heart Failure

European Study Group:

1. Evidence of CHF
2. Normal or mildly abnormal LV systolic function
3. Evidence of abnormal LV relaxation, filling, distensibility, or stiffness

Framingham Heart Study:

1. Definitive diagnosis of CHF (signs and symptoms; CXR; response to diuretics)
2. LVEF greater than or equal to 50% within 72 hr of episode
3. Objective evidence of LV diastolic dysfunction (abnormal LV relaxation/filling/distensibility indices by catheterization)

Abbreviations: CHF, chronic heart failure; LV, left ventricular; LVEF, left ventricular ejection fraction.
Source: From Refs. 53,270.

Table 11.6 Abnormalities Resulting in Diastolic Heart Failure

Extreme myocardial overload
Severe hypertension, aortic stenosis, mitral or aortic regurgitation)
Impaired myocardial relaxation
Ischemia, hypertrophy, hypothyroidism, aging, cardiomyopathy
Impaired ventricular filling
Mitral stenosis, endocardial fibroelastosis
Reduced ventricular distensibility
Constrictive pericarditis, pericardial tamponade, extrinsic compression
Increased ventricular stiffness
Age, ischemia, myocardial fibrosis or scarring, infiltrative cardiomyopathy, myocardial edema,
  microvascular congestion

Source: Adapted from Ref. 7.

circulatory pressure–volume loads (Table 11.6) (5). Cardiac output is maintained in such instances at rest with obligate elevation of ventricular filling pressures. Albeit normal at rest, the cardiac output either fails to rise appropriately with increased demand or does so with an abrupt rise in filling pressures, and the resultant precipitation of systemic or pulmonary venous and lymphatic congestion that causes limitation of exertion or symptoms.

There is increasing evidence that abnormalities of systolic function accompany most if not all instances of apparently "isolated" diastolic HF (54–56). In elderly patients, such systolic dysfunction not uncommonly results from the increased impedance to ventricular ejection into an increasingly stiffened arterial vascular circuit. Although a lesser degree of neurohormonal activation accompanies diastolic HF than systolic HF, exercise capacity in elderly patients with diastolic HF is comparably diminished as in patients with systolic HF (57). It is not possible on the basis of symptoms and signs alone to distinguish systolic HF from diastolic HF. Most patients with a history of HF and preserved ejection fraction at rest, evidence abnormal indexes of diastolic function by echocardiography, although such measures serve to confirm rather than establish the diagnosis of diastolic HF (58).

There have been few trials to date of lifestyle, pharmacologic or device therapies in this common clinical syndrome. Pharmacologic therapy is largely focused toward control of load, heart rate and rhythm, and symptomatic relief of episodic pulmonary congestion (50). To date, no therapies have been shown to reduce mortality in this common condition, although data from the CHARM study, suggest that therapy with angiotensin receptor blockers can reduce hospitalizations (therapy for diastolic heart failure is more extensively discussed in chap. 17). Although a time-honored therapeutic rubric is to maintain patients "…dry, slow,

Table 11.7   Sensitivity, Specificity and Predictive Value of Symptoms and Physical Signs in Diagnosing Chronic Heart Failure

Symptom or Sign	Sensitivity (%)	Specificity (%)	Predictive Accuracy (%)
Exertional dyspnea	66	52	23
Orthopnea	21	81	2
Paroxysmal nocturnal dyspnea	33	76	26
History of edema	23	80	22
Resting heart rate > 100 bpm	7	99	6
Rales	13	91	21
Third heart sound	31	95	61
Jugular venous distention	10	93	3
Edema (on examination)	10	93	3

Source: Adapted from Ref. 271.

normotensive and in sinus rhythm…," the clinical efficacy of this intuitively attractive rubric remains unproven. No currently available pharmacologic agent consistently or significantly improves intrinsic diastolic function or reliably reduces arterial stiffening. Results from the PhosphodiesteRasE-5 Inhibition to Improve Quality of Life And EXercise Capacity in Diastolic Heart Failure (RELAX) Trial will provide insights into whether increasing intracellular levels of cGMP with sildenafil improves outcomes specifically in diastolic HF.

In the absence of trial data specifically examining the entity of HF with preserved EF, many HF experts recommend application of the same stepwise pharmacologic therapies designed for systolic HF to patients with diastolic HF. Since over time progressive adverse ventricular remodeling also occurs in patients with predominant diastolic dysfunction, beta-blockers, angiotensin II inhibitors, and aldosterone inhibitors likely play an important role in attenuating disease progression (59).

DIAGNOSIS OF HEART FAILURE
Symptoms and Signs

The clinical syndrome of HF, whether systolic of diastolic, must be differentiated from other conditions resulting in dyspnea, fatigue, and exertional intolerance, including but not limited to pulmonary disease, chronic renal or hepatic failure, and anemia (2,7). Clinical HF rarely fulfills its classic "textbook" clinical profile in toto, that is, symptoms of exertional dyspnea, orthopnea, and paroxysmal nocturnal dyspnea, and signs of elevated jugular venous pressure, pulmonary rales, a third heart sound, and peripheral edema (60). No single symptom or sign is pathognomic for HF (61,62), and as previously stated, clinical parameters alone, including symptoms and signs, do not reliably distinguish patients with systolic HF from patients with diastolic HF (57,62–64).

In most observational studies, the symptoms most sensitive for HF include exertional dyspnea, orthopnea, and paroxysmal nocturnal dyspnea (65–69). The most specific symptoms include orthopnea and paroxysmal dyspnea. The sensitivity and specificity of common symptoms and signs is tabulated in Table 11.7. As is apparent, the sensitivity of common symptoms for HF ranges from 23% to 66%, and the specificity from 52% to 81%.

The signs of HF are also inherently nonspecific (70). Rales are absent in up to 80% of patients with chronic HF due to lymphatic hypertrophy (71). Edema occurs in only 25%

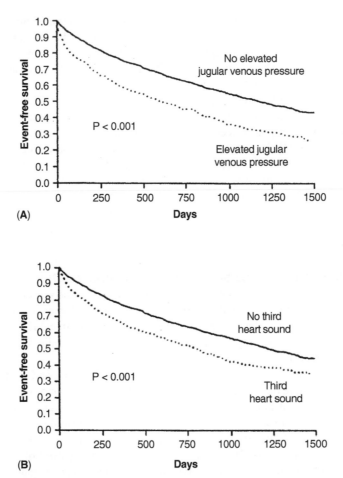

Figure 11.2 Kaplan–Meier analysis of event-free survival according to the presence or absence of elevated jugular venous pressure (*top panel*) and a third heart sound (*bottom panel*). The end-point was a composite of death or hospitalization for heart failure. *Source*: From Ref. 76.

of patients younger than 70 years with chronic HF (70). Evidence of right-sided HF is lacking in up to 50% of patients at the time of diagnosis with idiopathic dilated cardiomyopathy (7). In selected patients with severe HF, hepatojugular reflux (72,73) and the Valsalva maneuver (74,75) may provide ancillary evidence of elevated filling pressures (70). In a retrospective multivariate analysis of the 2569 participants of the SOLVD treatment trial, the presence of an elevated jugular venous pressure and third heart sound were both independently associated with increase risk of hospitalization for HF, death, or hospitalization for HF and death from pump failure (Fig. 11.2) (76). In an observational study of 1000 patients undergoing transplant evaluation, right atrial pressure at cardiac catheterization correlated reasonably well with pulmonary capillary wedge pressure ($r = 0.64$) (77). However, there is only fair interobserver agreement on clinician ascertainment of the jugular venous pressure (kappa statistic, 0.3–0.65) (78) and the presence of a third heart sound (79). A proportional pulse pressure less than 25% has a 91% sensitivity and 83% specificity for cardiac index less than 2.2 L/min/m² in patients with HF (70).

Given the lack of sensitivity and specificity of symptoms and signs, there exists no substitute for the performance of two-dimensional echocardiography to ascertain cardiac structure and function in all instances of suspected HF (2). Ascertainment of the presence or absence of depression of left ventricular ejection fraction (LVEF), left ventricular dimensions and wall thickness, valvular regurgitation, right ventricular dimension and function, and estimated pulmonary artery pressure are all crucial not only to accurate diagnosis but also the selection of appropriate therapy.

As emphasized earlier in this text, a large population of individuals with asymptomatic left ventricular dysfunction and high lifetime risk of evolving symptomatic HF exists (2). Since echocardiographic screening for asymptomatic ventricular dysfunction is not routinely performed, HF is typically diagnosed only once symptoms or signs supervene (3). The signs and symptoms of HF represent a quite advanced stage of ventricular dysfunction, appearing usually only after all compensatory hemodynamic, neurohormonal, and peripheral circulatory "counter-regulatory" homeostatic mechanisms have been overwhelmed. Earlier diagnosis of suspected asymptomatic or minimally symptomatic left ventricular dysfunction by echocardiography affords the opportunity to provide therapies that can retard ventricular remodeling and forestall morbidity and likely mortality.

Classification and Interpretation of the Clinical Presentation

The clinical diagnosis of HF remains largely empiric, based on the presence of symptoms, signs, radiographic evidence of pulmonary congestion or cardiomegaly, and echocardiographic evidence of ventricular dilatation and/or dysfunction. Clinical HF scoring systems have been developed for use in population-based epidemiologic studies but are rarely used in clinical practice (80).

Patients with HF present with a constellation of symptoms and signs referable to either a low output state during rest or exercise, systemic or pulmonary venous congestion, or some combination of both (2). As discussed, symptoms and signs bear an inconstant relationship to resting filling pressures, cardiac index, and ventricular function in individual patients. A clinically useful classification scheme of instances of decompensated HF has been proposed (Fig. 11.3) (71). In this scheme, patients occupy one of four "quadrants" depending on the presence or absence of symptoms and signs of inadequate cardiac output and systemic venous congestion. This "two-minute" hemodynamic assessment is helpful in the initial triage of patients and institution of initial therapy.

Accurate functional classification remains problematic for individual patients (2). The New York Heart Association (NYHA) classification scheme is limited by poor reproducibility, and relies exclusively on the presence and severity of symptoms rather than any marker of ventricular remodeling (81). Since the symptoms and signs of HF are inherently mutable and affected by the adequacy of pharmacologic therapies, any classification scheme based only on symptoms and signs must suffer from imprecision. Assessment of exercise tolerance (and cardiac reserve) during symptom-limited cardiopulmonary exercise testing, predicts prognosis more accurately than does classification based on symptoms and signs and demarcates disease severity more precisely (82).

Diagnostic Laboratory Modalities

Every patient with suspected or known HF requires an assessment of resting ventricular function and cardiac dimensions by two-dimensional echocardiography (2). Components of the diagnostic evaluation of newly diagnosed HF in the current ACC/AHA guidelines appear in Table 11.8. In all patients, the guidelines emphasize: (*i*) a careful history and physical examination; (*ii*) screening laboratories, including tests of renal and hepatic function, complete blood count, urinalysis, electrocardiogram and chest X-ray; (*iii*) a two-dimensional and Doppler echocardiogram; (*iv*) careful exclusion of coronary artery disease and thyroid disease in all patients; and (*v*) selective use of other diagnostic modalities,

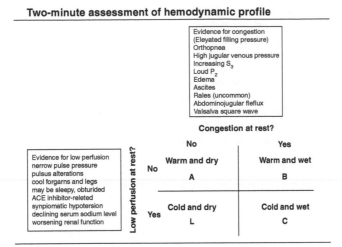

Figure 11.3 Diagram indicating clinically assessed hemodynamic profiles for patients presenting with heart failure. Most patients can be accurately classified in a 2-min assessment according to their presenting signs and symptoms. *Source*: From Ref. 71.

including serologic studies in some patients based on carefully elicited clinical characteristics, past medical and family history, and risk factors.

Plasma levels of B-type natriuretic peptides (BNP) or its amino terminal fragment (NT-proBNP) (83–85) have been used in the diagnosis of HF (86,87). Use of the BNP assay has been incorporated into consensus guidelines from the European Society of Cardiology and the ACC/AHA/ISHLT (88,89). BNP levels have been shown to distinguish between cardiac and noncardiac causes of dyspnea in patients presenting to emergency rooms, and appear to enhance the information provided by clinical assessment alone (90–93). Declines in BNP in response to beta-blockers are associated with improvements in symptoms and outcome (94,95). One study showed that titration of chronic pharmacologic therapy to BNP levels was superior to titration to global clinical assessment (96). BNP appears to be more limited as a screening tool for HF in populations (97) because BNP is elevated in diverse cardiovascular conditions (left ventricular hypertrophy, hypertension, acute coronary syndromes (98), and valvular heart disease) and its levels are age- and gender-dependent (99). BNP also provides prognostic value in chronic symptomatic HF populations (100–103).

Cardiac catheterization remains an important diagnostic tool to exclude significant coronary artery disease and define rest and exercise hemodynamics. Although patients with symptomatic HF may have normal resting hemodynamics, exercise hemodynamics are almost always abnormal, due to either an inadequate rise in cardiac output or an inappropriate rise in filling pressures.

COMMON CLINICAL FEATURES AND COMPLICATIONS
Certain clinical features and complications are common to the course of HF independent of disease etiology.

Arrhythmias
Atrial Fibrillation
Atrial fibrillation (AF) is an increasing public health problem in the United States (104). AF occurs in approximately 15–30% of patients with symptomatic HF (105–107) and in up

Table 11.8   Recommendations for the Evaluation of Patients with Heart Failure

Class I

Thorough history and physical examination

Initial and ongoing assessment of ability to perform routine and desired activities of daily living

Initial and ongoing assessment of volume status

Initial measurement of complete blood count, urinalysis, serum electrolytes, blood urea nitrogen,
  serum creatinine, blood glucose, liver function tests, thyroid-stimulating hormone

Serial monitoring of serum electrolytes and renal function

Initial 12-lead electrocardiogram and chest radiograph

Initial two-dimensional echocardiography with Doppler or radionuclide ventriculography to assess
  left ventricular systolic function

Cardiac catheterization with coronary angiography in patients with angina who are candidates for
  revascularization

Class IIa

Cardiac catheterization with coronary angiography in patients who are candidates for revascularization with:

• chest pain who have not had evaluation of their coronary anatomy
• known of suspected CAD but without angina

Noninvasive assessment of ischemia and viability in patients with known CAD without angina

Maximal exercise testing with measurement of respiratory gas exchange to determine:

• cause of exercise limitation
• candidacy for cardiac transplantation

Echocardiography in asymptomatic first-degree relatives of patients with IDCM

Repeat measures of ejection fraction in patients with change in clinical status

Screening for hemochromatosis

Measurement of ANA, RF, urinary VMA and metanephrines in selected patients

Class IIb

Noninvasive imaging to define likelihood of CAD

Maximal exercise testing to prescribe exercise program

Endomyocardial biopsy in patients with known or suspected inflammatory of infiltrative disorder

HIV testing

Class III

Endomyocardial biopsy in routine evaluation

Routine Holter-monitoring or signal-averaged electrocardiography

Repeat coronary angiography or noninvasive testing in patients in whom CAD has been excluded
  previously as the cause of left ventricular dysfunction

Routine measurement of norepinephrine

Abbreviations: CAD, coronary artery disease; IDCM, idiopathic dilated cardiomyopathy; ANA, antinuclear antibody; RF, rheumatoid factor; VMA, vanellylmandelic acid; HIV, human immunodeficiency virus.

to 50%of patients with class NYMA IV HF (108). Mechanisms leading to AF include atrial
electrical remodeling, atrial fibrosis, sinus node dysfunction, increased sympathetic activation, and elevated atrial filling pressures (109,110). The presence of AF is associated with
an increased all-cause mortality (105,108,111), including sudden cardiac death (112). AF
with rapid ventricular response (HR_110 bpm) may also be associated with rate related but
reversible deterioration in ventricular function (113). While it has not yet been proved that
maintenance of normal sinus rhythm improves mortality (114,115), most practitioners are
more aggressive in attempting to restore and maintain normal sinus rhythm in HF patients
with AF than in other patient populations. Although atrial pacing may reduce the number
of episodes of AF (116), right ventricular (RV) apical pacing in the DDDR mode more than

40% of the time may increase the frequency of HF decompensations and AF by inducing greater mechanical dyssynchrony (117). Cardiac resynchronization may be beneficial in AF, although studies to date remain few (118). Atrial defibrillators will be incorporated increasingly into implantable ventricular defibrillator devices in the future (119).

Ventricular Tachycardia
Nonsustained ventricular tachycardia is ubiquitous in symptomatic HF patients occurring in approximately 80% of patients during 24–48 hours of continuous ambulatory electrocardiogram monitoring (120,121). The risk of sudden cardiac death is closely related to both the severity of depression of ventricular function and the degree of ventricular enlargement rather than the demonstration of nonsustained ventricular tachycardia. Patients with ischemic cardiomyopathy and LVEFs less than 30% are at particularly high risk of sudden cardiac death, and their mortality can be reduced by empiric implantation of an implantable cardioverter defibrillator (ICD) (chap. 19).

Functional Limitation and Exercise Capacity
Mechanisms
Exercise limitation in chronic HF is multifactorial (82,122,123). Hemodynamic (cardiac output, left ventricular systolic and diastolic function, left ventricular filling pressures, and baroreceptor sensitivity), skeletal muscle (muscle mass, perfusion, histochemistry, capillary density, fiber composition, mitochondrial density and oxidative metabolism, and mechanoreceptor function), and pulmonary (respiratory drive and pattern, lung compliance, bronchial reactivity, alveolar–capillary diffusion and ventilatory response to exercise) factors all have varying effects on exercise capacity in individual patients with HF (82).

Cardiac
During exercise in normal subjects, cardiac output increases four- to sixfold due to a two- to fourfold increase in heart rate from basal levels and 20–50% augmentation of stroke volume (122). Both enhanced contractility and peripheral vasodilation effect greater ventricular emptying. Compared with normal subjects, patients with HF exhibit abnormally low maximal cardiac output due to both more modest increments in stroke volume and heart rate during exercise. The predominant mechanism to augment cardiac output in patients with HF is an increase in heart rate. Resting indices of ventricular function, such as ejection fraction, correlate poorly with maximal exercise capacity in patients with HF (124). The most important single factor in limiting exercise capacity in chronic HF is the inability of the left ventricle to augment work appropriately and deliver an adequate volume of oxygenated blood to metabolizing tissues in response to the increasing demand (122). Not surprisingly, left ventricular stroke work index was the single most potent predictor of prognosis in a study combining measurement of rest and exercise respiratory gas exchange, hemodynamics, and echocardiographic features during symptom-limited exercise testing in patients with advanced HF (125). In patients with similar ranges of peak oxygen uptake, dobutamine-stimulated left ventricular functional reserve has been shown to be a further discriminator of prognosis (126). In addition to left ventricular functional reserve, exercise-induced increases in mitral regurgitation limit stroke volume adaptation during exercise and limit exercise capacity as well (127).

Diastolic dysfunction is also exacerbated during exercise and contributes to exercise intolerance in patients with either systolic and diastolic HF (128). A reduction in cardiac cycle-dependent changes in the thoracic aortic area and distensibility are associated with exercise intolerance in elderly patients with apparently isolated diastolic HF (129).

Peripheral Blood Flow

Peripheral vasodilatory capacity is impaired in HF patients (130), particularly failure of exercise-induced vasodilation (131). Upregulation of multiple neurohormonal axes, including the sympathetic nervous, renin–angiotensin, and endothelin systems, likely account for this blunted vasodilatory reserve (122). There is evidence that at least a component of blunted reactivity results from "vascular deconditioning" that is partially reversible with training (132). Endothelial dysfunction, particularly attenuated nitric oxide-mediated endothelial-dependent vasodilation, contributes substantially to the altered distribution of cardiac output in HF patients (133,134). Exercise training improves endothelial function and may help to restore a more normal pattern of cardiac output distribution (135).

Skeletal Muscle

Skeletal muscle gross and ultrastructural morphology (136), fiber type (137), innervation, perfusion, and metabolism are abnormal in HF (138,139). Skeletal muscle mass predicts exercise capacity in noncachectic HF patients (140). Skeletal muscle adaptations may differ in men and women, with men exhibiting abnormalities not due to deconditioning alone (141). Apoptosis has been reported in the skeletal muscle of patients with HF, the magnitude of which is associated with the severity of exercise limitation and the degree of muscle atrophy (142). Metabolic abnormalities also occur in the skeletal muscle unrelated to blood flow (143) and are partly due to decreased levels of mitochondrial oxidative enzymes (144). The abnormality in skeletal muscle oxidative capacity in HF may also derive from nonmitochondrial abnormalities (145). Although studies are conflicting, reductions in capillary density are likely not an important mechanism resulting in skeletal muscle dysfunction (122). Patients with HF exhibit, however, a disproportionate reduction in the distribution of cardiac output to exercising muscle relative to normal subjects (146). Skeletal muscle training programs may partially offset this disproportionate reduction.

Ergoreflexes

Specific signals arising from exercising muscle may be abnormally enhanced in HF patients and contribute to the resultant abnormal integrated hemodynamic, autonomic, and ventilatory responses to exercise (122). Ergoreceptors in skeletal muscles are stimulated by metabolic acidosis leading to peripheral vasoconstriction and heart rate acceleration of (147). Centrally, these ergoreceptors mediate hyperventilation, increase sympathetic outflow, and lead to greater increases in vasoconstriction. Exercise training decreases this hyperresponsiveness (148).

Lungs

Ventilatory efficiency (the rate of increase of minute ventilation per unit of increase carbon dioxide production: VE/VCO_2 slope) is impaired and correlates with exercise limitation and survival (149). Assessment of ventilatory response to exercise improves risk stratification in patients with chronic HF compared with peak oxygen uptake alone (150), including in patients with preserved exercise capacity (151).

Effects of Gene Polymorphisms on Exercise Capacity

Gene polymorphisms may influence functional capacity in HF patients. Relative to patients with "wild-type" beta-adrenoreceptor genotypes, exercise capacity is reduced in HF patients with the Gly389 polymorphism of the beta1 allele (152), the Ile64 polymorphism of the beta2 receptor allele (153), and those homozygous for the angiotensin-converting enzyme deletion (DD) genotype (154).

Clinical Assessment of Functional and Exercise Capacity

New York Heart Association

The NYHA functional classification (155) is subject to considerable interobserver variation and is not sensitive to changes in exercise capacity (2). Correlations between NYHA class, six-walk test (six-WT) and peak oxygen uptake have been modest at best in HF populations, and within a given functional class large variations in mortality occur (156). Despite these limitations, NYHA classification remains a predictor of prognosis in broad HF populations. Specific activity scales have been developed that equate metabolic equivalents to activities of daily living (157). Other functional status instruments have been developed, but none have been as widely adopted for routine clinical practice as the NYHA classification (11, 158–160). The Minnesota Living with Heart Failure Questionnaire (MLHF) was developed to assess the patient's self-reported perceptions of the effects of heart failure and its treatment in daily life (161). This 21-question instrument incorporates both a physical domain (dyspnea, fatigue) and an emotional domain. At present, the MLHF is the most widely adopted instrument used in most interventional HF studies of pharmacologic agents and devices.

Six-Walk Test

The six-WT was developed for use in elderly, frail HF patients (162). In 898 patients from the SOLVD study, NYHA class and quartiles of six-WT results were only moderately correlated but the six-WT results were strongly and independently associated with morbidity and mortality in multivariate modeling (163). In the RESOLVD pilot study, test–retest reliability of the six-WT was very good (intraclass correlation coefficient 0.90), but six-WT results were only weakly inversely correlated to quality-of-life scores ($r = -0.26$) and NYHA class ($r = -0.43$) (164). In a study of 315 patients with moderate-to-severe HF, the six-WT did not correlate with resting hemodynamics, was only moderately correlated to exercise capacity, and was not selected as an independent predictor of prognosis in multivariate models, including NYHA class and peak oxygen uptake (165). In a study of severe HF, the six-WT distance was not a reliable surrogate of peak oxygen uptake or predictor of prognosis (166). In a separate study of 113 patients with severe HF (mean LVEF 21%), six-WT was weakly correlated to right atrial pressure ($r = -0.28$) and LVEF ($r = -033$) but not to pulmonary capillary wedge pressure or resting cardiac output, and was not an independent predictor of one-year survival in multivariate models (167). Even in elderly frail patients, the six-WT appears to be reasonably reproducible with an intraclass correlation coefficient of 0.91 reported (168). Peak oxygen uptake measured during the six-WT averages 15% lower than peak oxygen uptake measured during formal symptom-limited cardiopulmonary exercise testing in HF patients (169).

Cardiopulmonary Exercise Testing

Presently, symptom-limited cardiopulmonary exercise testing with simultaneous respiratory gas exchange assessment of peak oxygen uptake remains the most widely used method of determining the maximal exercise capacity and prognosis of patients with advanced HF (82,170,171). Peak oxygen uptake determination remains critically important in formulating the appropriateness and timing of cardiac transplantation (172). Accurate determination of peak oxygen uptake requires that patients exceed the anaerobic threshold during exercise. Peak oxygen uptake is 10–20% higher by treadmill compared with bicycle exercise protocols. Peak oxygen uptake correlates poorly with resting hemodynamics (125). Inclusion of additional variables to peak oxygen uptake in multivariate BNP levels were reported to predict exercise capacity in chronic HF (173).

Response to Pharmacologic Agents

Multiple therapies improve exercise capacity but are not necessarily associated with improved survival (e.g., enoximone) (174). Sildenafil has been reported to reduce the

Ve-VCO_2 slope during the exercise and modestly improve peak oxygen uptake in chronic HF patients (175). Controlled studies of coenzyme Q10 have not shown improvements in exercise capacity (176).

Exercise Training

Published studies suggest that peak oxygen uptake improves 12–31% during exercise training in HF patients (122). There are parallel improvements in six-WT performance and the ventilatory threshold (177). Long-term moderate exercise training in patients with HF results in improved quality of life and exercise capacity, and modest attenuation of left ventricular remodeling, including reductions in ventricular volumes (122,178,179). Improvement in LVEF is less consistently observed (122,178,179). Exercise training also improves endothelial function and partially attenuates sympathetic neural overactivity (180). Limited data suggest that exercise training is effective in older adults with HF (181). Training programs in carefully selected patients are safe and result in worthwhile improvements in exercise capacity (182). The duration, supervision, venue of training, volume of working muscle, intensity and mode of training, and concurrent medical therapies all effect the results of exercise training and benefits may not persist without ongoing maintenance (183). The effects of exercise training on survival are presently unknown and await longer-term trials (122).

Mitral Regurgitation

Mitral regurgitation (MR) frequently accompanies progressive ventricular dilatation without intrinsic pathology of the mitral valve apparatus (184,185). Such "functional" mitral regurgitation is most commonly due to lateral migration of the papillary muscles and inappropriate "tethering" of the mitral valve leaflets during systole (chap. 6) (186,187). Mitral annular dilation, papillary muscle, or subadjacent myocardial hypokinesis may also contribute (188,189). The regurgitant volume returned to the left ventricle increases preload and adversely affects ventricular remodeling (3). Not surprisingly, moderate to severe mitral regurgitation is associated with increased morbidity and mortality in chronic HF (190,191). Careful quantitation of the severity of regurgitation by resting Doppler echocardiography and myocardial "contractile reserve" are both critical in the assessment of the timing and appropriateness of isolated mitral valve repair or replacement in patients with chronic HF and severe mitral regurgitation (192,193). Increased mitral regurgitant volume during exercise echocardiography correlates well with reduced exercise tolerance (194,195) and higher risk of adverse events (196). Tailored hemodynamic therapy with optimization of filling pressures and volumes, cardiac resynchronization therapy, and positive inotropic pharmacologic agents all reduce the degree of functional mitral regurgitation (197–199). Encouraging intermediate-term results have been reported from select centers performing mitral valve repair in patients with advanced symptomatic HF and severe mitral regurgitation (chap. 22) (200–202). Although moderate MR frequently accompanies ischemic cardiomyopathy and marks a worse prognosis (203), most observational studies to date have been unable to demonstrate improved outcomes when mitral valve repair or replacement is routinely performed in addition to coronary artery bypass grafting (204).

Sleep Apnea

Central sleep apnea (CSA) afflicts approximately 33–40% of patients with symptomatic HF (205–209). In HF patients with CSA, the chronic hyperventilation resulting from pulmonary congestion is exacerbated by increased venous return in the supine position (205). Apnea is then induced by a greater degree of hyperventilation and further reduction in $PaCO_2$ until terminated by a rise in $PaCO_2$ above the ventilation stimulatory threshold. An enhanced sensitivity to carbon dioxide appears to predispose HF patients to CSA (210). Risk factors include male gender, hypocapnia, atrial fibrillation, and increasing age, but not obesity (211). CSA is distinctly less common in women with HF (205). In HF patients, sleep apnea (central or obstructive) increases blood pressure (212), atrial and ventricular dysrhythmias (213), sympathetic activation (214), filling pressures (215), and the risk of symptomatic deterioration. Since thoracic mechanics remain unaltered, ventricular after-load is not increased, and the effects of CSA on ventricular remodeling are less clear than for obstructive sleep apnea (OSA) (205). Therapy of OSA with continuous positive airway pressure (CPAP) during sleep improves symptoms and ventricular function (216,217).

Small observational studies have also reported lower mortality in patients with CSA treated with CPAP, but these studies await confirmation in larger trials. Nonetheless, most physicians recommend CPAP for HF patients with documented CSA. Empiric CPAP in the absence of documented CSA has not been studied in HF patients to date. Atrial overdrive pacing may reduce the number of episodes of sleep apnea (218). OSA afflicts approximately 10% of patients with heart failure (219). Given the prevalence, morbidity, and ready therapy of either type of sleep apnea in patients with HF, it is incumbent on the clinician to screen all patients with symptomatic heart failure for sleep apnea and provide appropriate therapy. Since long-term compliance with CPAP is only 50–80% (219), apparent treatment "failures" are commonly encountered in practice.

"Cardiorenal" Phenomena

In chronic HF, deterioration in renal function may result from diminished cardiac output and corresponding reduced glomerular filtration, alterations in the distribution of cardiac output, intrarenal vasoregulation, alterations in circulatory volume, the degree and type of neurohormonal activation, and the multiplicative toxic effects of medications (220). As a result, patients frequently exhibit altered renal function, including dysregulation of sodium and potassium homeostasis, a greater propensity to azotemia in response to vasodilators or diuretics, reduction in renal clearance of metabolic products or medications, and refractoriness to previously effective doses or schedules of oral or intravenous diuretic therapies (221). Approximately 25% of hospitalized HF patients exhibit deterioration in renal function despite appropriate medical therapy (222). In such hospitalized patients, a rise in serum creatinine of 0.1–0.5 mg/dL is associated with a longer hospital length of stay and increased inhospital mortality (223).

This constellation of poorly understood physiologic mechanisms and unpredictable clinical responsiveness to appropriate therapies has been termed the "cardiorenal" syndrome (71). Renal insufficiency is associated with increased mortality in both asymptomatic and symptomatic ambulatory HF patients (Fig. 11.4) (220,224,225). Patients with advanced HF often exhibit unexpected and unpredictable alterations in renal function, which render management challenging (71). Hyponatremia is an important prognostic marker in advanced HF and predicts mortality in ambulatory patients with symptomatic HF (226), advanced HF (227), and in patients hospitalized with HF (228). (For more detail, see chap. XX].

Cardiac Cachexia

Cardiac cachexia is usually defined as a nonintentional loss of greater than 7.5% of the "usual" weight of the patient (229). Cardiac cachexia is associated with increased mortality in chronic HF independent of age, NYHA class, and LVEF and peak oxygen consumption (230). Compared with noncachectic patients, cachectic HF patients evidence loss of lean muscle, adipose and bone tissue, and raised plasma levels of norepinephrine, epinephrine, cortisol, plasma renin activity, aldosterone, tumor necrosis factor-α (TNF-α) and

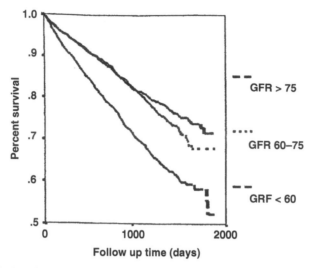

Figure 11.4   Kaplan–Meier survival analysis by level of glomerular filtration rate at presentation for ambulatory heart failure patients who participated in the Studies of Left Ventricular Dysfunction (SOLVD) trial. *Source*: From Ref. 272.

growth hormone, but reduced levels of insulin-like growth factor 1 and typically high levels of insulin resistance (229,231–234). Interestingly, levels of leptin, a hormone secreted in response to TNF-α that decreases food intake and increases energy expenditure, appear to be inappropriately low rather than high in cachectic HF patients (235). A poorly understood multifactorial process resulting from intersecting neurohormonal and inflammatory mediators, cardiac cachexia forebodes an ominous prognosis and bears appropriate recognition and response by practitioners (232). No specific therapy to counteract cardiac cachexia yet exists (236).

Anemia

Anemia occurs in up to 17% of patients with HF and is associated with a modest increase in all-cause mortality (Fig. 11.5) (237–240). Anemia is less prevalent in recent-onset HF (241). Potential mechanisms remain speculative but include the effects of chronic disease, excessive cytokine production, malnutrition, and plasma volume overload (242). Small trials to date have reported that therapy with subcutaneous erythropoietin and iron may not only restore red cell mass but also improve symptoms and exercise capacity in patients with moderate to severe chronic HF (242–244). There may be little benefit to normalization of the hematocrit via erythropoietin therapy in patients with HF receiving chronic hemodialysis (245). Elucidation of the role of erythropoietin therapy in patients with HF and anemia awaits larger randomized studies.

Psychiatric

In observational studies to date, approximately 30–60% of hospitalized HF patients (246,247) and 10–20% of ambulatory HF patients suffer from depression (248–250). Despite similar measures of objective functional capacity, depressed patients tend to report worse physical functional ability than nondepressed patients (251). Depression is also associated with reduced survival (249,252,253) and a 26–29% increase in the costs of care (254). Disease management programs for HF may also reduce symptoms of depression and improve quality of life (255). The prevalence of anxiety does not appear to be increased in

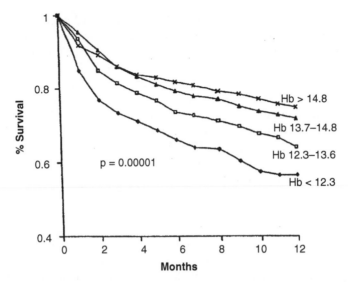

Figure 11.5 Kaplan–Meier survival analysis for ambulatory heart failure patients enrolled in a comprehensive disease management program stratified by quartile of hemoglobin (Hg) level. *Source*: From Ref. 238.

HF patients, although studies have been few (246). A sense of perceived control reduces emotional distress in HF patients, including depression and anxiety (256).

PROGNOSIS

Older studies from the Framingham Heart Study reported in excess of a 50% five-year mortality for patients with symptomatic HF, and no difference in survival among patients diagnosed between 1948 and 1974 compared with patients diagnosed between 1975 and 1988 (257). A study from the Framingham group, however, reported a reduction in 30-day, one-year, and five-year age-adjusted mortality rates in heterogenous cohorts of both men (from 12%, 30%, and 70% to 11%, 28%, and 59%, respectively) and women (from 18%, 28%, and 57% to 10%, 24%, and 45%, respectively) comparing the periods 1950–1969 to 1990–1999 (13).

Observational studies from selected academic centers have reported improved survival in patients with idiopathic dilated cardiomyopathy (258) and advanced HF (156,259). A large observational study from Scotland noted improved survival in HF patients hospitalized between 1986 and 1995, with declines in case-fatality rates in men and women of 26% and 17% at 30 days; and from 18% and 15% at one-year, respectively (260). An observational study of community-dwelling elderly persons found a substantial increase in death from HF with adjusted hazard ratios of 1.25 in patients with no HF and borderline LV function, 1.83 in patients with no HF and impaired LV function, 1.48 in patients with HF and normal LV function, 2.4 in patients with HF and borderline LV function, and 1.88 in patients with HF and impaired LV function (261). In a population-based observational study of 38,702 consecutive unselected community-dwelling patients hospitalized with HF between 1994 and 1997, the crude 30-day and one-year case-fatality rates after first admission for HF were 11.6% and 33.1%, respectively (262).

The contemporary combination of "triple" neurohormonal therapy with ACEI, beta-blockers, and aldosterone antagonists coupled with appropriate implantation of ICDs may reduce the annual mortality of advanced symptomatic heart failure by up to 75% (chronic therapy of heart failure is discussed in more detail in chaps. 12 and 13). In some clinical trials, including COPERNICUS, enrolling non–inotropic-dependent patients with NYHA IV heart failure, the one-year mortality in the placebo group was 18.5% (263). However, in a more fragile cohort of inotrope-dependent patients in the REMATCH trial, the mortality in the medical therapy group was 75% at one year (264). A comprehensive tabulation of the mortality results of clinical trials is summarized in Eichorn's comprehensive review (156).

Despite these gratifying results of chronic pharmacologic and device therapies, the number of deaths due to HF has increased in the United States, from 19,936 in 1979 to 43,010 in 1995, an increase of 116% (156). The improved survival reported in interventional pharmacologic trials compared with observational population-based studies in HF is likely due to differences in clinical characteristics (age, comorbidities, intensity of pharmacologic and device therapies), study exclusion criteria (recent infarction or revascularization, dementia, stroke, life-limiting illness), adherence to prescribed care and process of care (frequent study visits, for example). In particular, factors for improved survival include better dosing of ACI inhibitors, higher penetration of use of beta-blockers and aldosterone antagonists, increased use of aspirin and statin therapy in patients with coronary artery disease, decreased use of calcium channel blockers and type I antiarrhythmics, increasing indications for ICDs and amiodarone, biventricular pacing, ventricular assist devices and cardiac transplantation, specialized physician and nurse practitioners with expertise in heart failure, comprehensive HF centers, and use of HF disease management programs.

PREDICTION OF SURVIVAL

To date, no single study has simultaneously evaluated the more than 50 variables associated with prognosis in chronic HF (156). In his comprehensive review of published studies, Eichhorn identified norepinephrine levels, cardiac norepinephrine spillover, BNP levels, LVEF, peak oxygen uptake, advanced age, history of symptomatic ventricular arrhythmias or sudden cardiac death, and therapy with ACE inhibitors, beta-blockers, aldosterone antagonists, implantation of an ICD, and cardiac transplantation as the most important predictors of outcome in chronic HF (156).

Of particular note, LVEF may lose its predictive accuracy in patients with advanced HF symptoms (265,266) or in patients with an LVEF greater than 45% (267). Among hemodynamic variables measured during symptom-limited cardiopulmonary exercise testing, peak left ventricular stroke work index is the single most informative parameter (125). Patients admitted to the hospital with simultaneous signs of congestion and hypoperfusion have a higher adjusted hospital mortality (268). The presence of an S3 gallop and elevated jugular venous pressure upon enrollment into the SOLVD treatment and prevention trials predicted mortality (76,269).

The Seattle Heart Failure Model has been used to estimate survival and is widely used as a tool for risk evaluation and assessing the impact of treatment interventions in patients with CHF. Specific details about this model are covered elsewhere in chapter XX.

CONCLUSION

This chapter has focused on the epidemiology, pathophysiology, and clinical syndrome of HF with particular emphasis on clinical presentation and diagnosis. The last few decades have proved an exciting time in our understanding of the pathophysiology of HF and improvements of therapy. The rather impressive results of "antiremodeling" therapy with current "triple" neurohormonal antagonists (ACE inhibitors, beta-blockers, and aldosterone antagonists), coupled with that achieved with biventricular pacing and the decrease in sudden cardiac death risk with appropriate implantation of ICDs, has ushered in a new era of therapy for chronic HF. On the not too distant horizon, a more precise understanding of the pathophysiology and clinical course of HF, based in large part on elucidation of genetic determinants and interactions, may provide an opportunity for a more targeted and customized application of therapy than is now possible. The decades to come will undoubtedly witness a whole new era of mature, durable, and miniaturized devices and novel replacement therapies. It is not only conceivable, but indeed likely, that future therapeutic options will eventually render the all present, all-too-common clinical syndrome of HF a conquered disease of the past.

REFERENCES

1. Roger VL, Go AS, Lloyd-Jones DM, et al. Heart disease and stroke statistics, 2012 update: a report from the American heart association. Circulation 2012; 125: e2–e220.
2. Hunt SA, Baker DW, Chin MH, et al. ACC/AHA guidelines for the evaluation and management of chronic heart failure in the adult: a report of the American College of Cardiology/American Heart Association Task Force on practice guidelines (committee to review the 1995 guidelines for the evaluation and management of heart failure). Am Coll Cardiol 2001; [Available from: htpp://www.acc.org/clinical/guidelines/failure/hf_index.htm].
3. Jessup M, Brujena S. Heart failure. N Engl J Med 2003; 348: 2007–18.
4. Katz AM. Pathophysiology of heart failure: identifying targets for pharmacotherapy. Med Clin North Am 2003; 87: 303–16.
5. Angeja BG, Grossman W. Evaluation and management of diastolic heart failure. Circulation 2003; 107: 659–63.
6. Burkhoff D, Maurer MS, Pacher M. Heart failure with a normal ejection fraction: is it really a disorder of diastolic function? Circulation 2003; 107: 656–8.
7. Dec GW, Foster V. Idiopathic dilated cardiomyopathy. N Engl J Med 1994; 331: 1564–75.
8. Adams KF. New epidemiologic perspectives concerning mild-to-moderate heart failure. Am J Med 2001; 110:6S–13S.
9. Massie BM, Shah NB. Evolving trends in the epidemiology factors of heart failure: rationale for preventive strategies and comprehensive disease management. Am Heart J 1997; 133: 703–12.
10. Packer M, Cohn JN. Consensus recommendations for the management of heart failure. Am J Cardiol 1999; 83:1A–38A.
11. Ho KKL, Pinsky JL, Kannel WB, et al. The epidemiology of heart failure: the Framingham Study. J Am Coll Cardiol 1993; 22:6A–13A.
12. Lloyd-Jones D. The risk of congestive heart failure: sobering lessons from the Framingham heart study. Curr Cardiol Rep 2001; 3: 184–90.
13. Levy D, Kenchaiah S, Larson MG, et al. Long-term trends in the incidence and survival with heart failure. N Engl J Med 2002; 347: 1397–402.
14. Rich MW. Epidemiology, pathophysiology, and etiology of congestive heart failure in older adults. J Am Geriatr Soc 1997; 45: 968–74.
15. Wang TJ, Levy D, Benjamin EJ, et al. The epidemiology of "asymptomatic" left ventricular systolic dysfunction: implications for screening. Ann Intern Med 2003; 138: 907–16.
16. Redfield MM, Jacobsen SJ, Burnett JC, et al. Burden of systolic and diastolic ventricular dysfunction in the community: appreciating the scope of the heart failure epidemic. JAMA 2003; 289: 194–202.
17. O'Connell JB, Bristow MR. Economic impact of heart failure in the United States: time for a different approach. J Heart Lung Transplant 1994; 13: S107–12.
18. Boccuzzi SJ. Economics and cost-effectiveness in evaluating the value of cardiovascular therapies. Angiotensin-converting enzyme inhibitors in the management of congestive heart failure: a pharmaceutical industry perspective. Am Heart J 1999; 137: S120–2.
19. Towbin JA, Bowles NE. The failing heart. Nature 2002; 415: 227–33.
20. Hoshijima M, Chien KR. Mixed signal in heart failure: cancer rules. J Clin Invest 2002; 109: 849–55.
21. Fatkin D, MacRae C, Sasaki T, et al. Missense mutations in the rod domain of the lamin A/C gene as causes of dilated cardiomyopathy and conduction-system disease. N Engl J Med 1999; 341: 1715–24.
22. Kamisago M, Sharma SD, DePalma SR, et al. Mutations in sarcomere protein genes as a cause of dilated cardiomyopathy. N Engl J Med 2000; 342: 1688–96.
23. Dalakas MC, Park KY, Semino-Mora C, et al. Desmin myopathy, a skeletal myopathy with cardiomyopathy caused by mutations in the desmin gene. N Engl J Med 2000; 342: 770–80.
24. Franz WM, Muller M, Muller OJ, et al. Association of nonsense mutation of dystrophin gene with disruption of sarcoglycan complex in X-linked dilated cardiomyopathy. Lancet 2000; 355: 1781–5.

25. Mestroni L, Rocco C, Gregori D, et al. Familial dilated cardiomyopathy: evidence for genetic and phenotypic heterogeneity. J Am Coll Cardiol 1999; 34: 181–90.
26. Brodsky GL, Muntoni F, Miocic S, et al. Lamin A/C gene mutation associated with dilated cardiomyopathy with variable skeletal muscle involvement. Circulation 2000; 101: 473–6.
27. Kelly DP, Strauss AW. Inherited cardiomyopathies. N Engl J Med 1994; 330: 913–18.
28. Fadic R, Sunada Y, Waclawik AJ, et al. Brief report: deficiency of a dystrophin-associated glycoprotein (adhalin) in a patient with muscular dystrophy and cardiomyopathy. N Engl J Med 1996; 334: 362–6.
29. Muntoni F, Cau M, Ganau A, et al. Brief report: deletion of the dystrophin muscle-promoter region associated with X-linked dilated cardiomyopathy. N Engl J Med 1993; 329: 921–5.
30. Small KM, Wagoner LE, Levin AM, et al. Synergistic polymorphisms of beta-one and alpha2C-adrenergic receptors and the risk of congestive heart failure. N Engl J Med 2002; 347: 1135–42.
31. Exner DV, Dries DL, Domanski MJ, et al. Lesser response to angiotensin-converting-enzyme inhibitor therapy in black as compared with white patients with left ventricular dysfunction. N Engl J Med 2001; 344: 1351–7.
32. Yancy CW, Fowler MB, Colucci WS, et al. Race and the response to adrenergic blockade with carvedilol in patients with chronic heart failure. N Engl J Med 2001; 344: 1358–65.
33. Wood AJJ. Racial differences in the response to drugs—pointers to genetic differences. N Engl J Med 2001; 344: 1393–6.
34. Katz AM. Physiology of the Heart, 3rd edn. Philadelphia: PA. Lippincott, 2001.
35. Katz AM. Heart Failure: Pathophysiology, Molecular Biology, and Clinical Management, 1st edn. Philadelphia: PA. Lippincott, 2000.
36. Houser SR, Margulies KB. Is depressed myocyte contractility centrally involved in heart failure? Circ Res 2003; 92: 350–8.
37. Francis GS. Pathophysiology of chronic heart failure. Am J Med 2001; 101: 37S–46S.
38. Nadal-Ginard B, Kajstura J, Leri A, et al. Myocyte death, growth, and regeneration in cardiac hypertrophy and failure. Circ Res 2003; 92: 139–50.
39. Spinale FG. Matrix metalloproteinases: regulation and dysregulation in the failing heart. Circ Res 2002; 90: 520–30.
40. Mann DL. Inflammatory medicators and the failing heart: past, present and the foreseeable future. Circ Res 2002; 91: 988–98.
41. Bers DM. Cardiac excitation-contraction coupling. Nature 2002; 415: 198–205.
42. Lowes BD, Gilbert EM, Abraham WT, et al. Myocardial gene expression in dilated cardiomyopathy treated with betablocking agents. N Engl J Med 2002; 346: 1357–65.
43. Loh E, Rebbeck TR, Mahoney PD, et al. Common variant in AMPD1 gene predicts improved clinical outcome in patients with heart failure. Circulation 1999; 99: 1422–5.
44. McNamara DM, Holubkov R, Janosko K, et al. Pharmacogenetic interactions between beta-blocker therapy and the angiotensin-converting enzyme deletion polymorphism in patients with congestive heart failure. Circulation 2001; 103: 1644–8.
45. McNamara DM, Holubkov R, Postava L, et al. Effect of the Asp298 variant of endothelial nitric oxide synthase on survival for patients with congestive heart failure. Circulation 2003; 107: 1598–602.
46. Vasan RS, Larson MG, Benjamin EJ, et al. Congestive heart failure in subjects with normal versus reduced left ventricular ejection fraction: prevalence and mortality in a population-based cohort. J Am Coll Cardiol 1999; 33: 1948–55.
47. Senni M, Redfield MM. Heart failure with preserved systolic function: a different natural history? J Am Coll Cardiol 2001; 38: 1277–82.
48. Petrie MC, Caruana L, Berry C, McMurry JJ. "Diastolic heart failure" or heart failure caused by subtle left ventricular systolic dysfunction? Heart 2002; 87: 29–31.
49. Zile MR, Brutsgert DL. New concepts in diastolic dysfunction and diastolic heart failure: part I diagnosis, prognosis, and measurements of diastolic function. Circulation 2002; 105: 1387–93.
50. Zile MR, Brutsgert DL. New concepts in diastolic dysfunction and diastolic heart failure: diagnosis, prognosis, and measurements of diastolic function: part II causal mechanisms and treatment. Circulation 2002; 105: 1503–8.
51. Vasan RS, Benjamin EJ, Levy D. Congestive heart failure with normal left ventricular systolic function: clinical approaches to the diagnosis and treatment of diastolic heart failure. Arch Intern Med 1996; 156: 146–57.
52. Vasan RS, Levy D. Defining diastolic heart failure: a call for standardized diagnostic criteria. Circulation 2000; 101: 2118–21.
53. Lakatta EG. Arterial and cardiac aging: major shareholders in cardiovascular disease enterprises: part III: cellular and molecular clues to heart and arterial aging. Circulation 2003; 107: 490–7.

54. Kawaguchi M, Hay I, Fetics B, et al. Combined ventricular systolic and arterial stiffening in patients with heart failure and preserved ejection fraction: implications for systolic and diastolic reserve limitations. Circulation 2003; 107: 714–20.

55. Fitzgibbons TP, Meyer TE, Aurigemma GP, et al. Mortality in diastolic heart failure. Cardiol Rev 2009; 17: 51–5.

56. Yu CM, Lin H, Yang H, et al. Progression of systolic abnormalities in patients with "isolated" diastolic heart failure and diastolic dysfunction. Circulation 2002; 105: 1195–201.

57. Kitzman DW, Little WC, Brubaker PH, et al. Pathophysiological characterization of isolated diastolic heart failure in comparison to systolic heart failure. JAMA 2002; 288: 2144–50.

58. Zile MR, Gaasch WH, Carroll JD, et al. Heart failure with a normal ejection fraction: is measurement of diastolic function necessary to make the diagnosis of diastolic heart failure? Circulation 2001; 104: 779–82.

59. Brilla CG, Funck RC, Rupp H. Lisinopril-mediated regression of myocardial fibrosis in patients with hypertensive heart disease. Circulation 2000; 102: 1388–93.

60. Massie BM, Yamani MH. Chronic heart failure: diagnosis and management. In: Poole-Wilson PA, Colucci WS, et al., eds. Heart Failure. New York: Churchill Livingstone, 1997: 551–66.

61. Cheitlin MD. Can clinical evaluation differentiate diastolic from systolic heart failure? Is so, is it important? Am J Med 2002; 112: 496–7.

62. Badgett RG, Lucey CR, Mulrow CD. Can the clinical examination diagnose left-sided heart failure in adults? JAMA 1997; 277: 1712–19.

63. Thomas JT, Kelly RF, Thomas SJ, et al. Utility of history, physical examination, electrocardiogram, and chest radiograph for differentiating normal from decreased systolic function in patients with heart failure. Am J Med 2002; 112: 437–45.

64. Ghali JK, Kadakia S, Cooper RS, et al. Bedside diagnosis of preserved versus impaired left ventricular systolic function in heart failure. Am J Cardiol 1991; 67: 1002–6.

65. Harlan WR, oberman A, Grimm R, et al. Chronic congestive heart failure in coronary artery disease: clinical criteria. Ann Intern Med 1977; 86: 133–8.

66. Marantz PR, Tobin JN, Wassertheil-Smoller S, et al. The relationship between left-ventricular systolic function and congestive heart failure diagnosed by clinical criteria. Circulation 1988; 77: 607–12.

67. Mattleman SJ, Hakki AH, Iskandrian AS, et al. Reliability of bedside evaluation in determining left ventricular ejection function: correlation with left ventricular ejection fraction determined by radionuclide ventriculography. J Am Coll Cardiol 1983; 1: 417–20.

68. Gadsboll N, Høilund-Carlsen PF, Nielsen GG, et al. Symptoms and signs of heart failure in patients with myocardial infarction. reproducibility and relationship to chest x-ray, radionuclide ventriculography, and right heart catheterization. Eur Heart J 1989; 10: 1017–28.

69. Chakko C, Harlan WR, Harlan WR, et al. Clinical, radiographic, and hemodynamic correlations in chronic heart failure. Conflicting results may lead to inappropriate care. Am J Med 1991; 90: 353–9.

70. Stevenson LW, Perloff JK. The limited reliability of physical signs for estimating hemodynamics in chronic heart failure. JAMA 1989; 261: 884–8.

71. Nohria A, Lewis E, Stevenson LW. Medical management of advanced heart failure. JAMA 2002; 287: 628–40.

72. Ewy GA. The abdominojugular test: technique and hemodynamic correlates. Ann Intern Med 1988; 109: 456–60.

73. Butman SM, Ewy GA, Standen JR, et al. Bedside cardiovascular examination in patients with severe chronic heart failure: importance of rest of inducible jugular venous distention. J Am Coll Cardiol 1993; 22: 968–74.

74. Zema MJ, Restivo B, Sos T, et al. Left ventricular dysfunction: beside Valsalva manoeuvre. Br Heart J 1980; 44: 560–9.

75. Zema MJ, Caccovano M, Kligfield P. Detection of left ventricular dysfunction in ambulatory subjects with the bedside Valsalva maneuver. Am J Med 1983; 75: 241–8.

76. Drazner MH, Rame JE, Stevenson LW, et al. Prognostic importance of elevated jugular venous pressure and a third heart sound in patients with heart failure. N Engl J Med 2001; 345: 574–81.

77. Drazner MH, Hamilton MA, Fonarow G, et al. Relationship between right and left-sided filling pressures in 1000 patients with advanced heart failure. J Heart Lung Transplant 1999; 18: 1126–32.

78. McGee SR. Physical examination of venous pressure: a critical review. Am Heart J 1998; 136: 10–18.

79. Ishmail AA, Wing S, Ferguson J, et al. Interobserver agreement by auscultation in the presence of a third heart sound in patients with chronic heart failure. Chest 1987; 91: 870–3.

80. McKee PA, Castelli WP, McNamara PM, et al. The natural history of congestive heart failure. the Framingham study. N Engl J Med 1971; 285: 1441–6.

81. Criteria Committee of the New York Heart Association. Nomenclature and Criteria for Diagnosis of Diseases of the Heart and Great Vessels, 7th edn. Boston: Little, Brown, 1973.

82. Metra M, Nodari S, Raccagni D, et al. Maximal and submaximal exercise testing in heart failure. J Cardiovasc Pharm 1998; 32:S36–45.

83. Wilkins MR, Redondo J, Brown LA. The natriuretic-peptide family. Lancet 1997; 349: 1307–10.

84. Levin ER, Gardner DG, Stevenson WK. Natriuretic peptides. N Engl J Med 1998; 339: 321–8.

85. Burger MR, de Bold AJ. BNP in decompensated heart failure: diagnostic, prognostic and therapeutic potential. Curr Opin Investig Drug 2001; 2: 929–35.

86. Shapiro BP, Chen HH, Burnett JC, et al. Use of plasma brain natriuretic peptide concentration to aid in the diagnosis of heart failure. Mayo Clin Proc 2003; 78: 481–6.

87. Adams KF, Mathur VS, Chengheide M. B-type natriuretic peptide: from bench to bedside. Am Heart J 2003; 145: S34–46.

88. Dickstein K, Cohen-Solal A, Filippatos G, et al. ESC guidelines for the diagnosis and treatment of acute and chronic heart failure. Eur Heart J 2008; 29:2388–442.

89. Hunt SA, Abraham WT, Chin MH, et al. 2009 focused update incorporated into the ACC/AHA 2005 Guidelines for the Diagnosis and Management of Heart Failure in Adults: a report of the American College of Cardiology Foundation/American Heart Association Task Force on Practice Guidelines: developed in collaboration with the International Society for Heart and Lung Transplantation. Circulation 2009; 119: e391–479.

90. Maisel AS, Krishnaswamy P, Nowak RM, et al. Rapid measurement of B-type natriuretic peptide in the emergency diagnosis of heart failure. N Engl J Med 2002; 347: 161–7.

91. McCullough PA, Nowak RM, McCord J, et al. B-type natriuretic peptide and clinical judgment in emergency diagnosis of heart failure: analysis from Breathing Not Properly (BNP) Multinational Study. Circulation 2002; 106: 416–22.

92. Dao Q, Krishnaswamy P, Kazanegra R, et al. Utility of B-type natriuretic peptide in the diagnosis of congestive heart failure in an urgent-care setting. J Am Coll Cardiol 2001; 37: 379–85.

93. Collins SP, Ronan-Bentle S, Storrow AB. Diagnostic and prognostic usefulness of natriuretic peptides in emergency department patients with dyspnea. Ann Emerg Med 2003; 41: 532–45.

94. Richards AM, Doughty R, Nicholls MG, et al. Neurohumoral prediction of benefit from carvedilol in ischemic left ventricular dysfunction. Circulation 1999; 99: 786.

95. Stanek B, Frey B, Mismann M. Prognostic evaluation of neurohumoral plasma level before and during beta-blocker therapy in advanced left ventricular dysfunction. J Am Coll Cardiol 2001; 38: 436–42.

96. Troughton RW, Frampton CM, Yandle TG, et al. Treatment of heart failure guided by plasma amino-terminal brain natriuretic peptide (N-BNP) concentrations. Lancet 2000; 355: 1126–30.

97. Vasan RS, Benjamin EJ, Larson MG, et al. Plasma natriuretic peptides for community screening for left ventricular hypertrophy and systolic dysfunction: the Framingham Heart Study. JAMA 2002; 288: 1252–9.

98. de Lemos JA, Morrow DA, Bentley JH, et al. The prognostic value of B-type natriuretic peptide in patients with acute coronary syndromes. N Engl J Med 2001; 345: 1014–21.

99. Wang TJ, Larson MG, Levy D, et al. Impact of age and sex on plasma natriuretic peptide levels in healthy adults. Am J Cardiol 2002; 90: 254–8.

100. Tsutamoto T, Wada A, Maeda K, et al. Attenuation of compensation of endogenous cardiac natriuretic peptide system in chronic heart failure: prognostic role of plasma brain natriuretic peptide concentration in patients with chronic symptomatic left ventricular dysfunction. Circulation 1997; 96: 509–16.

101. Berger R, Huelsman M, Strecker K, et al. B-type natriuretic peptide predicts sudden death in patients with chronic heart failure. Circulation 2002; 105: 2392–7.

102. Anand IS, Fisher LD, Chiang YT, et al. Changes in brain natriuretic peptide and norepinephrine over time and mortality and morbidity in the Valsartan heart failure trial (Val-HeFT). Circulation 2003; 107: 1278.

103. Vrtovec B, Delgado R, Zewail A, et al. Prolonged QTc interval and high B-type natriuretic peptide levels together predict mortality in patients with advanced heart failure. Circulation 2003; 107: 1764–9.

104. Wattingney WA, Mensah GA, Croft JB. Increasing trends in hospitalization for atrial fibrillation in the United States, 1985 through 1999: implications for primary prevention. Circulation 2003; 108: 711–16.

105. Wang TJ, Larson MG, Levy D, et al. Temporal relations of atrial fibrillation and congestive heart failure and their joint influence on mortality: the Framingham heart study. Circulation 2003; 107: 2920–5.

106. Hynes BJ, Luck JC, Wolbrette DL, et al. Atrial fibrillation in patients with heart failure. Curr Opin Cardiol 2003; 18: 32–8.

107. Markides V, Prystowsky EN. Mechanisms underlying the development of atrial arrhythmias in heart failure. Heart Fail Rev 2002; 7: 243–53.
108. Maisel WH, Stevenson LW. Atrial fibrillation in heart failure: epidemiology, pathophysiology, and rationale for therapy. Amer J Cardiol 2003; 91: 2D–8D.
109. Sanders P, Morton JB, Davidson NC, et al. Electrical remodeling of the atria in congestive heart failure: electrophysiological and electroanatomical mapping in humans. Circulation 2003; 108: 1461–8.
110. Falk RH. Atrial fibrillation. N Engl J Med 2001; 344: 1067–78.
111. Dries DL, Exner DV, Gersh BJ, et al. Atrial fibrillation is associated with an increased risk for mortality and heart failure progression in patients with asymptomatic and symptomatic left ventricular systolic dysfunction: a retrospective analysis of the SOLVD trials. J Am Coll Cardiol 1998; 32: 695–703.
112. Cleland JG, Chattopadhyay S, Khand A, et al. Prevalence and incidence of arrhythmias and sudden death in heart failure. Heart Fail Rev 2002; 7: 229–42.
113. Shinbane JS, Wood MA, Jensen DN, et al. Tachycardia-associated cardiomyopathy: a review of animal models and clinical studies. J Am Coll Cardiol 1997; 29: 709–15.
114. Khand AU, Cleland JG, Deedwania PC. Prevention of and medical therapy for atrial arrhythmias in heart failure. Heart Fail Rev 2002; 7: 267–83.
115. Naccarelli GV, Wolbrette DL, Khan M, et al. Old and new antiarrhythmic drugs for converting and maintaining sinus rhythm in atrial fibrillation: comparative efficacy and results of trials. Am J Cardiol 2003; 91:15D–26D.
116. Lamas GA, Lee KL, Sweeney MO, et al. Ventricular pacing or dual-chamber pacing for sinus-node dysfunction. N Engl J Med 2002; 346: 1854–62.
117. Sweeney MO, Hellkamp AS, Ellenbogen KA, et al. Adverse effects of ventricular pacing on heart failure and atrial fibrillation among patients with normal baseline QRS duration in a clinical trial of pacemaker therapy for sinus node dysfunction. Circulation 2003; 107: 2932–7.
118. Leon AR, Greenberg JM, Kanuru N, et al. Cardiac resynchronization in patients with congestive heart failure and chronic atrial fibrillation: effect of upgrading to biventricular pacing after chronic right ventricular pacing. J Am Coll Cardiol 2002; 39: 1258–63.
119. Cooper JM, Katcher MS, Oz MV. Implantable devices for the treatment of atrial fibrillation. N Engl J Med 2002; 346: 206–68.
120. Stevenson WG, Epstein LM. Predicting sudden death risk for heart failure patients in the implantable cardioverter-defibrillator age. Circulation 2003; 107: 514–16.
121. Huikuri HV, Makikallio TH, Raatikainen MJ, et al. Prediction of sudden cardiac death: appraisal of the studies and methods assessing the risk of sudden arrhythmic death. Circulation 2003; 108: 110–15.
122. Pina IL, Apstein CS, Balady GJ, et al. American Heart Association Committee on exercise, rehabilitation, and prevention. Exercise and heart failure: a statement from the American Heart Association Committee on exercise, rehabilitation and prevention. Circulation 2003; 107:1210–25.
123. Sullivan MJ, Hawthorne MH. Exercise intolerance in patients with chronic heart failure. Prog Cardiovasc Dis 1995; 38: 1–22.
124. Franciosa JA, Park M, Levine TB. Lack of correlation between exercise capacity and indexes of resting left ventricular performance in heart failure. Am J Cardiol 1981; 47: 33–9.
125. Metra M, Faggiano P, D'Aloia A, et al. Use of cardiopulmonary exercise testing with hemodynamic monitoring in the prognostic assessment of ambulatory patients with chronic heart failure. J Am Coll Cardiol 1999; 33: 943–50.
126. Paraskevaidis IA, Adamopoulos S, Kremastinos DT. Dobutamine echocardiographic study in patients with nonischemic dilated cardiomyopathy and prognostically borderline values of peak exercise oxygen consumption: 18-month follow-up study. J Am Coll Cardiol 2001; 37: 1685–91.
127. Lapu-Bula R, Robert A, Van Craeynest D, et al. Contribution of exercise-induced mitral regurgitation to exercise stroke volume and exercise capacity in patients with left ventricular systolic dysfunction. Circulation 2002; 106: 1342–8.
128. Little WC, Kitzman DW, Cheng CP. Diastolic dysfunction as a cause of exercise intolerance. Heart Fail Rev 2000; 5: 310–16.
129. Hundley WG, Kitzman DW, Morgan TM, et al. Cardiac cycle-dependent changes in aortic area and distensibility are reduced in older patients with isolated diastolic heart failure and correlate with exercise intolerance. J Am Coll Cardiol 2001; 38: 796–802.
130. Zelis R, Mason DT, Braunwald E. A comparison of the effects of vasodilator stimuli on peripheral resistance vessels in normal subjects and in patients with congestive heart failure. J Clin Invest 1968; 47: 960–70.
131. LeJemtel TH, Maskin CS, Lucido D, et al. Failure to augment maximal limb blood flow in response to one-leg versus two-leg exercise in patients with severe heart failure. Circulation 1986; 74: 245–51.

132. Sinoway LI, Shenberger J, Wilson J, et al. A 30-day forearm work protocol increases maximal forearm blood flow. J Appl Physiol 1987; 62: 1063–7.

133. Kubo SH, Rector TS, Bank AJ, et al. Endothelium-dependent vasodilation is attenuated in patients with heart failure. Circulation 1991; 84: 1589–96.

134. Gilligan DM, Panza JA, Kilcoyne CM, et al. Contribution of endothelium-derived nitric oxide to exercise-induced vasodilation. Circulation 1994; 90: 2853–8.

135. Hambrecht R, Fiehn E, Weigl C, et al. Regular physical exercise corrects endothelial dysfunction and improves exercise capacity in patients with chronic heart failure. Circulation 1998; 98: 2709–15.

136. Sullivan MJ, Green HG, Cobb FR. Skeletal muscle biochemistry and histology in ambulatory patients with long-term heart failure. Circulation 1990; 81: 518–27.

137. Drexler H, Riede U, Munzel T, et al. Alterations of skeletal muscle in chronic heart failure. Circulation 1992; 85: 1751–9.

138. Minotti J, Christoph I, Oka R, et al. Impaired skeletal muscle function in patients with congestive heart failure: relationship to systemic exercise performance. J Clin Invest 1991; 88: 2077–82.

139. Piepoli MF, Scott AC, Capucci A, et al. Skeletal muscle training in chronic heart failure. Acta Physiol Scand 2001; 171: 295–303.

140. Cicoira M, Zanolla L, Franceschini L, et al. Skeletal muscle mass independently predicts peak oxygen consumption and ventilatory response during exercise in noncachectic patients with chronic heart failure. J Am Coll Cardiol 2001; 37: 2080–5.

141. Duscha BD, Annex BH, Green HJ, et al. Deconditioning fails to explain peripheral skeletal alterations in men with chronic heart failure. J Am Coll Cardiol 2002; 39: 1170–4.

142. Vescovo G, Volterrani M, Zennaro R, et al. Apoptosis in the skeletal muscle of patients with heart failure: investigation of clinical and biochemical changes. Heart 2000; 84:431–7.

143. Massie BM, Conway M, Rajagopalan B, et al. Skeletal muscle metabolism during exercise under ischemic conditions in congestive heart failure: evidence for abnormalities unrelated to blood flow. Circulation 1988; 78: 320–6.

144. Sullivan MJ, Green HJ, Cobb FR. Altered skeletal muscle metabolic responses to exercise in chronic hear failure: relation to skeletal muscle aerobic enzyme activity. Circulation 1991; 84: 1597–607.

145. Mettauer B, Zoll J, Sanchez H, et al. Oxidative capacity of skeletal muscle in heart failure patients versus sedentary or active control subjects. J Am Coll Cardiol 2001; 38: 947–54.

146. Sullivan MJ, Cobb FR. Central hemodynamic response to exercise in patients with chronic heart failure. Chest 1992; 101:340S–6S.

147. McCloskey DI, Mitchell JH. Reflex cardiovascular and respiratory responses originating in exercising muscle. J Physiol 1972; 224: 173–86.

148. Piepoli M, Clark AL, Volterrani M, et al. Contribution of muscle afferent to the hemodynamic, autonomic, and ventilatory responses to exercise in patients with chronic heart failure: effects of physical training. Circulation 1996; 93: 940–52.

149. Kleber FX, Vietzke G, Wernecke KD, et al. Impairment of ventilatory efficiency in heart failure: prognostic impact. Circulation 2000; 101: 2803–9.

150. Corra U, Mezzani A, Bosimini E, et al. Ventilatory response to exercise improves risk stratification in patients with chronic heart failure and intermediate functional capacity. Am Heart J 2002; 143: 418–26.

151. Ponikowski P, Francis DP, Piepoli MF, et al. Enhanced ventilatory response to exercise in patients with chronic heart failure and preserved exercise tolerance: marker of abnormal cardiorespiratory reflex control and predictor of poor prognosis. Circulation 2001; 103: 967–72.

152. Wagoner LE, Craft LL, Zengel P, et al. Polymorphisms of the beta-1 adrenergic receptor predict exercise capacity in heart failure. Am Heart J 2002; 144: 840–6.

153. Wagoner LE, Craft LL, Singh B, et al. Polymorphisms of the beta-2 adrenergic receptor determine exercise capacity in patients with heart failure. Circulation 2000; 86: 834–40.

154. Abraham MR, Olson LJ, Joyner MJ, et al. Angiotensin-converting enzyme genotype modulates pulmonary function and exercise capacity in treated patients with congestive stable heart failure. Circulation 2002; 106:1794–9.

155. The Criteria Committee of the New York Heart Association. Nomenclature and Criteria for Diagnosis, 9th edn. Boston: Little, Brown, 1994.

156. Eichhorn EJ. Prognosis determination in heart failure. Am J Med 2001; 110:14S–35S.

157. Goldman L, Hashimoto B, Cook EF, Luscalzo A. A comparative reproducibility and validity of systems for assessing cardiovascular functional class: advantages of a new specific activity scale. Circulation 1981; 64: 1227.

158. Green CP, Porter CB, Bresnahan DR, et al. Development and evaluation of the Kansas City cardiomyopathy questionnaire: a new health status measure for heart failure. J Am Coll Cardiol 2000; 35: 1245–55.

159. Guyatt GH, Nogradi S, Halcrow S, et al. Development and testing of a new measure of health status for clinical trials in heart failure. J Gen Intern Med 1989; 4: 101–7.

160. Feinstein AR, Fisher MB, Pigeon JG. Changes in dyspnea-fatigue ratings as indicators of quality of life in the treatment of congestive heart failure. Am J Cardiol 1989; 64: 50–5.

161. Rector TS, Kubo S, Cohn J. Patients self-assessment of their congestive heart failure. Part 2: content, reliability and validity of a new measure: the Minnesota Living with Heart Failure Questionnaire. Heart Fail 1987; 3: 198–209.

162. Guyatt GH, Sullivan MJ, Thompson PJ, et al. The 6-minute walk: a new measure of exercise capacity in patients with chronic heart failure. Can Med Assoc J 1985; 132: 919–23.

163. Bittner V, Weiner DH, Yusuf S, et al. Prediction of mortality and morbidity with a 6-minute walk test in patients with left ventricular dysfunction. JAMA 1993; 270: 1702–7.

164. Demers C, McKelvie RS, Negassa A, et al. Reliability, validity, and responsiveness of the six-minute walk test in patients with heart failure. Am Heart J 2001; 142: 698–703.

165. Opasich C, Pinna GD, Mazza A, et al. Six-minute walking performance in patients with moderate-to-severe heart failure: is it s useful indicator in clinical practice? Eur Heart J 2001; 22: 488–96.

166. Lucas C, Stevenson LW, Johnson W, et al. The 6-min walk and peak oxygen consumption in advanced heart failure: aerobic capacity and survival. Am Heart J 1999; 138: 618–24.

167. Woo MA, Moser DK, Stevenson LW, et al. Six-minute walk test and heart rate variability: lack of association in advanced stages of heart failure. Am J Crit Care 1997; 6: 348–54.

168. O'Keeffe ST, Lye M, Donnellan C, et al. Reproducibility and responsiveness of quality of life assessment and six minute walk test in elderly heart failure patients. Heart 1998; 80: 377–82.

169. Faggiano P, D'Aloia A, Gualeni A, et al. Assessment of oxygen uptake during the 6-minute walking test in patients with heart failure: preliminary experience with a portable device. Am Heart J 1997; 134: 203–6.

170. Lainchbury JG, Richards AM. Exercise testing in the assessment of chronic congestive heart failure. Heart 2002; 88: 538–43.

171. Beniaminovitz A, Mancini DM. The role of exercise-based prognosticating algorithms in the selection of patients for heart transplantation. Curr Opin Cardiol 1999; 14: 114–20.

172. Mancini DM, Eisen H, Kussmaul W, et al. Value of peak exercise oxygen consumption for optimal timing of cardiac transplantation in ambulatory patients with heart failure. Circulation 1991; 83: 778–86.

173. Kruger S, Graf J, Kunz D, et al. Brain natriuretic peptide levels predict functional capacity in patients with chronic heart failure. J Am Coll Cardiol 2002; 40: 718–22.

174. Lowes BD, Higginbotham M, Petrovich L, et al. Low-dose enoximone improves exercise capacity in chronic heart failure. Enoximone Study Group. J Am Coll Cardiol 2000; 36: 501–8.

175. Bocchi EA, Guimaraes G, Mocelin A, et al. Sildenafil effects on exercise, neurohormonal activation, and erectile dysfunction in congestive heart failure: a double-blind, placebo-controlled, randomized study followed by a prospective treatment for erectile dysfunction. Circulation 2002; 106: 1097–103.

176. Khatta M, Alexander BS, Krichten CM, et al. The effect of coenzyme Q10 in patients with congestive heart failure. Ann Intern Med 2000; 132: 636–40.

177. Hambrecht R, Niebauer J, Fiehn E, et al. Physical training in patients with stable chronic heart failure: effects on cardiorespiratory fitness and ultrastructural abnormalities in leg muscles. J Am Coll Cardiol 1995; 25: 1239–49.

178. Giannuzzi P, Temporelli PL, Corra U, et al. Antiremodeling effect of long-term exercise training in patients with stable chronic heart failure: results of the exercise in left ventricular dysfunction and chronic heart failure (ELVD-CHF) trial. Circulation 2003; 108: 554–9.

179. Sullivan MF, Higginbotham MB, Cobb FR. Exercise training in patients with severe left ventricular dysfunction: hemodynamic and metabolic effects. Circulation 1988; 78: 506–15.

180. Linke A, Schoene N, Gielen S, et al. Endothelial dysfunction in patients with chronic heart failure: systemic effects of lower-limb exercise training. J Am Coll Cardiol 2001; 37: 392–7.

181. Fleg JL. Can exercise conditioning be effective in older heart failure patients? Heart Fail Rev 2002; 7: 99–103.

182. Coats AJ. Exercise and heart failure. Cardiol Clin 2001; 19: 517–24.

183. Smart N, Fang ZY, Marwick TH. A practical guide to exercise training for heart failure patients. J Card Fail 2003; 9: 49–58.

184. Otto CM. Evaluation and management of chronic mitral regurgitation. N Engl J Med 2001; 345: 740–6.

185. Robbins JD, Maniar PB, Cotts W, et al. Prevalence and severity of mitral regurgitation in chronic systolic heart failure. Am J Cardiol 2003; 91: 360–2.

186. He S, Fontaine AA, Schwammenthal E, et al. Integrated mechanism for functional mitral regurgitation: leaflet restriction versus coapting force: in vitro studies. Circulation 1997; 96: 1826–34.
187. Otsuji Y, Gilon D, Jiang L, et al. Restricted diastolic opening of the mitral leaflets in patients with left ventricular dysfunction: evidence for increased valve tethering. J Am Coll Cardiol 1998; 32: 398–404.
188. Enriquez-Sarano M, Schaff HV, Frye RL. Mitral regurgitation: what causes the leakage is fundamental to the outcome of valve repair. Circulation 2003; 108: 253–6.
189. Karagiannis SE, Karatasakis GT, Koutsogiannis N, et al. Increased distance between mitral valve coaptation point and mitral annular plane: significance and correlations in patients with heart failure. Heart 2003; 89: 1174–8.
190. Trichon BH, Felker GM, Shaw LK, et al. Relation of frequency and severity of mitral regurgitation to survival among patients with left ventricular systolic dysfunction and heart failure. Am J Cardiol 2003; 91: 538–43.
191. Koelling TM, Aaronson KD, Cody RJ, et al. Prognostic significance of mitral regurgitation and tricuspid regurgitation in patients with left ventricular systolic dysfunction. Am Heart J 2002; 144: 373–6.
192. Thomas JD. Doppler assessment of valvular regurgitation. Heart 2002; 88: 651–7.
193. Enriquez-Sarano M. Timing of mitral valve surgery. Heart 2002; 87: 79–85.
194. Lebrun F, Lancellotti P, Pierard LA. Quantitation of functional mitral regurgitation during bicycle exercise in patients with heart failure. J Am Coll Cardiol 2001; 38: 1685–92.
195. Lapu-Baul R, et al. Quantitation of functional mitral regurgitation during bicycle exercise in patients with heart failure. Circulation 2002; 38: 1685–92.
196. Lancellotti P, Troisfontaines P, Toussaint AC, et al. Prognostic importance of exercise-induced changes in mitral regurgitation in patients with chronic ischemic left ventricular dysfunction. Circulation 2003; 108: 1713–17.
197. Stevenson LW. Tailored therapy to hemodynamic goals for advanced heart failure. Eur J Heart Fail 1999; 1: 251–7.
198. Saxon LA, Ellenbogan KA. Resynchronization therapy for the treatment of heart failure. Circulation 2003; 108: 1044–8.
199. Stevenson LW. Clinical use of inotropic therapy for heart failure: looking backward or forward? Circulation 2003; 108: 367–72; 492–497.
200. Bolling SF, Pagani FD, Deeb GM, et al. Intermediate-term outcome of mitral reconstruction in cardiomyopathy. J Thorac Cardiovasc Surg 1998; 115: 381–6.
201. Bolling SF. Mitral valve reconstruction in the patients with heart failure. Heart Fail Rev 2001; 6: 177–85.
202. Badhwar V, Bolling SF. Mitral valve surgery in the patients with left ventricular dysfunction. Semin Thorac Cardiovasc Surg 2002; 14: 133–6.
203. Grigioni F, Enriquez-Sarano M, Zehr KJ, et al. Ischemic mitral regurgitation: long-term outcome and prognostic implications with quantitative Doppler assessment. Circulation 2001; 103: 1759–64.
204. Trichon BH, Glower DD, Shaw LK, et al. Survival after coronary revascularization, with and without mitral valve surgery, in patients with ischemic mitral regurgitation. Circulation 2003; 108: II103–10.
205. Bradley TD, Floras JS. Sleep apnea and heart failure: I obstructive sleep apnea; II central sleep apnea. Circulation 2003; 107: 1822–1826.
206. Bradley TD, Floras JS. Pathophysiologic and therapeutic implications of sleep apnea in congestive heart failure. J Cardiac Fail 1996; 2: 223–40.
207. Wolk R, Kara T, Somers VK. Sleep-disordered breathing and cardiovascular disease. Circulation 2003; 108: 9–12.
208. Leung RST, Bradley TD. Sleep apnea and cardiovascular disease. Am J Respir Crit Care Med 2001; 164: 2147–65.
209. Kohnlein T, Welte T, Tan LB, et al. Central sleep apnea syndrome in patients with chronic heart disease: a critical review of the current literature. Thorax 2002; 57: 547–55.
210. Javaheri S. A mechanism of central sleep apnea in patients with heart failure. N Engl J Med 1999; 341: 949–54.
211. Sin DD, Fitzgerald F, Parker JD, et al. Risk factors for central and obstructive sleep apnea in 450 men and women with congestive heart failure. Am J Respir Crit Care Med 1999; 160: 1101–6.
212. Sin DD, Fitzgerald F, Parker JD, et al. Relationship of systolic BP to obstructive sleep apnea in patients with heart failure. Chest 2003; 123: 1536–43.
213. Javaheri S, Corbett WS. Association of low PaCO2 with central sleep apnea and ventricular arrhythmias in ambulatory patients with stable heart failure. Ann Intern Med 1998; 128: 204–7.
214. Narkiewicz K, Montano N, Cogliati C, et al. Altered cardiovascular variability in obstructive sleep apnea. Circulation 1998; 98: 1071–7.

215. Naughton MT, Rahman MA, Hara K, et al. Effect of continuous positive airway pressure on intrathoracic and left ventricular transmural pressures in patients with congestive heart failure. Circulation 1995; 91: 1725–31.
216. Sin DD, Logan AG, Fitzgerald FS, et al. Effects of continuous positive airway pressure on cardiovascular outcomes in heart failure patients with and without cheyne-stokes respiration. Circulation 2000; 102: 61–6.
217. Yan AT, Bradley TD, Lui PP. The role of continuous positive airway pressure in the treatment of congestive heart failure. Chest 2001; 120: 1675–85.
218. Garrigue S, Bordier P, Jais P. Benefit of atrial pacing in sleep apnea syndrome. NEJM 2002; 346: 404–12.
219. Flemons WW. Obstructive sleep apnea. N Engl J Med 2002; 347: 498–504.
220. Hillege HL, Girbes AR, de Kam PJ, et al. Renal function, neurohormonal activation and survival in patients with chronic heart failure. Circulation 2000; 102: 203–10.
221. Shlipak MG. Pharmacotherapy for heart failure in patients with renal insufficiency. Ann Intern Med 2003; 138: 917–24.
222. Weinfield MS, Chertow GM, Stevenson LW. Aggravated renal dysfunction during intensive therapy for advanced chronic heart failure. Am Heart J 1999; 138: 285–90.
223. Gottlieb SS, Abraham W, Butler J, et al. The prognostic importance of different definitions of worsening renal function in congestive heart failure. J Cardiac Fail 2002; 8: 136–41.
224. Dries DL, Exner DV, Domanski MJ, et al. The prognostic implications of renal insufficiency in asymptomatic and symptomatic patients with left ventricular dysfunction. J Am Coll Cardiol 2000; 35: 681–9.
225. Mahon NG, Blackstone EH, Francis GS, et al. The prognostic value of estimated creatinine clearance alongside functional capacity in ambulatory patients with chronic congestive heart failure. J Am Coll Cardiol 2002; 40: 1106–13.
226. Poole-Wilson PA, Uretsky BF, Thygesen K, et al. Mode of death in heart failure: findings from the ATLAS trial. Heart 2003; 89: 42–8.
227. Aaronson KD, Schwartz JS, Chen TM, et al. Development and prospective validation of a clinical index to predict survival in ambulatory patients referred for cardiac transplant evaluation. Circulation 1997; 95: 2660–267.
228. Chin MH, Goldman L. Correlates of major complications or death in patients admitted to the hospital with congestive heart failure. Arch Intern Med 1996; 156: 1814–20.
229. Anker SD, Chua TP, Ponikowski P, et al. Hormonal changes and catabolic/anabolic imbalance in chronic heart failure and their importance for cardiac cachexia. Circulation 1997; 96: 526–34.
230. Anker SD, Ponikowski P, Varney S, et al. Wasting as independent risk factor for mortality in chronic heart failure. Lancet 1997; 349: 1050–3.
231. Anker SD, Clark AL, Kemp M, et al. Tumor necrosis factor and steroid metabolism in chronic heart failure: possible relation to muscle wasting. J Am Coll Cardiol 1997; 30: 997–1001.
232. Anker SK, Sharma R. The syndrome of cardiac cachexia. Int J Cardiol 2002; 85: 51–66.
233. Neibauer J, Pflaum CD, Clark AL, et al. Deficient insulin-like growth factor 1 in chronic heart failure predicts altered body composition, anabolic deficiency, cytokine and neurohormonal activation. J Am Coll Cardiol 1998; 32: 393–7.
234. Swan JW, Anker SD, Walton C, et al. Insulin resistance in chronic heart failure: relation to severity and etiology of heart failure. J Am Coll Cardiol 1997; 30: 527–32.
235. Murdoch DR, Rooney E, Dargie HJ, et al. Inappropriately low plasma leptin concentration in the cachexia associated with chronic heart failure. Heart 1999; 82: 352–6.
236. Nagaya N, Kangawa K. Ghrelin improves left ventricular dysfunction and cardiac cachexia in heart failure. Curr Opin Pharmacol 2003; 3: 146–51.
237. Ezekowitz JA, McAlister FA, Armstrong PW. Anemia is common in heart failure and is associated with poor outcomes: insights from a cohort of 12,065 patients with new-onset heart failure. Circulation 2003; 107: 223–5.
238. Horwich TB, Fonarow GC, Hamilton MA, et al. Anemia is associated with worse symptoms, greater impairment in functional capacity and a significant increased in mortality in patients with advanced heart failure. J Am Coll Cardiol 2002; 39: 1780–6.
239. Mozaffarian D, Nye R, Levy WC. Anemia predicts mortality in severe heart failure: the prospective randomized amlodipine survival evaluation (PRAISE). J Am Coll Cardiol 2003; 41: 1933–9.
240. Kosiborod M, Smith GL, Radford MJ, et al. The prognostic importance of anemia in patients with heart failure. Am J Med 2003; 114: 112–19.
241. Kalra PR, Collier T, Cowie MR, et al. Hemoglobin concentration and prognosis in new cases of heart failure. Lancet 2003; 362: 211–12.

242. Mancini DM, Katz SD, Lang CC, et al. Effect of erythropoietin on exercise capacity in patients with moderate to severe chronic heart failure. Circulation 2003; 107: 294–9.

243. Silverberg DS, Wexler D, Blum M, et al. The use of subcutaneous erythropoietin and intravenous iron for the treatment of severe, resistant heart failure improves cardiac and renal function, functional cardiac class, and markedly reduces hospitalization. J Am Coll Cardiol 2000; 35: 1737–44.

244. Silverberg DS, Wexler D, Sheps D, et al. The effect of correction of mild anemia in severe, resistant congestive heart failure using subcutaneous erythropoietin and intravenous iron: a randomized controlled study. J Am Coll Cardiol 2001; 37: 1775–80.

245. Besarab A, Bolton WK, Browne JK, et al. The effects of normal as compared to low hematocrit values in patients with cardiac disease who are receiving hemodialysis and epoetin. N Engl J Med 1998; 339: 584–90.

246. MacMahon KMA, Lip GYH. Psychological factors in heart failure. Arch Intern Med 2002; 162: 509–16.

247. Guck TP, Elsasser GN, Kavan MG, et al. Depression and congestive heart failure. Congest Heart Fail 2003; 9: 163–9.

248. Krumholz HM, Butler J, Miller J, et al. Prognostic importance of emotional support for elderly patients hospitalized with heart failure. Circulation 1998; 97: 958–64.

249. Faris R, Purcell H, Henein MY, et al. Clinical depression is common and significantly associated with reduced survival in patients with non-ischemic heart failure. Eur J Heart Fail 2002; 4: 541–51.

250. Turvey CL, Schultz K, Arndt S, et al. Prevalence and correlates of depressive symptoms in a community sample of people suffering from heart failure. J Am Geriatr Soc 2002; 50: 2003–8.

251. Skotzko CE, Krichten C, Zietowski G, et al. Depression is common and precludes accurate assessment of functional status in elderly patients with congestive heart failure. J Card Fail 2000; 6: 300–5.

252. Rozzini R, Sabatini T, Frisoni GB, et al. Depression and major outcomes in older patients with heart failure. Arch Intern Med 2002; 162: 362–4.

253. Jiang W, Alexander J, Christopher E, et al. Relationship to depression to increased risk of mortality and rehospitalization in patients with congestive heart failure. Arch Intern Med 2001; 161: 1849–56.

254. Sullivan M, Simon G, Spertus J, et al. Depression-related costs in heart failure care. Arch Intern Med 2002; 162: 1860–6.

255. Benatar D, Bondmass M, Ghitelman J, et al. Outcomes of chronic heart failure. Arch Intern Med 2003; 163: 347–52.

256. Dracup K, Westlake C, Erickson VS, et al. Perceived control reduces emotional stress in patients with heart failure. J Heart Lung Transplant 2003; 22: 90–3.

257. Ho KKL, Anderson KM, Kannel WB, et al. Survival after the onset of congestive heart failure in Framingham heart study subjects. Circulation 1993; 88: 107–15.

258. Di Lenarda A, Secoli G, Perkan A, et al. Changing mortality in dilated cardiomyopathy. Br Heart J 1994; 72(Suppl): S46–51.

259. Stevenson WG, Stevenson LW, Middlekauff HR, et al. Improving survival for patients with advanced heart failure: a study of 737 consecutive patients. J Am Coll Cardiol 1995; 26: 1417–23.

260. MacIntyre K, Capewell S, Stewart S, et al. Evidence of improving prognosis in heart failure: trends in case fatality in 66,547 patients hospitalized between 1986 and 1995. Circulation 2000; 102: 1126–31.

261. Gottdeiner JS, McClelland RL, Marshall R, et al. Outcome of congestive heart failure in elderly persons: influence of left ventricular systolic function. Ann Intern Med 2002; 137: 631–9.

262. Jong P, Vowinckel E, Liu PP, et al. Prognosis and determinants of survival in patients newly hospitalized for heart failure. Arch Intern Med 2002; 162: 1689–94.

263. Packer M, Coats AJ, Fowler MB, et al. Effect of carvedilol on survival in severe chronic heart failure. N Engl J Med 2001; 344: 1651–8.

264. Rose EA, Gelijns AC, Moskowitz AJ, et al. Long-term use of a left ventricular assist device for end-stage heart failure. N Engl J Med 2001; 345: 1435–43.

265. Kao W, Constanzo MR. Prognosis determination in patients with advanced heart failure. J Heart Lung Transplant 1997; 16: S2–6.

266. Wilson JR, Schwartz JS, Sutton MS, et al. Prognosis in severe heart failure: relation to hemodynamic measurements and ventricular ectopic activity. J Am Coll Cardiol 1983; 2: 403–10.

267. Curtis JP, Sokol SI, Wang Y, et al. The association of left ventricular ejection fraction, mortality, and cause of death in stable outpatients with heart failure. J Am Coll Cardiol 2003; 42: 736–42.

268. Nohria A, Tsang SW, Fang JC, et al. Clinical assessment identifies hemodynamic profiles that predict outcomes in patients admitted with heart failure. J Am Coll Cardiol 2003; 41: 1797–804.

269. Drazner MH, Rame JE, Dris DL. Third heart sound and elevated jugular venous pressure as markers of the subsequent development of heart failure in patients with asymptomatic left ventricular dysfunction. Am J Med 2003; 114: 431–7.
270. Working Group Report. How to diagnose diastolic heart failure: European study group on diastolic heart failure. Eur Heart J 1998; 19: 990–1003.
271. Harlan WR, Oberman A, Crimm R, Roseti R. Heart failure. Ann Intern Med 1977; 56: 133–8.
272. Al-Ahmad A, Rand WM, Manjonath G, et al. Reduced kidney function and anemia as high factors for mortality in patients with left ventricular dysfunction. J Am Coll Cardiol 2001; 38: 955–62.

12
Clinical profiles and bedside assessment

Lynne Warner Stevenson

Each patient with heart failure presents a unique picture based on the etiology and time course of his cardiac disease, concomitant conditions, psychosocial factors, circulatory adaptations, and responses to therapy, all seen in the context of personal priorities for physical and social functioning and life goals. Recognizing that none of these pictures can be portrayed fully by categories, we nonetheless find classification schemes useful to describe clinical situations, to predict likely outcomes, and to target and titrate therapies with proven benefit. Aligned with the broader spectrum of disease progression, the classification schemes for patients with symptomatic disease include specific clinical assessments of symptoms and signs, and longitudinal integration of the clinical picture. In addition, the definition of profiles can enhance recognition of patients not well addressed by current therapies, which will inspire the development of new strategies.

DIFFERING PROFILES RELEVANT DURING DISEASE PROGRESSION

Multiple different clinical classification systems apply, depending upon where patients are in the course of disease (Fig. 12.1). The ACC/AHA stages define a one-way progression beginning with risk factors for heart failure (Stage A), then the abnormal left ventricular structure/function before symptoms develop (Stage B) (1). Patients who have ever had symptoms of heart failure cannot move backward from Stage C, even if symptoms resolve effectively with therapy. (Possible exceptions might be made for patients who might return to Stage B after a presumably reversible cause of cardiomyopathy, such as peripartum cardiomyopathy, tako-tsubo syndrome, or tachycardia-induced cardiomyopathy, but it seems unlikely that hearts who have ever experienced profound dysfunction could return to the naïve Stage A) . Patients within Stage C can include the entire symptomatic range from New York Heart Association Class I to Class IV symptoms. Unlike the stages, the New York Heart Classes allow patients frequent and unlimited movement in both directions. Patients who have predominantly Class IV symptoms despite rigorous maintenance of all recommended therapies within heart failure management are Stage D.

It is within Stage C and the Stage C-D interface that clinical assessment of the 4 resting hemodynamic profiles of wet-dry and warm-cold can guide adjustment of therapy to improve symptoms of heart failure (2). At the C-D interface and within Class IV, the 7 INTERMACS profiles of decompensation currently focus attention on the small minority of patients eligible for cardiac transplantation or mechanical ventricular support devices (3). As we gain further experience with these profiles, they may also help guide patients and physicians to recognize and adjust priorities for the remaining quality and length of life.

Clinical clcassification systems for hear failure

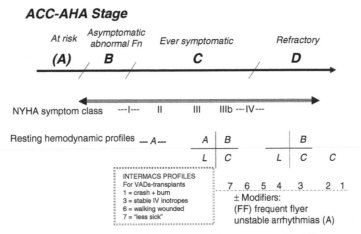

Figure 12.1 Comparison of various classification schemes to describe aspects of heart failure. The ACC-AHA system is designed to indicate the stages of disease, through which patients can move in only one direction, except perhaps for occasional reversal of underlying cause of disease, such as peripartum cardiomyopathy. The NYHA and other symptomatic classes describe the current clinical status; patients can increase and decrease their level of symptoms many times. The resting hemodynamic profiles describe the combination of congestion and perfusion, and are generally used to describe symptomatic heart failure, as resting hemodynamic status is expected to be near-normal in truly asymptomatic patients. The INTERMACS profiles, derived initially for patients considered for mechanical circulatory support, describe the clinical status of decompensation in advanced stages of disease (Table 12.3). In addition to moving back and forth between profiles, patients with advanced disease can be further described by modifiers such as "frequent flyer" for the patient with frequent readmissions for episodes of decompensation, and "arrhythmias" for the patient in whom recurrent ventricular tachyarrhythmias further compromise clinical stability. *Abbreviations*: NYHA, York Heart Association; VAD, ventricular assist device.

CLINICAL ASSESSMENT

Assessment of functional status, heart failure symptoms, and fluid status are ACC/AHA Level I recommendations during initial diagnosis of heart failure and during every subsequent evaluation (1). In addition to standard questions about specific activities from which functional status is determined using the New York Heart Association or Canadian classification, it is helpful to elicit from each patient their usual daily/weekly activities and the ability to perform them comfortably (4). For those who do not routinely go out to work, examples of common tasks to be tracked include pushing the grocery cart, walking the dog, folding the laundry, emptying the dishwasher, and going to the mailbox. These can then be queried serially to improve sensitivity for changes in functional capacity and symptoms. Measurement of the distance walked in 6 minutes along inside corridors may enhance detection of changes, particularly in the moderate-severe symptom range.

FOUR RESTING HEMODYNAMIC PROFILES BASED ON SYMPTOMS AND SIGNS

The "bedside" assessment of the hemodynamic profile takes place either in the outpatient clinic or during hospitalization. Patients are evaluated clinically to determine whether they are "wet or dry" based on evidence of congestion (elevated intra-cardiac filling pressures), and whether perfusion is likely to be adequate or critically reduced "warm or cold" (2).

Table 12.1 Utility of Physical Examination for Detecting PCW > 22 mmHg. In Patients Hospitalized with At Least One Symptom and One Sign of Congestion (On Chronic Therapy for Heart Failure LVEF ≤ 25%)

	Sensitivity (%)	Specificity (%)
Orthopnea > 2 pillows	86	25
Hepatojugular reflux	83	27
JVP ≥ 12 cmHg	65	64
Edema ≥ 2+	41	66
Ascites ≥ moderate	21	92
Hepatomegaly ≥ 4 fb	15	93
Rales ≥ 1/3 lung fields	15	89

Abbreviations: LVEF, left ventricular ejection fraction.
Source: Data adapted from Ref. 5.

Congestion

Symptoms of Congestion

Dyspnea is the most common symptom of heart failure but can reflect different hemodynamic contribution depending on the timing. When dyspnea occurs after prolonged or intensive exertion, the major likely cause is failure to increase peripheral oxygen delivery and distribution adequately to meet the increased skeletal muscle demands, leading to accumulation of lactate, buffered to carbon dioxide which accumulates to drive respiration until the buffering capacity is exhausted and respiratory drive increases further in response to acidemia. Filling pressures may or may not be elevated during this process. However, when the patient develops immediate dyspnea with light exertion (IDLE), such as with activities of daily living or walking from one room to another, the usual cause is resting elevation of pulmonary pressures that immediately increases further with exercise.

The most specific symptom of elevated filling pressures is *orthopnea*, dyspnea in the supine position Table 12.1 (5). In some patients, this may be manifest by a supine cough rather than by the sensation of shortness of breath. Orthopnea means elevated filling pressures until proven otherwise. However, other conditions that can potential limit supine respiration, such as obesity and chronic pulmonary disease, can render the interpretation of orthopnea less clear. Paroxysmal nocturnal dyspnea in a patient with no evidence of earlier orthopnea is more often an indication of intermittent events such as sleep apnea, arrhythmias, or myocardial ischemia.

While resting dyspnea suggests left-sided congestion, all of the other symptoms of congestion reflect systemic venous congestion, elevated right-sided cardiac filling pressures. Although not in the common litany of congestive symptoms, many patients describe, an uncomfortable feeling of fullness in their head or chest while bending over, particularly to put on socks, shoes, or to dig in the garden. This symptom, which might be termed *suffusion with socks*, often tracks with right-sided filling pressures, so may be the patient-performed equivalent of the abdomino-jugular reflex. *Gastro-intestinal symptoms*, once attributed to inadequate forward flow causing "gut ischemia", are usually due instead to hepato-splanchnic congestion from elevated right-sided filling pressures. This may cause anorexia, early satiety, and upper abdominal discomfort either generalized or localized to a tender, pulsatile liver. Ascites and peripheral edema can be either symptoms or signs depending on the observer, discussed below.

Signs of Congestion

A systematically focused physical examination remains the central diagnostic tool in the ongoing management of patients with symptomatic heart failure (6). The most common error in the general evaluation of chronic heart failure is failure to recognize elevated intracardiac filling pressures in the absence of pulmonary rales and peripheral edema (7). While acute elevations in pulmonary venous pressures frequently cause rales, such as in acute myocardial infarction, chronic elevation of elevated filling pressures leads to hypertrophy of the pulmonary lymphatics which continually clear the airspaces, while leaving residual interstitial fluid that causes the sensation of dyspnea, without hypoxia. Many patients, particularly those of young or middle age, do not demonstrate fluid retention as peripheral edema even when heart failure is severe.

Jugular Venous Distention

Jugular venous distention is clearly the most useful sign of elevated filling pressures. Experienced clinicians can identify elevation in jugular venous pressure with reasonable accuracy, as shown by comparison to right heart catheterization in patients hospitalized with heart failure (5). Discrepancies between the degree of elevation determined by different methods in some cases reflects rapid changes in actual pressures, which may occur during sedation and procedures. In most experiences, there are about 10–20% of patients in whom right-sided pressures cannot be assessed due to obesity or previous procedures. Nonetheless, the jugular venous pressure has been shown to be the most reliable sign for the detection of both right and left-sided filling pressure elevation in chronic heart failure (8).

Physical examination of the jugular veins has been underemphasized in recent training, but requires constant practice. A common practice is to assume that filling pressures are not elevated if the neck veins are not seen at all but this can lead to serious errors in diagnosis and management. Positioning of the patient should be at an angle that allows visualization of the top of the jugular venous pressure waves, in order to avoid missing very high and very low venous pressures. Patients with very high venous pressures may need to be examined sitting straight up, while patients with low filling pressures may need to be almost flat. The patient should generally be examined recumbent. A patient with high jugular venous pressures visible while sitting upright in a chair is accurately considered to have very high right-sided filling pressures, but the converse is not true. Due to abnormal vasoreactive reflexes with position, some patients will have sufficient venous pooling when sitting with the legs down that elevated filling pressures will not be detected. Jugular venous pressure cannot be reliably judged to be normal without evaluation in the recumbent position.

Two wave forms are usually evident in the venous pulse of the patient in sinus rhythm, which helps to distinguish the venous pulse from the arterial pulse. Additionally, the descents of the waves are accentuated by inspiration. Patients with severely elevated right-sided filling pressures may have increase in the heights with inspiration (positive Kussmaul's sign). Abdominal compression is another technique that helps to identify the venous pulsation. With the *abdomino-jugular reflex*, the jugular venous pressure may remain elevated for up to 10-15 seconds after abdominal compression, followed by a return to baseline during continued compression if there is normal systemic venous capacitance to accept the increased intravascular volume (9). Failure to return to baseline during continued compression provides evidence of at least mild reduction in systemic venous capacitance, evidence of increased venous volume.

The accuracy of jugular venous pressure assessment is often questioned in the presence of tricuspid regurgitation. In patients with chronic heart failure, the usual cause of increasing tricuspid regurgitation is right ventricular volume overload. Tricuspid regurgitation is thus itself a good marker for severely elevated right sided filling pressures, for which the exact level of elevation is less important than the presence of elevation.

Evaluation of the jugular venous pressure should be adequate to allow assessment of degrees of high and low filling pressures, not just "high or not". The patient with very high filling pressures requires different therapy than the patient with slight elevation. The patient with very low filling pressures may require adjustment of diuretics or other medications, or evaluation for other causes of low venous volumes, such as hemorrhage or sepsis. Once identified, the height of the jugular venous pressure is measured as the vertical distance between the top of the column and the sternal angle, generally about 5 cm above the right atrium in most positions. It is recommended that examiners measure the span of their hand in cm for calibration to avoid underestimating the actual height of the jugular venous pressure. The right atrial pressure in mmHg is commonly estimated as about ¾ of the jugular venous pressure in centimeters, but in practice, the numbers often appear to be closer.

Although a focal point for the standard cardiac examination, auscultation of the heart itself may not be as helpful as other signs for detecting elevated filling pressures in patients who are already known to have chronic heart failure. The new appearance or increasing intensity of *third heart sounds* suggests elevated filling pressures, but gallop rhythms may be audible all the time in some patients with known heart failure and never detected in others. New or increasing *murmurs of mitral and tricuspid regurgitation* are probably more specific for increasing filling pressures, but still not very sensitive. Moderate mitral regurgitation is present in most patients during decompensation in chronic dilated heart failure, but often is not heard in the dilated ventricle with diminished total stroke volume.

The cardiac examination should carefully locate the lateral-most area where the *pulmonic component of the second sound* is audible. Radiation of the split to the left of the sternal border suggests pulmonary artery systolic pressure >35–40 mmHg, which is most often due to elevated left-sided filling pressures in the chronic heart failure population. Ability to hear the second component at the mid-clavicular line suggests that the pulmonary artery systolic pressure may be in the range of 60-70 mmHg (personal communication, Robert Bourge M.D, University of Alabama, Birmingham). In chronic heart failure without complicating pulmonary disease, the pulmonary artery systolic pressure is generally about twice the pulmonary capillary wedge pressure (10).

Edema is the heart failure sign most familiar to patients. Peripheral fluid retention can be manifest as edema, ascites, or both. Pediatric patients and young adults with heart failure are more likely to develop ascites than peripheral edema. Fewer than half of adults referred to academic medical centers for evaluation for transplantation will have demonstrable peripheral edema. Edema due to elevated central venous pressures usually does not develop until at least 2–4 liters of fluid retention above optimal volume status. With increasing patient age and chronic venous insufficiency, particularly in the setting of obesity, many elderly patients can develop edema in the absence of heart failure. Patients with poor nutrition and hypo-albuminemia causing reduced oncotic pressures may have edema that develops or persists in the absence of elevated central venous pressure. Edema should in general not be attributed to high right-sided cardiac filling pressures unless there is accompanying elevation of jugular venous pressures.

Ascites is often difficult to assess. The characteristic flank bulge of ascites is usually obvious, but bedside diagnosis is often inadequate to distinguish adipose tissue from ascites. The search for shifting dullness is often unrewarding. Patients knowing their the heart failure diagnosis may over-estimate the contribution of ascites to the abdominal contour, and mistakenly increase diuretic dosing to reduce it. Abdominal ultrasound may be necessary to distinguish ascites from chronic fat accumulation.

The presence of a soft, or "boggy", enlarged liver in the absence of other cause provides relatively specific evidence for venous congestion. The inferior vena cava is the mirror of the superior vena cava transmitting into the jugular venous pressure. The presence of venous pulsations is additionally confirming. Some patients with dilated right ventricles may have transmission of the right ventricular impulse into the liver. Examination of the liver is particularly important in children or young adults, in whom the initial presentation of heart failure is often with gastro-intestinal complaints.

Familiarity with the blood pressure cuff technique for assessing the *Valsalva maneuver* can help distinguish between dyspnea of pulmonary and cardiac origin in patients able to cooperate (11). Examination of the lungs, even in the absence of rales, occasionally reveals *pleural effusions*, for which one cause may be elevated filling pressures; elevation of left-sided filling pressures leads to increased hydrostatic forces for fluid accumulation, while elevated right-sided filling pressures limit the ability for fluid reabsorption in the pleural cavities. The examiner should be alert to *periodic breathing* in the awake patient, which requires multiple levels of dysregulation, and often improves after effective diuresis (12).

Right – Left Mismatch for Congestion

Most of the clinical evidence for congestion derives from right-sided systemic venous congestion. However, left-sided filling pressures drive the dyspnea, which is the limiting symptom in over half of decompensation episodes. Furthermore, left-sided filling pressures may be more important in determining prognosis and the course of disease prior to the ominous onset of irreversible right ventricular failure.

Elevations in right-sided pressures match elevations in left-sided pressures in a consistent proportion of 75–80% of patients with chronic heart failure, when defined by a right atrial pressures < > 10 mmHg and a pulmonary capillary wedge pressure < > 22 mmHg (10). It has not been possible to define characteristics that identify patients with these mismatches prior to hemodynamic measurement. The possibility of right-left mismatch should be considered in patients in whom dyspnea typical of high filling pressures persists despite normal jugular venous pressure. However, other causes of such dyspnea include intermittent cardiac ischemia and unrecognized pulmonary disease. Conversely, when repeated attempts to reduce jugular venous pressure result in hypotension or renal dysfunction, the patient may have disproportionate elevation of right-sided filling pressures. Uncertainty about filling pressures or the failure of usual therapies should prompt consideration of direct hemodynamic measurement to determine the right-left relationship. However, the goals for treatment of patients with persistent right-left mismatches have not been established.

PERFUSION

After congestion, the other component of the hemodynamic profiles is the adequacy of resting perfusion (Fig. 12.2). Perfusion is more difficult to assess than congestion (5). The attributable symptoms are vague and ambiguous, including fatigue, trouble concentrating, and apathy. Some symptoms of hypoperfusion can be mimicked by symptoms occurring during uptitration of beta blockers. Cardiac output itself is less predictive of outcomes than filling pressures. However, cardiac output is a key contributor to activity tolerance and functional capacity, which are strong integrative predictors. An ominous symptom/sign is the inability to tolerate neurohormonal antagonists without crippling dizziness or fatigue, which often indicates that the resting cardiac output is low (13).

It should not be assumed that the patient with congestion necessarily has impaired resting perfusion. In fact, the majority of patients admitted to the hospital with symptomatic heart failure have reasonable perfusion at rest, whether ejection fraction is low or preserved (Fig. 12.3). Despite left ventricular ejection fractions as low as 1/3–¼ of normal, stroke volume is often preserved from a left ventricle dilated to 3–4 times normal. Relief and prevention of congestion is the major hemodynamic goal, but the lack

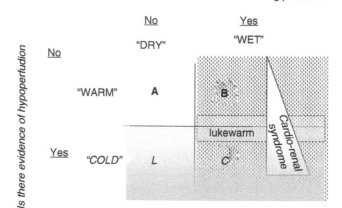

Figure 12.2 Depiction of the four hemodynamic profiles defining presence or absence of elevated filling pressures and adequacy or compromise of resting perfusion. The cardiorenal syndrome of worsening renal function despite excess circulating volume can occur in heart failure regardless of ejection fraction. Elevated right atrial filling pressures and elevated intraperitoneal pressures have recently been implicated in the cardiorenal syndrome, which can sometimes be addressed by therapies that improve cardiac output in order to effectively lower venous pressures. The difficulty in assessing adequacy of cardiac output may place some patients in an ambiguous "lukewarm" classification.

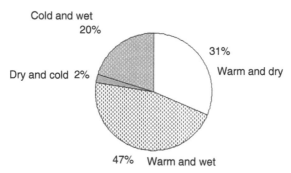

Figure 12.3 Pie graph showing the relative frequencies of the four hemodynamic profiles in 452 patients referred to a heart failure inpatient service, described by Nohria et al. (2). The relative proportion of warm to cold will be higher in a community population where more patients have heart failure with preserved ejection fraction and fewer patients with reduced ejection fraction have critically reduced perfusion.

of adequate perfusion can limit or prevent therapies. While a patient with systolic blood pressure 70 mmHg and obtundation is clearly suffering from critically reduced perfusion, more subtle degrees of hypoperfusion are often not appreciated.

Careful auscultation of the blood pressure is an essential part of every physical examination, and should not be relegated to assistants. Too often recorded from perfunctory measurement on an automated machine by a triage aide or medical assistant, casual blood pressures can be dangerously misleading, and can also miss crucial additional information appreciated by a careful examiner. The *systolic blood pressure* provides a robust indicator of prognosis and helps to guide chronic adjustment of ACEI and beta blockers as well as acute therapies during decompensation. A common error in automated measurement is the overestimation of systolic blood pressure, often by 10–30 mmHg, in patients with irregularity of atrial fibrillation and very frequent premature ventricular contractions. In these patients, it is important to listen for several minutes in order to determine where the majority of beats are heard.

The *proportional pulse pressure* is the difference between the systolic and diastolic blood pressure, divided by the systolic blood pressure (7). The curve relating prognosis and pulse pressure is "U"-shaped. A wide pulse pressure predicts poor outcome in a broad ambulatory population presumably due to its correlation with vascular disease and hypertension, while at the other end of the spectrum a very low pulse pressure indicates poor perfusion and poor prognosis in heart failure. The proportional blood pressure <25% raises concern that the cardiac index may be less than 2.2 L/min/m^2 (7). This threshold value has not been extensively validated, and may be misleading in elderly patients in whom stiff vasculature widens the pulse pressure. Despite the limited validation against absolute measurements, the breadth of the pulse pressure provides a useful metric for serial assessment of perfusion in a given patient during acute intervention or serially over time.

Other useful information provided by assessment of the blood pressure includes its pattern of variation. Patients with frequent premature contractions, particularly in a bigeminal pattern, may in some cases have absent pulsations during these beats, leaving the effective perfusion much lower than indicated by the systolic blood pressure detected. *Pulsus alternans* has been associated with alternating cycles of calcium entry and release. When this can be detected clinically, cardiac function may be more deranged than otherwise suspected. Pulsus alternans and paradoxical pulse can frequently be detected by palpation of the brachial pulse, where an experienced examiner can usually feel a difference of 10 mm or more.

Skin temperature provides a clue to the adequacy of perfusion. Warm feet provide reassurance of adequate peripheral perfusion. However, hands and feet nay be cold due to regional cutaneous sympathetic activation related to stress, despite good central circulation. The forearms and calves provide more reliable sites of assessment. The nomenclature of "cold" is used as a theoretical construct as well as a temperature; not all patients with resting hypoperfusion will have cold extremities (5). However, the detection of diffusely cool extremities despite a well-heated room should raise considerable doubt about the adequacy of perfusion.

Integration of all clinical information has yielded useful discrimination by experienced examiners of patients admitted with decompensated heart failure. Patients considered to be "cold" had markedly lower cardiac indices when measured than those considered "warm" (5). However, the estimated values of cardiac output did not correlate well with absolute values, which should be measured directly when the information is considered necessary for diagnosis or therapy (Table 12.2).

Table 12.2 Limited Utility of Clinical Assessment of Cardiac Index < 2.3 L/min/m^2. In Patients Hospitalized with At Least One Symptom and One Sign of Congestion (On Chronic Therapy for Heart Failure LVEF ≤ 25%)

	Sensitivity (%)	Specificity (%)
Fatigue	94	8
SBP < 100 mmHg	42	66
Physician "cold" profile	33	86
Cool extremities	20	88
SBP < 90 mmHg	12	84

Abbreviations: LVEF, left ventricular ejection fraction; SBP, systolic blood pressure.
Source: Data adapted from Ref. 5.

PREVALENCE AND PROGNOSIS OF FOUR HEMODYNAMIC PROFILES

The variations in congestion, perfusion, right and left ventricular function, the cardiorenal syndrome, and overall circulatory integration are not adequately summarized in the simple scheme of 4 hemodynamic profiles. However, they have proven useful for both triage and prognosis (2). The majority of patients hospitalized in trial centers demonstrate a "wet and warm" profile (Fig. 12.3), even when ejection fraction is low. The proportion with "wet and warm" is much higher among patients in community hospitals, where the average systolic blood pressure with low ejection fraction heart failure is over 130 mmHg. Patients with preserved EF heart failure usually fall in this category unless they have severe hypertrophic or restrictive disease with small LV cavity size.

The admission hemodynamic profile adds additional information. Patients admitted with heart failure symptoms who nonetheless appears to have neither congestion nor hypoperfusion may have symptoms due to another cardiac condition such as ischemia or arrhythmias, or a non-cardiac condition such as pulmonary disease or anemia. Overall, however, this profile of the warm and dry had the best one-year outcome among hospitalized patients, compared to which the "wet and warm" profile had a two-fold higher rate of death or urgent transplantation (2). The "wet and cold" had the worst outcome, with 3.7 fold higher risk, and a mortality of 40% at 6 months, comparable to the 46% seen in the control group on medical therapy in the medical arm of the REMATCH (Randomized Evaluation of Mechanical Assistance Trial in Chronic Heart Failure), the sickest population ever randomized in a heart failure trial (14).

Re-assessment of profiles provides further information. Patients achieving a "warm and dry" profile by the time of discharge have prognosis similar to patients considered "warm and dry" on admission (5). The one-month point after hospital discharge represents a crucial hinge point of prognosis. One study demonstrated that patients admitted with Class IV heart failure who at one month were without orthopnea, edema, weight gain, or recently increased diuretics had outcomes similar to patients with consistently Class III symptoms (15). In the more recent ESCAPE trial, re-evaluation at one month identified patients free from symptoms and signs of either congestion or hypoperfusion at one month, who had a mortality of 8% and readmission rate of 38% compared to 25% and 68% for patients who were either "wet" or "cold" at one month after discharge (16).

INTERMACS PROFILES FOR PATIENTS WITH LATE-STAGE DISEASE

"Refractory Class IV heart failure despite all accepted therapies" was once considered an adequate descriptor of the indication for cardiac transplantation. Selection and priority for cardiac transplantation have undergone major evolution since its approval for reimbursement as "best therapy" in 1984. However, the low ceiling of about 2200 hearts annually in the United States has created a large foyer of waiting candidates. The risk of death from irretrievable hemodynamic collapse while awaiting transplantation has been greatly reduced with the availability of mechanical circulatory support devices. This advancing technology has accelerated the evolution of a profile system to classify heart failure severity even within the late-stage disease (3). Although introduced initially to better understand outcomes in the INTERMACS database of approved mechanical circulatory support devices, these profiles are likely to find broader application in defining and addressing the many advanced heart failure patients who are not eligible for transplantation or implanted devices.

The INTERMACS system includes 7 clinical profiles and 3 situational modifiers (Table 12.3). Unlike previous classifications, implicit in this scheme is evaluation *after* systematic provision of all appropriate medical and standard surgical therapies. Over 80%

Table 12.3 INTERMACS Profiles

Profile 1: Critical Cardiogenic Shock *"Crash and burn"*
Patients with life-threatening hypotension despite rapidly escalating inotropic support, with critical organ hypoperfusion, often worsening lactate levels and acidosis

Profile 2: Progressive Decline *"Sliding on inotropes"*
Patient with declining function despite intravenous inotropic support, often manifested by worsening renal function, malnutrition, unresponsive volume overload. Also describes declining status in patients intolerant of inotropic therapy.

Profile 3: Stable but Inotrope Dependent *"Dependent stability"*
Patient with stable blood pressure, organ function, nutrition, and symptoms on continuous intravenous inotropic support (or a temporary circulatory support device or both), but demonstrating repeated failure to wean from support.

Profile 4: Resting Symptoms
Patients can be stabilized without progressive volume retention but experience daily experiences of symptoms of congestion at rest or during ADL. Doses of diuretics generally fluctuate at very high levels. Some patients may shuttle from 4 to 5.

Profile 5: Exertion Intolerant *"Housebound"*
Comfortable at rest and with ADL but unable to engage in any other activity, living predominantly within the house. Patients are comfortable at rest without congestive symptoms, but may have underlying refractory elevated volume status, often with renal dysfunction. If underlying nutritional status and organ function are marginal, patient may be more at risk than INTERMACS 4, and require definitive intervention.

Profile 6: Exertion Limited *"Walking wounded"*
Patient without evidence of fluid overload is comfortable at rest, with activities of daily living and minor activities outside the home but fatigues after the first few minutes of any meaningful activity.

Profile 7: Advanced NYHA III
A placeholder for more precise specification in future, this level includes patients who are without current or recent episodes of unstable fluid balance, living comfortably with meaningful activity limited to mild physical exertion.

Modifiers for Profiles

TCS-Temporary Circulatory Support can modify only patients in hospital with devices intended only for short-term in-hospital use

A - Arrhythmia –can modify any profile. Recurrent ventricular tachyarrhythmias contributing substantially to clinical compromise. This includes frequent appropriate ICD shocks

FF - Frequent Flyer – can modify only outpatients, designating a patient requiring frequent emergency visits or hospitalizations for diuretics, ultrafiltration, or intravenous vasoactive therapy.

Abbreviations: NYHA, New York Heart Association.
Source: Nomenclature condensed from Ref. 3.

of current device recipients are in Profiles 1 and 2, which have been associated with the highest rates of post-operative complications and death (3). Although approved indications for implanted devices currently include also Profiles 3–5 and sometimes 6, these states of lesser severity account for a small minority of current recipients. Profile 7 is a boundary state considered to describe a clinical severity that is "less sick" than currently considered to warrant mechanical circulatory support.

After initial experience with this classification for patients evaluated with late-stage disease, it has been modified to encompass a broader scope of common clinical situations in which some features are recurrent rather than continuous. The 3 modifiers are the use of temporary circulatory support (TCS) such as intra-aortic balloon or external centrifugal pump, which can append to profiles 1–3; arrhythmias (A) which can modify any profile, and frequent exacerbations of heart failure leading to emergency room visits or hospitalizations for therapy (FF for frequent flyer, can modify only outpatients).

SUMMARY

Heart failure as we currently perceive it can be visualized in broad stages, general symptom classes, and detailed symptomatic hemodynamic profiles. When the disease moves beyond standard medical and pacing device therapies, the integrated picture of decompensation can guide consideration of replacement therapies or design of therapies specifically to relieve symptoms for the lifetime remaining. At every stage, serial clinical assessment of both symptoms and physical signs is crucial to individualize care of the patient with therapies most likely to be effective. All systems of classification will leave some patients inadequately characterized by short-hand descriptions and other patients stranded between profiles. However, each system has helped to focus on the aspects of a patient's clinical presentation and course that place him/her in context with other patients from whom we have learned in the past. As the journey with heart failure continues to lengthen, there are ever more crossroads requiring recognition and sequential decisions. The differing classification systems guide these turns and point toward new unmet needs. They serve also as landmarks looking backward and forward to map our evolving therapies and understanding of the course of heart failure.

REFERENCES

1. Hunt SA, Abraham WT, Chin MH, et al. ACC/AHA guideline update for the diagnosis and management of chronic heart failure in the adult: a report of the American college of cardiology/American heart association task force on practice guidelines (writing committee to update the 2001 guidelines for the evaluation and management of heart failure): developed in collaboration with the American college of chest physicians and the international society for heart and lung transplantation: endorsed by the heart rhythm society. Circulation 2005; 112: e154–235.
2. Nohria A, Tsang SW, Fang JC, et al. Clinical assessment identifies hemodynamic profiles that predict outcomes in patients admitted with heart failure. J Am Coll Cardiol 2003; 41: 1797–804.
3. Kirklin JK, Naftel DC, Stevenson LW, et al. INTERMACS database for durable devices for circulatory support: first annual report. J Heart Lung Transplant 2008; 27: 1065–72.
4. Nohria A, Lewis E, Stevenson LW. Medical management of advanced heart failure. JAMA 2002; 287: 628–40.
5. Drazner MH, Hellkamp AS, Leier CV, et al. Value of clinician assessment of hemodynamics in advanced heart failure. The ESCAPE trial. Circ Heart Fail 2008; 1: 170–7.
6. Leier CV. Nuggets, pearls, and vignettes of master heart failure clinicians: part 2-the physical examination. Congest Heart Fail 2001; 7: 297–308.
7. Stevenson LW, Perloff JK. The limited reliability of physical signs for estimating hemodynamics in chronic heart failure. JAMA 1989; 261: 884–8.
8. Drazner MH, Yancy C, Shah MR, et al. Utility of the history and physical examination in assessing hemodynamics in patients with advanced heart failure: the ESCAPE trial (Abstract). Circulation (abstract) 2005; 112: II-640.
9. Butman SM, Ewy GA, Standen JR, et al. Bedside cardiovascular examination in patients with severe chronic heart failure: importance of rest or inducible jugular venous distension. J Am Coll Cardiol 1993; 22: 968–74.
10. Drazner MH, Hamilton MA, Fonarow G, et al. Relationship between right and left-sided filling pressures in 1000 patients with advanced heart failure. J Heart Lung Transplant 1999; 18: 1126–32.
11. Zema MJ, Restivo B, Sos T, et al. Left ventricular dysfunction-bedside valsalva manoeuvre. Br Heart J 1980; 44: 560–9.
12. Sobh JF, Lucas C, Stevenson LW, et al. Altered cardiorespiratory control in patients with severe congestive heart failure: a transfer function analysis approach. Comput Cardiol 1996; 1–4.

13. Kittleson M, Hurwitz S, Shah MR, et al. Development of circulatory-renal limitations to angiotensin-converting enzyme inhibitors identifies patients with severe heart failure and early mortality. J Am Coll Cardiol 2003; 41: 2029–35.

14. Rose EA, Gellijns AC, Moskowitz AJ, et al. Long-term use of a left ventricular assist device for end-stage heart failure. N Engl J Med 2001; 345: 1435–43.

15. Lucas C, Johnson W, Flavell C, et al. Freedom from congestion at one month predicts good two-year survival after hospitalization for class IV heart failure. Circulation 1996; 94: I-193.

16. Rogers JG, Hellkamp A, Young JB, et al. Low congestion score one month after hospitalization predicts better function and survival (Abstract). J Am Coll Cardiol 2007; 49; in press.

13
Prognosis in heart failure

J. Susie Woo and Wayne C. Levy

INTRODUCTION

As the incidence and diversity of heart failure has increased, so too has the complexity of therapy and variability in outcome. Mortality from heart failure has been reported to range from less than 5% to over 75% per year. The natural history of heart failure has changed dramatically as medical therapy has improved and physicians are armed with life-prolonging medications and devices to alter the course of the disease. These advancements, although welcome, have made it more complicated to predict the risk of death or other major cardio-vascular events in a given patient with heart failure.

The ability to predict prognosis may be helpful on multiple levels and situations. For primary care physicians, it may inform when to refer a patient for specialist care. For cardiologists, it may help anticipate the need and appropriate timing of aggressive therapies, such as devices or transplant. For the emergency physician, it may aid clinical decision making and risk stratification into patients who may be discharged home, admitted to the floor, or moved to more intensive care. For all providers, it helps educate patients about the chronicity of their disease and prepare them for the future. Often, heart failure patients are overly optimistic, expecting a lifespan based on their age and gender rather than one that reflects the severity of their disease. A survey of New York Heart Association (NYHA) Class IV outpatients revealed their unrealistic expectations of a 12-year life expectancy (1). As patients and their families are increasingly involved in clinical decisions, an objective assessment of prognosis can be invaluable in facilitating communication and discussion about risks and benefits of therapy or end-of-life care.

A list of some of the major independent predictors of heart failure morbidity and mortality that will be discussed in this chapter is provided in Table 13.1.

DEMOGRAPHIC AND CLINICAL FACTORS

As in most disease processes, mortality in heart failure increases with age, although the impact of age appears to be minor until after 60 years of age (2), and is generally overcome by the severity of heart failure as the disease progresses. Female gender has consistently been associated with a significantly lower risk of heart failure hospitalization and cardio-vascular mortality (2,3), irrespective of left ventricular ejection fraction (LVEF) or heart failure etiology (4).

The etiology of heart failure itself has some prognostic value, with increased mortality associated with infiltrative diseases, such as hemochromatosis and amyloidosis, HIV infection, doxorubicin therapy, and ischemic heart disease when compared with idiopathic dilated cardiomyopathy (5). These differences may reflect the presence of comorbidities,

Table 13.1 Prognostic Factors in Systolic Heart Failure

Clinical factors
  Age
  Gender
  Heart failure etiology
  Blood pressure
  Heart rate
  Signs and symptoms of decompensated heart failure
  BMI
Cardiac structure and function
  Left ventricular ejection fraction
  Left and right ventricular size
  Right ventricular function
  Mitral and tricuspid regurgitation
  Restrictive pattern of diastolic dysfunction
  Cardiomegaly on chest X-ray
  Bundle branch block
Functional capacity
  NYHA class
  Peak VO_2
  Ventilatory efficiency (VE/VCO_2)
  Six-minute walk test
Laboratory data
  Serum sodium
  Neurohormones
  BNP and NT-proBNP
  Troponin
  Anemia
  Renal dysfunction
Medications/devices

including liver or kidney dysfunction, immunosuppression, or vasculopathy, which are often associated with these conditions. In particular, there is evidence to suggest that ischemic heart disease and the presence of diabetes interact to accelerate the progression of myocardial dysfunction (6–8).

Clinical symptoms and signs, including elevated jugular venous pressure, rales, presence of a third heart sound, peripheral edema, and radiologic evidence of pulmonary edema, not only reflect patients' clinical status at a point in time, but can also predict future heart failure hospitalization and cardiovascular mortality (2,9). Tachycardia and hypotension also appear to portend poor outcomes, as the most obvious signs of sympathetic activation and decreasing cardiac output (2,6,10,11).

An ominous sign of decreased cardiac output is the presence of cardiac cachexia, which reflects the increased metabolic rate and catabolism of end-stage disease. Although elevated body mass index (BMI) is a major risk factor for the development of heart failure (12–16), an inverse association between BMI and mortality is seen when BMI is less than 30 in patients with established disease (2,6,17). Weight loss of 6% or more was found to be an especially powerful predictor of impaired survival (18).

CARDIAC STRUCTURE AND FUNCTION

LVEF has probably been the most universal measurement for estimating disease severity. It reflects the degree of left ventricular systolic dysfunction, which is the primary pathology in most cardiomyopathic patients with heart failure regardless of etiology. Lower LVEF has been found in multiple models to correlate with mortality (6,19,20), with a nearly linear relationship once the EF falls below 40–45% (2,21,22).

Left ventricular enlargement reflects the pathophysiologic remodeling process of heart failure and is also associated with a negative prognosis (19,23). Echocardiography may reveal additional predictors of mortality in patients with systolic heart failure, including right ventricular systolic dysfunction (24,25), right ventricular enlargement (26), the presence of tricuspid regurgitation (27), mitral regurgitation (2), or a restrictive pattern of diastolic dysfunction (20,28). Similarly, cardiomegaly, as defined by a cardiothoracic ratio greater than 50% on chest X-ray, reflects ventricular dilatation, and has been shown to have significant predictive value (2,6,22).

The presence of bundle branch block or QRS ≥ 120 milliseconds increases risk for both sudden cardiac death and all-cause mortality (2,29–32), presumably due to increased ventricular size, propensity for arrhythmia or as a marker of ventricular dyssynchrony resulting from the conduction defect. Correction of this dyssynchrony is the basis for the survival benefit seen with cardiac resynchronization therapy (biventricular pacing).

Despite its association with sudden cardiac death, nonsustained ventricular tachycardia does not appear to increase mortality after adjusting for other variables (33–35). The presence of atrial fibrillation at baseline also does not predict outcome (36,37), although new onset of the arrhythmia in patients with systolic heart failure may be associated with increased mortality (36,38,39). It remains uncertain whether aggressive attempts to maintain sinus rhythm are beneficial for clinical outcomes.

FUNCTIONAL CAPACITY

After ejection fraction, the single most important variable in determining therapy is NYHA functional class. Many treatment trials have defined their cohort based on this classification. However, the subjectiveness and inconsistency of this categorization between centers or physicians makes it less discerning than other objective measures of functional capacity.

Peak exercise oxygen consumption (VO_2) during maximal cardiopulmonary exercise testing has proved to be a useful, reproducible, noninvasive surrogate for maximal cardiac output and cardiac reserve. A peak VO_2 < 14 mL/min/kg was the first widely accepted measurement used to help identify patients who might be eligible for heart transplantation (40,41), but with interval changes in medical therapy and consequent improved survival, a peak VO_2 < 10 mL/min/kg may now be a more appropriate cutoff for transplant eligibility (42). Peak VO_2 is influenced by age, gender, body weight, conditioning status, motivation, and ability to exercise to anaerobic threshold, but continues to be a valuable prerequisite in the consideration for possible transplant.

Other cardiopulmonary exercise testing (CPET) parameters that are associated with prognosis include ventilatory efficiency (VE/VCO_2) (43), exercise duration and peak systolic blood pressure (44), and noninvasive measures of cardiac output reserve (45).

A simple submaximal 6-minute walk test has been shown to correlate with peak VO_2 and provide similar prognostic information about future heart failure hospitalization and mortality (46). It is inexpensive and can be measured serially in both the clinic and hospital setting, but is relatively time-consuming and has not demonstrated other clinical value or superiority over peak VO_2. Therefore, it has not gained widespread use in the evaluation of heart failure patients.

LABORATORY DATA AND NEUROHORMAL ACTIVATION

It is now understood that a fundamental component of heart failure pathophysiolog1y is the activation and interaction of the renin–angiotensin–aldosterone system (RAAS), sympathetic nervous system (SNS), and inflammatory systems. Hyponatremia is thought to be an indicator of the level of RAAS and SNS stimulation, is associated with higher diuretic doses, and has been a consistent prognostic factor in advanced heart failure (10,31,47).

Plasma norepinephrine levels are a direct measure of SNS activation and have in fact been shown to be a better predictor of mortality than serum sodium in patients with heart failure (21). However, its use in everyday practice has been hampered by limited availability of the test and its wide variability depending on patient activity, environment, anxiety and medical therapy, requiring supine rest and the withdrawal of certain medications prior to each measurement.

In a study by Latini et al, baseline levels of multiple neurohormones, including norepinephrine, renin activity, aldosterone, endothelin, and plasma brain natriuretic peptide (BNP) were compared in their ability to predict morbidity and mortality in over 4000 patients with stable chronic heart failure (48). BNP was found to be the most powerful predictor of poor outcomes. In a much smaller study of 142 patients with advanced heart failure, the N-terminal prohormone of BNP (NT-proBNP) was found to be a better prognostic marker for mortality or urgent transplantation than LVEF, peak VO_2, or the Heart Failure Survival Score (49). NT-proBNP has also been found to be strongly predictive of short-term mortality risk in patients presenting to the emergency department with acute heart failure, with a level greater than 5180 pg/mL conferring more than a fivefold increase in risk of death at 76 days (50). Although both peptides are released in equal ratios in response to ventricular wall tension or stretch, NT-proBNP levels can be 2–10 times higher than BNP due to its longer half-life, and thus, may be more sensitive in identifying lesser degrees of left ventricular dysfunction (51).

Evidence suggests that elevation of troponin may identify a different at-risk population than that of BNP, with elevations in both markers conferring the highest risk (52). Elevated cardiac troponin levels indicate ongoing myocardial damage, and have been associated with higher pulmonary capillary wedge pressures, lower cardiac indexes, and progressive decrease in LVEF over time (53). Serial measurements may be helpful, as an increase in troponin contributes additional risk for mortality in patients with stable chronic heart failure (54). A new highly sensitive troponin assay demonstrated preserved prognostic value at previously undetectable concentrations (55), increasing the marker's applicability to the general heart failure population.

Several other indirect markers of inflammation have been shown to have predictive value in heart failure and are easily measured with routine laboratory tests. These include a high uric acid level (56), low total cholesterol (57), low relative lymphocyte count (58), low albumin (59), and low hemoglobin/hematocrit (60–63). Correction of anemia has been proposed as a possible therapeutic target for patients with heart failure, and several large clinical trials are ongoing to determine whether treatment with iron or erythropoiesis-stimulating agents, such as darbepoeitin, may improve clinical outcomes in patients with heart failure (64–66).

Renal dysfunction may contribute to the anemia seen in heart failure patients and itself appears to be an independent risk factor for cardiovascular death and heart failure hospitalization, whether measured as blood urea nitrogen (BUN), creatinine, or creatinine clearance (CrCl) (67–69). The largest datasets included 2680 patients from the three CHARM trials and over 5800 patients in the SOLVD trials; both retrospective analyses found baseline estimated CrCl to be a strong continuous predictor of long-term survival regardless of LVEF (70,71).

CLINICAL PROGNOSTIC MODELS

Several models have sought to assimilate and condense this multitude of independent risk factors into a more convenient algorithm to aid in clinical decision making.

Four of these prediction models were compared in their ability to estimate inpatient death, inpatient death or complications, and 30-day mortality in over 33,500 patients

Table 13.2 The EFFECT Heart Failure Scoring System

Variable	30-Day Score	1-Year Score
Age	+ Age	+ Age
Respiratory rate, breaths/min (minimum of 20, maximum of 45)	+ Rate	+ Rate
Systolic blood pressure, mmHg		
≥180	−60	−50
160–179	−55	−45
140–159	−50	−40
120–139	−45	−35
100–119	−40	−30
90–99	−35	−25
<90	−30	−20
Urea nitrogen, mg/dL (maximum of 60)	+ Level	+ Level
Sodium concentration <136 mEq/L	+10	+10
Cerebrovascular disease	+10	+10
Dementia	+20	+20
Chronic obstructive pulmonary disease	+10	+10
Hepatic cirrhosis	+25	+35
Cancer	+15	+15
Hemoglobin <10.0 g/dL	N/A	+10

The EFFECT heart failure scoring system was developed to estimate a patient's risk of death at 30 days and one year based on information obtained within hours of initial hospital presentation for a primary diagnosis of heart failure. The 30-day and one-year risk scores are calculated from the sum of the points assigned in each column, stratifying patients into very low risk (total score ≤60), low risk (61–90), intermediate risk (91–120), high risk (121–150), or very high-risk (>150) categories. The 30-day risk score was found to correlate with an approximate mortality rate of <1% in the very low-risk group, 12% in the intermediate risk group, and over 30% in the very high-risk group. The one-year risk score predicts a mortality rate of approximately 10% in the very low risk group, 30% in the intermediate risk group, and over 65% in the very high risk group. An online and Pocket PC version of the model is available at http://www.ccort.ca/Research/CHFRiskModel.aspx.
Source: From Ref. 10.

admitted with a diagnosis of heart failure (72). The ADHERE risk tree was designed to be a bedside tool, requiring only systolic blood pressure (SBP), BUN, and creatinine to stratify patients into one of five risk groups (73). The ADHERE logistic regression (LR) model uses these same variables to calculate a log odds of mortality (= $0.0212 \times$ BUN − $0.0192 \times$ SBP + $0.0131 \times$ HR + $0.0288 \times$ age − 4.72). The EFFECT model uses very similar clinical variables but adds the effect of comorbidities to stratify patients into five risk groups (10). The Brigham and Women's Hospital (BWH) prediction rule uses SBP, respiratory rate, serum sodium, and ST-T wave changes on electrocardiogram to assign 0–5 points to estimate risk (74). The ADHERE LR and EFFECT models were found to have equal or greater discriminatory power than the ADHERE Tree and BWH rule for all outcomes.

The EFFECT model may also be used to predict survival of these acutely decompensated patients at one year, and remains unique in its inclusion of major comorbid conditions (cancer, dementia, cerebrovascular disease, cirrhosis, and chronic obstructive pulmonary disorder) and its exclusion of a measure of left ventricular function (Table 13.2). It has been validated in large outpatient clinical trial databases (75) as well as a hospitalized Veterans Affairs population (76).

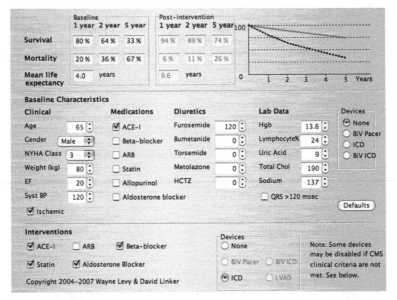

Figure 13.1 The Seattle Heart Failure Model Calculator. This web-based calculator, as well as free Palm, PocketPC, Mac, and PC versions of the Seattle Heart Failure Model are available online for health care providers at SeattleHeartFailureModel.org. A given patient's clinical variables, medications, diuretic dose, laboratory data, and the presence or absence of devices are input into the calculator, which provides estimates of 1-, 2-, and 5-year survival as well as a mean life expectancy. The effect of interventions, in the form of medica tions or devices, is seen with parallel postintervention estimates of survival and mortality. In this example, an NYHA III patient on an ACE inhibitor and furosemide is found to have an estimated 20% 1-year mortality, which improves to 6% with the addition of a beta-blocker, statin, aldosterone blocker and ICD. Estimated life expectancy correspondingly increases by more than 5 years. Conversely, the withdrawal of the ACE inhibitor (unchecking the ACE intervention box) would increase his mortality to 25%. In this manner, the SHFM may encourage the use of lifesaving medications and devices. *Abbreviations*: NYHA, New York Heart Association; ACE, angiotension-converting enzyme; ICD, implantable cardioverter-defibrillator; SHFM, Seattle Heart Failure Model.

The Heart Failure Survival Score was the first multivariate heart failure model to be prospectively validated in a separate heart failure population and was originally published in 1997 to assist in the risk stratification of ambulatory patients referred for cardiac transplantation (31). The variables in this model (ischemic etiology, LVEF, mean blood pressure, heart rate, QRS width $\geq$120 milliseconds, serum sodium, and peak VO_2) are used to stratify patients into low-, moderate-, or high-risk groups. Subsequent changes in heart failure therapy, especially the use of beta-blockers (77), has required modification of this model (77) and has raised the question of whether it remains useful in our current era of medical therapy (42).

The DIG model uses age, LVEF, NYHA class, BMI, cardiomegaly, the number of heart failure signs or symptoms, creatinine, blood pressure, nitrate use, and the interaction of diabetes with ischemic etiology to provide a useful absolute estimate of one- and three-year survival (6), but has yet to be validated in another dataset and requires a cumbersome calculation.

The CHARM model has likewise not been validated in a separate dataset, and uses 24 variables with their coefficients to calculate an individual risk score (2). Using the published nomogram, one can then convert the risk score into an estimate of two-year survival or survival free of heart failure hospitalization. No laboratory data is included in this model,

Table 13.3   Summary/Comparison of Heart Failure Survival Models

Variables	HFSS (31)	EFFECT (10)	ADHERE LR (73)	DIG (6)	CHARM (2)	SHFM (75)
Age		✓	✓	✓	✓	✓
Gender					✓	✓
BMI or weight				✓	✓	✓
Blood pressure	✓	✓	✓	✓	✓	✓
Heart rate	✓		✓		✓	
Respiratory rate		✓				
NYHA class					✓	✓
LVEF	✓			✓	✓	✓
Cardiomegaly				✓	✓	
Ischemic etiology/MI	✓			✓	✓	✓
Comorbidities		✓			✓	
Diabetes				✓	✓	
HF signs/symptoms				✓	✓	
Bundle branch block	✓				✓	
Peak VO$_2$	✓					
Sodium	✓	✓				✓
Renal function		✓	✓	✓		
Hemoglobin						✓
Lymphocytes, %						✓
Uric acid						✓
Total cholesterol						✓
HF medications				1 (nitrates)	1 (candesartan)	7
HF devices (ICD, CRT)						✓
Output	Risk groups for 1-yr event-free survival	Risk groups for 30-day and 1-yr mortality	In-hospital mortality	12-mo and 36-mo survival	2-yr event-free and total survival	1- to 5-yr survival and life expectancy

Abbreviations: BMI, body mass index; CRT, cardiac resynchronization therapy; ICD, implantable cardioverter-defibrillator; HF, heart failure; LVEF, left ventricular ejection fraction; NYHA, New York Heart Association.

as they were measured in only a subset of patients in the derivation cohort; however, the model includes several unique variables including the presence of atrial fibrillation, mitral regurgitation, current smoking, prior heart failure hospitalization, and diagnosis more than two years prior to presentation.

Another multivariate model for ambulatory heart patients is the Seattle Heart Failure Model (SHFM), which was derived using data from the PRAISE-1 trial of amlodipine in patients with severe heart failure (NYHA IIIB or IV with EF ≤ 30%). It remains distinctive in its inclusion of multiple medications and devices, in addition to more common variables, in its calculation of risk. It has been validated in multiple cohorts totaling more than 14,000 patients, who encompass a wide range of ages, ejection fractions, severity of heart failure symptoms, and countries of origin (75,78). It provides an estimate of average life expectancy and one- to five-year survival, and displays how this estimate may be altered by adding or subtracting heart failure medications or devices. The model may also help predict the potential mode of death (pump failure vs sudden death) (79). The addition of BNP (but not BUN or creatinine) has been shown to significantly improve the predictive value of the SHFM (78). The need for complex or time-consuming calculations is circumvented by its easy accessibility in multiple formats at SeattleHeartFailureModel. org (Fig. 13.1).

A summary of these multivariate heart failure risk models is provided in Table 13.3.

CONCLUSION

Historically and in general practice, prognosis in heart failure continues to be estimated from a gestalt of a patient's age, signs and symptoms of heart failure, functional status, LVEF, response to therapy, and comorbid conditions. This estimate may be improved by knowledge and assessment of additional independent prognostic factors that have been detailed above. However, the increasing complexity of heart failure patients and their medical therapy, combined with the shortage of cardiac transplant donors but availability of left ventricular assist devices as destination therapy, has highlighted the need for a more sophisticated and objective quantification of prognosis.

This need has been met by the development of several multivariate risk models for the assessment of patients presenting with both inpatient decompensated and outpatient stable disease. The ADHERE Tree model is the simplest in application and can effectively risk stratify patients in the Emergency Room. The slightly more complex EFFECT model, which includes comorbidities, has an online calculator and provides greater gradations of risk than the ADHERE model as well as a longer-term prediction of mortality at one year. The SHFM has not yet been validated in hospitalized patients, but provides estimates of one- to five-year survival and may be recalculated at any time in the outpatient setting to reflect changes in clinical status or medical treatment. It is the only model that allows users to modify patients' risk by accounting for the survival benefits of heart failure medications and devices. All models will need to be modified as new knowledge and therapeutics become available and must be convenient to use if they are to remain relevant, helpful tools to both physicians and their patients.

REFERENCES

1. Allen LA, Yager JE, Funk MJ, et al. Discordance between patient-predicted and model-predicted life expectancy among ambulatory patients with heart failure. JAMA 2008; 299: 2533–42.
2. Pocock SJ, Wang D, Pfeffer MA, et al. Predictors of mortality and morbidity in patients with chronic heart failure. Eur Heart J 2006; 27: 65–75.
3. Frazier CG, Alexander KP, Newby LK, et al. Associations of gender and etiology with outcomes in heart failure with systolic dysfunction: a pooled analysis of 5 randomized control trials. J Am Coll Cardiol 2007; 49: 1450–8.
4. O'Meara E, Clayton T, McEntegart MB, et al. Sex differences in clinical characteristics and prognosis in a broad spectrum of patients with heart failure: results of the candesartan in heart failure: assessment of reduction in mortality and morbidity (CHARM) program. Circulation 2007; 115: 3111–20.
5. Felker GM, Thompson RE, Hare JM, et al. Underlying causes and long-term survival in patients with initially unexplained cardiomyopathy. N Engl J Med 2000; 342: 1077–84.

6. Brophy JM, Dagenais GR, McSherry F, Williford W, Yusuf S. A multivariate model for predicting mortality in patients with heart failure and systolic dysfunction. Am J Med 2004; 116: 300–4.
7. Bart BA, Shaw LK, McCants CB Jr, et al. Clinical determinants of mortality in patients with angiographically diagnosed ischemic or nonischemic cardiomyopathy. J Am Coll Cardiol 1997; 30: 1002–8.
8. Dries DL, Sweitzer NK, Drazner MH, Stevenson LW, Gersh BJ. Prognostic impact of diabetes mellitus in patients with heart failure according to the etiology of left ventricular systolic dysfunction. J Am Coll Cardiol 2001; 38: 421–8.
9. Drazner MH, Rame JE, Stevenson LW, Dries DL. Prognostic importance of elevated jugular venous pressure and a third heart sound in patients with heart failure. N Engl J Med 2001; 345: 574–81.
10. Lee DS, Austin PC, Rouleau JL, et al. Predicting mortality among patients hospitalized for heart failure: derivation and validation of a clinical model. JAMA 2003; 290: 2581–7.
11. Bouvy ML, Heerdink ER, Leufkens HG, Hoes AW. Predicting mortality in patients with heart failure: a pragmatic approach. Heart 2003; 89: 605–9.
12. Chen YT, Vaccarino V, Williams CS, et al. Risk factors for heart failure in the elderly: a prospective community-based study. Am J Med 1999; 106: 605–12.
13. He J, Ogden LG, Bazzano LA, et al. Risk factors for congestive heart failure in US men and women: NHANES I epidemiologic follow-up study. Arch Intern Med 2001; 161: 996–1002.
14. Lee DS, Massaro JM, Wang TJ, et al. Antecedent blood pressure, body mass index, and the risk of incident heart failure in later life. Hypertension 2007; 50: 869–76.
15. Kenchaiah S, Evans JC, Levy D, et al. Obesity and the risk of heart failure. N Engl J Med 2002; 347: 305–13.
16. Wilhelmsen L, Rosengren A, Eriksson H, Lappas G. Heart failure in the general population of men; morbidity, risk factors and prognosis. J Intern Med 2001; 249: 253–61.
17. Kenchaiah S, Pocock SJ, Wang D, et al. Body mass index and prognosis in patients with chronic heart failure: insights from the candesartan in heart failure: assessment of reduction in mortality and morbidity (CHARM) program. Circulation 2007; 116: 627–36.
18. Anker SD, Negassa A, Coats AJ, et al. Prognostic importance of weight loss in chronic heart failure and the effect of treatment with angiotensin-converting-enzyme inhibitors: an observational study. Lancet 2003; 361: 1077–83.
19. Wong M, Staszewsky L, Latini R, et al. Severity of left ventricular remodeling defines outcomes and response to therapy in heart failure: valsartan heart failure trial (Val-HeFT) echocardiographic data. J Am Coll Cardiol 2004; 43: 2022–7.
20. Rihal CS, Nishimura RA, Hatle LK, Bailey KR, Tajik AJ. Systolic and diastolic dysfunction in patients with clinical diagnosis of dilated cardiomyopathy: relation to symptoms and prognosis. Circulation 1994; 90: 2772–9.
21. Cohn JN, Levine TB, Olivari MT, et al. Plasma norepinephrine as a guide to prognosis in patients with chronic congestive heart failure. N Engl J Med 1984; 311: 819–23.
22. Cohn JN, Johnson GR, Shabetai R, et al. Ejection fraction, peak exercise oxygen consumption, cardiothoracic ratio, ventricular arrhythmias, and plasma norepinephrine as determinants of prognosis in heart failure. The V-HeFT VA Cooperative Studies Group. Circulation 1993; 87: VI5–16.
23. Grayburn PA, Appleton CP, DeMaria AN, et al. Echocardiographic predictors of morbidity and mortality in patients with advanced heart failure: the beta-blocker evaluation of survival trial (BEST). J Am Coll Cardiol 2005; 45: 1064–71.
24. de Groote P, Millaire A, Foucher-Hossein C, et al. Right ventricular ejection fraction is an independent predictor of survival in patients with moderate heart failure. J Am Coll Cardiol 1998; 32: 948–54.
25. Gavazzi A, Berzuini C, Campana C, et al. Value of right ventricular ejection fraction in predicting short-term prognosis of patients with severe chronic heart failure. J Heart Lung Transplant 1997; 16: 774–85.
26. Sun JP, James KB, Yang XS, et al. Comparison of mortality rates and progression of left ventricular dysfunction in patients with idiopathic dilated cardiomyopathy and dilated versus nondilated right ventricular cavities. Am J Cardiol 1997; 80: 1583–7.
27. Hung J, Koelling T, Semigran MJ, et al. Usefulness of echocardiographic determined tricuspid regurgitation in predicting event-free survival in severe heart failure secondary to idiopathic-dilated cardiomyopathy or to ischemic cardiomyopathy. Am J Cardiol 1998; 82: 1301–3, A10.
28. Giannuzzi P, Temporelli PL, Bosimini E, et al. Independent and incremental prognostic value of Doppler-derived mitral deceleration time of early filling in both symptomatic and asymptomatic patients with left ventricular dysfunction. J Am Coll Cardiol 1996; 28: 383–90.
29. Baldasseroni S, Opasich C, Gorini M, et al. Left bundle-branch block is associated with increased 1-year sudden and total mortality rate in 5517 outpatients with congestive heart failure: a report from the Italian network on congestive heart failure. Am Heart J 2002; 143: 398–405.

30. Hawkins NM, Wang D, McMurray JJ, et al. Prevalence and prognostic impact of bundle branch block in patients with heart failure: evidence from the CHARM programme. Eur J Heart Fail 2007; 9: 510–17.

31. Aaronson KD, Schwartz JS, Chen TM, et al. Development and prospective validation of a clinical index to predict survival in ambulatory patients referred for cardiac transplant evaluation. Circulation 1997; 95: 2660–7.

32. Iuliano S, Fisher SG, Karasik PE, Fletcher RD, Singh SN. Department of veterans affairs survival trial of antiarrhythmic therapy in congestive heart failure. QRS duration and mortality in patients with congestive heart failure. Am Heart J 2002; 143: 1085–91.

33. Doval HC, Nul DR, Grancelli HO, et al. Nonsustained ventricular tachycardia in severe heart failure: independent marker of increased mortality due to sudden death. GESICA-GEMA investigators. Circulation 1996; 94: 3198–203.

34. Teerlink JR, Jalaluddin M, Anderson S, et al. Ambulatory ventricular arrhythmias in patients with heart failure do not specifically predict an increased risk of sudden death. PROMISE (Prospective Randomized Milrinone Survival Evaluation) investigators. Circulation 2000; 101: 40–6.

35. Singh SN, Fisher SG, Carson PE, Fletcher RD. Prevalence and significance of nonsustained ventricular tachycardia in patients with premature ventricular contractions and heart failure treated with vasodilator therapy. Department of veterans affairs chf stat investigators. J Am Coll Cardiol 1998; 32: 942–7.

36. Carson PE, Johnson GR, Dunkman WB, et al. The influence of atrial fibrillation on prognosis in mild to moderate heart failure. The V-HeFT Studies. The V-HeFT VA Cooperative Studies Group. Circulation 1993; 87: VI102–10.

37. Crijns HJ, Tjeerdsma G, de Kam PJ, et al. Prognostic value of the presence and development of atrial fibrillation in patients with advanced chronic heart failure. Eur Heart J 2000; 21: 1238–45.

38. Swedberg K, Olsson LG, Charlesworth A, et al. Prognostic relevance of atrial fibrillation in patients with chronic heart failure on long-term treatment with beta-blockers: results from COMET. Eur Heart J 2005; 26: 1303–8.

39. Wang TJ, Larson MG, Levy D, et al. Temporal relations of atrial fibrillation and congestive heart failure and their joint influence on mortality: the Framingham Heart Study. Circulation 2003; 107: 2920–5.

40. Mancini DM, Eisen H, Kussmaul W, et al. Value of peak exercise oxygen consumption for optimal timing of cardiac transplantation in ambulatory patients with heart failure. Circulation 1991; 83: 778–86.

41. Costanzo MR, Augustine S, Bourge R, et al. Selection and treatment of candidates for heart transplantation. A statement for health professionals from the Committee on Heart Failure and Cardiac Transplantation of the Council on Clinical Cardiology, American Heart Association. Circulation 1995; 92: 3593–612.

42. Butler J, Khadim G, Paul KM, et al. Selection of patients for heart transplantation in the current era of heart failure therapy. J Am Coll Cardiol 2004; 43: 787–93.

43. Arena R, Myers J, Aslam SS, Varughese EB, Peberdy MA. Peak VO2 and VE/VCO2 slope in patients with heart failure: a prognostic comparison. Am Heart J 2004; 147: 354–60.

44. Williams SG, Jackson M, Ng LL, et al. Exercise duration and peak systolic blood pressure are predictive of mortality in ambulatory patients with mild-moderate chronic heart failure. Cardiology 2005; 104: 221–6.

45. Williams SG, Jackson M, Cooke GA, et al. How do different indicators of cardiac pump function impact upon the long-term prognosis of patients with chronic heart failure? Am Heart J 2005; 150: 983.

46. Zugck C, Kruger C, Durr S, et al. Is the 6-minute walk test a reliable substitute for peak oxygen uptake in patients with dilated cardiomyopathy? Eur Heart J 2000; 21: 540–9.

47. Klein L, O'Connor CM, Leimberger JD, et al. Lower serum sodium is associated with increased short-term mortality in hospitalized patients with worsening heart failure: results from the Outcomes of a Prospective Trial of Intravenous Milrinone for Exacerbations of Chronic Heart Failure (OPTIME-CHF) study. Circulation 2005; 111: 2454–60.

48. Latini R, Masson S, Anand I, et al. The comparative prognostic value of plasma neurohormones at baseline in patients with heart failure enrolled in Val-HeFT. Eur Heart J 2004; 25: 292–9.

49. Gardner RS, Ozalp F, Murday AJ, Robb SD, McDonagh TA. N-terminal pro-brain natriuretic peptide; a new gold standard in predicting mortality in patients with advanced heart failure. Eur Heart J 2003; 24: 1735–43.

50. Januzzi JL, van Kimmenade R, Lainchbury J, et al. NT-proBNP testing for diagnosis and short-term prognosis in acute destabilized heart failure: an international pooled analysis of 1256 patients: the International Collaborative of NT-proBNP Study. Eur Heart J 2006; 27: 330–7.

51. Godkar D, Bachu K, Dave B, Niranjan S, Khanna A. B-type natriuretic peptide (BNP) and proBNP: role of emerging markers to guide therapy and determine prognosis in cardiovascular disorders. Am J Ther 2008; 15: 150–6.

52. Taniguchi R, Sato Y, Nishio Y, Kimura T, Kita T. Measurements of baseline and follow-up concentrations of cardiac troponin-T and brain natriuretic peptide in patients with heart failure from various etiologies. Heart Vessels 2006; 21: 344–9.

53. Horwich TB, Patel J, MacLellan WR, Fonarow GC. Cardiac troponin I is associated with impaired hemodynamics, progressive left ventricular dysfunction, and increased mortality rates in advanced heart failure. Circulation 2003; 108: 833–8.

54. Miller WL, Hartman KA, Burritt MF, et al. Serial biomarker measurements in ambulatory patients with chronic heart failure: the importance of change over time. Circulation 2007; 116: 249–57.

55. Latini R, Masson S, Anand IS, et al. Prognostic value of very low plasma concentrations of troponin T in patients with stable chronic heart failure. Circulation 2007; 116: 1242–9.

56. Anker SD, Doehner W, Rauchhaus M, et al. Uric acid and survival in chronic heart failure: validation and application in metabolic, functional, and hemodynamic staging. Circulation 2003; 107: 1991–7.

57. Rauchhaus M, Clark AL, Doehner W, et al. The relationship between cholesterol and survival in patients with chronic heart failure. J Am Coll Cardiol 2003; 42: 1933–40.

58. Huehnergarth KV, Mozaffarian D, Sullivan MD, et al. Usefulness of relative lymphocyte count as an independent predictor of death/urgent transplant in heart failure. Am J Cardiol 2005; 95: 1492–5.

59. Horwich TB, Kalantar-Zadeh K, MacLellan RW, Fonarow GC. Albumin levels predict survival in patients with systolic heart failure. Am Heart J 2008; 155: 883–9.

60. Steinborn W, Doehner W, Anker SD. Anemia in chronic heart failure; frequency and prognostic impact. Clin Nephrol 2003; 60: S103–7.

61. Szachniewicz J, Petruk-Kowalczyk J, Majda J, et al. Anaemia is an independent predictor of poor outcome in patients with chronic heart failure. Int J Cardiol 2003; 90: 303–8.

62. O'Meara E, Clayton T, McEntegart MB, et al. Clinical correlates and consequences of anemia in a broad spectrum of patients with heart failure: results of the Candesartan in Heart Failure: Assessment of Reduction in Mortality and Morbidity (CHARM) Program. Circulation 2006; 113: 986–94.

63. Mozaffarian D, Nye R, Levy WC. Anemia predicts mortality in severe heart failure: the prospective randomized amlodipine survival evaluation (PRAISE). J Am Coll Cardiol 2003; 41: 1933–9.

64. Beck-da-Silva L, Rohde LE, Pereira-Barretto AC, et al. Rationale and design of the IRON-HF study: a randomized trial to assess the effects of iron supplementation in heart failure patients with anemia. J Card Fail 2007; 13: 14–17.

65. van Veldhuisen DJ, McMurray JJ, RED-HF Executive Committee. Are erythropoietin stimulating proteins safe and efficacious in heart failure? Why we need an adequately powered randomised outcome trial. Eur J Heart Fail 2007; 9: 110–12.

66. Levy WC. Anemia in heart failure: marker or mediator of adverse prognosis? J Am Coll Cardiol 2008; 51: 577–8.

67. Al-Ahmad A, Rand WM, Manjunath G, et al. Reduced kidney function and anemia as risk factors for mortality in patients with left ventricular dysfunction. J Am Coll Cardiol 2001; 38: 955–62.

68. Mahon NG, Blackstone EH, Francis GS, et al. The prognostic value of estimated creatinine clearance alongside functional capacity in ambulatory patients with chronic congestive heart failure. J Am Coll Cardiol 2002; 40: 1106–13.

69. McAlister FA, Ezekowitz J, Tonelli M, Armstrong PW. Renal insufficiency and heart failure: prognostic and therapeutic implications from a prospective cohort study. Circulation 2004; 109: 1004–9.

70. Hillege HL, Nitsch D, Pfeffer MA, et al. Renal function as a predictor of outcome in a broad spectrum of patients with heart failure. Circulation 2006; 113: 671–8.

71. Dries DL, Exner DV, Domanski MJ, Greenberg B, Stevenson LW. The prognostic implications of renal insufficiency in asymptomatic and symptomatic patients with left ventricular systolic dysfunction. J Am Coll Cardiol 2000; 35: 681–9.

72. Auble TE, Hsieh M, McCausland JB, Yealy DM. Comparison of four clinical prediction rules for estimating risk in heart failure. Ann Emerg Med 2007; 50: 127–35, 135.e1–2.

73. Fonarow GC, Adams KF Jr, Abraham WT, Yancy CW, Boscardin WJ, ADHERE Scientific Advisory Committee, Study Group, and Investigators. Risk stratification for in-hospital mortality in acutely decompensated heart failure: classification and regression tree analysis. JAMA 2005; 293: 572–80.

74. Chin MH, Goldman L. Correlates of major complications or death in patients admitted to the hospital with congestive heart failure. Arch Intern Med 1996; 156: 1814–20.

75. Levy WC, Mozaffarian D, Linker DT, et al. The seattle heart failure model: prediction of survival in heart failure. Circulation 2006; 113: 1424–33.

76. Rector TS, Ringwala SN, Ringwala SN, Anand IS. Validation of a risk score for dying within 1 year of an admission for heart failure. J Card Fail 2006; 12: 276–80.

77. Koelling TM, Joseph S, Aaronson KD. Heart failure survival score continues to predict clinical outcomes in patients with heart failure receiving beta-blockers. J Heart Lung Transplant 2004; 23: 1414–22.

78. May HT, Horne BD, Levy WC, et al. Validation of the seattle heart failure model in a community-based heart failure population and enhancement by adding B-type natriuretic peptide. Am J Cardiol 2007; 100: 697–700.

79. Mozaffarian D, Anker SD, Anand I, et al. Prediction of mode of death in heart failure: the seattle heart failure model. Circulation 2007; 116: 392–8.

14

Biomarkers in heart failure

Ravi V. Shah and Thomas J. Wang

INTRODUCTION

The clinical diagnosis of heart failure (HF) relies primarily on signs and symptoms of congestion, complemented by radiographic and echocardiographic studies. Unfortunately, most physical and historical criteria for the diagnosis of HF (e.g., jugular venous distension, rales, peripheral edema, and dyspnea) are variably present and may only modestly increase the likelihood of a correct diagnosis (1,2). In the past decade, a number of circulating biomarkers have been identified that are elevated in individuals with cardiac overload or overt HF, raising the hope that measurement of these biomarkers could assist in acute diagnosis of HF, as well as the determination of prognosis.

There are several features that characterize a clinically useful biomarker (3,4). Such a biomarker should (*i*) track with disease severity, (*ii*) change during administration of therapies known to be beneficial in the disease, (*iii*) be incrementally superior or additive to currently available prognostic indices, and (*iv*) have pathophysiologic plausibility. Furthermore, any novel biomarker must convey insight into prognosis, disease mechanism, or patient management beyond currently available biomarkers for HF. In addition, biomarkers should provide "orthogonal" information to currently available biomarkers to allow for improved diagnostic and prognostic discrimination (5).

Biomarkers in chronic HF have been divided into pathophysiologically distinct subgroups, including markers reflecting hemodynamic stress, neurohormonal activation, inflammation, and necrosis (4). In this chapter, we will review evidence supporting the role for different cardiovascular biomarkers in the diagnosis, prognosis, and subsequent management of patients with acute and chronic HF. We will comment on the utility of different biomarkers in patients with HF, and describe selected biomarkers that are currently under investigation (Table 14.1).

HEMODYNAMIC STRESS
Natriuretic Peptides

B-type natriuretic peptide (BNP) and N-terminal pro-BNP are the only two FDA-approved biomarkers for the diagnosis of HF (6). BNP exists in a family of structurally similar peptides (with atrial natriuretic peptide [ANP] and C-type natriuretic peptide [CNP]) synthesized in cardiomyocytes and released during conditions of pressure or volume overload (7). Physiologically, BNP induces vasodilatation and natriuresis (7). BNP is secreted initially in a pre-pro-BNP form, which is subsequently cleaved into the physiologically inactive but longer-lasting N-terminal pro-BNP and the active but more transient BNP fragment (7).

Table 14.1 Summary of Selected Cardiovascular Biomarkers in HF and Their Use for Diagnostic and Prognostic Purposes, and to Guide Therapy in Acute HF

Biomarker	Diagnosis	Prognosis	Guided Therapy
BNP	++ (8–13)	++ (14–20)	+/- (109,110)
NT-proBNP	++ (9–13)	++ (14–20)	+/- (109,110)
ST2	+ (47)	++ (44–47)	No evidence
Adrenomedullin	No evidence	+ (48–52)	No evidence
Cardiac troponin	No evidence	++ (54–57)	No evidence
Renin-angiotensin system markers	No evidence	+ (63–67)	No evidence
Matrix metalloproteinases	No evidence	+ (84–88)	No evidence
C-reactive protein	No evidence	+ (91,92)	No evidence
IL-6	No evidence	+ (94–96)	No evidence
TNFα	No evidence	+ (94–96)	No evidence

Note: ++, Strongly supported; +, Supported; +/–, Weakly supported.

BNP has a proven role in the exclusion of HF as a cause of dyspnea, but may be of limited value as a confirmatory test. In the Breathing Not Properly (BNP) study (8), Maisel and coworkers measured BNP in 1586 patients presenting to an emergency ward with undifferentiated acute dyspnea, subsequently diagnosed clinically as dyspnea due of HF or non-HF origin. Higher BNP levels were present in patients with HF and correlated with disease severity as indicated by New York Heart Association (NYHA) functional class. Although a BNP level >100 pg/mL was associated with a 30-fold higher risk of HF beyond other clinical markers of HF, BNP had a poor specificity (76%) and positive predictive value (79%) at this level, suggesting that the utility of BNP may be in "ruling-out" HF in patients presenting with acute dyspnea. In patients without a prior BNP measurement, reliance on a single elevated BNP alone for the diagnosis of HF may therefore lead to inaccurate diagnosis.

These results were extended by Januzzi et al. in the N-terminal Pro-BNP Investigation of Dyspnea in the Emergency Department (PRIDE) study (9). The presence of an elevated NT-proBNP was strongly associated with a HF diagnosis in patients with acute dyspnea. A cutoff value of <300 pg/mL to exclude HF had excellent operating characteristics, regardless of age (sensitivity and negative predictive value 99%). Furthermore, in patients with clinical HF and preserved left ventricular (LV) function, use of NT-proBNP to guide diagnosis led to a lower false-negative rate (missed HF diagnoses) as compared with BNP (10). Similar results have been reported in other studies of BNP and NT-proBNP (11–13).

Elevations in BNP and NT-proBNP may also have implications beyond diagnosis. In a study from patients enrolled in the Acute Decompensated Heart Failure National Registry (ADHERE), BNP elevations on admission predicted in-hospital mortality after LV function, renal function, systolic blood pressure, and other traditional risk markers were taken into account (14). Although single measurements of BNP and NT-pro-BNP are weakly correlated with filling pressures (15), serial increases in BNP during HF hospitalization and prior to discharge predict an elevated risk of mortality or readmission for HF (16–18). Similar data have been reported with NT-pro-BNP (19). Furthermore, increases in BNP over 12 months are prognostically informative (20). In addition, an NT-pro-BNP-guided strategy reduced 60-day re-hospitalization for HF by 35% and nearly $5,000 per patient in costs for subsequent outpatient and emergency visits over standard care (13).

BNP has been studied in a variety of other clinically important settings, including HF with preserved ejection fraction (diastolic HF) and asymptomatic LV dysfunction. BNP is elevated in patients with diastolic HF (21) and may correlate with the degree of diastolic abnormalities as assessed by echocardiography (22). Although BNP cannot be used to differentiate between normal and depressed LV function reliably, BNP levels are highest in the presence of both systolic and diastolic abnormalities (23). With regard to asymptomatic LV dysfunction, results from the Framingham Heart Study suggest that BNP may not detect asymptomatic LV dysfunction with high sensitivity (24). However, a later study suggested that use of BNP for whole population screening followed by echocardiography for validation may still be cost-effective (25).

Therapies for chronic HF have been shown to affect BNP and NT-proBNP. For instance, increases in BNP have been shown to be attenuated by valsartan (20) or enalapril (26). Patients with a higher NT-pro-BNP had a poorer survival at one year, with a nonsignificant trend toward lower mortality in patients receiving carvedilol (27). Accordingly, outpatient management of patients with stable HF targeted to lowering BNP levels may promote higher utilization of neurohormonal blockade (beta-blockers and angiotensin-converting enzyme inhibitors) and a lower risk for HF mortality or hospitalization (28). Declines in NT-pro-BNP level are significant and sustained at 18 months after implementation of cardiac resynchronization therapy (29), and elevated levels prior to implantation may even be predictive of response to resynchronization therapy (30). Finally, BNP may be a potent, independent predictor of sudden cardiac death in patients with advanced HF (31). In addition, there is ongoing investigation into the potential for natriuretic peptide-guided therapy in chronic and acute HF states (see "Potential for Biomarker-Guided Therapy In Acute HF" section below).

Despite their widespread utility in the diagnosis, prognosis, and potentially in the management of patients with chronic and acute HF, there are several limitations in the use of BNP or NT-pro-BNP in the diagnosis and management of HF. Natriuretic peptides can be elevated in a variety of other circumstances, including pulmonary embolism, sepsis, acute coronary syndrome, anemia, and atrial fibrillation (32). Other clinical characteristics that may lead to lower or higher natriuretic peptide levels, independent of heart failure, are obesity (lower) (33–37), renal dysfunction (higher) (38–40), female gender (higher), and advanced age (higher) (41,42). Although these factors do not appear to diminish the prognostic value of BNP or NT-proBNP measurements, there is controversy about whether cutpoints should be altered in certain situations.

ST2

ST2, an interleukin-1 (IL-1) receptor with both soluble and transmembrane forms, was shown to be overexpressed during mRNA microarray analysis of cultured cardiomyocytes exposed to biomechanical stress (43). ST2 is expressed both in a soluble isoform (measured in serum) and as a transmembrane receptor for which IL-33 serves as a ligand (43). IL-33 signaling via the transmembrane ST2 receptor has been shown to limit LV hypertrophy in response to pressure overload in mice, and soluble ST2 competitively inhibits the antihypertrophic action of IL-33 (43). In an aortic constriction model of cardiac pressure overload, ST2-deficient mice experience a greater increase in LV hypertrophy and decrement in LV function, effects that could not be rescued by treatment with IL-33 (43). This evidence suggests that the ST2/IL-33 system may serve as a self-regulating system to limit cardiac injury and remodeling.

A study on patients with HF has suggested a relationship between ST2 and cardiac structure and function, as well as prognosis. Shah et al. reported a significant relationship between higher ST2 levels during index admission for HF and larger LV dimension, and poorer LV and RV function (44). Furthermore, in a Cox regression model, including echocardiographic indices of cardiac structure and function, natriuretic peptides, ST2 independently predicted death at four years [hazard ratio (HR) = 2.70; P = 0.003] (44). The soluble form of ST2 can be detected in patients with LV dysfunction postmyocardial infarction (45). Interestingly, in patients with acute myocardial infarction, ST2 was predictive of cardiovascular mortality or HF independent of NT-proBNP level, and was additive to NT-proBNP in a model of risk prediction, even when other traditional clinical markers of disease severity were taken into account (46). In a study of 161 patients with advanced HF, ST2 level was modestly correlated with BNP and predicted death or need for cardiac transplantation (45). In the PRIDE study, ST2 levels were measured in patients with acute HF, with elevated ST2 levels higher in patients with HF and predictive of mortality at one year (47).

Although both ST2 and NT-proBNP are induced by myocyte stretch, the prognostic independence of these biomarkers suggests that there may be additional, distinct pathways for induction of ST2 yet undiscovered. Further studies to clarify the role of ST2 in diastolic HF and the utility of ST2-guided therapy above conventional clinical judgment and BNP-guided strategies are future areas of investigation.

ADRENOMEDULLIN

Adrenomedullin (ADM) is a widely expressed peptide hormone that increases cyclic AMP bioavailability with subsequent potent vasodilator and natriuretic effects (48,49). ADM has been primarily studied as a prognostic biomarker in acute and chronic HF. ADM is produced in the heart in proportion to severity of HF and LV dysfunction (50) and predicts mortality and hospitalization (48). Carvedilol attenuates the impact of high adrenomedullin levels on mortality (48), in agreement with the role of ADM in increasing cAMP activity, a pathway hindered by beta-blockade. Interestingly, adrenomedullin may also correlate with the presence of diastolic dysfunction (51).

Although the role of ADM in prognostication is clear, the difficulty with measuring ADM in plasma (due to protein binding and rapid metabolism (49)) limits its widespread clinical applicability. ADM is secreted in prohormone form as preproadrenomedullin (49). Of note, a midregional fragment of the prohormone, MR-proADM, is more stably measured, and has been shown to predict hospitalization or HF postmyocardial infarction independent of NT-proBNP (49). In a study of patients with acute HF, MR-proADM level was strongly associated with death at 90 days even after adjustment for concomitant NT-proBNP levels (52). Although ADM is a predictor of outcomes, ADM has not been widely investigated as a diagnostic marker.

CARDIAC TROPONIN

Cardiac troponins, routinely used as a sensitive marker of myocardial necrosis in acute coronary syndromes, are potent short- and long-term prognostic markers in acute and chronic HF. Persistent elevation in troponin T is associated with a greater degree of LV remodeling, lower ejection fraction, and worse long-term survival (53). In patients with chronic HF analyzed with a high-sensitivity troponin T assay (with a lower detection threshold 0.001 ng/mL), both positive troponin T and high-sensitivity troponin T predicted mortality and HF hospitalization in a dose-dependent fashion (54). However, when added to natriuretic peptides, troponins only modestly improved risk prediction (55), suggesting that these biomarkers may capture similar prognostic information.

The value of troponin in risk stratification has been extended to acute HF syndromes. In a substudy of the ADHERE registry, Peacock and coworkers examined the relationship between a positive cardiac troponin and short-term events (56). Patients with positive troponin (T or I) had more decompensated hemodynamics on admission (lower ejection fraction and systolic blood pressure) and higher mortality during the index hospitalization. Patients with a positive troponin also had a higher requirement for escalated therapies, including mechanical ventilation, need for and time in an intensive care unit, and mechanical circulatory support. In a different study, development or persistence of a positive troponin during therapy in the hospital was associated with higher mortality (57).

The pathophysiologic basis for elevated troponins in individuals with HF remains unclear. The troponins are found in two locations in the cardiomyocyte: cytosolic (<5%) and sarcomeric (>95%). It has been proposed that the troponin release occurs secondary to progressive cardiomyocyte loss from apopotosis or necrosis. Subendocardial "demand" ischemia leading to a troponin elevation has also been suggested, but largely unsupported. In a study of 71 patients with advanced nonischemic HF with normal coronary angiography, patients with a positive troponin I had more diastolic dysfunction and LV remodeling, with a similar overall ejection fraction as patients without a positive troponin (58). Other proposed mechanisms include oxidative stress, neurohormonal activation, microvascular ischemia, and enhanced cardiomyocyte protein turnover (55).

NEUROHORMONAL ACTIVATION

Early studies in patients with HF suggested that higher norepinephrine levels are associated with more severe HF (59,60). Renin, norepinephrine, and arginine vasopressin are elevated in patients with both asymptomatic LV dysfunction and symptomatic HF, with higher levels present in symptomatic patients (61). Higher norepinephrine levels are related to higher filling pressures and systemic vascular resistance and lower cardiac index (62). In addition to a relationship with hemodynamics and symptoms, higher levels of norepinephrine, aldosterone, angiotensin II, and endothelin have been linked to sudden death in patients with advanced HF (63–66). In patients with asymptomatic LV dysfunction, neurohormonal activation predicts incident HF as well as mortality (67). Angiotensin-converting enzyme inhibitors and angiotensin II receptor antagonists decrease neurohormonal activation in a sustained and significant fashion (63,68–70). Although the mechanistic and therapeutic insights provided by neurohormones in acute and chronic HF syndromes have heralded significant advances in HF, the short half-life of these molecules in the circulation, as well as the need for measurement under controlled conditions (e.g., morning supine collection, with minimization of the effect of intravenous catheter placement on neurohormone levels) have limited their widespread applicability in the management of patients with HF.

EXTRACELLULAR MATRIX REMODELING

Markers of collagen turnover, including matrix metalloproteinases (MMP), tissue inhibitors of MMP (TIMP), and procollagen type I and type III fragments (71–73), are also associated with prognosis in chronic HF. Increased MMP activity (particularly MMP-9, MMP-2, and MMP-3) has been consistently related to LV dilatation, poorer ejection fraction, functional status, and increased risk for mortality or HF hospitalization in patients postmyocardial infarction or with HF (74–79). Similarly, higher levels of TIMP-1 are associated with poorer LV function and mortality postmyocardial infarction (77) and with higher mortality in stable HF (80).

The critical feature of the MMP/TIMP system is a balance between extracellular matrix synthesis and degradation that produces ventricular remodeling in HF. It has been suggested that higher collagen turnover stimulated by higher MMP activity during myocardial infarction may stimulate TIMP activity to limit matrix disruption (77). Accordingly, TIMP and MMP expression is upregulated at the mRNA level in dilated cardiomyopathy (81), and both serum TIMP and MMP track with markers of neurohor-monal activation (82). In addition, the ratio of MMP-9 to TIMP-1 or TIMP-2 is markedly elevated in patients with HF, although this relationship does not hold for other isoforms of MMP (79). A higher ratio of MMP-1 to TIMP-1 expression has been associated with extensive LV remodeling and is higher in patients with systolic as compared with diastolic HF (83).

MMP levels respond to therapies for advanced HF, further suggesting a mechanistic link between matrix remodeling and prognosis in HF. In patients with chronic HF, spirono-lactone reduces collagen turnover, improving clinical outcomes in patients with elevated markers of collagen turnover (84). In addition, MMP-9 levels decrease in patients who exhibit reverse remodeling after cardiac resynchronization therapy (85). MMP-1 and MMP-8 expression is elevated in the myocardium of patients who need LV assist device support for advanced HF (86), and implantation of a LV assist device leads to higher TIMP-1 (87) and TIMP-3 expression (88) and lower MMP-1 and MMP-9 expression (88). Future research will be aimed at clarifying the role of these biomarkers in prognosis in and severity of diastolic HF (71) and at discovering novel markers of ventricular stiffness (e.g., advanced glycosylation endproducts (89)) in chronic HF.

INFLAMMATION
C-Reactive Protein
Inflammatory cytokines are important in the pathogenesis of HF and can serve as biomark-ers for HF progression (90). Levels of C-reactive protein (CRP) are correlated with symp-toms, neurohormonal activation, and prognosis (independent of BNP), and decrease with therapy in patients with HF (91,92). In addition, elevated levels of tumor necrosis factor-α (TNFα) are associated with more renal insufficiency, hyponatremia, and cardiac cachexia, markers of poor prognosis in HF (93). Both TNFα levels and IL-6 are related to symptom severity (94) and poorer hemodynamics (95), and IL-6 levels decline significantly after optimization of HF therapy (96).

Growth differentiation factor-15, a member of the transforming growth factor-β fam-ily, is induced in conditions of pressure overload and has been shown to limit hypertrophy when expressed in an in vivo animal model (97). GDF-15 has been shown to correlate with symptom class and mortality independent of classical markers, including NT-pro-BNP (98), in patients with HF.

In spite of their ability to forecast a poorer prognosis, the pathophysiologic signifi-cance of TNFα and IL-6 elaboration in HF remains unclear. Myocardial TNFα receptor expression was lower and soluble TNFα receptor expression was higher in a study of patients with dilated cardiomyopathy (99), suggesting that higher levels of soluble TNFα receptor may bind circulating TNFα and protect the myocardium from its effects (99,100). Alternatively, circulating TNFα–TNFα receptor complexes may liberate a steady state of serum TNFα, reinforcing its deleterious effects (100). In addition, TNFα appears to be expressed exclusively in the myocardium of patients with HF (not in normal myocardium), suggesting that cardiac TNFα may have a pathogenic role in the progression of HF (99). Unfortunately, TNFα antagonists have not proven useful in reduction of hard clinical end-points (death, HF hospitalization) in patients with chronic HF (101). Further work is neces-sary to clarify the significance of inflammatory biomarkers in the pathogenesis of HF, and the role for these biomarkers remains limited.

OXIDATIVE STRESS
Increasing evidence suggests that oxidative stress may be an important factor in the progres-sion of HF (102). In a study of patients with advanced HF, plasma levels of lipid peroxides

correlated with the clinical severity of HF (103). Elevated levels of 8-iso-prostaglandin $F_2\alpha$ in the pericardium of patients with advanced HF were associated with worse NYHA functional class and a greater extent of adverse LV remodeling (104). Further studies revealed that MMP-2 and MMP-9 levels were increased in patients with high levels of pericardial 8-iso-prostaglandin $F_2\alpha$ and chronic coronary artery disease without HF, and correlated with a more dilated LV (105), suggesting a link between oxidative stress and extracellular matrix remodeling in the pathogenesis of HF. Myeloperoxidase (106) and uric acid (107,108) are other markers of oxidative stress that have been correlated with symptom severity, hemodynamic severity, or survival. Further studies targeting markers of oxidative stress (e.g., allopurinol therapy for uric acid lowering) will clarify the therapeutic relevance of these biomarkers.

POTENTIAL FOR BIOMARKER-GUIDED THERAPY IN ACUTE HF

Aside from the role of cardiovascular biomarkers in the initial diagnosis and long-term prognosis of patients with acute HF, there has been considerable interest in the utility of serial biomarker testing to guide therapy in acute HF, specifically using natriuretic peptides. Troughton et al. (109) randomized 69 outpatients with advanced HF (LV ejection fraction <40%) to standard vs NT-proBNP-guided care, with a primary composite endpoint of cardiovascular death, worsening HF, or HF admission. Patients in the NT-proBNP-guided arm had a significantly lower NT-proBNP level on discharge and a lower composite endpoint in the NT-proBNP-guided cohort.

These results with NT-proBNP have been recapitulated with BNP in larger populations with ambulatory HF, including the BATTLESCARRED study. In BATTLES-CARRED, 364 patients with symptomatic HF were managed to NT-proBNP-guided versus non-natriuretic peptide (normal and "intensive" therapy)-guided groups and followed for a median 2.8 years with an endpoint of mortality and HF hospitalization (110). Use of NT-proBNP decreased all-cause mortality compared with usual care, but not the intensive care arm. Interestingly, younger patients (<75 years) enjoyed a greater benefit in terms of the primary endpoint with natriuretic peptide-guided therapy as compared with their older counterparts. Similar results were attained with BNP-guided therapy in the STARS-BNP trial (a reduction in HF mortality or hospitalization at a median of 15 months follow-up) (111) and the STARBRITE trial (higher hospitalization-free survival in BNP-guided arm at 90 days) (112).

The Trial of Intensified versus Standard Medical Therapy in Elderly Patients With Congestive Heart Failure (TIME-CHF) investigated a predominantly elderly (mean age 76 years) male cohort with systolic HF randomized to symptom-guided versus symptom- plus NT-proBNP-guided therapy (113) followed for 18 months for hospitalization and quality of life. There was no difference between NT-proBNP versus symptom-guided approach in all-cause hospitalization, but a lower rate of HF hospitalization in the NT-proBNP arm. In a cohort of patients younger than 75 years, there was a significant benefit in the overall survival with an NT-proBNP-guided strategy, in agreement with prior clinical evidence that a strategy targeting biomarker levels may be useful in younger patients.

There has been some concern regarding the generalizability of the TIME-CHF results. The older age cohort (>75 years old) were different from the younger cohort: more female, poorer renal function, and more atrial fibrillation, coronary disease, hypertension, with a higher LV ejection fraction and lower incidence of dilated cardiomyopathy. There is concern regarding the applicability of most neurohormonal therapies to older patients, given difficulties with tolerability with dose titration and inadequate evidence of benefit in this older population. In fact, fewer patients were on optimal HF therapy at target doses (e.g., beta-blockade and spironolactone). It is possible, therefore, that these patients may have been phenotypically distinct (e.g., more diastolic HF) from the typical ambulatory HF patient, with less latitude for achieving target medication doses.

The Pro-BNP-Guided Therapy of Chronic Heart Failure to Improve Heart Failure Morbidity and Mortality (PRIMA) study randomized 345 patients after index admission for HF to symptom- or NT-proBNP-guided therapy (targeting a postdischarge natriuretic peptide level) with a maximal follow-up of one year (114). Again, the mean age was over 70 years in both groups with systolic HF. Although there was no effect on mortality or HF hospitalization overall, patients in the NT-proBNP-guided arm who actually attained their target natriuretic peptide level enjoyed a significantly lower mortality as compared with patients in the clinical only arm. These results suggest that patients who can maintain a lower NT-proBNP level in follow-up may have better outcomes than patients who are managed with usual care alone.

In a meta-analysis of six trials, including the study by Troughton et al. (109), STARS-BNP (111), STARBRITE (112), TIME-CHF (113), BATTLESCARRED (110), and PRIMA (114), Felker et al. found a statistically significant 31% reduction in the risk of death with BNP or NT-proBNP-guided HF management (115). Although routine NT-proBNP-guided therapy in the inpatient or outpatient setting cannot be routinely advocated based on randomized evidence, these results suggest that in select populations (younger individuals with systolic HF), a natriuretic peptide-guided approach may offer clinical benefit. The PROTECT study was published a year or two ago (PMID: 22018299) and NORTHSTAR (116), we should have a clearer picture of the role of serial measurement of natriuretic peptides in the management of acute HF.

CURRENT ISSUES IN BIOMARKER RESEARCH: LIMITATIONS AND FUTURE DIRECTIONS

Despite their widespread use in the diagnosis and prognosis assessment in acute and chronic HF states, certain issues surrounding the broader clinical utility of biomarkers remain. Any proposed biomarker must add to diagnosis or prognosis independent of other markers of clinical risk. Natriuretic peptides and ST2 concentrations, for example, have been found to be related to risk independent of traditional clinical or echocardiographic indices (14,44). Nevertheless, the majority of clinical risk is determined by these traditional risk factors, and thus novel biomarkers lead to only modest changes in discrimination between individuals who achieve an outcome and those who do not. For example, in Val-HeFT, the addition of high-sensitivity troponin to clinical risk factors only effected a small change in C statistic (54). In addition, models of clinical risk that include traditional risk factors and biomarker measurements must accurately predict the actual risk faced by these patients, referred to as calibration. As an example, in the Val-HeFT cohort, addition of high-sensitivity troponin did not improve the calibration of an already well-calibrated model that included traditional risk factors, e.g. addition of troponin did not improve how closely the model estimated the actual rate of mortality (54).

In order to improve discrimination, several groups have attempted a multiple biomarker strategy in the diagnosis and prognosis of HF. For example, Januzzi et al. found addition of elevated ST2 concentrations to elevated NT-proBNP levels identified a cohort of patients with HF who were at a significantly higher risk of death at four years, when compared with elevated ST2 or NT-proBNP concentration alone (117).

Newer technologies that systematically profile large numbers of molecules may facilitate the identification of new HF biomarkers (5). For instance, a microarray analysis of total RNA isolated from endomyocardial biopsies of patients with advanced HF discovered a panel of 45 transcripts that identified patients who had a poorer prognosis (death, need for mechanical circulatory support, or transplantation), with a sensitivity of 74% (118). Mass spectrometry and nuclear magnetic resonance are other tools that have been used to generate molecular signatures in plasma or serum in individuals with cardiovascular disease (119).

CONCLUSION

Biomarkers of HF could serve as prognostic and diagnostic adjuncts to standard clinical and laboratory assessment. Ideal biomarkers are rapidly and reproducibly assessed, and can provide incremental information above traditional risk factors. Although natriuretic peptides remain the benchmark for biomarkers in HF, other markers of myocardial stretch, inflammation, oxidative stress, and remodeling also appear to provide prognostic information and insights into mechanisms involved in HF progression.

New technologies for biomarker discovery, including genome-wide transcriptional analysis and real-time analysis of metabolic byproducts, may provide a way to identify novel biomarkers for diagnosing acute and chronic HF. Future methods to integrate metabolic, genomic, and serum biomarkers to produce a composite prognostic index in chronic HF and asymptomatic LV dysfunction may allow early targeting of high-risk populations and more aggressive therapies in patients with established HF.

REFERENCES

1. Gheorghiade M, Zannad F, Sopko G, et al. Acute heart failure syndromes: current state and framework for future research. Circulation 2005; 112: 3958–68.
2. Wang CS, FitzGerald JM, Schulzer M, Mak E, Ayas NT. Does this dyspneic patient in the emergency department have congestive heart failure? JAMA 2005; 294: 1944–56.
3. Morrow DA, de Lemos JA. Benchmarks for the assessment of novel cardiovascular biomarkers. Circulation 2007; 115: 949–52.
4. Braunwald E. Biomarkers in heart failure. N Engl J Med 2008; 358: 2148–59.
5. Gerszten RE, Wang TJ. The search for new cardiovascular biomarkers. Nature 2008; 451: 949–52.
6. Hunt SA, Abraham WT, Chin MH, et al. ACC/AHA 2005 Guideline Update for the Diagnosis and Management of Chronic Heart Failure in the Adult: summary article. Circulation 2005; 112: 1825–52.
7. Daniels L, Maisel A. Natriuretic peptides. JACC 2007; 50: 2357–68.
8. Maisel A, Krishnaswamy P, Nowak RM, et al. Rapid measurement of B-type natriuretic peptide in the emergency diagnosis of heart failure. N Engl J Med 2002; 347: 161–7.
9. Januzzi J, Camargo CA, Anwaruddin S, et al. The N-terminal pro-BNP investigation of dyspnea in the emergency department (PRIDE) study. Am J Cardiol 2005; 95: 948–54.
10. O'Donoghue M, Chen A, Baggish AL, et al. The effects of ejection fraction on N-terminal ProBNP and BNP levels in patients with acute CHF: analysis from the PRIDE study. J Card Fail 2005; 11: S9–S14.
11. Lee S, Stevens TL, Sandberg SM, et al. The potential of brain natriuretic peptide as a biomarker for New York Heart Association class during the outpatient treatment of heart failure. J Card Fail 2002; 8: 149–54.
12. Morrison LK, Harrison A, Krishnaswamy P, et al. Utility of a rapid B-natriuretic peptide assay in differentiating congestive heart failure from lung disease in patients presenting with dyspnea. JACC 2002; 39: 202–9.
13. Moe G, Howlett J, Januzzi JL, et al. N-terminal pro-B-type natriuretic peptide testing improves the management of patients with suspected acute heart failure. Circulation 2007; 115: 3103–10.
14. Fonarow G, Peacock WF, Phillips CO, et al. Admission B-type natriuretic peptide levels and in-hospital mortality in acute decompensated heart failure. JACC 2007; 49: 1943–50.
15. Forfia P, Watkins SP, Rame JE, et al. Relationship between B-type natriuretic peptides and pulmonary capillary wedge pressure in the intensive care unit. JACC 2005; 45: 1667–71.
16. Logeart D, Thabut G, Jourdain P, et al. Predischarge B-type natriuretic peptide assay for identifying patients at high risk for re-admission after decompensated heart failure. JACC 2004; 43: 635–41.

17. Cheng V, Kazanagra R, Garcia A, et al. A rapid bedside test for B-type peptide predicts treatment outcomes in patients admitted for decompensated heart failure: a pilot study. JACC 2001; 37: 386–91.

18. Bettencourt P, Ferreira S, Azevedo A, et al. Preliminary data on the potential usefulness of B-type natriuretic peptide levels in predicting outcome after hospital discharge in patients with heart failure. Am J Med 2002; 113: 215–19.

19. Januzzi J, van Kimmenade R, Lainchbury J, et al. NT-proBNP testing for diagnosis and short-term prognosis in acute destabilized heart failure: an international pooled analysis of 1256 patients. Eur Heart J 2006; 27: 330–7.

20. Anand I, Fisher LD, Chiang YT, et al. Changes in brain natriuretic peptide and norepinephrine over time and mortality and morbidity in the Valsartan Heart Failure trial (Val-HeFT). Circulation 2003; 107: 1278–83.

21. Yamaguchi H, Yoshida J, Yamamoto K, et al. Elevated of plasma brain natriuretic peptide is a hallmark of diastolic heart failure independent of ventricular hypertrophy. JACC 2004; 43: 55–60.

22. Lubien E, DeMaria A, Krishnaswamy P, et al. Utility of B-natriuretic peptide in detecting diastolic dysfunction: comparison with Doppler velocity recordings. Circulation 2002; 105: 595–601.

23. Krishnaswamy P, Lubien E, Clopton P, et al. Utility of B-natriuretic peptide levels in identifying patients with left ventricular systolic or diastolic dysfunction. Am J Med 2001; 111: 274–9.

24. Vasan R, Benjamin EJ, Larson MG, et al. Plamsa natriuretic peptides for community-based screening for left ventricular hypertrophy and systolic dysfunction: the Framingham heart study. JAMA 2002; 288: 1252–9.

25. Heidenreich PA, Gubens MA, Fonarow GC, et al. Cost-effectiveness of screening with B-type natriuretic peptide to identify patients with reduced left ventricular ejection fraction. JACC 2004; 43: 1019–26.

26. Yoshimura M, Mizuno Y, Nakayama M, et al. B-type natriuretic peptide as a marker of the effects of enalapril in patients with heart failure. Am J Med 2002; 112: 716–20.

27. Hartmann F, Packer M, Coats AJ, et al. Prognostic impact of plasma N-terminal pro-brain natriuretic peptide in severe chronic congestive heart failure: a substudy of the Carvedilol Prospective Randomized Cumulative Survival (COPERNICUS) trial. Circulation 2004; 110: 1780–6.

28. Jourdain P, Jondeau G, Funck F, et al. Plasma brain natriuretic peptide-guided therapy to improve outcome in heart failure: the STARS-BNP Multicenter Study. JACC 2007; 49: 1733–9.

29. Fruhwald F, Fahrleitner-Pammer A, Berger R, et al. Early and sustained effects of cardiac resynchronization therapy on N-terminal pro-B type natriuretic peptide in patients with moderate to severe heart failure and cardiac dyssynchrony. Eur Heart J 2007; 28: 1592–7.

30. Lellouche N, De Diego C, Cesario DA, et al. Usefulness of preimplantation B-type natriuretic peptide level for predicting response to cardiac resynchronization therapy. Am J Cardiol 2007; 99: 242–6.

31. Berger R, Huelsman M, Strecker K, et al. B-type natriuretic peptide predicts sudden death in patients with chronic heart failure. Circulation 2002; 105: 2392–7.

32. Omland T. Advanced in congestive heart failure management in the intensive care unit: B-type natriuretic peptides in evaluation of acute heart failure. Crit Care Med 2008; 36: 17–27.

33. Krauser D, Lloyd-Jones DM, Chae CU, et al. Effect of body mass index on natriuretic peptide levels in patients with acute congestive heart failure: a ProBNP Investigation of Dyspnea in the Emergency Department (PRIDE) substudy. Am Heart J 2005; 149: 744–50.

34. Wang T, Larson MG, Levy D, et al. Impact of obesity on plasma natriuretic peptide levels. Circulation 2004; 109: 594–600.

35. Das S, Drazner MH, Dries DL, et al. Impact of body mass and body composition on circulating levels of natriuretic peptides: results from the Dallas Heart Study. Circulation 2005; 112: 2163–8.

36. Daniels L, Clopton P, Bhalla V, et al. How obesity affects the cut-points for B-type natriuretic peptide in the diagnosis of acute heart failure. Results from the Breathing Not Properly Multinational Study. Am Heart J 2006; 151: 999–1005.

37. Horwich T, Hamilton M, Fonarow G. B-type natriuretic peptide levels in obese patients with advanced heart failure. JACC 2006; 47: 85–90.

38. Anwaruddin S, Lloyd-Jones DM, Baggish A, et al. Renal function, congestive heart failure, and amino-terminal pro-brain natriuretic peptide measurement: results from the ProBNP Investigation of Dyspnea in the Emergency Department (PRIDE) Study. JACC 2006; 47: 91–7.

39. Tsutamoto T, Wada A, Sakai H, et al. Relationship between renal function and plasma brain natriuretic peptide in patients with heart failure. JACC 2006; 47: 582–6.

40. McCullough PA, Duc P, Omland T, et al. B-type natriuretic peptide and renal function in the diagnosis of heart failure: an analysis from the Breathing Not Properly Multinational Study. Am J Kidney Dis 2003; 41: 571–9.

41. Wang T, Larson MG, Levy D, et al. Impact of age and sex on plasma natriuretic peptide levels in healthy adults. Am J Cardiol 2002; 90: 254–8.

42. Redfield M, Rodeheffer RJ, Jacobsen SJ, et al. Plasma brain natriuretic peptide concentration: impact of age and gender. JACC 2002; 40: 976–82.

43. Sanada S, Hakuno D, Higgins LJ, et al. IL-33 and ST2 comprise a critical biomechanically induced and cardioprotective signaling system. J Clin Invest 2007; 117: 1538–49.

44. Shah R, Chen-Tournoux AA, Picard MH, et al. Serum levels of the interleukin-1 receptor family member ST2, cardiac structure and function, and long-term mortality in patients with acute dyspnea. Circ Heart Fail 2009; 2: 311–19.

45. Weinberg E, Shimpo M, Hurwitz S, et al. Identification of serum soluble ST2 receptor as a novel heart failure biomarker. Circulation 2003; 107: 721–6.

46. Sabatine M, Morrow DA, Higgins LJ, et al. Complementary roles for biomarkers of biomechanical strain ST2 and N-terminal prohormone B-type natriuretic peptide in patients with ST-elevation myocardial infarction. Circulation 2008; 117: 1936–44.

47. Januzzi JL Jr, Peacock WF, Maisel AS, et al. Measurement of the interleukin family member ST2 in patients with acute dyspnea: results from the PRIDE (Pro-Brain Natriuretic Peptide Investigation of Dyspnea in the Emergency Department) study. JACC 2007; 50: 607–13.

48. Richards AM, Doughty R, Nicholls MG, et al. Plasma N-terminal pro-brain natriuretic peptide and adrenomedullin: prognostic utility and prediction of benefit from carvedilol in chronic ischemic left ventricular dysfunction. JACC 2001; 37: 1781–7.

49. Khan SQ, O'Brien RJ, Struck J, et al. Prognostic value of midregional pro-adrenomedullin in patients with acute myocardial infarction: the LAMP study. JACC 2007; 49: 1525–32.

50. Jougasaki M, Rodeheffer RJ, Redfield MM, et al. Cardiac secretion of adrenomedullin in human heart failure. J Clin Invest 1996; 97: 2370–6.

51. Yu C, Cheung BM, Leung R, et al. Increase in plasma adrenomedullin in patients with heart failure characterized by diastolic dysfunction. Heart 2001; 86: 155–60.

52. Anker S. BACH trial. In: American Heart Association Annual Scientific Sessions. New Orleans, LA: 2008.

53. Sato Y, Yamada T, Taniguchi R, et al. Persistently increased serum concentrations of cardiac troponin T in patients with idiopathic dilated cardiomyopathy are predictive of adverse outcomes. Circulation 2001; 103: 369–74.

54. Latini R, Masson S, Anand IS, et al. Prognostic value of very low plasma concentrations of troponin T in patients with stable chronic heart failure. Circulation 2007; 116: 1242–9.

55. Wang T. Significance of circulating troponin in heart failure: if these walls could talk. Circulation 2007; 116: 1217–20.

56. Peacock W, De Marco T, Fonarow GC, et al. Cardiac troponin and outcome in acute heart failure. N Engl J Med 2008; 358: 2117–26.

57. Del Carlo C, Pereira-Barretto AC, Cassaro-Strunz C, et al. Serial measure of cardiac troponin T levels for prediction of clinical events in decompensated heart failure. J Card Fail 2004; 10: 43–8.

58. Logeart D, Beyne P, Cusson C, et al. Evidence of cardiac myolylsis in severe nonischemic heart failure and the potential role of increased wall strain. Am Heart J 2001; 141: 247–53.

59. Chidsey C, Braunwald E, Morrow A. Stores of norepinephrine in congestive heart failure. Am J Med 1965; 30: 442–51.

60. Thomas J, Marks B. Plasma norepinephrine in congestive heart failure. Am J Cardiol 1978; 41: 233–43.

61. Francis G, Benedict C, Johnstone DE, et al. Comparison of neuroendocrine activation in patients with left ventricular dysfunction with and without congestive heart failure. A substudy of the Studies of Left Ventricular Dysfunction (SOLVD). Circulation 1990; 82: 1724–9.

62. Levine T, Francis GS, Goldsmith SR, et al. Activity of the sympathetic nervous system and renin-angiotensin system assessed by plasma hormone levels and their relation to hemodynamic abnormalities in congestive heart failure. Am J Cardiol 1982; 49: 1659–66.

63. Swedberg K, Eneroth P, Kjekshus J, et al. Hormones regulating cardiovascular function in patients with severe congestive heart failure and their relation to mortality. CONSENSUS Trial Study Group. Circulation 1990; 82: 1730–6.

64. Masson S, Latini R, Anand IS, et al. The prognostic value of big endothelin-1 in more than 2,300 patients with heart failure enrolled in the Valsartan Heart Failure Trial (Val-HeFT). J Card Fail 2006; 12: 375–9.

65. Anand I, Fisher LD, Chiang YT, et al. Changes in brain natriuretic peptide and norepinephrine over time and mortality and morbidity in the Valsartan Heart Failure Trial (Val-HeFT). Circulation 2003; 107: 1278–83.

66. Hulsmann M, Stanek B, Frey B, et al. Value of cardiopulmonary exercise testing and big endothelin plasma levels to predict short-term prognosis of patients with chronic heart failure. JACC 1998; 32: 1695–700.
67. Benedict C, Shelton B, Johnstone DE, et al. Prognostic significance of plasma norepinephrine in patients with asymptomatic left ventricular dysfunction. Circulation 1996; 94: 690–7.
68. Benedict C, Francis GS, Shelton B, et al. Effect of long-term enalapril therapy on neurohormones in patients with left ventricular dysfunction. Am J Cardiol 1995; 75: 1151–7.
69. Cohn J, Anand IS, Latini R, et al. Sustained reduction of aldosterone in response to the angiotensin receptor blocker valsartan in patients with chronic heart failure: results from the Valsartan Heart Failure trial. Circulation 2003; 108: 1306–9.
70. Latini R, Masson S, Anand I, et al. Effects of valsartan on circulating brain natriuretic peptide and norepinpehrine in symptomatic chronic heart failure: the Valsartan Heart Failure trial (Val-HeFT). Circulation 2002; 106: 2454–8.
71. Cicoira M, Rossi A, Bonapace S, et al. Independent and additional prognostic value of aminoterminal propeptide of type III procollagen circulation levels in patients with chronic heart failure. J Card Fail 2004; 10: 403–11.
72. Spinale F, Coker ML, Krombach SR, et al. Matrix metalloproteinase inhibition during the development of congestive heart failure: effects on left ventricular dimensions and function. Circulation Res 1999; 85: 364–76.
73. Martos R, Baugh J, Ledwidge M, et al. Diastolic heart failure: evidence of increased myocardial collagen turnover linked to diastolic dysfunction. Circulation 2007; 115: 888–95.
74. Ohtsuka T, Nishimura K, Kurata A, et al. Serum matrix metalloproteinase-3 as a novel marker for risk stratification of patients with nonischemic dilated cardiomyopathy. J Card Fail 2007; 13: 752–8.
75. George J, Patal S, Wexler D, et al. Circulating matrix metalloproteinase-2 but not matrix metalloproteinase-3, matrix metalloproteinase-9, or tissue inhibitor of metalloproteinase-1 predicts outcomes in patients with congestive heart failure. Am Heart J 2005; 150: 484–7.
76. Yan A, Yan RT, Spinale FG, et al. Plasma matrix metalloproteinase-9 level is correlated with left ventricular volumes and ejection fraction in patients with heart failure. J Card Fail 2006; 12: 514–19.
77. Kelly D, Khan SQ, Thompson M, et al. Plasma tissue inhibitor of metalloproteinase-1 and matrix metalloproteinase-9: novel indicators of left ventricular remodeling and prognosis after acute myocardial infarction. Eur Heart J 2008; 29: 2116–24.
78. Squire I, Evans J, Ng LL, et al. Plasma MMP-9 and MMP-2 following acute myocardial infarction in man: correlation with echocardiographic and neurohormonal parameters of left ventricular dysfunction. J Card Fail 2004; 10: 328–33.
79. Wilson E, Gunasinghe HR, Coker ML, et al. Plasma matrix metalloproteinase and inhibitor profiles in patients with heart failure. J Card Fail 2002; 8: 390–8.
80. Frantz S, Stork S, Michels K, et al. Tissue inhibitor of metalloproteinases levels [sic] in patients with chronic heart failure: an independent predictor of mortality. Eur J Heart Fail 2008; 10: 388–95.
81. Sivakumar P, Gupta S, Sarkar S, et al. Upregulation of lysyl oxidase and MMPs during cardiac remodeling in human dilated cardiomyopathy. Mol Cell Biochem 2008; 307: 159–67.
82. Yan A, Yan RT, Spinale FG, et al. Relationships between plasma levels of matrix metalloproteinases and neurohormonal profile in patients with heart failure. Eur J Heart Fail 2008; 10: 125–8.
83. Lopez B, Gonzalez A, Querejeta R, et al. Alterations in the pattern of collagen deposition may contribute to the deterioration of systolic function in hypertensive patients with heart failure. JACC 2006; 48: 89–96.
84. Zannad F, Alla F, Dousset B, et al. Limitation of excessive extracellular matrix turnover may contribute to survival benefit of spironolactone therapy in patients with congestive heart failure: insights from the randomized aldactone evaluation study (RALES). Circulation 2000; 102: 2700–6.
85. Hessel M, Bleeker GB, Bax JJ, et al. Reverse ventricular remodeling after cardiac resynchronization therapy is associated with a reduction in serum tenascin-C and plasma matrix metalloproteinase-9 levels. Eur J Heart Fail 2007; 9: 1058–63.
86. Felkin L, Birks EJ, George R, et al. A quantitative gene expression profile of metalloproteinases (MMPS) and their inhibitors (TIMPS) in the myocardium of patients with deteriorating heart failure requiring left ventricular assist device support. J Heart Lung Transplant 2006; 25: 1413–19.
87. Klotz S, Foronjy RF, Dickstein ML, et al. Mechanical unloading during left ventricular assist device support increases left ventricular collagen cross-linking and myocardial stiffness. Circulation 2005; 112: 364–74.
88. Li Y, Feng Y, McTiernan CF, et al. Downregulation of matrix metalloproteinases and reduction in collagen damage in the failing human heart after support with left ventricular assist devices. Circulation 2001; 104: 1147–52.

89. Shapiro B, Owan TE, Mohammed SF, et al. Advanced glycation end products accumulate in vascular smooth muscle and modify vascular but not ventricular properties in elderly hypertensive canines. Circulation 2008; 118: 1002–10.

90. Seta Y, Shan K, Bozkurt B, et al. Basic mechanisms in heart failure: the cytokine hypothesis. J Card Fail 1996; 2: 243–9.

91. Elster S, Braunwald E, Wood H. A study of C-reactive protein in the serum of patients with congestive heart failure. Am Heart J 1956; 51: 533–41.

92. Anand I, Latini R, Florea VG, et al. C-reactive protein in heart failure: prognostic value and the effect of valsartan. Circulation 2005; 112: 1428–34.

93. Levine B, Kalman J, Mayer L, et al. Elevated circulating levels of tumor necrosis factor in severe chronic heart failure. N Engl J Med 1990; 323: 236–41.

94. Torre-Amione G, Kapadia S, Benedict C, et al. Proinflammatory cytokine levels in patients with depressed left ventricular ejection fraction: a report from the Studies of Left Ventricular Dysfunction (SOLVD). JACC 1996; 27: 1201–6.

95. Tsutamoto T, Hisanaga T, Wada A, et al. Interleukin-6 spillover in the peripheral circulation increases with the severity of heart failure, and the high plasma level of interleukin-6 is an important prognostic predictor in patients with congestive heart failure. JACC 1998; 31: 391–8.

96. Maeda K, Tsutamoto T, Wada A, et al. High levels of plasma brain natriuretic peptide and interleukin-6 after optimized treatment for heart failure are independent risk factors for morbidity and mortality in patients with congestive heart failure. JACC 2000; 36: 1587–93.

97. Xu J, Kimball TR, Lorenz JN, et al. GDF15/MIC-1 functions as a protective and antihypertrophic factor released from the myocardium in association with SMAD protein activation. Circulation Res 2006; 98: 342–50.

98. Kempf T, von Haehling S, Peter T, et al. Prognostic utility of growth differentiation factor-15 in patients with chronic heart failure. JACC 2007; 50: 1054–60.

99. Torre-Amione G, Kapadia S, Lee J, et al. Tumor necrosis factor-α and tumor necrosis factor receptors in the failing human heart. Circulation 1996; 93: 704–11.

100. Packer M. Is tumor necrosis factor an important neurohormonal mechanism in chronic heart failure? Circulation 1995; 92: 1379–82.

101. Anker SD, Coats AJ. How to RECOVER from RENAISSANCE? The significance of the results of RECOVER, RENAISSANCE, RENEWAL and ATTACH. Int J Cardiol 2002; 86:123–30.

102. Grieve D, Shah A. Oxidative stress in heart failure: more than just damage. Eur Heart J 2003; 24: 2161–3.

103. Keith M, Geranmayegan A, Sole MJ, et al. Increased oxidative stress in patients with congestive heart failure. JACC 1998; 31: 1352–6.

104. Mallat Z, Philip I, Lebret M, et al. Elevated levels of 8-iso-prostaglandin F2α in pericardial fluid of patients with heart failure: a potential role for in vivo oxidant stress in ventricular dilatation and progression to heart failure. Circulation 1998; 97: 1536–9.

105. Kameda K, Matsunaga T, Abe N, et al. Correlation of oxidative stress with activity of matrix metalloproteinase in patients with coronary artery disease: possible role for left ventricular remodeling. Eur Heart J 2003; 24: 2180–5.

106. Tang W, Brennan ML, Philip K, et al. Plasma myeloperoxidase levels in patients with chronic heart failure. Am J Cardiol 2006; 98: 796–9.

107. Anker S, Doehner W, Rauchhaus M, et al. Uric acid and survival in chronic heart failure: validation and application in metabolic, functional, and hemodynamic staging. Circulation 2003; 107: 1991–7.

108. Kittleson MM, St Jhon ME, Bead V, et al. Increased levels of uric acid predict hemodynamic compromise in patients with heart failure independently of B-type natriuretic peptide levels. Heart 2007; 93: 365–7.

109. Troughton RW, Frampton CM, Yandle TG, et al. Treatment of heart failure guided by plasma aminoterminal brain natriuretic peptide (N-BNP) concentrations. Lancet 2000; 355: 1126–30.

110. Richards AM, Lainchbury JG, Troughton RW, et al. NT-proBNP-Guided treatment for chronic heart failure: results from the battlescarred trial (abstract 5946). Circulation 2008; 118S: 1035–6.

111. Jourdain P, Jondeau G, Funck F, et al. Plasma brain natriuretic peptide-guided therapy to improve outcome in heart failure: the STARS-BNP Multicenter Study. J Am Coll Cardiol 2007; 49: 1733–9.

112. Shah M. STARBRITE: a randomized pilot trial of BNP-guided therapy in patients with advanced heart failure. Circulation 2006; 114: II528.

113. Pfisterer M, Buser P, Rickli H, et al. BNP-guided vs symptom-guided heart failure therapy: the trial of intensified vs standard medical therapy in elderly patients with congestive heart failure (TIME-CHF) randomized trial. JAMA 2009; 301: 383–92.

114. Cleland J, Coletta AP, Clark AL, et al. Clinical trials update from the American College of Cardiology 2009: ADMIRE-HF, PRIMA, STICH, REVERSE, IRIS, partial ventricular support, FIX-HF-5, vagal stimulation, REVIVAL-3, pre-RELAX-AHF, ACTIVE-A, HF-ACTION, JUPITER, AURORA, and OMEGA. Eur J Heart Fail 2009; 11: 622–30.
115. Felker G, Hasselblad V, Hernandez AF, et al. Biomarker-guided therapy in chronic heart failure: a meta-analysis of randomized controlled trials. Am Heart J 2009; 158: 422–30.
116. Schou M, Gustafsson F, Videbaek L, et al. Design and methodology of the NorthStar Study: NT-proBNP stratified follow-up in outpatient heart failure clinics – a randomized Danish multicenter study. Am Heart J 2008; 156: 649–55.
117. Rehman S, Januzzi J, Mueller T. Characteristics of the novel interleukin family biomarker ST2 in patients with acute heart failure. J Am Coll Cardiol 2008; 52: 1458–65.
118. Heidecker B, Kasper EK, Wittstein IS, et al. Transcriptomic biomarkers for individual risk assessment in new-onset heart failure. Circulation 2008; 118: 238–46.
119. Lewis G, Asnani A, Gerszten R. Application of metabolomics to cardiovascular biomarker and pathway discovery. JACC 2008; 52: 117–23.

15

Noninvasive imaging modalities for the evaluation of heart failure

Kimberly A. Parks, Malissa J. Wood, Ian S. Rogers, and Godtfred Holmvang

INTRODUCTION

Noninvasive imaging plays an important role in the diagnosis and management of heart failure. It is critical in determining the etiology of heart failure and is useful in assessing response to treatment and in monitoring progression of disease. The advent of new technology has brought about many novel techniques in the assessment of cardiac structure as well as mechanical and physiologic function. With the increasing armamentarium of imaging tools available, it is important for the clinician to discern which modality to choose in a given clinical scenario.

The oldest, most widely accepted technique is echocardiography, and it remains the "test of choice" for the initial evaluation of heart failure. Radionuclide methods, computed tomography, magnetic resonance imaging (MRI) and positron emission tomography (PET) have become more widely recognized techniques for evaluation of cardiac structure and function.

This chapter provides an overview of the current technologies available for noninvasive imaging in the heart failure patient, including their strengths and limitations, and role in the diagnosis and management of heart failure.

PART 1: ECHOCARDIOGRAPHY

Ultrasound has been used in the diagnosis of cardiac disease for over half a century. It was first studied as a medical diagnostic tool in the 1950s by German physicist Wolf-Deiter Keidel who discovered a method for recording cardiac rhythmic volume variations. The first clinical use of echocardiography was in the diagnosis of pericardial effusion and mitral valve disease in the early 1950s using M-Mode echocardiography (1). This discovery led to the development of Doppler, two-dimensional (2-D) echocardiography, contrast echocardiography and transesophageal imaging. Findings that left ventricular (LV) wall thickness, internal dimensions, stroke volume, ejection fraction, and valvular regurgitation could all be measured by ultrasonography were reported in the 1960s (2–4). Newer techniques include three-dimensional (3-D) imaging, tissue Doppler, Strain, tissue synchronization, vector imaging, and tissue tracking imaging.

Echocardiography remains a first line tool for the diagnosis and treatment of heart failure and the cardiomyopathies. It is safe, easy, and accurate. There is no radiation exposure and there have been no patient injuries reported to date from the use of ultrasound. It can identify structural abnormalities and can be used to provide valuable information about hemodynamics, such as cardiac output and pulmonary artery pressures. Echocardiography is an excellent means for assessing a patient's response to therapy and can provide important prognostic information.

One of the first heart failure trials to use echocardiography as a means to provide prognostic information was the SAVE trial, which demonstrated that increased LV size after myocardial infarction was associated with adverse cardiac events (5). The next landmark trial was the BEST trial, which showed that the strongest predictors of survival in patients with an ejection fraction of 35% or less were severity of mitral regurgitation, LV end-diastolic volume, and deceleration time of early diastolic mitral inflow velocity (6). There have been numerous subsequent trials using echocardiography to assess prognosis in patients with heart failure.

Left Ventricular Structure and Function

Echocardiography provides a means to evaluate structural and physiologic data during the entire cardiac cycle, providing meaningful information during systole and diastole. The following section will discuss quantitative and qualitative measures of both systolic and diastolic performance, as each contribute to interpreting the diagnosis and assessing symptomatology in the heart failure patient.

Systolic performance can be assessed using M-Mode, 2-D, 3-D, and Doppler methods.

ASSESSMENT OF VENTRICULAR MASS AND VOLUME

As pathologic conditions develop in the myocardium, there are complex changes in contractile function and in loading conditions to the ventricle. Morphologic changes occur as a result and LV mass increases.

Mass and volume can be assessed using M-mode, 2-D, and 3-D echocardiography.

3-D echocardiography with harmonic imaging is the most accurate ultrasound technique for measuring LV mass and has been shown to have significantly less intraobserver variability compared with 2-D imaging (7). When contrast agents are used during 2-D echo assessment of LV volume, however, accuracy is comparable to measurements obtained with 3-D, noncontrast imaging (8).

Ventricular volume, mass, and shape can be accurately assessed using M-Mode echocardiography. A single line is obtained at the level of the mitral valve chordae in the parasternal long and short axes. Measurements are made from leading edge to leading edge beginning from anterior to posterior. The septal wall thickness (IVS), posterior wall thickness (PWT), and the diastolic LV internal dimension are all measured during end diastole. The systolic LV internal dimension is measured during end systole. Respiratory shifts in position of the heart as the diaphragm flattens in diastole and malalignment of the M-mode beam during acquisition of data can both lead to errors in measurements. LV mass is calculated using a cube formula, thus small errors in acquisition of data can lead to large errors in the calculation of LV mass. LV hypertrophy (LVH) in general is defined by echo as an LV mass greater than 224 g in men and greater than 162 g in women. The ASE-recommended cube formula for determining LV mass can be used with LV linear dimensions and is defined as (9):

$$\text{LV mass} = 0.8 \times \{1.04\,[(\text{IVS} + \text{LVID} + \text{PWT})^3 - \text{LVID}^3]\} + 0.6\,\text{g}$$

As LV mass increases and the LV cavity becomes enlarged, wall thickness may remain the same. In these cases, determining relative wall thickness (RWT) is more accurate in determining those who have hypertrophy and is defined by:

$$RWT = 2 \times (PWT/LVID)$$

Linear derived LV volumes can be estimated using the Teichholz equation:

$$V_{diastole} = [7/(2.4 + LVID)] \times [LVID^3]$$

Linear formulas used to assess LV volume rely on geometric assumptions, therefore, these formulas are not recommended for use in clinical practice. The preferred method for measurement of LV volume is 2-D echocardiography, from which stroke volume and ejection fraction can be calculated. LV volume is best calculated using the method of disk summation or "Simpson method" (Fig. 15.1). To perform this technique, orthogonal apical views are obtained of the apical two-chamber and apical four-chamber views. Alternatively, the apical five-chamber and apical four-chamber view can be used. The endocardial border is then outlined in both systole and diastole and can be done manually or detected automatically using sophisticated software packages that include automated border detection. The accuracy of this method thus relies on the precision of identification of the endocardial border. The left ventricle is then divided along its axis into multiple cylinders of equal height. The volume of each cylinder is then calculated as height × disk area, where height is the length of the LV long axis. This value is then divided by the number of segments or disks. The surface area of each disk is determined and the ventricular volume can be calculated. This technique is demonstrated in the figure below. Once the LV volume is calculated in both end systole and end diastole, stroke volume and ejection fraction can be calculated. Biplane measurements are most accurate and are preferred, as segmental wall motion abnormalities in a single plane view can lead to under or overestimation of ejection fraction, but single plane measurements can be made.

ASSESSMENT OF SYSTOLIC FUNCTION

Ejection fraction is the most widely accepted means to define global LV systolic function. Left ventricular ejection fraction (LVEF) is the percentage of volume that is ejected at the end of LV systole compared with the volume present at end diastole, that is, stroke volume divided by LV end diastolic volume. It can be measured using single plane linear methods as well as by 2-D and 3-D echocardiography. Often the LVEF is determined by visual inspection. Although this method can be quite accurate when interpreted by the experienced reader, considerable intraobserver variability remains, thus it is preferable to use volumetric measurements to determine ejection fraction. M-mode calculations can be easily reproduced, but they are limited to the patient with normal geometry and calculations can be inaccurate in the presence of regional wall motion variability. Reference values for ejection fraction are listed in Table 15.1.

ADDITIONAL INDICES IN ASSESSING LEFT VENTRICULAR PERFORMANCE
Fractional Shortening

Fractional shortening (FS) is another method of assessing LV performance and is defined as the percentage change in diameter of the left ventricle from diastole to systole (i.e., with each contraction). It is expressed by the following equation:

$$(LVIDd - LVIDs)/LVIDd$$

The reference range for normal fractional shortening is greater than 0.25–0.45 (see Table 15.1). This measurement should not be used in patients with regional wall motion

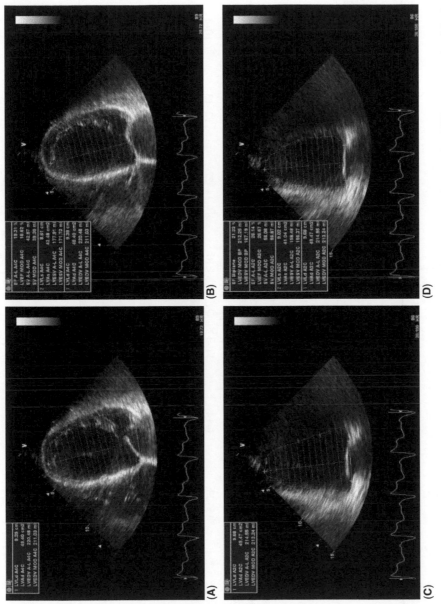

Figure 15.1 Determination of left ventricular volumes and LVEF using the biplane disk summation method (Simpson method) in the apical four chamber (**A,B**) and apical two chamber (**C,D**) views at end-diastole (**A,C**) and end-systole (**B,D**). The LV cavity has been divided into 15 segments of equal height. Individual disk volume is calculated, the ventricular volume is the sum of the individual disk volumes.

Table 15.1 Quantification of Cardiac Chamber Size, Ventricular Mass and Function: Reference Limits and Partition Values

Method/Measure	Women				Men			
	Reference Range	Mildly Abnormal	Moderately Abnormal	Severely Abnormal	Reference Range	Mildly Abnormal	Moderately Abnormal	Severely Abnormal
Linear method								
LV mass, g	67–162	163–186	187–210	>211	88–224	225–258	259–292	>293
Relative wall thickness, cm	0.22–0.42	0.43–0.47	0.48–0.52	>0.53	0.24–0.42	0.43–0.46	0.47–0.51	>0.52
Septal wall thickness, cm	0.6–0.9	1.0–1.2	1.3–1.5	>1.6	0.6–1.0	1.1–1.3	1.4–1.6	>1.7
Posterior wall thickness, cm	0.6–0.9	1.0–1.2	1.3–1.5	>1.6	0.6–1.0	1.1–1.3	1.4–1.6	>1.7
Endocardial fractional shortening, %	27–45	22–26	17–21	<16	25–43	20–24	15–19	<14
Midwall fractional shortening, %	15–23	13–14	11–12	<10	14–22	12–13	10–11	<10
2-d method								
LV mass, g	66–150	151–171	172–182	>193	96–200	201–227	228–254	>255
LV diastolic diameter, cm	3.9–5.3	5.4–5.7	5.8–6.1	>6.2	4.2–5.9	6.0–6.3	6.4–6.8	>6.9
LV diastolic volume, mL	56–104	105–117	118–130	>131	67–155	156–178	179–201	>201
LV systolic volume, mL	19–49	50–59	60–69	>70	22–58	59–70	71–82	>83
Ejection fraction, %	>55	45–54	30–44	<30	>55	45–54	30–44	<30

Source: Adapted from Tables 4 and 5 of Ref. 9.

abnormalities for the reasons mentioned above. FS can be overestimated when afterload is reduced such as in the case of mitral valve regurgitation, ventricular septal defect or peripheral vasodilatation. In patients with LV hypertrophy, midwall fractional shortening rather than endocardial fractional shortening is more useful in assessing for systolic dysfunction.

E-point Septal Separation

The E-point is the maximum mitral valve early diastolic excursion point (see Fig. 15.2). The normal distance between the E point and the LV septum in less than 6 mm. When systolic function is reduced, this distance is increased (see Fig. 15.2).

dP/dt

LV contractility can be assessed by measuring the rate of LV pressure change during isovolumic contraction. A normal LV dP/dt is >1200 mmHg/sec, a dP/dt <600 mmHg/sec has been associated with a poor prognosis in patients with systolic heart failure (10). Techniques for Doppler-derived dP/dt have been well validated (11–13) and in some studies have shown to correlate with postoperative systolic function in patients with mitral regurgitation (14) and can be a predictor of survival in patients with chronic CHF. dP/dt is derived using the continuous wave Doppler velocity spectrum of mitral regurgitation and assumes that there is no significant change in left atrial pressure during isovolumic contraction. The rate of change in pressure between 1 m/sec and 3 m/sec measured by continuous Doppler signal of the mitral regurgitant jet during isovolumic contraction has been substantiated with invasive measurements of dP/dt.

Right ventricular dP/dt can be derived using the tricuspid regurgitant jet and using a dP interval between 1m/sec and 2m/sec.

Index of Myocardial Performance, "Tei" Index

Index of myocardial performance (IMP) is a method to evaluate global ventricular function using systolic and diastolic time intervals, which are easily obtained using Doppler echo. The IMP incorporates the isovolumic contraction time (IVCT), isovolumic relaxation time

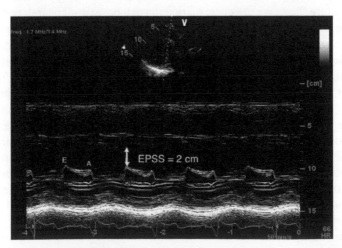

Figure 15.2 M-Mode echocadiogram in a patient with reduced systolic function. The E point to septal separation (EPSS) is increased at 2 cm, normal is <0.6 cm.

(IVRT), and the LV ejection time (ET). In systolic dysfunction, the IVCT and the IVRT are prolonged, and the ejection time is shortened. IMP can also be used in assessing right ventricular (RV) performance and can be used to assess patients with pulmonary hypertension.

Despite novel technologies such as 3-D echo, strain, vector, and tissue Doppler imaging, 2-D echocardiography remains the primary means for assessing LV systolic function and for chamber quantification.

ASSESSMENT OF RIGHT VENTRICULAR STRUCTURE AND FUNCTION

Echocardiographic evaluation of the right ventricle remains challenging because of its complex shape and geometry. The RV is a thin-walled, crescent-shaped structure, which wraps around the left ventricle. It cannot be visualized completely using any single 2-D image and it should be emphasized that accurate assessment requires images acquired from multiple planes including the parasternal long and short axis views, the RV inflow tract view, apical four chamber and subcostal views. Quantification of RV volumes and systolic function is generally estimated visually as there is no standard method for accurate assessment of RV volumes. RV fractional area change, tissue Doppler tricuspid annular velocity, Tricuspid annular plane systolic excursion and IMP are ways that systolic performance can be estimated in a more quantitative manner.

ASSESSMENT OF DIASTOLIC FUNCTION

Analysis of the Acute Decompensated Heart Failure National Registry (ADHERE), which assessed more than 100,000 patients hospitalized for heart failure revealed that in patients who had in hospital assessment of LV function, 50.4% had preserved LV systolic function (LVEF $\geq$ 40%), so called diastolic heart failure or, later termed, "heart failure with preserved ejection fraction." This study emphasizes the value of our understanding of the pathophysiology and diagnostic evaluation of this prevalent disease. It is important to understand that "diastolic dysfunction" describes a structural condition, and does not necessarily translate to the clinical syndrome of heart failure. The presence of abnormalities in diastolic function can occur with or without symptoms of congestion, and with normal or abnormal systolic function. Almost all conditions which impair systolic function will also impair diastolic function.

This section is not intended to review the pathophysiology or etiologies of diastolic heart failure, however, it is necessary to have a basic understanding of the cardiac cycle and the components of diastole. Diastole comprises approximately two-third of the duration of the cardiac cycle and consists of three phases. The initial phase consists of isovolumic relaxation and rapid early filling, which is an "active" process. In the normal healthy heart, most of diastolic filling is complete in the initial phase. In the healthy heart, a wide range of volumes can be introduced to the left ventricle without elevation in filling pressures. As ventricular relaxation and compliance becomes impaired, the left ventricle can no longer accept a wide shift in volumes and LV filling pressure becomes elevated. During diastole, LV end diastolic pressure is transmitted to the left atrium and pulmonary veins. Because it comprises a longer portion of the cardiac cycle than systole, it has a much greater contribution of transmission of elevated pressures to the LA and pulmonary veins than during systole. Thus, in the patient with systolic dysfunction, the assessment of diastolic parameters can be helpful in predicting clinical symptoms.

There are many methods to assess diastolic function by echocardiography. The most widely used are assessment of mitral inflow by pulsed Doppler, pulmonary venous flow by pulsed Doppler, and mitral annular tissue Doppler assessment. Grading systems have been developed to classify the degree of diastolic dysfunction present. LVH, reduced longitudinal motion of the mitral annulus, and a dilated left atrium (in the absence of significant mitral regurgitation) are all findings suggestive of diastolic dysfunction. When these findings are present, one should be prompted to make a more detailed assessment of diastolic indices. This includes isovolumic relaxation time (IVRT), Doppler measurement of early (E) and late (A) diastolic mitral inflow velocities, early velocity of the mitral annulus via tissue Doppler (Ea or E') and color M-mode measurement of mitral inflow propagation velocity (Vp).

Echo Findings Specific to the Cardiomyopathies
Amyloidosis

Cardiac amyloidosis can be associated with all forms of amyloidosis, the general etiologies include immunocytic dyscrasias, systemic reactive type, and familial and senile amyloidosis. The most typical echocardiographic feature in patients with amyloid deposition within the myocardium is diffuse myocardial thickening with a granular or "speckled" appearance of the myocardium. Hypertrophy is usually pronounced and involves both ventricles. Ventricular chamber size is small while atrial size may be markedly enlarged due to chronically elevated filling pressures. There will be a restrictive pattern of diastolic filling and systolic function may be decreased, but the ventricular cavity will not be dilated. There may be valvular thickening and thickening of the intraatrial septum. Pericardial effusions and or pleural effusions may be present.

Cardiac Sarcoidosis

There is no current consensus for the optimal test in diagnosing cardiac sarcoidosis and the diagnosis of cardiac sarcoid cannot be made by 2-D echo alone. Echocardiographic findings have been reported to be present in 14–41% of patients with sarcoidosis (15–17). The myocardium may appear hyperechogenic in areas of granulomatous infiltration (18). There may be pericardial involvement, pericardial effusions, ventricular aneurysms, valvular regurgitation, or decreased ejection fraction. Focal wall motion abnormalities may be present that are not within the distribution of a coronary artery. Other features include ventricular wall thickening or wall thinning, ventricular dilation, papillary muscle dysfunction, chamber enlargement, and diastolic dysfunction (19,20).

Left Ventricular Noncompaction

LV noncompaction (LVNC) syndrome is a primary genetic cardiomyopathy that occurs when there is intrauterine arrest of compaction of the spongy meshwork of the interwoven myocardial fibers within the LV endocardium. Echocardiographic features include prominent ventricular trabeculations with deep intertrabecular recesses. Color Doppler will often reveal flow within these trabeculations and this provides a substrate for thrombus formation. The myocardium is thickened and consists of two layers, "compacted" and "noncompacted" myocardium (21,22). It can be associated with other congenital anomalies, thus careful inspection for other congenital defects, such as bicuspid aortic valve or ventricular septal defect should be made. There may be associated systolic dysfunction, cavity dilation and currently there is no accepted unifying criteria for the diagnosis of LVNC, however, the following criteria have been validated when all three features are present: (*i*) A maximum ratio of >2:1 of noncompacted to compacted myocardium at end-systole in the parasternal short-axis view; (*ii*) prominent flow within the deep intertrabecular recesses by color Doppler; (*iii*) prominent trabeculations in the LV apex or midventricular segments (inferior and lateral wall) (23,24).

Arrhythmogenic Right Ventricular Cardiomyopathy

ARVC is difficult to diagnose using echocardiography and often the RV will appear normal in this condition. There may be mild or marked dilation of the RV with hypokinesis. There is increased echogenicity of the RV moderator band and often prominent RV trabeculations. Other features include small aneurismal projections from the RV free wall during diastole and in its advanced form, there will be biventricular dilation and biventricular systolic dysfunction (25).

Endomyocardial Fibroelastosis

Endomyocardial fibroelastosis can be congenital or can be acquired. It is also associated with the hypereosinophilic syndrome and has been called Loeffler's or Davies disease in North Africa. Typical features include increased reflectivity of the apex suggesting patchy calcification, obliteration of the apex (one or both ventricles) with dense fibrous tissue and thrombus, increased thickening of the basal papillary muscle, and posterior atrio ventricular valves. Systolic function is typically preserved and ventricular cavity size is normal, with markedly enlarged atria (26,27). There is restrictive physiology due to progressive obliteration of the ventricular cavity.

Iron Overload Cardiomyopathy

Iron overload can occur as a result of hemochromatosis, massive increase in oral iron intake, frequent blood transfusions or increased iron absorption, resulting in iron deposition within the myocardial cells. It is difficult to differentiate from other forms of cardiomyopathy by echocardiography. The typical findings are increased wall thickness, increased myocardial mass, ventricular dilation, and ventricular dysfunction. There may be biatrial enlargement due to chronically elevated filling pressures.

Strain and Strain Rate Imaging

Strain imaging is a form of tissue Doppler imaging that can assess regional ventricular function by assessing myocardial velocity gradients. Strain is thought to be superior to tissue Doppler imaging in evaluating systolic and diastolic function given the inability of tissue Doppler imaging to differentiate tissue contraction from translation or tethering motion. It can be used to assess regional systolic and diastolic function. Strain reflects deformation of a structure and thus can characterize contraction and relaxation patterns of the myocardium, and as such can detect areas of intraventricular dyssynchrony. Systolic dysfunction, may, in fact, be present in individuals with mild cardiomyopathy even in the setting of preserved LVEF. Tissue Doppler techniques have been demonstrated to be superior to measurement of LVEF when subtle changes in LV function are present (28)

$$SR = \varepsilon - \frac{L - L_0}{L_0} - \frac{\Delta L}{L_0}$$

Strain is a dimensionless index that is representative of the degree of shortening or lengthening of myocardium following the application of stress. Strain represents the total deformation of myocardium relative to its resting length. Lagrangian strain is represented by the figure above. Given the complex myocardial fiber orientation it is helpful to measure strain in the three directions in which contraction occurs, including rotational, translational, and longitudinal axis shortening. During systolic shortening of normally contracting myocardium longitudinal and circumferential strain are represented by a negative curve when measured by longitudinal or circumferential strain (Fig. 15.3). Radial strain is

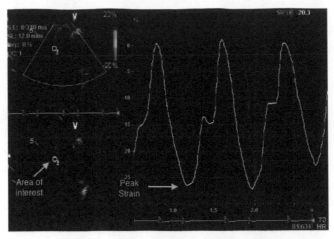

Figure 15.3 Peak Doppler-derived systolic strain.

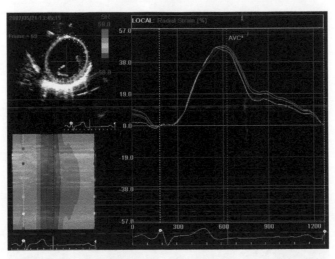

Figure 15.4 2D speckle derived radial left ventricular strain.

normally represented by a positive curve, which is reflective of the relative myocardial lengthening (Fig. 15.4). Advantages of strain imaging over tissue Doppler imaging include absence of tethering effects, precise localization of myocardial shortening, and lengthening rather than translation of the myocardium with respect to the transducer, and lack of dependence on endocardial boundary detection for quantification of contractile function.

Strain can be derived from both Doppler and 2D speckle tracking methods. Doppler derived strain requires imaging at a high frame rate (>130–140 frames per second) and the data acquired is highly angle-dependent. Strain derived from speckle tracking is determined by tracking the motion of unique myocardial speckles throughout the cardiac cycle. This method is advantageous in that lower frame rates can be utilized to acquire data (50–70 frames per second) and it is angle independent (Fig. 15.5).

Sophisticated mathematical algorithms are applied to the 2D derived data collected and the resultant strain and SR values are derived. The intra and inter-observer variability are superior with 2D as compared to tissue Doppler-derived strain (Fig. 15.6) (29).

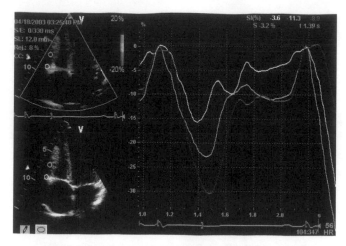

Figure 15.5 RV strain as measured in the basal, mid and apical regions demonstrating higher strain in the mid and apical regions relative to the base.

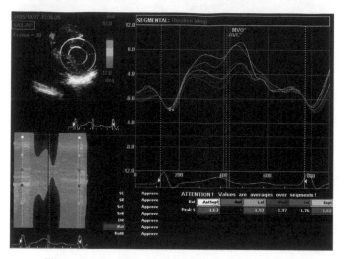

Figure 15.6 2D derived rotation of the LV apex.

Strain and strain rate imaging are useful in the evaluation of patients with cardiomyopathies and appear to be helpful both in determining the etiology and suitability for potential cardiac resynchronization therapy. Strain imaging has been studied and found to be of value in determining diagnosis and response to therapy in cardiac amyloidosis, hypertrophic cardiomyopathy LV noncompaction, Fabry's disease, and Freidrich's ataxia (30–32).

Myocardial contraction and relaxation not only consists of the piston-like shortening and lengthening along the long axis of the heart but also includes a twisting of the basal and apical segments. The base of the heart rotates in a clockwise motion while the apex twists in a counterclockwise motion. Rotation can be measured using 2-D speckle tracking and torsion can be calculated. LV torsion results from contraction of obliquely oriented myocardial fibers and is characterized by rotation of the apex and base in opposite directions. Studies examining LV torsion in healthy and myopathic hearts have demonstrated the integration of systolic and diastolic function. There appears to be an interdependent relationship between systolic LV twisting and diastolic untwisting. LV untwisting is an important determinant of LV filling (33,34). Torsion is the maximal difference between rotation angles of the base and apex. Torsion is reduced in patients with systolic heart failure. As LV systolic dysfunction progresses the LV cavity dilates and assumes a more spherical shape. LV torsion decreases proportionally as the LV dilates and sphericity increases (35).

The assessment of LV torsion may be helpful in the heart failure population following therapeutic interventions including cardiac resynchronization (CRT) and cardiac transplantation. An acute improvement in LV torsion following CRT has proved useful in predicting overall response to cardiac resynchronization (36). Haykowsky and colleagues examined changes in LV rotation in heart transplant recipients and healthy donor and recipient age matched controls prior to and following submaximal exercise. The heart transplant recipients and recipient controls demonstrated blunted LV peak torsion and untwisting compared with donor matched controls. This response likely contributes to the impaired diastolic filling found in transplant recipients and suggests accelerated aging of the allograft (37).

Three-Dimensional Echocardiography

The latest ultrasound systems are capable of producing live 3-D images. This relatively new technique allows for visualization of complex anatomy and can accurately provide quantitative and qualitative measurements. Reconstruction of images after acquisition can be rather time consuming, thus 3-D imaging is not routinely used in clinical practice. The main advantage conferred by 3-D echo is that it does not rely on geometric assumptions and is therefore the echocardiographic "gold standard" for the measurement of ventricular volumes and ejection fraction. In contrast to 2-D imaging, 3-D imaging can make an accurate assessment of RV volume and ejection fraction (38). When compared with MRI, quantitative measurements of the RV have been found to have good interobserver and intraobserver agreement and low test-retest variation (39–41). One exception is in individuals with marked RV dilation; the sector angle is unable assess the inflow and outflow tracts in one full sweep, and thus an accurate assessment cannot be made. It may be useful in the future in identifying cardiomyopathies and can be used for accurate visualization during interventional procedures, such as RV biopsy.

PART 2: RADIONUCLIDE IMAGING METHODS

There are a variety of radionuclide methods, which are useful in the assessment of the heart failure patient using single photon emission computed tomography (SPECT), PET, and radionuclide ventriculography (RNV). Using these modalities, precise measurements of myocardial structure, function, perfusion, and viability can be made and prognostic information can be obtained. Newer methods are emerging, which assess sympathetic autonomic changes that occur in the diseased heart. The current available techniques, including their clinical significance and limitations are reviewed here.

ASSESSMENT OF VENTRICULAR FUNCTION: ECG-GATED SPECT IMAGING

Electrocardiogram (ECG)-gated SPECT (GSPECT) imaging uses the image subject's ECG to guide image acquisition such that myocardial contraction can be viewed in over a series of R–R intervals in the resultant images. Technetium-99m based radiotracers are typically used because of their ability to provide high count statistics. Regional wall motion, degree of myocardial thickening, and measurement of global LVEF can all be performed using quantitative measures. Images can be obtained over an 8-frame gating technique (8 R–R intervals) or a 16-frame. Overestimation on LVEF can occur in the setting of a small LV cavity size, likely due to overestimation of ventricular volumes (42). Conversely, the 8-frame gating technique can underestimate the LVEF due to oversampling of the time–volume curve. Accuracy of GSPECT imaging in determining LVEF has been compared with echocardiography, contrast ventriculography, RNV, and MRI and has shown close correlation and reproducibility compared with these other modalities (43–45). GSPECT is typically not used in the evaluation of LVEF alone, but rather in when simultaneous assessment of ventricular perfusion and function is desired.

ASSESSMENT OF BLOOD FLOW: MYOCARDIAL PERFUSION IMAGING

An important step in the initial evaluation of the patient with heart failure is determining its etiology. Because of its high negative predictive value, radionuclide myocardial perfusion imaging (MPI) is an excellent noninvasive means to distinguish patients with nonischemic cardiomyopathy from those with ischemic disease and is thus reasonable in the initial evaluation of the heart failure patient. Gated techniques allow for accurate assessment of LV function in addition to evaluation for ischemia as an underlying etiology. Several studies have assessed the sensitivity of MPI in the patient with systolic dysfunction and these studies have correlated with a 100% negative predictive value (46–49). False positive studies are quite frequent, likely owing to the fact that there may be nonhomogenous areas of fibrosis in the patient with non ischemic cardiomyopathy as well as abnormalities in microvascular blood flow. It should be noted that the positive predictive value of MPI in the patient with LV dysfunction is only 40–50%. Unfortunately, a positive test is not useful in distinguishing ischemic disease from nonischemic disease, and those with an abnormal test should be referred for more definitive testing. MPI has been shown to predict long term cardiovascular outcomes in heart failure patients with ischemic disease (48,49), however the gold standard for assessing for presence of coronary artery disease is through invasive coronary angiography. Coronary angiography should be performed when an abnormal perfusion study is present to determine whether an ischemic cardiomyopathy is present.

PERFUSION IMAGING IN SPECIFIC CARDIOMYOPATHIES

Nuclear imaging can be helpful in distinguishing ischemic vs. nonischemic cardiomyopathies, as a normal perfusion test has a 100% negative predictive value. An abnormal test, however, can be present in an array of etiologies other than ischemia.

Patients with hypertrophic cardiomyopathy (HCM) will frequently have evidence of abnormal myocardial perfusion and ischemia on stress testing in the absence of macrovascular coronary disease. This is due to the presence of a mismatch in "supply" and "demand" owing to the degree of myocardial hypertrophy relative to perfusion. Myocardial bridging resulting in compression of intramural vessels, small vessel disease, myocardial fibrosis and microvascular dysfunction may also contribute to the abnormalities seen during perfusion imaging in patients with HCM (50–53).

Specific radiotracers can be helpful in the diagnosis of particular cardiomyopathies, for example, 99mTcDPD may be able to distinguish between transthyretin-related cardiac amyloidosis and AL related cardiac amyloidosis.

RADIONUCLIDE VENTRICULOGRAPHY

Since the 1970s, radionuclide ventriculography has been recognized as a highly accurate technique for assessing LV function. Radionuclide angiography (RNA), Radionuclide cine angiography (RNCA), multiple gated cardiac blood pool imaging (MUGA), and equilibrium radionuclide angiography are all synonymous with radionuclide ventriculography

(RVG). RVG, in addition to cardiac magnetic resonance imaging, is the modality of choice (ACC/AHA class IA recommendation) when precise measurements of LV function are necessary or when slight changes of LV function are important such as during administration of cardiotoxic drugs. It can be useful when less precise modalities produce conflicting data and a management decision needs to be made based on the LVEF, such as placement of a prophylactic internal cardiac defibrillator. It can be done safely in patients who have metal prosthesis who would not be candidates for cardiac magnetic resonance imaging (CMR). Its use has largely been replaced by more cost effective and more sophisticated competing technologies such as SPECT MPI and CMR.

There are currently two techniques that are applied in radionuclide ventriculography, first-pass and equilibrium. Both methods require "blood pool labeling," whereby the patients red blood cells are labeled with technetium 99m (tc99m) either through the in vivo method in which tc99m is directly injected intravenously, or via the in vitro method in which a sample of the patients blood is labeled and subsequently injected. In first pass imaging, systolic function is measured over only a few heartbeats while the equilibrium method involves 800 to 1000 seconds thus exposing the patient to a greater amount of radiation.

First-Pass Radionuclide Angiography

First-pass radionuclide angiography (FPRNA) can be used to assess both LV and RV function at rest and during stress. When used in combination with exercise, it can be used to assess for reversible perfusion abnormalities in the case of coronary artery disease. The standard radionuclide used in FPRNA is Technetium 99m diethylamine triamine pentaacetic acid (DTPA), but Tc-99m pertechnetate can also be used. DTPA is renally excreted and minimizes the patient's radiation exposure. The technique requires that a rapid bolus of radionuclide be injected while the patient remains in upright position and acquisition of straight anterior views are obtained. Multicrystal or single-crystal gamma camera can be used for imaging, however multicrystal cameras are preferred because of their high count rate capability. Systolic emptying rates, diastolic filling rate, ventricular volumes and shunt detection can all be determined using FPRNA.

Equilibrium Method

In clinical practice, the most widely used scintographic method to evaluate ventricular function is the equilibrium multiple gated blood pool scintigraphy method. Red blood cells are radiolabeled and images are then acquired and performed in synchrony with or gated to the patients electrocardiogram. Wall motion is assessed and ejection fraction is calculated using geographic assumptions. By using this gated technique, intra and inter-observer variability is extraordinarily low. Additionally, diastolic filling time, systolic and diastolic volumes can be accurately assessed. Intraventricular dyssynchrony can be observed using phase analysis of ECG gated SPECT MPI (54).

POSITRON EMISSION TOMOGRAPHY (PET)

PET imaging works by detecting gamma rays that are emitted indirectly by a positron emitting biologically active radiotracer. Imaging can be performed using several different isotopes and has vast clinical applications. It can be used to assess perfusion, myocardial oxygen uptake, metabolism and cardiac adrenergic innervation. It quantifies absolute rather than relative myocardial perfusion defects and thus may be technologically more accurate than SPECT imaging. Myocardial beta-adrenreceptor density can be measured using positron emission tomography (PET) with the radioisotope 11C-CGP-12177. When imaging is performed shortly after myocardial infarction, down-regulation of myocardial beta-adrenoceptor has been shown to be predictive of LV dilatation at follow-up (55). In patients with HF due to dilated cardiomyopathy, myocardial beta-adrenoceptor density is reduced. Down-regulation of myocardial beta-adrenoceptor is even more pronounced in patients with hypertrophic cardiomyopathy who progress to development of LV dilation and HF (56). It's current use in clinical practice is mainly limited to assessment of ischemia and myocardial viability. It is helpful in distinguishing patients those patient with ischemic cardiomyopathy who may benefit from revascularization versus those who should be referred for cardiac transplantation.

RADIONUCLIDE CARDIAC NEURONAL IMAGING

The imaging methods discussed thus far have focused on evaluation of cardiac structure and function. Newer radionuclide modalities can evaluate neurohormonal changes and changes in cardiac innervation that occur in heart failure via radionuclide cardiac neuronal imaging. Neuronal imaging can provide valuable information on prognosis and response to treatment.

Cardiac neuronal innervation is of critical importance in cardiac function, as sympathetic and parasympathetic input work closely with circulating catecholamines to regulate cardiac output. Parasympathetic function is mediated by acetylcholine, while sympathetic function is mediated by norepinephrine. In patients with heart failure, there is significant decrease in uptake of norepinephrine in pre-synaptic receptors as disease progresses, as well as an overall down regulation of myocardial beta-adrenoreceptor density (57,58). Radiotracer imaging is an excellent method for assessment of sympathetic autonomic function. Current available radiotracers are applicable to the sympathetic system, as there are no available parasympathetic tracers in use in humans as of this writing. Imaging focuses on the synaptic junction, where reduced sympathetic activity can be revealed. Evaluation of cardiac innervation can be performed using PET or SPECT imaging and can assess presynaptic and postsynaptic sympathetic innervation. Presynaptic PET radiotracers available for clinical and experimental use include C-11 metahydroxyephedrine (HED), C-11 epinephrine, C-11 phenylephrine, F-18 6-fluorodopamine, F-18 6-flurometaraminol, F-18-6-fluoronorepinephrine, F-18 para-fluorobenzylguanidine (PFBG), F-18 fluoroido-benzylguanidine, Br-76 metabromobenzylguanidine. The radiotracer used with SPECT imaging is iodine-meta-iodobenzylguanidine (^{123}I-MIBG). SPECT imaging using ^{123}I-MIBG will be the focus of this section as it is the most studied and most widely used in clinical practice. Hybrid imaging techniques which incorporate the use of SPECT, PET and CT are currently under investigation such that integrated information can be obtained with respect to function, viability and ischemia.

MIBG

The most studied radiotracer for neuronal imaging is radioactive iodine-meta-iodobenzylguanidine (^{123}I-MIBG). Meta-iodobenzylguanidine (MIBG) is an analog of norepinephrine and guanethidine and can be used to assess physiologic progression of heart failure and can provide prognostic information to predict mortality in the heart failure patient. A radiolabeled iodine-123 MIBG compound can thus be administered to a patient and imaging can provide visualization of the number of receptors present. While this modality does not provide morphologic information, it is excellent in assessing the changes that occur to the autonomic nervous system during heart failure, and can be used as an adjunct to other imaging modalities to assist in prognostication.

Imaging is rather simple. The patient is injected with the radiolabled compound and planar or topographic images are then obtained using SPECT imaging. A ratio of radiotracer activity is then calculated using the heart and mediastinal windows. A calculation is generated as the heart to mediastinum ratio (HMR), the average value in normal individuals has been reported around 1.9 to 2.8. Studies are underway to develop and validate a standard quantitative index for the for assessment of cardiac MIBG uptake.

In early studies of ^{123}I-MIBG imaging, impaired cardiac adrenergic innervation was an independent predictor of cardiac mortality regardless of etiology, and reduced late HMR was the strongest long-term prognostic indicator compared to other indicators such as LVEF, age and New York Heart Association Class (59–64). Initial reports demonstrated in patients with an LVEF <45%, a HMR less than 1.2 correlated with a 6th month and 1 year survival of 60% and 40% respectively and that patients with higher ratios demonstrated 100% survival at 1 year. Recently reported results of the ADMIRE-HF phase III clinical trial demonstrated that patients with a HMR <1.6 had a significantly higher rate of adverse cardiac events, including arrhythmia, progression of heart failure and cardiac deaths (65).

In addition to being a useful prognostic indicator, other potential uses for ^{123}I-MIBG imaging include prediction of response to cardiac resynchronization therapy (CRT), monitoring cardiotoxic effects of chemotherapy agents, and assessment of response to treatment with neurohormonal blocking agents. Lower ratios of MIBG uptake has been shown to predict nonresponders to CRT and may become an important imaging modality in the future when determining patients who are appropriate for specific device therapies, including AICD selection and CRT. A decrease in MIBG will precede a subsequent decrease in LVEF after therapy with cardiotoxic chemotherapy agents (66–68) and thus could potentially identify patients in whom chemotherapy should be discontinued as well as identify patients who are candidates for therapy with neurohormonal blocking agents. Studies have consistently shown improvement in HMR after therapy with -blocking agents as well as with agents that affect the renin angiotensin system (69–74) thus ^{123}I-MIBG imaging may be used to assess response to treatment for heart failure.

PART 3: PRINCIPLES OF CARDIAC MAGNETIC RESONANCE AND CARDIAC COMPUTED TOMOGRAPHPY

CARDIAC MAGNETIC RESONANCE

Distinct from the mechanisms of tissue attenuation of x-ray beams used in radiography and computed tomography, the detection of high-energy photons generated by radioactive isotopes used in nuclear imaging, and the tissue reflection of ultrasound waves used in ultrasound techniques, magnetic resonance images water and fat in human tissues by transiently altering the energy state of hydrogen nuclei in these molecules. Hydrogen nuclei can effectively receive radio signals of the appropriate frequency when placed in a strong external magnetic field, such as the fields currently used for clinical magnetic resonance imaging (MRI). This begins the resonance process by causing a transition to a higher energy state. As the nuclei subsequently return to their normal state of energy, a radiofrequency signal is generated. This signal can then be received by the scanner ("antennas"), known as coils, placed over the body area being imaged. Signals received by the coils are ultimately converted into images.

While MRI has been used clinically for imaging of the brain and other static organs since the early to mid 1980s, cardiac MRI (CMR) required a more extensive development process as the heart is a constantly moving object. As a result of major technical advances, CMR can now accurately provide information about cardiac structure, function, flow, perfusion, myocardial viability, and tissue characterization. Magnetic resonance angiography (MRA) of the coronary arteries remains under development and is currently utilized mainly for the identification of congenital anomalies of the coronary arteries, and for evaluation and follow-up of coronary artery aneurysms.

By adjusting some of the scan parameters, various imaging pulse sequences, for example spin echo or fast spin echo sequences, can be used to bring out image contrast between different types of tissues by decreasing the signal intensity of water relative to fat in T1-weighted images, or alternatively, by high-lighting signal from nonflowing fluid or tissue edema in T2-weighted images. Steady state free precession (SSFP) sequences provide elements of both T1 and T2 weighting, as they highlight structures with high water content and high fat content, and provide cine images as well. Additionally, images can be obtained 10 to 30 minutes after the administration of intravenous gadolinium to assess for the presence of delayed contrast enhancement. Gadolinium distribution is increased into, and wash-out is delayed from, areas of injury, infarction and fibrosis, causing these areas to appear hyperintense relative to surrounding normal myocardium in T1-weighted images, a phenomenon appropriately termed "late Gadolinium enhancement" or "delayed hyperenhancement." These types of images can show unique delayed enhancement "signature" patterns for several different forms of cardiomyopathy (see below).

CMR is a safe and generally well tolerated imaging modality. As with echocardiography, CMR does not involve exposure to ionizing radiation. However, the high quality images obtained without exposure to radiation are balanced by the expense of an exam as well as the expertise and the time duration required to perform an exam. Most CMR exams take an hour or more to complete, during which the patient must lie still on his/her back on the exam table and must strictly adhere to breathing instructions, which commonly include serial breath holds of 10 up to 30 seconds in duration. Patients with symptomatic heart failure from a cardiomyopathy may have difficulty tolerating these requirements. Patients should be screened for other potential contraindications, such as claustrophobia and metallic implants. Prosthetic heart valves, intracoronary stents, and sternal wires are generally compatible with MRI. Implanted pacemakers and defibrillators remain a strong relative contraindication, although ongoing research and development has lead to wider compatibility. Finally, administration of gadolinium is restricted in patients with renal insufficiency depending on severity, due to the risk for nephrogenic systemic fibrosis.

INDICATIONS FOR CMR IN THE EVALUATION OF CARDIOMYOPATHY

The 2006 Appropriateness Criteria for Cardiac Computed Tomography and Cardiac Magnetic Resonance Imaging endorse CMR for a number of indications pertaining to cardiomyopathy evaluation (75). These indications have been developed further in the 2010 Multi-Society Expert Consensus Document on CMR (76) and include:

- Evaluation of LV or RV function following myocardial infarction or in heart failure patients when only technically limited images are available from echocardiography
- Quantification of LV or RV function when functional assessment on prior testing yields discordant information
- Evaluation for specific cardiomyopathies, usually with delayed enhancement imaging, including infiltrative (such as amyloid and sarcoid), hypertrophic, noncompaction, dilated and iatrogenic from cardiotoxic agents
- Evaluation for arrythmogenic right ventricular cardiomyopathy (ARVC) in patients presenting with syncope or ventricular arrhythmia
- Evaluation of myocarditis or myocardial infarction in patients with positive cardiac enzymes but without obstructive atherosclerosis on angiography
- Evaluation of pericardial conditions, such as constrictive pericarditis
- Determination of location and extent of myocardial necrosis post-acute myocardial infarction using late gadolinium enhancement

- Determination of viability prior to revascularization to establish the likelihood of recovery of function, or when viability assessment by SPECT or dobutamine echo has provided "equivocal or indeterminate" results.
- Identification of myocardial iron overload and monitoring chelation therapy.

The committee felt that use of CMR for the evaluation of LV function following myocardial infarction or in heart failure patients was of uncertain appropriateness when adequate assessment can be obtained from echocardiography, as echocardiography-derived values of function are typically sufficient for clinical management and can be obtained without the expense of CMR. Also important to note is that the committee inclusion of a history of syncope or ventricular arrhythmia reflects a higher threshold for ARVC evaluation with CMR, suggesting that CMR in patients at very low risk for ARVC is likely not cost effective. First-degree relatives of patients with an established diagnosis of ARVC are at increased risk, and may be screened by MRI even in the absence of syncope or ventricular ectopy.

CMR FOR STRUCTURAL AND FUNCTIONAL EVALUATION

CMR is regarded by many as the "gold standard" for the assessment of left and right ventricular function and volumes. For this purpose, most protocols currently acquire cine images with an SSFP technique in long axis (2 chamber and 4 chamber) views and in a multi-slice series of short axis images. The SSFP technique provides for sharp definition of the myocardium and the endocardial border, and the gated acquisition provides for accurate measurement of chamber dimensions in both systolic and diastolic phases of the cardiac cycle.

The cine images allow for qualitative assessment of both global and regional LV and RV function. For quantitative assessment, calculation of end-diastolic and end-systolic volumes for both ventricular cavities is commonly performed by applying Simpson's rule to the stack of short axis cine images. This rule derives the volume of a chamber from the sum of the cross sectional areas of the chamber in each short axis slice in a series of contiguous slices, multiplied by the slice thickness. While Simpson's calculation can be performed by hand, many vendors offer semi-automated software packages. Even with semi-automated software, experience is still necessary to correctly identify end-systole and end-diastole, locate the valve planes that separate the ventricles from the atria and the great vessels, define and edit the endocardial contours, and distinguish the endocardial borders from adjacent papillary muscles, the inconsistent inclusion of which can alter accuracy.

Delineation of the LV epicardial contour in addition to the endocardial contour permits calculation of LV mass and measures of wall thickening. Following delineation of the epicardial and endocardial borders on each short axis slice, the total volume of the LV myocardium can be derived as the summation of the area of myocardium for each slice multiplied by the interslice distance. LV mass can then be calculated as the product of the LV myocardial volume (mL) and the density, 1.05 g/mL. Semi-automated software packages can also use these contours to calculate end-diastolic and end-systolic wall thickness, providing for the calculation of percent thickening in each ventricular segment. Due to the thin myocardium of the RV, calculations of RV mass and wall thickening are not routinely performed.

Several imaging pulse sequences are available for more advanced analysis of cardiac function and flow. Examples include quantitation of regional myocardial strain, and evaluation of diastolic function by methods analogous to those used in cardiac ultrasound. Discussion of details of these techniques falls outside the scope of this chapter on heart failure and the underlying myopathic processes. Phase contrast cine acquisitions are a well established tool for mapping flow velocities over time during the cardiac cycle throughout the heart chambers and great vessels. The velocity information at every point in the image is encoded by the pulse sequence into the phase of the MRI signal. The measured velocity distribution can then be averaged over the region of interest in space, and integrated over time through the cardiac cycle to measure flow volumes at different locations in the heart. If done carefully this allows accurate and reproducible quantitation of shunt lesions, and of valvular regurgitation severity during monitoring over extended follow-up.

ISCHEMIC CARDIOMYOPATHY

CMR can assess both rest and stress myocardial perfusion, the latter when pharmacologic stress CMR protocols are utilized. First pass perfusion protocols use rapidly updating T1-weighted images to follow the passage of an injected bolus of gadolinium from the systemic veins through the right heart, pulmonary vessels, left heart, coronary arteries, and myocardium, noting the increase in signal intensity as the gadolinium arrives. The resulting myocardial "blush" will be nonuniform in proportion to regional myocardial hypoperfusion. Assessment of myocardial perfusion is generally performed qualitatively, although semi-quantitative and quantitative methods do exist. A unique feature of CMR is its ability to detect subendocardial perfusion abnormalities in patients who are symptomatic but found to be free of epicardial coronary disease on invasive angiography (77). Pharmacologic stress protocols utilize dobutamine, adenosine, regadenoson or dipyridamole.

Delayed enhancement sequences examine for myocardial hyperenhancement, which can identify the location (i.e., vascular territory) and extent of recent or remote myocardial infarction (78). Unlike nonischemic cardiomyopathies, which typically demonstrate mid-myocardial or subepicardial hyperenhancement, ischemic cardiomyopathy is characterized by subendocardial extending to transmural hyperenhancement (Fig. 15.7).

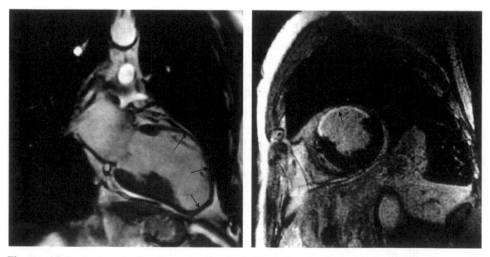

Figure 15.7 Ischemic Cardiomyopathy. Left: End-systolic frame from SSFP cine in the paraseptal long axis view of the left ventricle showing large LAD-territory myocardial infarction (arrows) with marked wall thinning and akinesis extending from the base to around the apex which is dyskinetic. The calculated LV ejection fraction is 24%. Right: Short axis delayed enhancement image from the same patient showing the typical appearance of old transmural myocardial infarction with strong delayed enhancement of the severely thinned anterior wall infarct segment (arrow) consistent with chronic, nonviable scar.

Research has shown that myocardial segments demonstrating significant dysfunction but 25% or less transmural hyperenhancement are likely to be viable and have a good chance of recovery of systolic function following revascularization if there is a flow-limiting lesion in the epicardial coronary artery supplying the area, whereas recovery is increasingly unlikely in segments demonstrating 50–75% or greater transmural hyperenhancement (79). Viability imaging with CMR can also utilize low dose dobutamine to assess for improvement in contractile function during dobutamine infusion, and thus confirm potential for recovery. Combining late gadolinium enhancement imaging with functional cine MRI prior to and during low dose dobutamine infusion provides the best accuracy for identifying hibernating myocardium and predicting the likelihood of recovery of function following revascularization (80).

DILATED CARDIOMYOPATHY

Many myopathic pathways ultimately converge to a late-stage appearance of dilated cardiomyopathy with greatly enlarged ventricular volumes, often with thin walls and with global severe impairment of systolic function. The process is most commonly idiopathic, but infectious (late stage of myocarditis), hemodynamic (long-standing volume overload), toxic (such as post chemotherapy) and familial causes can frequently be recognized. In addition to accurate quantitation of ventricular volumes and of the depressed ejection fraction to establish the need for anticoagulation and prophylactic implantation of an ICD, CMR will identify associated hazards such as the presence of intracardiac thrombus, may allow recognition of other entities such as noncompaction or "burnt-out" hypertrophic cardiomyopathy, and may identify patterns of late gadolinium enhancement that could suggest an underlying mechanism (ischemic, myocarditis, sarcoid). Importantly, a characteristic pattern of linear mid-myocardial delayed enhancement which may be seen most commonly in the interventricular septum but which may extend circumferentially (Fig. 15.8), correlates with a layer of mid-wall fibrosis and has been linked to adverse prognosis (81).

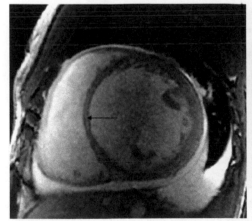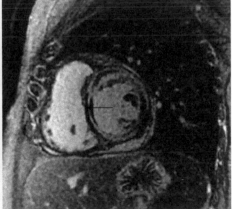

Figure 15.8 Dilated Cardiomyopathy. Two patients with idiopathic dilated cardiomyopathy. Left: Short axis end-systolic SSFP cine frame showing massively dilated left ventricle with small pericardial and pleural effusions. The calculated LV EF = 10%. The cine images were acquired shortly after IV Gadolinium administration, and a mid-wall layer with stronger enhancement can be discerned in the interventricular septum (arrow), consistent with mid-wall fibrosis. Right: Delayed enhancement image in the short axis view showing a relatively thin left ventricular wall with a central layer of nearly complete circumferential delayed enhancement consistent with mid-wall fibrosis.

INFILTRATIVE CARDIOMYOPATHY

Myocardial deposition of amyloid fibrils is the most common model for infiltrative cardio-myopathy. This can be screened for by CMR, which can visualize a pattern of homogenous thickening of both the atrial and ventricular walls with normal or reduced ventricular cav-ity size. The myocardial wall thickening seen with amyloid can, in fact, mimic hypertro-phic cardiomyopathy (82) and thickening of the papillary muscles and valve leaflets can also be seen. Reasonable specificity for amlyoidosis has previously been described from the concomitant observation of atrial septal thickening, right atrial free wall thickening, depressed contractility of a thickened myocardium, and a reduction in the myocardial sig-nal intensity ratio (83). While most of the structural findings can also be seen on echocar-diography, the key finding on MRI is delayed hyperenhancement, which is often in a global patchy to diffuse circumferential pattern with subendocardial predominance (Fig. 15.9). One trial involving 30 patients with tissue proven amlyoidosis yielded 87% accuracy for the detection of cardiac amlyoidosis when a reduced subendocardial T1 value combined with a pattern of global subendocardial late gadolinium enhancement were observed; this improved to 97% when the difference in T1 between the subendocardium and the blood was considered (84).

Other forms of infiltrative cardiomyopathy also lead to increased interstitial volume due to the abnormal infiltrate, into which the extracellular gadolinium contrast will distribute,

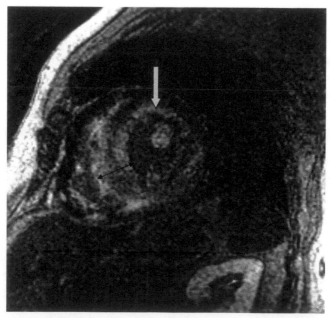

Figure 15.9 Infiltrative cardiomyopathy due to amyloid. Short axis delayed enhancement image at a mid-ventricular level showing diffusely increased wall thickness (double-headed arrow in the infero-septal segment of the LV) with circumferential subendocardial delayed enhancement (solid arrow, anterior segment). Delayed enhancement is also evident in the papillary muscles and along the RV endocardial aspect of the interventricular septum. The signal intensity of the blood pool is characteristically low (dark) in delayed enhancement images from amyloid patients due to a reduced difference in T1 values between blood and myocardium (higher Gadolinium content in the myocardium, faster Gadolinium clearance from the blood), such that inversion time settings that null myocardial signal intensity will likely also null the signal from the blood.

resulting in a higher tissue gadolinium concentration compared to normal myocardium, greater T1 shortening and thus higher T1 signal intensity with potential abnormal delayed enhancement. This includes glycogen storage disease as well as Fabry disease; the latter tends to display a characteristic pattern of mid-wall delayed enhancement affecting the infero-lateral segments at basal to mid-ventricular levels (85).

CARDIAC SARCOIDOSIS

Cardiac infiltration of sarcoid is believed to occur in as many as 20% to 30% or more of patients with systemic sarcoidosis (86) and may be detected as areas of myocardial edema on T2-weighted sequences and more reliably as areas of fibrosis in a pattern of patchy hyper-enhancement that does not correspond to any specific vascular territory on delayed enhancement sequences (87) (Fig. 15.10). Increased LV wall thickness and impact on global and regional LV function can also be observed on SSFP sequences. Response to systemic steroid therapy may be possible to assess with CMR, as regression of myocardial delayed enhancement has been observed in responders to therapy (88).

MYOCARDITIS

CMR is useful to support the diagnosis in cases of suspected myocarditis. The myocardial edema associated with myocardial inflammation causes a prolonged T2-relaxation time, such that affected myocardium may show regional signal hyperintensity relative to surrounding normal myocardium on T2-weighted images. The T2 signal intensity in the myocardium is also compared with the T2 signal intensity of skeletal muscle to yield a signal intensity ratio which, if greater than 1.9, suggests diffuse myocardial edema. Similarly, the ratio of the early signal intensity enhancement of the myocardium relative to the enhancement of skeletal muscle is calculated from T1-weighted spin echo images acquired before and immediately following administration of a standard dose of intravenous Gadolinium. A ratio of 4.0 or higher is consistent with myocarditis and reflects the increased distribution of Gadolinium into the myocardium due to the vascular hyperemia, increased capillary permeability, and increased interstitial fluid space associated with myocardial inflammation.

Delayed hyperenhancement is a less sensitive but more specific CMR finding for myocarditis and likely indicates irreversible myocardial injury under the premise that

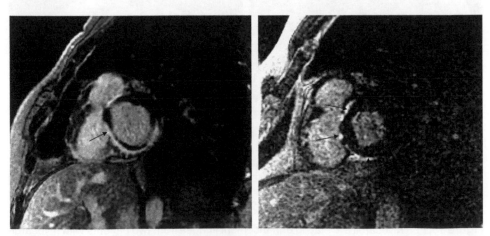

Figure 15.10 Sarcoid. Short axis delayed enhancement images from two patients with cardiac sarcoid, showing multiple areas of late Gadolinium enhancement (arrows) consistent with sarcoid infiltration and fibrosis.

myocytes damaged from the inflammatory process of myocarditis will have increased cell membrane permeability and accumulate gadolinium intracellularly. One trial found the lateral wall most frequently involved, with areas of hyperenhancement occurring most often in the outer (subepicardial to midwall) myocardial layers, sparing the subendocardium (89), and thereby differentiating myocarditis from ischemic injury (Fig. 15.11). Another trial found a cutoff value of 4.0 for the T1 global early enhancement ratio relative to skeletal muscle to have a sensitivity, specificity, and accuracy of 80%, 68%, and 74.5%, respectively. A threshold value of 1.9 for the T2 signal intensity ratio relative to skeletal muscle had a sensitivity of 84%, specificity of 74%, and accuracy of 79%, and the presence of delayed hyperenhancement had a sensitivity, specificity, and accuracy of 44%, 100%, and 71%, respectively (90). In a recent large trial (91) CMR performed well against endomyocardial biopsy for the diagnosis of acute myocarditis (symptom duration up to 14 days) when 2 of the above 3 parameters were required to be abnormal (sensitivity 81%, specificity 71%, accuracy 79%), but performed less well in patients with symptom duration >14 days (chronic myocarditis). Use of CMR in myocarditis has been extensively reviewed (92).

IRON OVERLOAD CARDIOMYOPATHY

Identification of iron overload cardiomyopathy, which results in systolic and/or diastolic dysfunction secondary to increased deposition in cardiac myocytes, is a unique indication for CMR. Cardiac iron deposition is seen primarily in patients with primary hemochromatosis, or secondary to transfusion-related iron overload, such as in thalassemia and sickle cell anemia. CMR can detect the increases in LV wall thickness, increases in LV end diastolic chamber diameter, and functional impairments that can be seen with iron deposition, but can also quantitate the T2 relaxation time (the time constant for the decay of the MRI signal that can be recovered from the myocardium following an excitation pulse). Iron deposition in the heart shortens the myocardial T2 value in relation to the severity of the iron overload in the tissue. Thus abnormal myocardial T2 relaxation time is considered by

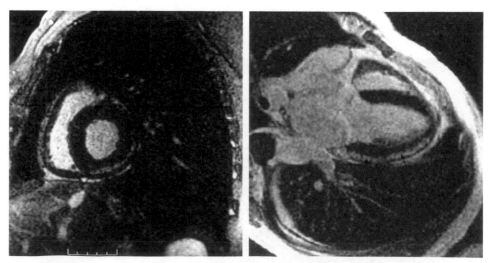

Figure 15.11   Myocarditis. Delayed enhancement images from two patients with myocarditis. *Left panel*: Short axis view showing typical subepicardial delayed enhancement in the basal infero-lateral wall (arrows). *Right panel*: 4-chamber view showing subepicardial delayed enhancement extending from base to apex in the lateral wall (arrows).

some to be the best noninvasive predictor of cardiac iron deposition (93). In current practice the measure used is the myocardial T2* (pronounced T2 star) relaxation time, which is derived from the signal intensity decay at increasing echo times using gradient echo pulse sequences that have increased sensitivity to local magnetic field inhomogeneities resulting from the presence of microscopic iron deposits in the myocardium. A T2* value which falls below the normal value (52 ± 16 msec) provides an opportunity to initiate chelation therapy before the onset of ventricular dysfunction, which correlates with myocardial T2* values <20 msec (94).

ARRYTHMOGENIC RIGHT VENTRICULAR CARDIOMYOPATHY

The diagnostic criteria for the diagnosis of ARVC are classified into six categories and into minor and major criteria according to the original ARVC Task Force (95) as well as the recently proposed modification (96). To establish a definite diagnosis of ARVC, two major criteria, one major plus two minor criteria, or four minor criteria from different categories must be present. If the number of minor criteria that are present is reduced by one or two, the diagnosis becomes borderline or possible, respectively. CMR can detect any of the diagnostic criteria related to global and/or regional dysfunction and structural alterations:

- Regional RV akinesia or dyskinesia or dyssynchronous RV contraction plus one of the following:
  For major criterion:
      RV end-diastolic volume index ≥110 mL/m² (male) or ≥100 mL/m² (female)
      or RV ejection fraction ≤40%
  For minor criterion:
      RV end-diastolic volume index ≥100 to <110 mL/m² (male) or ≥90 to <100 mL/m²
      (female) or RV ejection fraction >40% to ≤45%

One additional major criterion for ARVC, fibrofatty replacement of myocardium on endomyocardial biopsy, (the pathologic substrate for the disease,) can also be identified using CMR (Fig. 15.12). However, it has been found that fat infiltration is seldom the only abnormal finding on CMR and may be less sensitive than RV regional dysfunction for the diagnosis of ARVC (97). The relatively poor specificity of fat visualized by CMR has been repeatedly observed (98,99). The presence of delayed hyperenhancement consistent with myocardial scar is likely to prove useful in the CMR evaluation of ARVC. In a study of 30 patients with potential ARVC, Tandri et al. found 12 patients who met the diagnostic criteria for ARVC; eight of the 12 patients (67%) had delayed hyperenhancement on CMR, whereas none (0%) of the patients without ARVC had delayed hyperenhancement (p < 0.001) (100).

HYPERTROPHIC CARDIOMYOPATHY

CMR provides for the accurate characterization of asymmetric septal hypertrophy, apical hypertrophy, and other variants of pathologic hypertrophy. CMR can be of particular value where ultrasound imaging is limited by poor acoustic windows, or where the myocardial hypertrophy localizes to areas that may be less well visualized by echocardiography, such as at the LV apex. SSFP cine sequences allow accurate measurement of end-diastolic wall thickness of all myocardial segments to define distribution and severity of hypertrophy, quantitation of myocardial mass and assessment of the influence of any observed hypertrophy on global and regional LV and RV function. Cine SSFP sequences also allow septal forms of hypertrophy to be characterized as obstructive or nonobstructive, both from visual inspection for systolic anterior motion of the mitral valve, by detection of signal voids due

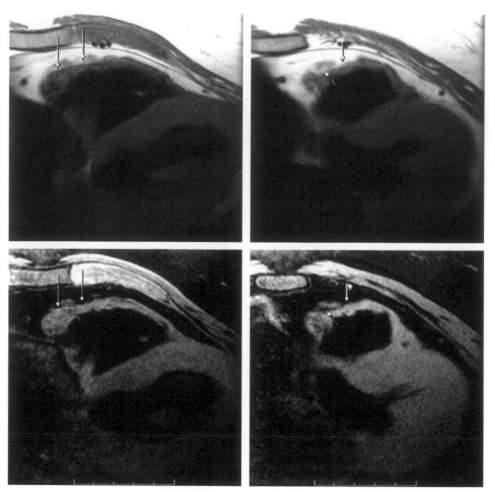

Figure 15.12   Arrhythmogenic Right Ventricular Cardiomyopathy. Oblique axial T1-weighted spin echo images acquired without (top row) and with (bottom row) fat suppression, from a patient with Arrhythmogenic Right Ventricular Cardiomyopathy. The images show subepicardial bright signal (arrows) consistent with intramyocardial fatty change centrally in the RV anterior free wall (left) and at the base of the RV outflow tract (right). In the corresponding fat-suppressed images this bright signal has become hypointense with respect to the myocardium, proving the presence of intramyocardial fat. Cine acquisitions through the area demonstrated a wall motion deficit that co-localized with the intramyocardial fatty change.

to high-velocity complex flow in the LV outflow tract during systole (101) and from quantitation of peak systolic velocity and gradient in the left ventricular outflow tract (LVOT) using phase contrast cine velocity mapping. Also of note, T2-weighted imaging can identify associated myocardial injury/ edema, and delayed enhancement sequences can identify ensuing myocardial fibrosis, which is commonly seen in the LV in a patchy intramyocardial pattern in the interventricular septum near the RV insertion sites (52), and also deep within the regions of hypertrophy (Fig. 15.13). The extent of scarring may find an important role in risk stratification for sudden cardiac death. Pending availability of larger studies with longer follow-up and greater statistical power, however, late gadolinium enhancement imaging was given a Class IIb recommendation in the 2011 ACCF/AHA Guidelines for the Diagnosis and Treatment of Hypertrophic Cardiomyopathy, to use as an

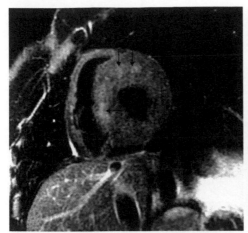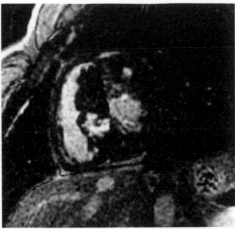

Figure 15.13 Hypertrophic Cardiomyopathy. *Left panel:* Fat-suppressed T2-weighted image in the short axis view from a patient with hypertrophic cardiomyopathy showing asymmetric hypertrophy affecting the anterior, septal and inferior segments with focal areas of T2 signal hyperintensity deep within the hypertrophied regions (arrows) suggesting injury/edema. *Right panel:* Short axis delayed enhancement image through the same region showing co-localizing areas of late Gadolinium enhancement consistent with injury with fibrous scar.

"arbitrator" when sudden cardiac death risk stratification is inconclusive based on the conventional risk factors (102).

NONCOMPACTION CARDIOMYOPATHY

Ventricular noncompaction is believed to result from arrested endomyocardial morphogenesis (103) and is usually limited to the left ventricle, most commonly involving the apical and midventricular segments of the anterior and lateral walls (Fig. 15.14). A ratio of noncompacted to compacted myocardium ≥2.3 at end-diastole on SSFP cine CMR sequences has been found to have a sensitivity, specificity, PPV, and NPV of 86%, 99%, 75%, and 99%, respectively, for the diagnosis of noncompaction, with noncompacted myocardium of some degree observed in 10 ± 3 of 17 LV segments in patients with pathologic noncompaction (104). The use of delayed enhancement imaging has been proposed to evaluate for the myocardial fibrosis that can also occur with noncompaction (105).

OTHER CARDIOMYOPATHIES

Other forms of cardiomyopathy where delayed enhancement imaging may identify characteristic features (in addition to the functional impairments) include hypereosinophilic syndromes where the delayed enhancement is typically subendocardial, tending to be circumferential and not confined to a specific vascular territory, often with overlying thrombus adherent to the injured endocardial surface. Characteristic delayed enhancement findings have also been described in Chagas' disease (predominantly midwall and subepicardial, encompassing multiple coronary territories with a preference for LV apical and inferolateral regions) (106). Typical patterns of delayed enhancement consistent with fibrosis are also recognized in systemic vasculitis (Churg-Strauss) and systemic sclerosis syndromes (incomplete or complete circumferential subendocardial involvement, not limited to specific coronary territories), and in cardiomyopathy related to cocaine abuse (both ischemic and non-ischemic patterns of fibrosis) (107). Patterns of myocardial fibrosis in the muscular dystrophies have recently been

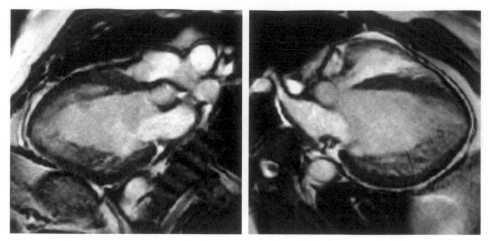

Figure 15.14 Noncompaction Cardiomyopathy. End-diastolic frames from radially oriented long axis SSFP cine views showing deep layer of LV hypertrabeculation extending almost to the base, partially sparing the interventricular septum. Along the lateral wall at the mid-ventricular level the ratio of noncompacted to compacted myocardial wall thickness is 22 mm : 7 mm = 3.1 (see measurements in right-hand panel).

comprehensively reviewed (108). Scattered patchy or diffuse myocardial fibrosis is also a feature of multiple other forms of heart disease that can lead to heart failure, including diabetic cardiomyopathy and pressure overload states such as aortic stenosis; this can be evaluated semi-quantitatively using myocardial T1 mapping techniques (109,110). In general for all the forms of cardiomyopathy, the more extensive the delayed enhancement and myocardial fibrosis, the less favorable the prognosis tends to be.

PERICARDIAL DISEASE
CMR allows direct visualization of the pericardium, which is generally 2 mm or less in thickness in normal individuals. This modality can be particularly useful for the detection of the pericardial thickening (4 mm or greater) that is usually (although not always) associated with noncalcified constrictive pericarditis. Cine sequences with myocardial tagging, which essentially place a grid of magnetic reference lines over the myocardium, pericardium, and adjacent tissue, can assess whether there is abnormal pericardial function as a result of adhesions between the pericardial surfaces (111). Postgadolinium delayed enhancement images can demonstrate pericardial fibrosis/scarring (Fig. 15.15), and real-time cine acquisition during deep breathing can evaluate ventricular interdependence due to constrictive physiology by demonstrating respirophasic shifts in the diastolic position of the interventricular septum (112). The above combination of imaging sequences allows surgically correctable pericardial constriction to be differentiated from heart failure with preserved systolic function in patients with restrictive forms of cardiomyopathy.

CARDIAC COMPUTED TOMOGRAPHY
The field of cardiac computed tomography (CCT) imaging has benefited from dramatic technical advancements in CT technology over the past decade. Scanners that boast as many as 320 detector rows, spatial resolutions approaching that of invasive angiography, or breath holds of 2 seconds or less have replaced scanners that only recently contained just

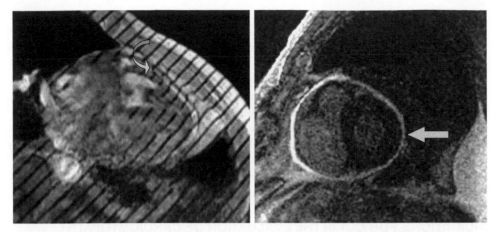

Figure 15.15 Pericardial constriction. *Left panel*: Late systolic frame from a cine acquired with myocardial tagging in a modified 4-chamber view in a patient with constrictive pericarditis. The parallel tag lines which are perpendicular to the pericardial profile over the anterior surface of the heart, were straight when deposited at end-diastole, but show deformation (mostly at the level of the more pliable epicardial fat layer) as the RV myocardium descends towards the apex during systole. The absence of a discontinuity in the tag lines at the level of the thickened pericardial contour indicates abnormal pericardial function with pericardial adhesion (curved arrow). *Right panel*: Short axis delayed enhancement image from the same patient shows strong abnormal delayed enhancement of the thickened pericardial layer circumferentially, consistent with pericardial fibrosis (heavy arrow).

4 detector rows, had spatial resolutions of over 1mm, and required breath holds of 30 seconds or more. While cardiac CT has its roots in coronary computed tomography angiography (CTA), additional applications of CT are validating the modality as more than just a noninvasive angiogram.

Historically, cardiac CT studies have been conducted on two distinct types of scanners: Electron beam computed tomography (EBCT) scanners and multidetector computed tomography (MDCT) scanners. MDCT scanners, however, represent the vast majority of scanners currently in clinical use. In CT, X-rays are projected by one or more X-ray tubes through the anatomic area being imaged, are attenuated to different degrees as they pass through varying tissues in the body, and are received by detectors on the opposite side (or 180 degrees from the tube).

Many cardiac CT protocols acquire images in a helical, or spiral, mode of operation in which the ring that contains the tube(s) and detectors, called the gantry, continually rotates around the patient, acquiring several simultaneous channels of data during continuous advancement of the CT table, with the pitch of the helix defined by the distance of table travel per gantry rotation, relative to the X-ray beam width. Tube current is delivered throughout the cardiac cycle, and the images are processed using retrospective ECG gating, which can permit dataset reconstruction at multiple time points in the cardiac cycle (e.g., 35%, 65%, and 70% of the R–R interval), and allow review of the data in cine mode. Prospective ECG triggering, also known as the "step and shoot" mode of acquisition, acquires axial images only at fixed points in the R–R interval, such as at 65% of the R–R interval. After acquiring an axial image at one level, the table is advanced over the next heart beat, permitting axial acquisition in a narrow window of the cardiac cycle every other heart beat for a lower total radiation dose. Substantial reductions of X-ray dose can be achieved using high pitch helical scanning in combination with prospective ECG triggering.

While a 2007 article in the Journal of the American Medical Association by Einstein et al. focused attention on the risks of radiation exposure from CCT (113), it is important to consider that cardiac CT, cardiac SPECT, cardiac PET, and invasive angiography all expose patients to radiation. At the time of publication of Einstein et al., radiation exposure from retrospectively gated 64-slice CT studies typically ranged from 7–14 mSv when dose modulation strategies were employed (114). This exposure was higher than the effective radiation dose from an invasive coronary angiogram (5–7 mSv) but comparable to stress SPECT (9–12 mSv) and lower than a thallium myocardial perfusion scan (18–21 mSv) (115,116). However, as scanner technology has continued to develop, the radiation exposure to patients from CCT has been dramatically reduced. Radiation exposure is commonly in the vicinity of 1 mSv or less with state-of-the-art CCT scanners and acquisition protocols (117).

INDICATIONS FOR CCT IN THE EVALUATION OF CARDIOMYOPATHY

Overall, the most common appropriate use of CCT is for the evaluation of patients with chest pain and an intermediate pre-test probability of coronary artery disease. Additionally, the 2010 Appropriate Use Criteria for Cardiac Computed Tomography (118) endorse CCT for a number of indications related to evaluation of cardiomyopathy with newly diagnosed heart failure. These indications include the following:

- Evaluation of coronary arteries in patients with new onset heart failure to assess for ischemic heart disease as the etiology.
- Quantitative evaluation of LV and RV function if images from other noninvasive methods are inadequate.
- Evaluation of native or prosthetic valve dysfunction if images from other noninvasive methods are inadequate.
- Evaluate suspected mass/ thrombus if images from other noninvasive methods are inadequate.
- Assessment of complex adult congenital heart disease including anomalies of coronary circulation, great vessels, cardiac chambers and valves.
- Evaluation of pericardial conditions (constrictive pericarditis, or complications of cardiac surgery) in patients with technically limited images from echocardiogram, MRI, or trans-esophageal echocardiogram (TEE).
- Noninvasive coronary vein mapping prior to placement of biventricular pacemaker for cardiac resynchronization therapy.
- Suspected arrhythmogenic right ventricular dysplasia.

EXCLUSION OF ISCHEMIC CARDIOMYOPATHY

Numerous studies have been published that have investigated the accuracy of CCT to detect significant coronary artery stenosis. Overall, the results on a per patient basis demonstrate that CT performs with an excellent sensitivity and negative predictive value for the detection of significant stenosis, however, the specificity and positive predictive value results have been more modest (119). A systematic review that pooled available data from 2045 patients derived a per-patient sensitivity of 98%, specificity of 88%, NPV of 96%, and PPV of 93% (120). These results indicate that CCT can safely exclude the presence of significant stenosis.

In the evaluation of patients with a newly diagnosed cardiomyopathy, the strength of CCT lies in its ability to noninvasively distinguish an ischemic from a nonischemic etiology. In patients in whom obstructive CAD is not suspected as the etiology following clinical assessment, CCT may offer an alternative to the "obligatory cath." Ghostine and colleagues reported a prospective trial of 93 patients without a known history of CAD or MI who underwent both CCT and invasive angiography for the evaluation of symptomatic heart failure with LV dilatation and LV systolic dysfunction (121). On a per patient basis, CT demonstrated a sensitivity, specificity, PPV, and NPV of 98%, 92%, 91%, and 98%, respectively, for the detection of significant stenosis, as compared with invasive angiography.

In patients with cardiomyopathy, CCT can accurately evaluate global and regional LV function and can visualize aortic and mitral valvular function. However, given the exposure to iodinated contrast and radiation required for CCT, this modality should not be routinely performed solely for functional assessment, as echocardiography and CMR can provide this data without these exposures.

NONISCHEMIC CARDIOMYOPATHIES

CCT provides exquisite images of morphology in patients with structural cardiomyopathies, such as hypertrophic or noncompaction cardiomyopathy, and structural anomalies, such as congenital heart disease. CCT is particularly valuable when there is a specific need to exclude obstructive coronary artery disease, obtain anatomic images with high spatial resolution, and when the primary imaging modality may have left questions unresolved or yielded inadequate images, such as poor ultrasound windows.

Formal trial data to systematically assess the use of CCT for the evaluation of heart failure associated with any of the nonischemic cardiomyopathies, such as cardiac amlyoidosis or cardiac sarcoidosis, is limited given that CMR can make these assessments without radiation exposure. However, CCT may prove to be helpful when CMR is absolutely or relatively contraindicated. Achenbach and colleagues have reported cases using dual source cardiac CT to demonstrate the typical amyloid pattern of subendocardial, circumferential delayed enhancement in all four cardiac chambers in a patient with biopsy proven amyloid (122), and patchy, subepicardial areas of delayed enhancement in the apical region and lateral wall in a patient with suspected cardiac sarcoid who could not undergo CMR due to an implanted cardioverter defibrillator (ICD) (123). Use of cardiac CT for evaluation of cardiac sarcoidosis has also been described by others (124,125).

Dambrin and colleagues reported a case series of 12 patients with suspected acute myocarditis that underwent cardiac CT (126). Contrast-enhanced CMR was consistent with the diagnosis of myocarditis in 11 of the patients (one patient could not tolerate CMR due to claustrophobia). The authors reported that delayed CT images revealed areas of persistence of contrast in the myocardium in a focal pattern in six patients and in a multifocal pattern in the remaining six patients. The location and extent seen on CT correlated well with the location and extent of delayed hyperenhancement seen on CMR.

Bomma and colleagues reported on 31 patients with known or suspected ARVC who underwent CCT, 29 of whom already had an ICD in place, and thus were not candidates for CMR (127). They found that increased RV trabeculation, RV intramyocardial fat, and RV scalloping on CCT were significantly associated with the final diagnosis of ARVC. They also reported that RV volumes, RV inlet dimensions, and RV outflow tract surface area were found to be increased on CT in patients diagnosed with ARVC. Soh and colleagues similarly reported a case of a patient subsequently diagnosed with ARVC who was found to have RV enlargement, excessive trabeculations, fatty infiltration, and marked RV hypokinesia on CCT (128).

REFERENCES
1. Edler I, Lindström K. The history of echocardiography. Ultrasound Med Biol 2004; 30: 1565–644.
2. Feigenbaum H, Popp RL, Chip JN, Haine CL. Left ventricular wall thickness measured by ultrasound. Arch Intern Med 1968; 121: 391–5.

3. Popp RL, Wolfe SB, Hirata T, Feigenbaum H. Estimation of right and left ventricular size by ultrasound. A study of the echoes from the interventricular septum. Am J Cardiol 1969; 24: 523–30.

4. Feigenbaum H, Zaky A, Nasser WK. Use of ultrasound to measure left ventricular stroke volume. Circulation 1967; 35: 1092–9.

5. Sutton M, Pfeller M, Palppert T, et al. Quantitative two-dimensional echocardiographic measurements are major predictors of adverse cardiovascular events after acute myocardial infarction. The protective effects of Captopril. Circulation 1994; 89: 68–75.

6. Grayburn P, Appleton C, DeMaria A, et al. Echocardiographic predictors of morbidity and mortality in patients with advanced heart failure. The Beta-blocker Evaluation of Survival Trial (BEST). J Am Coll Cardiol 2005; 45: 1064–71.

7. Mor-Avi V, Sugeng L, Weinert L, et al. Fast measurement of left ventricular mass with real-time three-dimensional echocardiography: comparison with magnetic resonance imaging. Circulation 2004; 110: 1814–18.

8. Jenkins C, Moir S, Chan J, et al. Left ventricular volume measurement with echocardiography: a comparison of left ventricular opacification, three-dimensional echocardiography, or both with magnetic resonance imaging. Eur Heart J 2009; 30: 98–106.

9. Lang RM, Bierig M, Devereux RB, et al. Recommendations for chamber quantification: a report from the American Society of Echocardiography's Guidelines and Standards Committee and the Chamber Quantification Writing Group, developed in conjunction with the European Association of Echocardiography, a branch of the European Society of Cardiology. J Am Soc Echocardiogr 2005; 18: 1440–63.

10. Kolias T, Aaronson K, Armstrong W. Doppler-derived dP/dt and –dP/dt predict survival in congestive heart failure. J Am Coll Cardiol 2000; 36: 1594–9.

11. Chen C, Rodriguez L, Lethor JP, et al. Continuous wave Doppler echocardiography for the noninvasive assessment of left ventricular dP/dt and relaxation time constant from mitral regurgitant spectra in patients. J Am Coll Cardiol 1994; 23: 970–6.

12. Chen C, Rodriguez L, Levine RA, Weyman AE, Thomas JD. Noninvasive measurement of the time constant of left ventricular relaxation using the continuous-wave Doppler velocity profile of mitral regurgitation. Circulation 1992; 86: 272–8.

13. Nishimura RA, Schwartz RS, Tajik AJ, Holmes DR. Noninvasive measurement of rate of left ventricular relaxation by Doppler echocardiography: validation with simultaneous cardiac catheterization. Circulation 1993; 88: 146–55.

14. Pai RG, Bansal RC, Shah PM. Doppler-derived rate of left ventricular pressure rise: its correlation with the postoperative left ventricular function in mitral regurgitation. Circulation 1990; 82: 514–20.

15. Fahy GJ, Marwick T, McCreery CJ, et al. Doppler echocardiographic detection of left ventricular diastolic dysfunction in patients with pulmonary sarcoidosis. Chest 1996; 109: 62–6.

16. Burstow DJ, Tajik AJ, Bailey KR, et al. Two-dimensional echocardiographic findings in systemic sarcoidosis. Am J Cardiol 1989; 63: 478–82.

17. Friart A, Philippart C, Bruart J. Echocardiography in systemic sarcoidosis. Lancet 1987; 1: 513.

18. Sharma OP, Maheshwari A, Thaker K. Myocardial sarcoidosis. Chest 1993; 103: 253–8.

19. Yazaki Y, Isobe M, Hiramitsu S, et al. Comparison of clinical features and prognosis of cardiac sarcoidosis and idiopathic dilated cardiomyopathy. Am J Cardiol 1998; 82: 537–40.

20. Lewin RF, Mor R, Spitzer S, et al. Echocardiographic evaluation of patients with systemic sarcoidosis. Am Heart J 1985; 110: 116–22.

21. Ritter M, Oechslin E, Sütsch G, et al. Isolated noncompaction of the myocardium in adults. Mayo Clin Proc 1997; 72: 26.

22. Weiford BC, Subbarao VD, Mulhern KM. Noncompaction of the ventricular myocardium. Circulation 2004; 109: 2965.

23. Jenni R, Oechslin E, Schneider J, et al. Echocardiographic and pathoanatomical characteristics of isolated left ventricular non-compaction: a step towards classification as a distinct cardiomyopathy. Heart 2001; 86: 666.

24. Frischknecht BS, Attenhofer Jost CH, Oechslin EN, et al. Validation of noncompaction criteria in dilated cardiomyopathy, and valvular and hypertensive heart disease. J Am Soc Echocardiogr 2005; 18: 865.

25. Kjaergaard J, Hastrup Svendsen J, Sogaard P, et al. Advanced quantitative echocardiography in arrhythmogenic right ventricular cardiomyopathy. J Am Soc Echocardiogr 2007; 20: 27.

26. Acquatella H, Schiller NB, Puigbó JJ, et al. Value of two-dimensional echocardiography in endomyocardial disease with and without eosinophilia. A clinical and pathologic study. Circulation 1983; 67: 1219.

27. Acquatella H, Schiller NB. Echocardiographic recognition of Chagas' disease and endomyocardial fibrosis. J Am Soc Echocardiogr 1988; 1: 60.

28. Gorcsan J, Deswal A, Mankad S, et al. Quantification of the myocardial response to low-dose dobutamije using tissue Doppler echocardiographic measures of velocity and velocity gradient. Am J Cardiol 1998; 81: 615–23.

29. Hanekom L, Cho GMY, Leano R, et al. Comparison of two-dimensional speckle and tissue Doppler strain measurement during dobutamine stress echocardiography: an angiographic correleation. Eur Heart J 2007; 28: 1765–72.

30. Falk R. Diagnosis and management of the cardiac amyloidoses. Circulation 2005; 112: 2047–60.

31. Bellavia D, Pellikka P, Abraham T, et al. Evidence of impaired left ventricular systolici function in cardiac amyloidosis with strain rate echocardiography. J Am Soc Echocardiogr 2007; 20: 1194–202.

32. Kato TS, Noda A, Izawa H, et al. Discrimination of nonobtructive hypertrophic cardiomyopathy from hypertensive left ventricular hypertrophy on the basis of strain rate imaging by tissue Doppler ultrasonography. Circulation 2004; 110: 3808–14.

33. Burns AT, La Gerche A, Prior DL, Macisaac AI. Left ventricular untwisting is an important determinant of early diastolic function. JACC Cardiovasc Imaging 2009; 2: 709–16.

34. Bertini M, Marsan NA, Delgado V, et al. Effects of cardiac resynchronization therapy on left ventricular twist. J Am Coll Cardiol 2009; 54: 1317–25.

35. Saraiva R, Dermikol S, Greenberg N, et al. Left ventricular torsional mechanics worsen with left ventricular remodeling in heart failure. Circulation 2009; 120: S339.

36. Corrado D, Fontaine G, Marcus FI, et al. Arrhythmogenic right ventricular dysplasia/cardiomyopathy: need for an international registry. Study group on Arrhythmogenic Right Ventricular Dysplasia/Cardiomyopathy of the Writing Groups on Myocardial and Pericardial Disease and Arrhythmias of the European Society of Cardiology and of the Scientific Council of Cardiomypathies of the World Heart Federation. Circulation. 2000; 101: E101–6.

37. Esch BT, Scott JM, Warburton DER, et al. Left ventricular torsion and untwisting during exercise in heart transplant recipients. J Physiol 2009; 587: 2375–86.

38. Chen G, Sun K, Huang G. In vitro validation of right ventricular volume and mass measurement by realtime three-dimensional echocardiography. Echocardiography 2006; 23: 395–9.

39. Kjaergaard J, Petersen CL, Kjaer A, et al. Evaluation of right ventricular volume and function by 2D and 3D echocardiography compared to MRI. Eur J Echocardiogr 2006; 7: 430–8.

40. Gopal AS, Chukwu EO, Iwuchukwu CJ, et al. Normal values of right ventricular size and function by real-time 3-dimensional echocardiography: comparison with cardiac magnetic resonance imaging. J Am Soc Echocardiogr 2007; 20: 445–55.

41. Jenkins C, Chan J, Bricknell K, et al. Reproducibility of right ventricular volumes and ejection fraction using real-time three-dimensional echocardiography: comparison with cardiac MRI. Chest 2007; 131: 1844–51.

42. Khalil MM, Elgazzar A, Khalil W, Omar A, Ziada G. Assessment of left ventricular ejection fraction by four different methods using 99mTc tetrofosmin gated SPECT in patients with small hearts: correlation with gated blood pool. Nucl Med Commun 2005; 26: 885–93.

43. Williams KA, Taillon LA. Left ventricular function in patients with coronary artery disease assessed by gated tomographic myocardial perfusion images. Comparison with assessment by contrast ventriculography and first-pass radionuclide angiography. J Am Coll Cardiol 1996; 27: 173.

44. Germano G, Kiat H, Kavanagh PB, et al. Automatic quantification of ejection fraction from gated myocardial perfusion SPECT. J Nucl Med 1995; 36: 2138.

45. Ioannidis JP, Trikalinos TA, Danias PG. Electrocardiogram-gated single-photon emission computed tomography versus cardiac magnetic resonance imaging for the assessment of left ventricular volumes and ejection fraction: a meta-analysis. J Am Coll Cardiol 2002; 39: 2059.

46. Bourque JM, Velazquez EJ, Borges-Neto S, et al. Radionuclide viability testing: should it affect treatment strategy in patients with cardiomyopathy and significant coronary artery disease? Am Heart J 2003; 145: 758–67.

47. Neglia D, Michelassi C, Trivieri MG, et al. Prognostic role of myocardial blood flow impairment in idiopathic left ventricular dysfunction. Circulation 2002; 105: 186–93.

48. Wallis DE, O'Connell JB, Henkin RE, et al. Segmental wall motion abnormalities in dilated cardiomyopathy: a common finding and good prognostic sign. J Am Coll Cardiol 1984; 4: 674–9.

49. Dori YL, Chikamori T, Takata J, et al. Prognostic value of thallium-201 perfusion defects in idiopathic dilated cardiomyopathy. Am J Cardiol 1991; 67: 188–93.

50. Kyriakidis MK, Dernellis JM, Androulakis AE, et al. Changes in phasic coronary blood flow velocity profile and relative coronary flow reserve in patients with hypertrophic obstructive cardiomyopathy. Circulation 1997; 96: 834.

51. Posma JL, Blanksma PK, van der Wall EE, et al. Assessment of quantitative hypertrophy scores in hypertrophic cardiomyopathy: magnetic resonance imaging versus echocardiography. Am Heart J 1996; 132: 1020.

52. Choudhury L, Mahrholdt H, Wagner A, et al. Myocardial scarring in asymptomatic or mildly symptomatic patients with hypertrophic cardiomyopathy. J Am Coll Cardiol 2002; 40: 2156.

53. Moon JC, McKenna WJ, McCrohon JA, et al. Toward clinical risk assessment in hypertrophic cardiomyopathy with gadolinium cardiovascular magnetic resonance. J Am Coll Cardiol 2003; 41: 1561.

54. Chen J, Henneman MM, Trimble MA, et al. Assessment of left ventricular mechanical dyssynchrony by phase analysis of ECG-gated SPECT myocardial perfusion imaging. J Nucl Cardiol 2008; 15: 127–36.

55. Spyrou N, Rosen SD, Fath-Ordoubadi F, et al. Myocardial beta-adrenoceptor density one month after acute myocardial infarction predicts left ventricular volumes at six months. J Am Coll Cardiol 2002; 40: 1216–24.

56. Merlet P, Delforge J, Syrota A, et al. Positron emission tomography with 11C CGP-12177 to assess beta-adrenergic receptor concentration in idiopathic dilated cardiomyopathy. Circulation 1993; 87: 1169–78.

57. Ungerer M, Bohm M, Elce JS, et al. Altered expression of beta-adrenergic receptor kinase and beta 1-adrenergic receptors in the failing human heart. Circulation 1993; 87: 454–63.

58. Caldwell JH, Link JM, Levy WC, et al. Evidence for pre to postsynaptic mismatch of the cardiac sympathetic nervous system in ischemic congestive heart failure. J Nucl Med 2008; 49: 234–41.

59. Merlet P, Valette H, Dubois-Rande JL, et al. Prognostic value of cardiac metaiodobenzylguanidine imaging in patients with heart failure. J Nucl Med 1992; 33: 471–7.

60. Merlet P, Benvenuti C, Moyse D, et al. Prognostic value of MIBG imaging in idiopathic dilated cardiomyopathy. J Nucl Med 1999; 40: 917–23.

61. Cohen-Solal A, Esanu Y, Logeart D, et al. Cardiac metaiodobenzylguanidine uptake in patients with moderate chronic heart failure: relationship with peak oxygen uptake and prognosis. J Am Coll Cardiol 1999; 2: 759–66.

62. Nakata T, Miyamoto K, Doi A, et al. Cardiac death prediction and impaired cardiac sympathetic innervation assessed by MIBG in patients with failing and nonfailing hearts. J Nucl Cardiol 1998; 5: 579–90.

63. Wakabayashi T, Nakata T, Hashi-moto A, et al. Assessment of underlying etiology and cardiac sympathetic innervation to identify patients at high risk of cardiac death. J Nucl Med 2001; 42: 1757–67.

64. Kyuma M, Nakata T, Hashimoto A, et al. Incremental prognostic implications of brain natriuretic peptide, cardiac sympathetic innervation, and noncardiac disorders in patients with heart failure. J Nucl Med 2004; 45: 155–63.

65. Jacobson AF, Lombard J, Banerjee G, et al. 123-I-mIBG scintigraphy to predict risk for adverse cardiac outcomes in heart failure patients: design of two prospective multicenter international trials. J Nucl Cardiol 2009; 16: 113–21.

66. Wakasugi S, Fischman AJ, Babich JW, et al. Metaiodobenzylguanidine: evaluation of its potential as a tracer for monitoring doxorubicin cardiomyopathy. J Nucl Med 1993; 34: 1282–6.

67. Valdé s Olmos RA, ten Bokkel Huinink WW, ten Hoeve RFA, et al. Assessment of anthracycline-related myocardial adrenergic derangement by [123I]Metaiodobenzylguanidine scintigraphy. Eur J Cancer 1995; 31: 26–31.

68. Carrió I, Estorch M, Bernaet al. Assessment of anthracycline-related myocardial adrenergic Indium-111-antimyosin and iodine-123-MIBG studies in early assessment of doxorubicin cardiotoxicity. J Nucl Med 1995; 36: 2024–49.

69. Lotze U, Kaepplinger S, Kober A, et al. Recovery of the cardiac adrenergic nervous system after long-term b-blocker therapy in idiopathic dilated cardiomyopathy: assessment by increase in myocardial 123I-metaiodobenzylguanidine uptake. J Nucl Med 2001; 42: 49–54.

70. Cohen-Solal A, Rouzet F, Berdeaux A, et al. Effects of carvedilol on myocardial sympathetic innervation in patients with chronic heart failure. J Nucl Med 2005; 46: 1796–803.

71. Gerson MC, Craft LL, McGuire N, et al. Carvedilol improves left ventricular function in heart failure patients with idiopathic dilated cardiomyopathy and a wide range of sympathetic nervous system function as measured by iodine 123 metaiodobenzylguanidine. J Nucl Cardiol 2002; 9: 608–15.

72. Takeishi Y, Atsumi H, Fujiwara S, et al. ACE inhibition reduces cardiac iodine-123-MIBG release in heart failure. J Nucl Med 1997; 38: 1085–9.

73. Toyama T, Aihara Y, Iwasaki T, et al. Cardiac sympathetic activity estimated by 123I-MIBG myocardial imaging in patients with dilated cardiomyopathy after b-blocker or angiotensin-converting enzyme inhibitor therapy. J Nucl Med 1999; 40: 217–23.

74. Kasama S, Toyama T, Kumakura H, et al. Addition of valsartan to an angiotensin-converting enzyme inhibitor improves cardiac sympathetic nerve activity and left ventricular function in patients with congestive heart failure. J Nucl Med 2003; 44: 884–90.

75. Hendel RC, Patel MR, Kramer CM, et al. ACCF/ACR/SCCT/SCMR/ASNC/NASCI/SCAI/SIR 2006 appropriateness criteria for cardiac computed tomography and cardiac magnetic resonance imaging: a report of the American College of Cardiology Foundation Quality Strategic Directions Committee Appropriateness Criteria Working Group, American College of Radiology, Society of Cardiovascular Computed Tomography, Society for Cardiovascular Magnetic Resonance, American Society of Nuclear

Cardiology, North American Society for Cardiac Imaging, Society for Cardiovascular Angiography and Interventions, and Society of Interventional Radiology. J Am Coll Cardiol 2006; 48: 1475–97.

76. Hundley WG, Bluemke DA, Finn JP, et al. ACCF/ACR/AHA/NASCI/SCMR 2010 expert consensus document on cardiovascular magnetic resonance. J Am Coll Cardiol 2010; 55: 2614–62.

77. Panting JR, Gatehouse PD, Yang GZ, et al. Abnormal subendocardial perfusion in cardiac syndrome X detected by cardiovascular magnetic resonance imaging. N Engl J Med 2002; 346: 1948.

78. Kim RJ, Albert TS, Wible JH, et al. Performance of delayed-enhancement magnetic resonance imaging with gadoversetamide contrast for the detection and assessment of myocardial infarction: an international, multicenter, double-blinded, randomized trial. Circulation 2008; 117: 629.

79. Hillenbrand HB, Kim RJ, Parker MA, et al. Early assessment of myocardial salvage by contrast-enhanced magnetic resonance imaging. Circulation 2000; 102: 1876–682.

80. Romero J, Xue X, Gonzalez W, et al. CMR imaging assessing viability in patients with chronic ventricular dysfunction due to coronary artery disease. JACC Cardiovasc Imaging 2012; 5: 494–508.

81. Assomull RG, Prasad SK, Lyne J, et al. Cardiovascular magnetic resonance, fibrosis, and prognosis in dilated cardiomyopathy. J Amer Coll Cardiol 2006; 48: 1977–85.

82. Siqueira-Filho AG, Cunha CL, Tajik AJ, et al. M-mode and two-dimensional echocardiographic features in cardiac amyloidosis. Circulation 1981; 63: 188–96.

83. Celletti F, Fattori R, Napoli G, et al. Assessment of restrictive cardiomyopathy of amyloid or idiopathic etiology by magnetic resonance imaging. Am J Cardiol 1999; 83: 798–801.

84. Maceira AM, Joshi J, Prasad SK, et al. Cardiovascular magnetic resonance in cardiac amyloidosis. Circulation 2005; 111: 186–93.

85. De Cobelli F, Esposito A, Belloni E, et al. Delayed-Enhancement cardiac MRI for differentiation of Fabry's disease from symmetric hypertrophic cardiomyopathy. AJR 2009; 192: W97–W102.

86. Silverman KJ, Hutchins GM, Bulkley BH. Cardiac sarcoid: a clinicopatholoic study of 84 unselected patients with systemic sarcoidosis. Circulation 1978; 58: 1204–11.

87. Mahrholdt H, Wagner A, Judd RM, et al. Delayed enhancement cardiovascular magnetic resonance assessment of non-ischaemic cardiomyopathies. Eur Heart J 2005; 26: 1461.

88. Vignaux O, Dhote R, Blancge P, et al. Myocardial MRI in sarcoidosis: 3-years follow-up and evaluation of the effects of steroid therapy. J Cardiovasc Magn Reson 2004; 6: 44.

89. Mahrholdt H, Goedecke C, Wagner A, et al. Cardiovascular magnetic resonance assessment of human myocarditis: a comparison to histology and molecular pathology. Circulation 2004; 109: 1250–8.

90. Abdel-Aty H, Boyé P, Zagrosek A, et al. Diagnostic performance of cardiovascular magnetic resonance in patients with suspected acute myocarditis: comparison of different approaches. J Am Coll Cardiol 2005; 45: 1815–22.

91. Lurz P, Eitel I, Adam J, et al. Diagnostic performance of CMR imaging compared with EMB in patients with suspected myocarditis. JACC Cardiovasc Imaging 2012; 5: 513–24.

92. Friedrich M, Sechtem U, Schulz-Menger J, et al. Cardiovascular magnetic resonance in myocarditis: a JACC White Paper. J Am Coll Cardiol 2009; 53: 1475–87.

93. Liu P, Oliveri N, Sullivan H, et al. Magnetic resonance imaging in beta-thalassemia: detection of iron content and association with cardiac complications. J Am Coll Cardiol 1993; 21: 491.

94. Anderson LJ, Holden S, Davis B, et al. Cardiovascular T2-star (T2*) magnetic resonance for the early diagnosis of myocardial iron overload. Eur Heart J 2001; 22: 2171–9.

95. McKenna WJ, Thiene G, Nava A, et al. Diagnosis of arrhythmogenic right ventricular dysplasia/cardiomyopathy. Task Force of the Working Group Myocardial and Pericardial Disease of the European Society of Cardiology and of the Scientific Council on Cardiomyopathies of the International Society and Federation of Cardiology. Br Heart J 1994; 71: 215.

96. Marcus FI, McKenna WJ, Sherrill D, et al. Diagnosis of arrhythmogenic right ventricular cardiomyopathy/dysplasia: proposed modification of the task force criteria. Eur Heart J 2010; 31: 806–14.

97. Tandri H, Macedo R, Calkins H, et al. Role of magnetic resonance imaging in arrhythmogenic right ventricular dysplasia: insights from the North American arrhythmogenic right ventricular dysplasia (ARVD/C) study. Am Heart J 2008; 155: 147–53.

98. Fontaliran F, Fontaine G, Fillette F, et al. Nosologic frontiers of arrhythmogenic dysplasia. Quantitative variations of normal adipose tissue of the right heart ventricle. Arch Mal Coeur Vaiss 1991; 84: 33–8.

99. Globits S, Kreiner G, Frank H, et al. Significance of morphological abnormalities detected by MRI in patients undergoing successful ablation of right ventricular outflow tract tachycardia. Circulation 1997; 96: 2633–40.

100. Tandri H, Saranathan M, Rodriguez ER, et al. Noninvasive detection of myocardial fibrosis in arrhythmogenic right ventricular cardiomyopathy using delayed-enhancement magnetic resonance imaging. J Am Coll Cardiol 2005; 45: 98–103.

101. Park JH, Kim YM, Chung JW, et al. MR imaging of hypertrophic cardiomyopathy. Radiology 2002; 185: 441–6.

102. Gersh BJ, Maron BJ, Bonow RO, et al. ACCF/AHA guideline for the diagnosis and treatment of hypertrophic cardiomyopathy: a report of the American College of Cardiology Foundation/American Heart Association Task Force on Practice Guidelines. Circulation 2011; 124: 2761–96.

103. Pignatelli RH, McMahon CJ, Dreyer WJ, et al. Clinical characterization of left ventricular noncompaction in children: a relatively common form of cardiomyopathy. Circulation 2003; 108: 2672–8.

104. Petersen SE, Selvanayagam JB, Wiesmann F, et al. Left ventricular non-compaction: insights from cardiovascular magnetic resonance imaging. J Am Coll Cardiol 2005; 46: 101–5.

105. Alsaileek AA, Syed I, Seward JB, et al. Myocardial fibrosis of left ventricle: magnetic resonance imaging in noncompaction. J Magn Reson Imaging 2008; 27: 621–4.

106. Rochitte CE, Oliveira PF, Andrade JM, et al. Myocardial delayed enhancement by magnetic resonance imaging in patients with Chagas' disease. J Amer Coll Cardiol 2005; 46: 1553–58.

107. Aquaro GD, Gabutti A, Meini M, et al. Silent myocardial damage in cocaine addicts. Heart 2011; 97: 2056–62.

108. Verhaert D, Richards K, Rafael-Fortney JA, et al. Cardiac involvement in patients with muscular dystrophies. Circ Cardiovasc Imaging 2011; 4: 67–76.

109. Iles L, Pfluger H, Phrommintikul A, et al. Evaluation of diffuse myocardial fibrosis in heart failure with magnetic resonance contrast-enhanced T1 mapping. J Amer Coll Cardiol 2008; 52: 1574–80.

110. Mewton N, Liu CY, Croisille P, et al. Assessment of myocardial fibrosis with cardiovascular magnetic resonance. J Amer Coll Cardiol 2011; 57: 891–903.

111. Holmvang G, Dinsmore RE. Magnetic resonance imaging with tagging in constrictive pericarditis. J Am Coll Cardiol 1997; 29(2, Suppl. A): 24A.

112. Francone M, Dymarkowski S, Kalantzi M, et al. Assessment of ventricular coupling with real-time cine MRI and its value to differentiate constrictive pericarditis from restrictive cardiomyopathy. Euro Radiol 2006; 16: 944–51.

113. Einstein AJ, Henzlova MJ, Rajagopalan S. Estimating risk of cancer associated with radiation exposure from 64-slice computed tomography coronary angiography. JAMA 2007; 298: 317–23.

114. Einstein AJ, Moser KW, Thompson RC, et al. Radiation dose to patients from cardiac diagnostic imaging. Circulation 2007; 116: 1290–305.

115. Budoff MJ, Cohen MC, Garcia MJ, et al. ACCF/AHA clinical competence statement on cardiac imaging with computed tomography and magnetic resonance. Circulation 2005; 112: 598–617.

116. Coles DR, Smail MA, Negus IS, et al. Comparison of radiation doses from multislice computed tomography coronary angiography and conventional diagnostic angiography. J Am Coll Cardiol 2006; 47: 1840–5.

117. Achenbach S, Marwan M, Ropers D, et al. Coronary computed tomography angiography with a consistent dose below 1 mSv using prospectively electrocardiogram-triggered high-pitch spiral acquisition. Eur Heart J 2010; 31: 340–6.

118. Taylor AJ, Cerqueira M, Hodgson JM, et al. ACCF/SCCT/ACR/AHA/ASE/SCAI/SCMR 2010 appropriate use criteria for cardiac computed tomography. J Am Coll Cardiol 2010; 56: 1864–94.

119. Budoff MJ, Achenbach S, Blumenthal RS, et al. Assessment of coronary artery disease by cardiac computed tomography: a scientific statement from the American Heart Association Committee on Cardiovascular Imaging and Intervention, Council on Cardiovascular Radiology and Intervention, and Committee on Cardiac Imaging, Council on Clinical Cardiology. Circulation 2006; 114: 1761–91.

120. Stein PD, Yaekoub AY, Matta F, Sostman HD. 64-slice CT for diagnosis of coronary artery disease: a systematic review. Am J Med 2008; 121: 715–25.

121. Ghostine S, Caussin C, Habis M, et al. Non-invasive diagnosis of ischaemic heart failure using 64-slice computed tomography. Eur Heart J 2008; 29: 2133–40.

122. Marwan M, Pflederer T, Ropers D, et al. Cardiac amyloidosis imaged by dual-source computed tomography. J Cardiovasc Comput Tomogr 2008; 2: 403–5.

123. Muth G, Daniel WG, Achenbach S. Late enhancement on cardiac computed tomography in a patient with cardiac sarcoidosis. J Cardiovasc Comput Tomogr 2008; 2: 272–3.

124. Kanao S, Tadamura E, Yamamuro M, et al. Demonstration of cardiac involvement of sarcoidosis by contrast-enhanced multislice computed tomography and delayed-enhanced magnetic resonance imaging. J Comput Assist Tomogr 2005; 29: 745–8.

125. Smedema JP, Truter R, de Klerk PA, et al. Cardiac sarcoidosis evaluated with gadolinium-enhanced magnetic resonance and contrast-enhanced 64-slice computed tomography. Int J Cardiol 2006; 112: 261–3.

126. Dambrin G, Laissy JP, Serfaty JM, et al. Diagnostic value of ECG-gated multidetector computed tomography in the early phase of suspected acute myocarditis. A preliminary comparative study with cardiac MRI. Eur Radiol 2007; 17: 331–8.

127. Bomma C, Dalal D, Tandri H, et al. Evolving role of multidetector computed tomography in evaluation of arrhythmogenic right ventricular dysplasia/cardiomyopathy. Am J Cardiol 2007; 100: 99–105.

128. Soh EK, Villines TC, Feuerstein IM. Sixty-four-multislice computed tomography in a patient with arrhythmogenic right ventricular dysplasia. J Cardiovasc Comput Tomogr 2008; 2: 191–2.

16

Role of invasive monitoring in heart failure: Pulmonary artery catheters in the post-ESCAPE era

W. H. Wilson Tang and Gary S. Francis

Hemodynamic derangement is a consistent finding in patients presenting with congestive heart failure. Elevated intracardiac pressure as a result of impaired ejection or filling of the left ventricle is associated with poor long-term prognosis, even in the contemporary era of heart failure management (1). It is now recognized that reduction of these pressures may improve symptoms, decrease valvular regurgitation, and can actually improve forward cardiac output. Clinical assessment of filling pressures provides reasonable targets for therapy in the hospital, although more precise measurement may lead to further reduction of valvular regurgitation and symptom improvement. Hence over the past decades, many attempts have been made to facilitate safe and accurate quantification of hemodynamic derangements across the spectrum of heart failure. The technique of bedside pulmonary artery catheterization (PAC) introduced in the early 1970s has evolved to routine clinical use. This advancement has led to many insights regarding acute myocardial infarction, cardiogenic shock, and acute heart failure.

HISTORICAL PERSPECTIVES

Forssmann, a urology trainee working in Germany in 1929 was the first to insert a catheter into the right atrium in a human (himself) for the purpose of infusing medications, for which he was later awarded the Nobel Prize (2). Cournand, a mentor to Eugene Braunwald, also shared the Nobel Prize in later years for developing techniques for right heart catheterization for diagnostic purposes in humans in the 1940s (3). Louis Dexter, for years a fixture at Peter Bent Brigham Hospital, measured the first capillary wedge pressure in 1949 during an attempt to catheterize the renal veins to measure renal vein rennin (4). However, it was Swan, Ganz, and colleagues who really developed bedside hemodynamic monitoring at Cedars-Sinai Hospital in the 1970s (5). It served us well for 35–40 years with predominantly the same technique and design. The importance of the PAC to the development of the specialty of cardiology cannot be overstated. Many of the variables measured by PAC have not changed over the decades, except for perhaps a few enhancements such as the installation of the operator-controlled balloon-tip, using temperature difference of injectate (thermodilution technique) or the arterial-mixed venous oxygen saturation gradient (utilizing the Fick equation) to estimate cardiac output rather than the "green dye" technique, and additional options (such as pacing electrodes or continuous cardiac output sensors).

A large panel of calculated derivatives from measured hemodynamic variables have been created and tested at the bedside in an attempt to better describe the physiologic state of the congested patient with heart failure or with other conditions leading to profound hemodynamic deterioration. Many important concepts linked to the cardiocirculatory model of heart failure were constructed with the help of hemodynamic observations made in parallel to the broad utilization of vasodilators, inotropic drugs, and loop diuretics (so-called "hemodynamically-guided" or "tailored" medical therapy). In fact, some drugs approved during this period were due to demonstration of their hemodynamic benefits using precise invasive measurements by the PAC. The use of the beside PAC moved the field of hemodynamics forward and provided a rich venue to help us understand cardiogenic shock, heart failure, and pharmacologic interventions designed to treat these serious medical conditions.

Skeptics began to criticize the overzealous use of PACs in the late 1980s. The primary concern was the unverified safety record, the potential overutilization of the PAC, and the lack of sophistication by some operators when interpreting. There were observational retrospective data published suggesting that PAC use might be associated with adverse outcomes in critically ill patients (6,7). Two retrospective studies in particular demonstrates that PAC use in the setting of post-myocardial infarction complicated by shock or heart failure was associated with a longer hospital stay, higher in-hospital mortality, and no difference in long-term mortality compared with those without PAC guidance (8,9). Data available in the critical care literature suggested neutral effects with higher complication rates in a wide range of non–heart failure settings (10–13). These concerns eventually prompted equipoise or even skepticism about the use of PACs in the medical community. A large meta-analysis of the major published work on the use of PAC in the critical care setting suggested that a routine use of PAC to guide therapy may not improve long-term clinical outcomes (14). Following a consensus workshop (10), the Evaluation Study of Congestive Heart Failure and Pulmonary Artery Catheterization Effectiveness (ESCAPE) was designed and conducted to prospectively examine the safety and efficacy of such invasive procedure was launched (15). The purpose of this chapter is to put the PAC and results of the ESCAPE into the perspective of today's contemporary management of patients with advanced heart failure.

THE ESCAPE TRIAL

The ESCAPE trial was a multicenter, randomized controlled trial of 433 patients at 26 sites conducted from January 2000 to November 2003. Patients were randomly allocated to receive therapy guided by clinical assessment and a PAC or clinical assessment alone. In ESCAPE, 218 patients were managed with clinical assessment alone and 215 were managed with clinical assessment and a PAC. The two groups were well matched: mean left ventricular ejection fraction of 19% and 20%, mean blood urea nitrogen of 34 mg/dL and 36 mg/dL, mean serum creatinine of 1.5 mg/dL in both groups, and mean B-type natriuretic peptide (BNP) of 974 pg/mL and 1018 pg/mL, respectively (16). In the PAC group, the mean right atrial pressure was 14 mmHg, mean pulmonary capillary wedge pressure was 25, and the mean cardiac index was 1.9 L/min/m^2.

The primary results as well as some substudy analyses have been published. Overall outcomes including the primary endpoint (the number of days that patients were hospitalized or the number of patients died during the 6-month period after randomization) were essentially similar between the two groups (Fig. 16.1). Complications related to the PAC were observed in 4.2% in the PAC group, with an overall frequency of adverse events being 22% in the PAC group and 11% in the control group. A consistent trend for improved cardiac function and exercise ability was observed in patients in the PAC group.

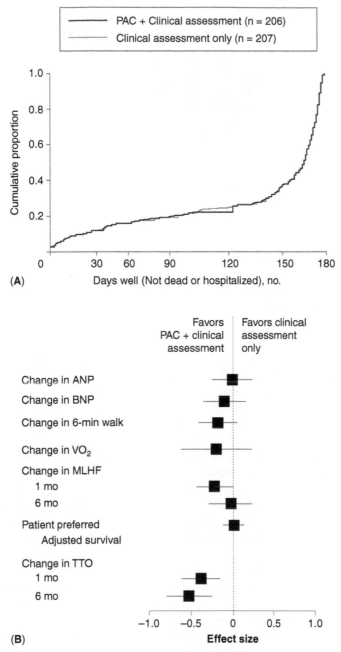

Figure 16.1 **(A)** Primary and **(B)** secondary results of the ESCAPE trial. *Abbreviations*: ANP, atrial natriuretic peptide; BNP, brain natriuretic peptide; MLHF, Minnesota Living with Heart Failure questionnaire; PAC, pulmonary artery catheterization; TTO, time trade-off score; VO_2, peak oxygen consumption.

We also learned that the use of the PAC plus careful clinical assessment allowed better anticipation (but not overall incidence) of adverse events such as worsening renal function (17), but it did not affect mortality or overall hospitalization. Biomarker analysis also indicated that there may be a correlation, albeit loose, between hemodynamic

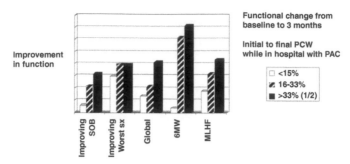

Figure 16.2 Relationship of reduction in pulmonary capillary wedge pressures (PCW) during hospitalization to improvement in symptoms (Sx) measured at 3 months after discharge, from the ESCAPE trial. *Abbreviations*: 6MW, 6-minute walk; MLHF, Minnesota Living with Heart Failure; PAC, pulmonary artery catheterization; SOB, shortness of breath.

measurements and cardiac biomarkers such as BNP or cardiac troponin (18). Preliminary data from another substudy with impedance cardiography measurements also failed to demonstrate a strong correlation between non-invasive versus invasive hemodynamic assessment (Fig. 16.2) (19).

LESSONS FROM ESCAPE

What are the major clinical implications of ESCAPE? It is clear that the primary conclusion from ESCAPE has been that *routine* use of PAC is not indicated in patients who are being considered for hemodynamically guided therapy. However, patients judged to be *in need* of invasive monitoring with a PAC were excluded from the study. Such a statement does not imply that one should not use a PAC to guide diagnosis and therapy in those who may be clinically judged to benefit from a PAC. This is evident in the ESCAPE Registry data trial that demonstrate that those who were not randomized to the trial had greater baseline severity of disease and a higher risk for adverse clinical outcomes during and after hospitalization (20). Hence, for them there was a perceived need to use the PAC. The challenge is now to define which subset of patients needs PAC monitoring. It is those patients whose initial therapy fails to relieve symptoms of clinical congestion or have end-organ dysfunction despite conventional therapeutic interventions that may benefit from PAC monitoring.

There are several commonly overlooked points from the ESCAPE trial that may warrant some discussion. First, it is important to recognize that the lack of harm is convincingly shown in a prospective randomized trial manner. These findings may ward off those who are skeptical of the use of PAC and who may believe that recognition of hemodynamic measurements may in some way cause inappropriate and overzealous treatments. In fact, further reassurance has been provided by data from ambulatory implantable hemodynamic monitoring trials where treatment guided by hemodynamic measurements can restore hemodynamic balance without significant adverse consequences (21). Safe and proficient placement of the PAC in ESCAPE, although not absolute, was very impressive. However, placement of the PAC was overseen by experienced investigators in large medical centers. Today, bedside fluoroscopy is commonly used in our coronary care unit when placing a PAC, providing a further margin of safety regarding placements. It is not clear whether such a remarkably safe procedure in experienced hands is equally safe when used by less experienced operators.

Second, a major drawback to these studies is the perception that whether treatment was similar in both the PAC group and the non-PAC group, could one realistically expect the PAC group to do better? After all, PAC use is not a treatment. There may be vastly different interventions in response to the same PAC measurements from different study sites, and it is clear that even from these highly selected (primarily academic) investigational sites from ESCAPE, there was a wide variety of practice patterns and therapeutic selections (22). These observations highlight the limitations of unifying current therapeutic approaches when patients present in the decompensated state of advanced heart failure, and this can lead to heterogeneous findings even if the measurements were beneficial.

Third, preliminary data have suggested that filling pressures estimated clinically by careful physical examination is surprisingly consistent with direct invasive measurements. This is likely due to the fact that experienced investigators in ESCAPE were savvy regarding clinical assessment, biomarkers, renal function, and judgment regarding pathophysiology and treatment. However, a similar argument may not hold for less experienced individuals who may falsely interpret hemodynamic data, swaying them away from what would have been appropriate management strategies. While the primary endpoint did not reach significant differences between the two groups, there were indicators that favored the PAC arm in terms of reduced risk of developing renal insufficiency (17). Interestingly, other noninvasive or biochemical substitution of hemodynamic measurement tools failed to predict hemodynamic values similar to those derived from the PAC.

WHO SHOULD HAVE A PAC PLACED IN TODAY'S SETTING?

We, like others, have observed that the use of the PAC has decreased in the United States over the past decade (23). The data collected to date do not support "routine use" of PAC in any patient group. If anything, they vindicate Eugene Robin's warning of over 20 years ago that "... physicians should limit catheter use to circumstances in which there is a large probability that the data will result in more effective management" (24) However, one should remember that the overall impact of the PAC was neutral (and not negative) on patient outcomes (14). The neutral outcome may have more to do with our inability to treat acute heart failure effectively than the PAC per se. The main indications of assessing central hemodynamics using PAC remain (*i*) its ability to distinguish various forms of circulatory shock; (*ii*) its ability to provide short- and long-term risk prediction; and (*iii*) its potential to identify those patients who may benefit from specific effective therapies.

DIAGNOSTIC CONSIDERATION

The role of the PAC in the setting of worsening or acute heart failure when there is uncertainty regarding preloading conditions and perfusion to vital organs has not been refuted, especially when initial attempts of stabilization have failed (e.g., fluid resuscitation, diuretic therapy). It is still common to see critically ill patients with poor perfusion in whom assessment of filling pressure is ambiguous despite careful clinical assessment. The contribution of pulmonary insufficiency versus cardiac failure to syndrome of acute respiratory distress, pulmonary edema, or pulmonary arterial hypertension can be vexing problems that sometimes can only be distinguished by invasive measurements. There is no simple bedside test to measure effective circulating volume. Shock, pulmonary hypertension, portopulmonary hypertension, and inadequate organ perfusion can occur outside the setting of elevated LV filling pressure. Occasionally, contractile reserve must be assessed in the setting of severe valvular heart disease. In these situations, acute assessment of central hemodynamics is necessary.

Risk Stratification

It has been recognized for years that "congestion" is a more accurate predictor of short-term risk than cardiac output. We have confirmed this in our own experience, where high filling pressures more fully predicted short-term and long-term outcomes than cardiac output itself (1). Patients who leave the intensive care unit who are not yet fully decongested are at a greater risk throughout their hospital stay and more likely to be readmitted sooner (25). Clearly, certain characteristics of central hemodynamics (especially in the form of elevated right-sided filling pressures and pulmonary vascular resistance) may have important implications on candidacy of cardiac transplantation status and/or implantation of mechanical circulatory support devices.

Guiding Management

The decision to increase filling pressure versus giving intravenous diuretic therapy can be difficult even in experienced hands. The determination that inotropic support or intravenous vasodilators such as sodium nitroprusside should be used and the accurate titration of such therapy are based to a large extent on hemodynamic monitoring. The initial titration of drugs, such as epoprostenol for pulmonary arterial hypertension, is largely determined by response (or the lack of) to therapy using a PAC. It is therefore a natural extension for regulatory agencies to mandate hemodynamic characterization in the research and development of therapeutic agents for critical care setting. In turn, assessing response to therapy is particularly useful, and the PAC can help guide treatment decisions in specific patients.

CONCLUSIONS

The rise and fall in the clinical utilization of PAC to some extent underlines the changes in the perception of how to best use a diagnostic device when managing patients who are critically ill from their circulatory compromise. We have seen similar trends in other medical devices such as recalled pacemaker or defibrillator leads, drug-eluting coronary stents, when early enthusiasm was followed by skepticisms following broad use. PAC was slightly different–the diagnostic and prognostic data derived from PAC has yet to provide demonstrable benefit in the overall patient population presenting with acute decompensated heart failure, even though there are specific clinical scenarios when physicians may still find value in understanding central hemodynamics in the care of their patients. In the final analysis, the physician caring for the patient with ADHF will have to evaluate the individual patient risks and benefits, and proceed with PAC for hemodynamic monitoring if the benefit outweighs the risk. To this end, we have suggested certain scenarios where PAC monitoring may be quite helpful. To generally dismiss the use of PAC in all such patients is tantamount to misinterpretation of the very important ESCAPE trial. Neither nihilism nor unbridled enthusiasms is prudent when making such decisions.

REFERENCES

1. Mullens W, Abrahams Z, Skouri HN, et al. Prognostic evaluation of ambulatory patients with advanced heart failure. Am J Cardiol 2008; 101:1297–302.
2. Forssmann W. The catheterization of the right side of the heart. Klin Wochenschr 1929; 45: 2085–7.
3. Cournand A, Lauson H, Bloomfield R, Breed E, Baldwin E. Recording of right heart pressures in man. Proc Soc Exp Biol Med 1944; 55: 34–6.
4. Hellems H, Haynes F, Dexter L. Pulmonary "capillary" pressure in man. J Appl Physiol 1949; 2: 24–9.
5. Swan HJ, Ganz W, Forrester J, et al. Catheterization of the heart in man with use of a flow-directed balloon-tipped catheter. N Engl J Med 1970; 283: 447–51.
6. Dalen JE, Bone RC. Is it time to pull the pulmonary artery catheter? JAMA 1996; 276: 916–18.
7. Connors AF Jr, Speroff T, Dawson NV, et al. The effectiveness of right heart catheterization in the initial care of critically ill patients. support investigators. JAMA 1996; 276: 889–97.

8. Cohen MG, Kelly RV, Kong DF, et al. Pulmonary artery catheterization in acute coronary syndromes: insights from the GUSTO IIb and GUSTO III trials. Am J Med 2005; 118: 482–8.

9. Gore JM, Goldberg RJ, Spodick DH, Alpert JS, Dalen JE. A community-wide assessment of the use of pulmonary artery catheters in patients with acute myocardial infarction. Chest 1987; 92: 721–7.

10. Bernard GR, Sopko G, Cerra F, et al. Pulmonary artery catheterization and clinical outcomes: national heart, lung, and blood institute and food and drug administration workshop report: consensus statement. JAMA 2000; 283: 2568–72.

11. Richard C, Warszawski J, Anguel N, et al. Early use of the pulmonary artery catheter and outcomes in patients with shock and acute respiratory distress syndrome: a randomized controlled trial. JAMA 2003; 290: 2713–20.

12. Harvey S, Harrison DA, Singer M, et al. Assessment of the clinical effectiveness of pulmonary artery catheters in management of patients in intensive care (PAC-Man): a randomised controlled trial. Lancet 2005; 366: 472–7.

13. Wheeler AP, Bernard GR, Thompson BT, et al. Pulmonary-artery versus central venous catheter to guide treatment of acute lung injury. N Engl J Med 2006; 354: 2213–24.

14. Shah MR, Hasselblad V, Stevenson LW, et al. Impact of the pulmonary artery catheter in critically ill patients: meta-analysis of randomized clinical trials. JAMA 2005; 294: 1664–70.

15. Shah MR, O'Connor CM, Sopko G, et al. Evaluation Study of Congestive Heart Failure and Pulmonary Artery Catheterization Effectiveness (ESCAPE): design and rationale. Am Heart J 2001; 141: 528–35.

16. Binanay C, Califf RM, Hasselblad V, et al. Evaluation study of congestive heart failure and pulmonary artery catheterization effectiveness: the ESCAPE trial. JAMA 2005; 294: 1625–33.

17. Nohria A, Hasselblad V, Stebbins A, et al. Cardiorenal interactions: insights from the ESCAPE trial. J Am Coll Cardiol 2008; 51: 1268–74.

18. Shah MR, Hasselblad V, Tasissa G, et al. Rapid assay brain natriuretic peptide and troponin i in patients hospitalized with decompensated heart failure (from the evaluation study of congestive heart failure and pulmonary artery catheterization Effectiveness Trial). Am J Cardiol 2007; 100: 1427–33.

19. Yancy C, Rogers J, Pauly DF. Diagnostic implications of impedance cardiography in the setting of severe acute decompensated heart failure: results of the bioimpedance cardiography (BIG) substudy in the ESCAPE trial [Abstract]. Circulation 2005; 112(Suppl II): II–639.

20. Allen LA, Rogers JG, Warnica W, et al. Who escaped randomization to receive a pulmonary artery catheter? the escape registry [abstract]. J Card Fail 2007; 13(6 Suppl 2): S134.

21. Bourge RC, Abraham WT, Adamson PB, et al. Randomized controlled trial of an implantable continuous hemodynamic monitor in patients with advanced heart failure: the COMPASS-HF study. J Am Coll Cardiol 2008; 51: 1073–9.

22. Elkayam U, Tasissa G, Binanay C, et al. Use and impact of inotropes and vasodilator therapy in hospitalized patients with severe heart failure. Am Heart J 2007; 153: 98–104.

23. Wiener RS, Welch HG. Trends in the use of the pulmonary artery catheter in the United States, 1993–2004. JAMA 2007; 298: 423–9.

24. Robin ED. The cult of the Swan-Ganz catheter. overuse and abuse of pulmonary flow catheters. Ann Intern Med 1985; 103: 445–9.

25. Stevenson LW, Tillisch JH. Maintenance of cardiac output with normal filling pressures in patients with dilated heart failure. Circulation 1986; 74: 1303–8.

17

Conventional therapy of chronic heart failure: Diuretics, vasodilators, and digoxin

G. William Dec

TREATMENT GOALS

Heart failure treatment goals should include improvement in symptoms, increased functional capacity, prevention or partial amelioration of left ventricular remodeling, and improvement in survival (1,2). Obese patients should lose weight, smokers should discontinue tobacco use, and low-level aerobic physical activity should be encouraged. Every effort should be made to identify and correct reversible causes for heart failure. Specific treatment should be initiated for anemia, thyrotoxicosis, or other causes of high output failure. Systemic hypertension should be aggressively treated, and surgical correction of significant valvular or congenital cardiac lesions should be considered. Withdrawal of any cardiac depressants, such as alcohol ($\geq$2 drinks/day) should be encouraged.

Heart failure that persists, after correction of reversible causes, should be treated with dietary sodium restriction (2–3 g daily), diuretics for volume overload, vasodilator therapy [particularly angiotensin-converting enzyme inhibitors (ACEIs)], and β-adrenergic blockers (Fig. 17.1) (2). A sodium restriction below 3 g/day is generally indicated for patients with New York Heart Association (NYHA) class III/IV heart failure symptoms (2). Restriction of daily fluid intake to less than 2 L should be considered for patients with both severe hyponatremia (Na$^+$ <130 mEq/L) and who demonstrated a volume overload despite high doses of diuretics and an appropriate sodium restriction (2).

PHARMACOLOGIC THERAPY FOR SYSTOLIC HEART FAILURE
Diuretics

Diuretics remain the mainstay of treatment for "congestive" symptoms, but have not been shown to improve survival. Diuretics interfere with sodium retention by inhibiting the resorption of sodium or chloride in the renal tubules. Although most agents further activate the renin-angiotensin system by lowering afferent glomerular renal blood flow, neurohormonal activation (renin, angiotensin II, endothelin-1, and brain natriuretic peptide) often acutely decreases among patients with acute decompensated heart failure (ADHF) (3). All diuretics except spironolactone reach luminal transport sites within the kidney through the tubular fluid. Two pharmacological classes of agents are available: loop diuretics and agents that act in the distal tubule (4). Thiazides and distal diuretics have sufficiently long half-lives that they can be administered once or twice daily. Loop diuretics have shorter half-lives that range from one hour for bumetanide to three to four hours for torsemide. The relationship between the arrival of a diuretic at its site of action in the kidney and

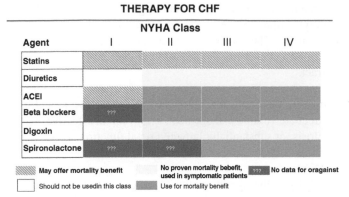

Figure 17.1 Standard pharmacological approach to heart failure based on the agent and severity of clinical heart failure symptoms *Abbreviations*: ACEIs, angiotensin-converting enzyme inhibitors; CHF, congestive heart failure; NYHA, New York Heart Association. *Source*: From Ref. 34.

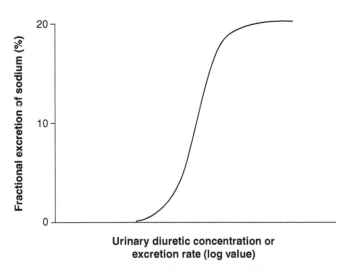

Figure 17.2 Pharmacodynamic effect of a loop diuretic. The relationship between the natriuretic response and the amount of diuretic reaching the site of action is represented by a sigmoid-shaped curve. *Source*: From Ref. 4.

the natriuretic response determines the pharmacodynamics of the drug (Fig. 17.2). This relationship indicates that a threshold quantity of drug must be achieved at the site of action in order to produce a diuretic response. Thus, diuretic dosing must be individualized in order to determine that dose which will be sufficient to achieve the steep portion of this curve, as shown in Figure 17.2 (i.e., the effective dose).

Loop Diuretics

Loop diuretics (bumetanide, ethacrynic acid, furosemide, and torsemide) are the most potent diuretics currently available and inhibit tubular reabsorption of sodium chloride in the ascending limb of the loop of Henle (the diluting segment). Recent data suggest that torsemide and bumetanide may be more effective than furosemide in advanced heart failure (4,5). While the oral availability of furosemide varies widely (10–100%), absorption of torsemide and bumetanide is nearly complete (ranging from 80% to 100% (4). Torsemide may also reduce myocardial fibrosis due to decreased procollagen type I carboxy-terminal proteinase activation (5). These newer drugs are particularly effective in the presence of right-sided heart failure, which may substantially impair absorption of the agent from the gastrointestinal tract.

Retrospective observational studies suggest an independent dose-association between high doses of loop diuretics and worse survival (6). Nonetheless, loop diuretics continue to be essential for adequate volume management. They remain effective, even in the presence of metabolic alkalosis, or substantially impaired renal function.

Thiazide Diuretics

Thiazides act mainly by inhibiting reabsorption of sodium and chloride in the distal convoluted tubules of the kidney. They also increase potassium secretion in the distal convoluted tubules and collecting ducts, resulting in potassium depletion. Thiazide-induced diuresis is generally relatively modest; these agents are ineffective when the glomerular filtration rate falls below 40 mL/min (4). Chlorothiazide and hydrochlorothiazide are the most commonly prescribed agents. Thiazides often precipitate or exacerbate hyperglycemia, worsen hyperuricemia, and decrease sexual function. Further, thiazides can adversely affect lipid metabolism, producing up to an 8% elevation of LDL cholesterol and a 15–20% increase in triglyceride levels. Fortunately, many of these adverse effects on lipids resolve within 12–24 months of therapy.

Metolazone is a member of the quinazoline-sulfonamide group; it exerts its effects primarily by inhibiting sodium reabsorption at the cortical diluting site and in the proximal convoluting tubule. The drug's prolonged duration of action is due to protein binding and enterohepatic recycling.

Potassium-Sparing Diuretics

Spironolactone, triamterene, and amiloride are relatively weak diuretics but enhance the action and counteract the kaliuretic effects of the more potent loop diuretics. The spirono-lactones are steroid analogs of the mineralocorticoids, and work by inhibiting the effects of aldosterone in the distal tubule. These agents should be used in heart failure patients whose creatinine failure is below 2.5 mg/dL, and potassium level is below 5.0 mEq/L. Both spironolactone and eplerenone have been shown to improve survival in advanced heart failure and following acute myocardial infarction (MI), respectively. A recent trial demonstrated that aldosterone-inhibiting agents can also benefit patients with mild heart failure (6a).

Diuretic Tolerance

Lack of response to diuretic therapy may be caused by excessive sodium intake, use of agents that antagonize their effects (e.g., nonsteroidal anti-inflammatory drugs), worsening renal dysfunction, or impaired renal blood flow. Further, long-term administration of a loop diuretic is associated with hypertrophy of the distal nephron segments, with concomitant increases in reabsorption of sodium (7). Sodium that escapes from the loop of Henle is, therefore, actively reabsorbed at more distal sites, decreasing overall diuresis. This phenomenon results in long-term tolerance to loop diuretics. Thiazide diuretics block the nephron sites at which this hypertrophy occurs. Thus, the combination of a loop diuretic plus a thiazide may create a synergistic response and should be considered for patients who do not have an adequate response to an optimal dose of a loop diuretic. Metolazone exacts a markedly additive response when administered with furosemide. High-dose furosemide when administered as a continuous infusion may also be more effective than when given as bolus administration for hospitalized patients with ADHF and impaired renal function (8). In cases of advanced (NYHA class III/IV) heart failure, patients should be instructed to follow a flexible diuretic program, whereby they adjust their daily diuretic dose to maintain a desired prespecified "dry" body weight.

Preserving renal function while affecting appropriate diuresis remains a therapeutic challenge. Several new classes of drugs are undergoing clinical trials. Vasopressin receptor antagonists remove water by increasing aquaporin-2 activity in the renal collecting ducts. Controlled studies with lixivaptan and tolvaptan have shown significant improvements in hyponatremia and dyspnea index among ADHF patients. However, the EVEREST (Efficacy of Vasopressin Antagonism in Heart Failure Outcome Study with Tolvaptan) trial failed to demonstrate a survival benefit (9). Similarly, while preliminary phase II studies with selective adenosine-receptor antagonists demonstrated dose-dependent increases in urine output, reduction in loop diuretic dosing, and improvement in glomerular filtration rate during treatment for ADHF, controlled trial results have been disappointing (10).

VASODILATOR THERAPY

Vasodilator therapy remains a cornerstone of heart failure treatment (Fig. 17.1). Its mechanisms of action vary and include a direct effect on venous capacitance vessels (nitrates) and arterioles (hydralazine), or a balanced venous and arterial effect (sodium nitroprusside, α-adrenergic blocking agents, angiotensin-converting enzyme (ACE) inhibitors, and angiotensin II receptor blocker).

Nitrates, as primary venodilators, can effectively reduce pulmonary congestion, while having little effect on systemic blood pressure. Conversely, agents that primarily dilate the arterioles, reduce systemic vascular resistance and improve cardiac output, but produce little change in ventricular filling pressures. Balanced vasodilators should generally be chosen as first-line outpatient therapy since most heart failure patients have elevated preload and afterload that requires pharmacologic modulation.

The ACE inhibitors play a crucial initial role in the treatment of heart failure by altering the vicious cycle of hemodynamic abnormalities and neurohormonal activation. ACE inhibitors decrease the formation of angiotensin II that inhibits the breakdown of bradykinin. In turn, increased bradykinin levels result in the formation of nitric oxide and other important endogenous vasodilators. Although tissue affinities differ between drugs, this property has not been shown to impact clinical outcomes.

Randomized, controlled clinical trials have demonstrated the beneficial effects of ACE inhibitors on functional status, neurohormonal activation, quality of life, and survival in patients with chronic systolic heart failure (11). ACE inhibitors reduce the risk of death due to heart failure, sudden cardiac death, and MI; similar mortality benefits have been demonstrated with multiple agents in a broad range of patients (Table 17.1) (11). In patients with NYHA class III or IV heart failure symptoms, captopril has been shown to increase survival to a greater extent than hydralazine when doses are titrated to achieve similar hemodynamic goals (12).

A variety of well-designed prospective, placebo-controlled studies, particularly Cooperative New Scandinavian Enalapril Study I (CONSENSUS I), Vasodilator Heart Failure Trial (V-He FT), Studies of Left Ventricular Dysfunction (SOLVD) trials, and the Munich Mild Heart Failure Trial (MHFT) have shown improvement in symptoms and survival in patients with heart failure symptoms, ranging from NYHA class I–IV (12). A survival benefit was evident for at least 12 years among patients who participated in the SOLVD trial (Fig. 17.3) (13). Thus, ACE inhibitors have a class I indication from the Heart Failure Society of America and the American Heart Association/American College of Cardiology guidelines committees for the routine use in symptomatic and asymptomatic patients with left ventricular systolic dysfunction and left ventricular ejection fraction <40% (1,2).

Important racial differences may also exist in pharmacological responsiveness to different vasodilator agents. Retrospective analyses of both the V-HeFT and SOLVD

Table 17.1   Effect of ACE Inhibitors on Mortality in Patients with Heart Failure

Trial	Mortality		RR (95% CI)
	ACE Inhibitors	**Controls**	
Chronic CHF			
CONSENSUS I	39%	54%	0.56 (0.34–0.91)
SOLVD (Treatment)	35%	40%	0.82 (0.70–0.97)
SOLVD (Prevention)	15%	19%	0.92 (0.79–1.08)
Post MI			
SAVE	20%	25%	0.81 (0.68–0.97)
AIRE	17%	23%	0.73 (0.60–0.89)
TRACE	35%	42%	0.78 (0.67–0.91)
SMILE	10%	14%	0.71 (0.49–0.94)

Abbreviations: ACE, angiotensin-converting enzyme; AIRE, Acute Infarction Ramipril Effect; SAVE, Survival and Ventricular Enlargement; TRACE, Trandolapril Cardiac Evaluation; CHF, congestive heart failure; CONSENSUS, Cooperative New Scandinavian Enalapril Study I; MI, myocardial infarction; RR, risk ratio; SOLVD, Studies of Left Ventricular Dysfunction; SMILE, Survival of Myocardial Infarction Long-term Evaluation.

populations have confirmed that although enalapril was effective in decreasing mortality and hospitalizations among white patients, it was ineffective in black patients with heart failure of comparable severity (14,15). In contrast, hydralazine and isosorbide dinitrate therapy appears effective in lowering all-cause mortality in blacks (16). It is effective in both men and women and has also been shown to produce further regression of abnormal left ventricular remodeling when added to background therapy with an renin-angiotensin antagonist and beta blocker (17,18). These differences may be related to genetic polymorphisms in key genes such as the angiotensin-converting enzyme or due to differences in endothelial function, particularly diminished release of nitric oxide or increased inactivation of nitric oxide caused by increased oxidative stress (17).

Dosing

The Assessment of Treatment with Lisinopril And Survival (ATLAS) trial demonstrated that high doses of lisinopril (32.5 to 35 mg daily) were better than low dosages (2.5–5 mg daily) in reducing the risk of hospitalization, but the two dosages had similar effects on symptoms and mortality (19). Nanes et al. found no significant differences in survival and clinical or hemodynamic variables, between patients who received standard- versus high-dose enalapril (20). A study by Tang and colleagues could not demonstrate any difference between high- and low-dose enalapril on serum aldosterone or plasma angiotensin II suppression, despite a dose-dependent reduction in serum ACE activity (21). While dosing should be guided by randomized clinical trial data, even low doses confer a significant benefit, and dose adjustments may be necessary in order to permit the use of other agents, particularly β-blockers, in patients when marginal blood pressure is present.

ACE Inhibitors in Post-Myocardial Infarction Management

Post-MI trials have now randomized over 100,000 patients and have demonstrated that ACE inhibitor treatment results in a 10–27% reduction in all-cause mortality, and a 20–50% reduction in the risk of developing symptomatic heart failure (Table 17.1) (22). Pooled mortality data from the SAVE, AIRE, and TRACE studies found an odds ratio for ACE inhibitor therapy versus placebo of 0.74 (95% CI: 0.66–0.83, p < 001) (23). For every 1000

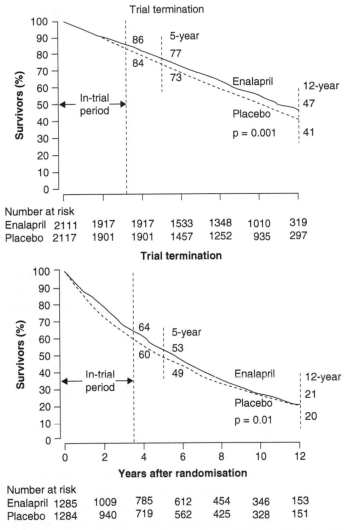

Figure 17.3 Long-term survival for patients who participated in the Studies of Left Ventricular Dysfunction (SOLVD) Prevention (upper panel) and Treatment (lower panel) trial. Survival analysis extends to 12 years. Numbers beside the curves denote the percentage of survival at trial termination, 5 years, and 12 years after randomization, calculated by the Kaplan–Meier method. *Source*: From Ref. 13.

patients treated, approximately 60 deaths will be avoided (or, to avoid one death, 15 patients will need to be treated for about 30 months). Oral ACE inhibitors, begun within 24 hours of acute MI, are safe and appear most beneficial for patients whose LVEFs are reduced below 40–45%.

ACE Inhibitor–Aspirin Interaction

Two retrospective analyses of large-scale clinical trials have suggested that aspirin decreases the beneficial effects of ACE inhibitors on survival and cardiovascular morbidity (24). Despite these concerning post-hoc findings, prospective studies have not evaluated their possible adverse interactions. It is possible that the potential interaction between aspirin and ACE inhibitors may be dose-related; a meta-analysis of hypertensive and heart failure patients suggested that aspirin at doses less than 100 mg showed no interaction with ACE inhibitors (25).

ACE inhibitors are known to augment bradykinin, which in turn stimulates synthesis of key prostaglandins that may contribute to vasodilatation. In the presence of aspirin, the bradykinin-induced increases in prostaglandins may be attenuated, thereby potentially reducing the benefits of ACE inhibition. Heart Failure Society of America practice guidelines indicate that there is currently insufficient evidence to warrant withholding either agent when indications exist for their administration (2).

DIGITALIS

Digitalis inhibits sarcolemmal Na^+-K^+-ATPase activity, thereby restricting the transport of sodium and potassium across the plasma membrane (26). This enzymatic inhibitor property leads to an increase in the intracellular sodium and an efflux of potassium from the cell. Coupled with the influx of sodium is an increase in calcium uptake, which is then made available to the contractile elements of the myofibrils.

Abnormalities of carotid baroreceptor function and excess sympathetic nervous system activity are both important components of chronic heart failure. Digitalis can partially restore the inhibitory effects of the cardiac baroreceptor system on sympathetic efferent outflow from the central nervous system (26,27). Digoxin also partially restores the impaired circadian pattern of heart rate variability that is prominent in heart failure patients (27).

Clinical Trials of Digoxin Efficacy in Chronic Heart Failure

Short- and long-term controlled and uncontrolled clinical trials have provided unequivocal evidence that chronic digoxin administration can increase LVEF, improve exercise capacity, decrease heart failure symptoms, and reduce heart failure-associated hospitalizations and emergency room visits (26). An elegant study by Lee et al. reported beneficial effects of chronic digoxin therapy as assessed by a summated clinical heart failure score that consisted of a dyspnea index, presence or absence of pulmonary rales, heart rate, signs of right-sided congestion, and chest X-ray findings of left-sided heart failure (28). A multivariate analysis showed that the presence of a third heart sound was the strongest predictor of improvement during digoxin treatment in that study (28).

The Randomized Assessment of Digoxin on Inhibitors of Angiotensin Converting Enzyme (RADIANCE) examined the outcome of digoxin withdrawal in patients with stable heart failure (NYHA functional class II or III) and systolic dysfunction (LVEF <35%) (29). Following digoxin withdrawal, 40% of patients demonstrated worsening of heart failure symptoms (defined as increased diuretic requirement, need for emergency room visit or hospital treatment). Treadmill exercise tolerance and quality of life measures also substantially worsened over the next three months. Although no clinical trial has specifically examined digoxin's efficacy in patients with NYHA class IV symptoms, there is strong evidence that the agent works across the spectrum of left ventricular systolic dysfunction.

A retrospective analysis from the Digitalis Investigator's Group (DIG) trial examined the effect of digoxin discontinuation on outcome. Among 1699 patients who discontinued digoxin during the trial, a significant increase in all-cause hospitalizations (adjusted hazard ratio (AHR): 1.18; 95% CI: 1.09–1.28; $p < 0.0001$) and heart failure hospitalizations (AHR: 1.35; 95% CI: 1.20–1.51; $p < 0.0001$) was observed (30). However, no effect on mortality was noted (AHR: 1.06; 95 CI: 0.95–1.19; $p = 0.272$) (30).

Effects on Mortality

The DIG trial examined the effect of digoxin on survival in over 6500 patients with mild to moderate heart failure. At a mean follow-up of 37 months, no differences were noted in all-cause or cardiovascular mortality (31). However, substantially fewer patients who received digoxin were hospitalized for worsening heart failure (26.8% *vs.* 34.7%; odds ratio, 0.72; 95% CI: 0.66–0.79; p < 0.001) (31). The relative risk reduction was greatest among patients with more advanced heart failure symptoms, particularly those whose LVEFs were below 25% at study entry (31). One cautionary note has arisen since publication of this trial. Retrospective subgroup analysis has suggested an increased risk of all-cause mortality among women who received digoxin during the DIG trial (32). It has been speculated that this increased risk may have been related to higher mean digoxin levels among women compared with men. A post-hoc analysis of this trial has reported a significant reduction in all-cause mortality rates (AHR: 0.75; 95% CI: 0.63–0.90, p = 0.002), all-cause hospitalizations (AHR: 0.80; 95% CI: 0.70–0.91, p = 0.001), and hospitalizations for heart failure (AHR: 0.60; 95% CI: 0.50–0.73, p < 0.0001) among patients whose serum digoxin concentration was below 1.0 ng/mL (30). Further, women did not appear to have an increased mortality risk as long as their serum digoxin concentration level did not exceed 1.0 ng/mL (33).

Digoxin Dosing

Recent data suggest that the target dose of digoxin should be lower than what is traditionally assumed (Fig. 17.4). Although higher doses may be necessary for maximum hemodynamic improvement, beneficial neurohormonal and functional effects appear to be achieved at a relatively low serum digoxin concentration, typically that associated with a dose of 0.125 mg daily (31,33). For patients with reduced renal function, the elderly, those small in

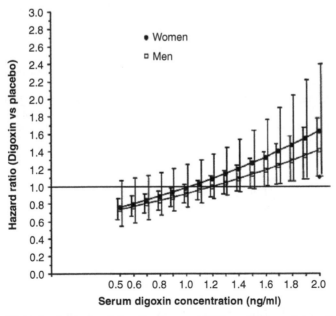

Figure 17.4 Plot of adjusted point estimates and 95% confidence intervals for men and women for the hazard rate of death on digoxin versus placebo at various serum digoxin concentrations (ng/mL) with concentration modeled as a continuous variable. *Source*: From Ref. 33.

stature, or those with substantial conduction defects on ECG, the initial starting dose may be less than 0.125 mg daily, and can be uptitrated as necessary to achieve a trough level less than 1.0 ng/dL.

Consensus Guidelines on Digoxin Use

Heart Failure Society of America and the American College of Cardiology/ American Heart Association clinical practice guidelines provide the following recommendations on digoxin administration (1,2):

1. Digoxin should be considered for outpatient treatment of patients who have persistent heart failure symptoms (NYHA class III–IV) despite standard pharmacologic therapy with diuretics, an ACE inhibitor, and a beta blocker, when the heart failure is caused by systolic dysfunction (strength of evidence = A for NYHA class II–III; B for NYHA class IV).
2. Digoxin should not be used for primary treatment of acutely decompensated heart failure (strength of evidence = B); rather it should be initiated prior to discharge as part of a long-term maintenance program.

REFERENCES

1. Jessup M, Abraham WT, Casey DE, et al. 2009 Focused update: ACCF/AHA guidelines for the diagnsosis and management of heart failure in the adult. J Am Coll Cardiol 2009; 53: 1343–82.
2. Lindenfeld J, Albert N, Boehmer JP, et al. Executive summary: HFSA 2010 comprehensive heart failure practice guidelines. J Cardiac Fail 2010; 16: 475–539.
3. Johnson W, Omland T, Hall C, et al. Neurohormonal activation rapidly decreases after intravenous therapy with diuretics and vasodilators for class IV heart failure. J Am Coll Cardiol 2002; 39: 1623–9.
4. Brater DC. Diuretic therapy. N Engl J Med 1998; 339: 397–5.
5. Lopez B, Gonzalez A, Beaumont J, et al. Identification of a potential cardiac anti-fibrotic mechanism of torsemide in patients with chronic heart failure. J Am Coll Cardiol 2007; 50: 859–67.
6. Eshaghian S, Horwich TB, Fonarow GC. Relationship of loop diuretic dose to mortality in advance heart failure. Am J Cardiol 2006; 97: 1759–64.
6a. Butler J, Ezekowitz JA, Collins SP, et al. Update on aldosterone antagonist use in heart failure with reduced ejection fraction-Heart Failure Society of America Guidelines Committee. J Cardiac Fail 2012; 18; 265–81.
7. Loon NR, Wilcox CS, Unswin RJ. Mechanism of impaired natriuretic response to furosemide during prolonged therapy. Kidney Int 1989; 83: 113–16.
8. Dormans TPJ, VanMeyel JJM, Gerlag DGG, et al. Diuretic efficacy of high dose furosemide in severe heart failure: bolus infusion versus continuous infusion. J Am Coll Cardiol 1996; 28: 376–82.
9. Konstam MA, Gheorghiade M, Burnett JC, et al. Effects of oral tolvaptan in patients hospitalized for worsening heart failure. The EVEREST outcome trial. JAMA 2007; 291: 1319–31.
10. Givertz MM. Adenosine A1 receptor antagonists at a fork in the road. Circulation Heart Fail 2009; 2: 519–22.
11. Givertz MM. Manipulation of the renin-angiotensin system. Circulation 2001; 104: e14–18.
12. Fonarow GC, Chelimsky-Fallich C, Stevenson LW. Effect of direct vasodilation with hydralazine versus angiotensin-converting-enzyme inhibition with captopril on mortality in advanced heart failure. J Am Coll Cardiol 1992; 19: 842–50.
13. Jong P, Yusuf S, Rousseau MF, Ahn SA, Bangdiwala SI. Effect of enalapril on 12-year survival and life-expectancy in patients with left ventricular systolic dysfunction: a follow-up study. Lancet 2003; 361: 1843–8.
14. Exner DV, Dries DL, Domanski MJ, et al. Lesser response to angiotensin-converting enzyme inhibitor therapy in black compared to white patients with left ventricular dysfunction. N Engl J Med 2001; 344: 1351–7.
15. Shekelle PG, Rich MW, Morton SC, et al. Efficacy of angiotensin-converting enzyme inhibitors and beta-blockers in the management of left ventricular systolic dysfunction according to race, gender, and diabetic status. a meta-analysis of major clinical trials. J Am Coll Cardiol 2003; 41: 1529–38.
16. Ferdinand KC. African american heart failure trial. role of endothelial dysfunction and heart failure in African Americans. Am J Cardiol 2007: 99(Suppl): 3D–6D.

17. Taylor AL, Lindenfeld JA, Ziesche S, et al. Outcomes by gender in the african-american heart failure trial. J Am Coll Cardiol 2006; 48: 2263–7.
18. Cohn JN, Tam SW, Anand IS, et al. Isosorbide dinitrate and hydralazine in a fixed–dose combination produces further regression of left ventricular remodeling in a well-treated black population with heart failure: results from A-HeFT. J Cardiac Fail 2007; 13: 331–9.
19. Packer M, Poole-Wilson PA, Armstrong PW, et al. The ATLAS study group. Comparative effects of low and high doses of the angiotensin-converting-enzyme inhibitor, lisinopril, on morbidity and mortality in chronic heart failure. Circulation 1999; 100: 2312–18.
20. Nanas JK, Alexopoulos G, Anastansiou-Nana MI, et al. Outcome of patients with congestive heart failure treated with standard versus high doses of enalapril: a multi-center study. J Am Coll Cardiol 2000; 36: 2090–5.
21. Tang WHW, Vagelos RH, Yee Y-G, et al. Neurohormonal and clinical responses to high-versus low-dose enalapril therapy in chronic heart failure. J Am Coll Cardiol 2002; 39: 70–8.
22. ACE Inhibitor Myocardial Infarction Collaborative Group. Indications for ACE inhibitors in the early treatment of acute myocardial infarction: systematic overview of individual data from 100,000 patients in randomized trials. Circulation 1991; 97: 2202–12.
23. Flather MD, Yusuf S, Kuber L, et al. For the ACE Inhibitor Collaborative Group. Long-term ACE inhibitor therapy in patients with heart failure or left ventricular dysfunction: a systemic overview of data from individual patients. Lancet 2000; 355: 1575–81.
24. Al-Khadra SS, Salem DN, Rand WM, et al. Anti-platelet agents and survival: a cohort analysis of the Studies of Left Ventricular Dysfunction (SOLVD) trial. J Am Coll Cardiol 1998; 31: 419–25.
25. Nawarskas JJ, Spinler AS. Does aspirin interfere with the therapeutic efficacy of angiotensin-converting enzyme inhibitors in hypertension or heart failure? Pharmacotherapy 1998; 18: 1041–52.
26. Gheorghiade M, vanVeldhuisen DJ, Colucci WS. Contemporary use of digoxin in the management of cardiovascular disorders. Circulation 2006; 113: 2556–64.
27. Newton GE, Tong JH, Schofield AM, et al. Digoxin reduces cardiac sympathetic activity in severe heart failure. J Am Coll Cardiol 1996; 28: 155–61.
28. Lee DCS, Johnson RA, Bingham JB, et al. Heart failure in outpatients. A randomized trial of digoxin versus placebo. N Engl J Med 1988; 306: 699–705.
29. Packer M, Gheorghiade M, Young JB, et al. Withdrawal of digoxin from patients with chronic heart failure treated with angiotensin-converting-enzyme inhibitors. N Engl J Med 1993; 329: 1–7.
30. Ahmed A, Gambassi G, Weaver MT, et al. Effect of discontinuation of digoxin versus continuation at low serum digoxin concentrations in chronic heart failure. Am J Cardiol 2007; 100: 280–4.
31. The Digitalis Investigation Group. The effect of digoxin on mortality and morbidity in patients with heart failure. N Engl J Med 1997; 336: 525–33.
32. Rathorne SS, Wang Y, Krumholz HM. Sex-based differences in the effect of digoxin for the treatment of heart failure. N Engl J Med 2002; 347: 1403–11.
33. Adams KF, Patterson JH, Gattis WA, et al. Relationship of serum digoxin concentration to mortality and morbidity in women in the Digoxin Investigation Group trial. a retrospective analysis. J Am Coll Cardiol 2005; 46: 497–504.
34. Eichhorn EJ. Experience with beta blockers in heart failure mortality trials. Clin Cardiol 1999; 22(Suppl): V21–29.

18

Conventional therapy of chronic heart failure: Beta-adrenergic blockers

G. William Dec

In the failing heart, beta-adrenergic signal transduction is reduced, secondary to desensitization of both the β_1 and β_2 receptors, inhibitory G protein (G_i), an enzyme responsible for modulating receptor activity by phosphorylation of β–adrenergic receptor kinase (BARK) is increased, and adenyl cyclase activity is altered (1). In end-stage heart failure, 50–60% of the total signal transducing potential of the myocardium is lost; nonetheless, substantial signaling capacity remains present (1,2). Beta blocker therapy helps restore partially the efficacy of this all important adrenergic signaling pathway. Long-term therapy results in improvement in cellular, hemodynamic, and clinical parameters.

BENEFICIAL EFFECTS OF BETA-ADRENERGIC BLOCKERS

The long-term effects of beta blockade on myocardial function are diametrically opposite to their short-term negative inotropic effects (1,2). Table 18.1 summarizes the potential cellular and hemodynamic beneficial effects of these agents. Improvement in left ventricular ejection fraction (LVEF) (typically 5–8 EF units) has been one of the most consistent long-term effects of these agents, seen with both cardioselective and nonselective agents (Fig. 18.1A). The observed rise in ejection fraction has been shown to be dose-related (3). Treatment with beta blockers generally leads to improvement in heart failure symptoms, as manifested by a decrease in New York Heart Association (NYHA) functional class and Minnesota Living with Heart Failure scores (4).

Exercise Tolerance

Data from a variety of clinical trials suggest only modestly favorable results for cardioselective agents, as opposed to predominantly neutral effects for nonselective beta blockers. The likely explanation for this apparent paradox is the blunted maximum heart rate response during exercise under the influence of full beta-adrenergic blockade. This effect may offset the favorable hemodynamic improvements achieved by enhanced myocardial contractility.

Ventricular Remodeling

By preventing excessive adrenergic exposure, beta blockers retard the effects of norepinephrine on myocardial necrosis and apoptosis, alter genetic expression, and promote reverse ventricular remodeling in chronic heart failure. Hall and colleagues have convincingly shown regression of left ventricular hypertrophy, a decrease in left ventricular mass,

330

Table 18.1 Potential Beneficial Cellular Effects of β-Adrenergic Blocker Therapy in Heart Failure

Cellular

Upregulation of β_1-receptors

Correction of G_s and G_i abnormalities

Protection against cytosolic calcium overload

Shift in metabolic substrate utilization from fatty acids to glucose

Decrease in renin release

Prevention of myocyte hypertrophy

Antioxidant effects

Decrease in apoptosis

Anti-arrhythmic effects

Hemodynamic

Alterations in loading conditions of the ventricles

Negative chronotropic effects

Improved myocardial contractility

Improved lusitropy

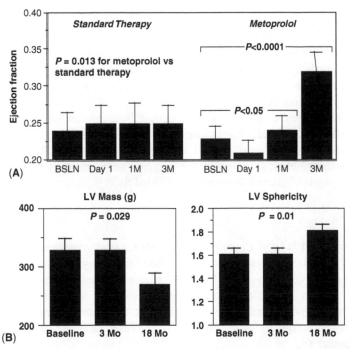

Figure 18.1 (A) Time course of changes in left ventricular function during beta-blocker therapy. A transient fall in ejection fraction was observed on day 1 of treatment with metoprolol but was not observed in the control group. Ejection fraction had risen by month 3 in the metoprolol group. BSLN: baseline measurement; M: month. **(B)** Time course for changes in left ventricular mass and sphericity during beta-blocker therapy. A fall in left ventricular mass was evident at 18 months of treatment with metoprolol; no such change was observed for the control group (data not shown). Likewise, an improvement in left ventricular sphericity was evident at 18 months of metoprolol therapy but was not seen for the control population (data not shown). *Abbreviations*: LV, left ventricular; Mo, months. *Source*: From Ref. 5.

and partial restoration of the elliptical ventricular shape (as quantified by an increased sphericity index) (Fig. 18.1B) (5). Further, findings from the Carvedilol Post-Infarct Control in Left Ventricular Dysfunction (CAPRICORN) trial confirmed beneficial effects on ventricular remodeling among patients with new-onset systolic dysfunction after acute myocardial infarction, treated with an angiotensin-converting enzyme (ACE) inhibitor (6).

TYPES OF BETA BLOCKERS

Propranolol and other "first-generation" compounds, such as timolol, are nonselective agents with equal affinity for blocking the β_1 and β_2 receptors; they have no pharmacologic properties beyond beta-adrenergic blockade (1,7). Second-generation agents, particularly metoprolol and bisoprolol, are "cardioselective" compounds that block the $\beta_1 \gg \beta_2$ receptor. Third-generation compounds (e.g., labetalol, carvedilol, and bucindolol) block both β_1 and β_2 receptors and also have ancillary effects, including α_1 blockade (labetalol and carvedilol), antioxidant properties, (carvedilol) and intrinsic sympathomimetic (bucindolol) activity. Labetalol has been studied extensively in hypertensive heart disease, but has not been prospectively validated for use in heart failure populations. Carvedilol is a slightly β_1 selective agent (approximately sevenfold) that becomes nonselective at higher target doses (7). Carvedilol has a two- to threefold selectivity for β_1-versus α_1-receptors. This degree of α_1 blockade is responsible for its moderate vasodilator properties.

EFFECTS ON MORTALITY

The most persuasive outcome measure in heart failure therapy remains all-cause mortality. Combined clinical endpoints, including mortality plus hospitalizations, or mortality and heart failure hospitalizations have also emerged as key measures. These combined clinical endpoints represent a more comprehensive assessment of the influence of therapy on disease progression. A substantial beneficial effect of beta blocker therapy on both mortality and combined endpoints has been demonstrated in randomized clinical trials of patients with NYHA class II–IV symptoms who received treatment with metoprolol controlled released/extended release (CR/XL), bisoprolol, and carvedilol (Table 18.2). Large scale, well-designed clinical trials with these agents were generally performed on stable patients receiving background therapy that included ACE inhibitors (>90%) and diuretics (>90%) (7).

Metoprolol

The Metoprolol and Dilated Cardiomyopathy (MDC) trial compared metoprolol tartrate with placebo in 383 patients with idiopathic dilated cardiomyopathy (8). All patients had NYHA class II/III symptoms and LVEF <40%. Metoprolol reduced the primary composite endpoint by 34%, a finding of marginal significance (p = 0.058) (4). The benefit was entirely due to a reduction in the morbidity endpoint. Importantly, metoprolol did improve ventricular function, quality of life measures, decreased hospitalizations, and improved exercise tolerance (8).

The Metoprolol CR/XL Randomized Intervention Trial in Congestive Heart Failure (MERIT-HF) was the first large scale, randomized, placebo-controlled mortality trial. The trial included 3991 patients; 96% of whom had NYHA functional class II/III symptoms (9). The average dose of metoprolol achieved in the MERIT-HF trial was larger than in MDC (159 mg vs. 108 mg daily). The study was prematurely discontinued after an interim analysis that revealed a 34% reduction in all-cause mortality in the metoprolol group (relative risk: 0.66; 95% confidence interval, 0.53–0.81, p = 0.006). Significantly, sudden death mortality and progressive heart failure deaths were both reduced (9). Further, the mortality reductions were observed across most demographic groups, including older versus younger

Table 18.2   Overview of Major β-Blocker Clinical Trials

FEATURE	USCS	CIBIS-II	MERIT-HF	BEST	COPERNICUS	COMET	
Drug	CRV	bisoprolol	MET[a]	bucindolol	CRV	CRV	MET[b]
Starting dose (mg)	6.25 bid	1.25 qd	12.5 qd	3 qd	3.125 bid	3.125 bid	5 bid
Target dose (mg)	25–50 bid	10 qd	200	100–200 qd	25 bid	25 bid	50 bid
No. of patients	1094	2647	3991	2708	2289	1511	1518
Mean age (yrs)	58	61	64	60	64	62	62
Mean LVEF (%)	22	27	28	23	20	26	26
NYHA class	II–IV	III–IV	III–IV	III–IV	IV	II–IV	II–IV
RR in mortality (%)	65	34	34	10	35	CRV 17% relative to MET	
P value	0.0001	0.0005	0.00009	0.11	0.00014	0.0017	

[a]Metoprolol succinate;
[b]metoprolol tartarate.
Abbreviations: CRV, carvedilol; LVEF, left ventricular ejection fraction; MET, metoprolol; NYHA, New York Heart Association; RR, relative reduction; USCS, United States Carvedilol Studies

patients, non-ischemic versus ischemic etiologies for heart failure, and lower versus higher ejection fractions (9,10). However, there was almost no reduction in the mortality rate in the relatively small number (23%) of female patients.

Bisoprolol

The Cardiac Insufficiency Bisoprolol Study (CIBIS-I) randomized 641 patients with left ventricular systolic dysfunction and NYHA class III/IV symptoms (Table 18.2) (11). Although under-powered, the trial demonstrated a moderate but significantly insignificant 20% reduction in mortality (11). The risk of hospitalization was significantly reduced by 34% (p < 0.01) (11). The favorable trends observed in the CIBIS-I trial led investigators to undertake a larger study. CIBIS-II enrolled 2647 patients with NYHA class III/IV heart failure symptoms (12). Treatment with bisoprolol reduced annual mortality by 34% (13.2% placebo *vs.* 8.8% bisoprolol; hazard ratio: 0.66; 95% confidence interval 0.54–0.81, p < 0.001) (12). Hospitalizations for worsening heart failure were also decreased by 32%. *Post-hoc* analysis from CIBIS-I had suggested benefits might be greater in patients with non-ischemic cardiomyopathy; this finding was not confirmed in the larger CIBIS-II trial (12).

Carvedilol

Four separate clinical trials that enrolled 1094 patients were combined to evaluate the effect of carvedilol on disease progression, defined as worsening heart failure leading to death, hospitalization, or a sustained increase in background medications (in one trial) (8). The patients included in the trial had an LVEF <35% and NYHA class II to IV symptoms, and had tolerated carvedilol 6.25 mg twice daily during an open run-in phase. They were then randomized based on the results of a 6-minute walk test into mild, moderate, or severe trials. The overall trial was prematurely based on a significant reduction in mortality. The combined trials demonstrated an all-cause mortality risk reduction of 65% compared with placebo (p < 0.0001) (3,8). Further, the combined risk of hospitalization or death was also reduced by 38% (20% for placebo vs. 14% for carvedilol; (p < 0.001) (Table 18.2) (8). Two component trials, Multicenter Oral Carvedilol Heart Failure Assessment (MOCHA) (13) and Prospective Randomized Evaluation of Carvedilol on Symptoms and Exercise (PRECISE) (14), were completed while the mild (15) and severe trials were terminated prematurely. The MOCHA study provided strong evidence for increased benefit from higher doses (25 mg twice daily) versus lower doses (6.25 mg twice daily) of carvedilol; thus, uptitration of the drug to 25 mg twice daily is generally recommended. Nonetheless, favorable effects were noted even at the 6.25 mg twice daily dose. The mild trial demonstrated a significant reduction in the primary combined endpoint of total mortality, cardiovascular hospitalizations, or increasing heart failure medications (15).

The Australia-New Zealand carvedilol trial enrolled 415 patients with ischemic cardiomyopathy and an LVEF <45% (16). The majority of patients enrolled were NYHA class I (30%) or II (54%). During an average follow-up of 19 months, carvedilol reduced the combined risk of all-cause mortality or any hospitalization by 26% (relative risk 0.74; 95% confidence interval 0.57–0.95, p = 0.02).

The mortality benefit of beta blocker therapy in patients with advanced (NYHA class IV) heart failure symptoms has also been established. Prior trials have generally included only a small minority (3–16%) of patients with advanced heart failure (17). The Carvedilol Prospective Randomized Cumulative Survival (COPERNICUS) trial randomized 2289 patients with heart failure symptoms at rest or on minimal exertion, and an LVEF <25% to treatment with either carvedilol or placebo, in addition to conventional therapy (18). Carvedilol therapy reduced all-cause mortality by 35%. In addition, carvedilol reduced the combined risk of death or hospitalization for cardiovascular causes by 27% (p < 0.001), and the combined risk of death or hospitalization for heart failure by 31% (p < 0.001) (18). Further, patients who received carvedilol treatment spent 40% fewer days in the hospital for decompensated heart failure (p < 0.001) (18). A subgroup analysis from the COPERNICUS trial confirmed carvedilol to be efficacious when added to background therapy that included the aldosterone antagonist, spironolactone (19).

Bucindolol

The Beta Blocker Evaluation of Survival Trial (BEST) randomized 2708 patients with advanced heart failure (NYHA class III/IV) symptoms to placebo or bucindolol (Table 18.2) (20). Bucindolol produced a nonsignificant 10% reduction in total mortality (p = 0.10) and a favorable reduction in most secondary endpoints (20). Retrospective analysis of BEST findings indicated that the majority of the study population (non-black patients with NYHA class III symptoms) experienced a mortality reduction consistent with results of other major beta blocker trials in similar populations (20). The overall efficacy was statistically insignificant, as mortality reductions were not observed among patients with NYHA class IV symptoms or blacks in this trial. Whether the lack of overall mortality benefit was due to the population demographics or the drug's intrinsic sympathomimetic activity is uncertain.

BETA BLOCKER USE IN SPECIAL POPULATIONS

Data on the benefit of beta blockers among women and minorities are limited. Ghali and colleagues performed a retrospective analysis of female patients enrolled in the MERIT-HF trial (21). Treatment with metoprolol CR/XL resulted in a 21% reduction in the primary combined endpoint of all-cause mortality and hospitalizations (p = 0.04) (21). Further, the number of cardiovascular hospitalizations was reduced by 29% and hospitalizations for heart failure were reduced by 42%. Shekelle et al. also performed a meta-analysis of the effect of gender on beta blocker responsiveness in major clinical trials (22). Pooling data from CIBIS-II, U. S. carvedilol trials, MERIT-HF, and COPERNICUS yielded a total of

2134 treated female patients. The relative risk reduction for women receiving beta blockers was 0.63 (95% confidence interval, 0.44–0.91). These findings were virtually identical to the results observed in men who experienced a risk reduction of 0.66 (95% confidence interval 0.59–0.75) (21).

The lack of efficacy of bucindolol among black heart failure patients has raised the question of whether differences in the racial background may influence the response to specific agents. Pooled data from the MERIT-HF, US carvedilol, COPERNICUS, and BEST trials included 1,172 blacks and more than 8,000 white patients (22). The risk reduction among black patients was only 0.97 (95% confidence interval 0.68 to 1.37), whereas for white patients, it was 0.69 (95% confidence interval 0.55 to 0.85) (22). However, after excluding BEST results, the risk reduction on mortality for black patients in the remaining 3 trials was 0.67 (95% confidence interval 0.38 to 1.16), similar to that observed for non-black patients. These authors concluded that black patients may experience the same risk reduction as white patients when treated with currently approved beta blockers: bisoprolol, metoprolol, or carvedilol. However, other investigators remain less convinced.

A growing body of data on differences in genetic polymorphisms in α- and β-adrenergic receptors among races may have clinical relevance to therapeutic response to beta blockade. Small et al. reported that a double adrenergic receptor polymorphism, specifically α_{2c} deletion-loss of function genotype (α_{2c} Del 322–325), combined with a high functioning α_1 receptor genotype (β_1 Arg 389), conferred a tenfold increased risk for the development of heart failure (23). Importantly, this α_{2c} polymorphism is enriched in black populations and may provide a partial explanation for the poorer cardiac function and prognosis observed among black heart failure patients (23). It is conceivable that the α_{2c} polymorphism may have predisposed black patients who received bucindolol to the adverse effects of enhanced sympatholysis (24). McNamara et al. also confirmed the pharmacogenetic interactions between beta blocker therapy and polymorphisms in the ACE gene among heart failure recipients (25). Ultimately, more precise pharmacogenetic profiling may be used to better predict response to specific beta-blocking agents; this more careful profiling should allow selection of the optimum drug based on age, gender, and racial background.

CLINICAL CONSIDERATIONS IN SELECTION OF A SPECIFIC BETA BLOCKER

Given the beneficial effects of metoprolol, bisoprolol, and carvedilol, clinicians are often confronted with selecting the most appropriate beta blocker for their patients. Studies by DiLenarda et al. and a meta-analysis by Packer et al. have demonstrated that carvedilol produces greater increases in left ventricular ejection fraction than metoprolol (26,27). Conversely, some but not all studies show that metoprolol improves maximum exercise capacity to a greater degree than carvedilol (28,29). It has been postulated that these differences may be partially explained by carvedilol's ability to improve post-receptor events, most notably by downregulation of BARK, which leads to pre-sensitization of the beta receptors. The Carvedilol Or Metoprolol European Trial (COMET) remains the only large-scale study to *directly* compare the effects of carvedilol to metoprolol on mortality and morbidity (30). This multicenter, double-blind study enrolled 3029 patients with chronic heart failure (NYHA class II–IV) and ejection fractions below 35%. All-cause mortality was 34% for carvedilol compared with 40% for metoprolol (hazard ratio 0.83; 95% confidence interval 0.74 to 0.93; p = 0.0017) (Fig. 18.2) (30). However, the composite endpoint of mortality or all-cause hospitalizations did not differ between treatment groups (74% for carvedilol, 76% for metoprolol, p = 0.12). A *post-hoc* analysis reported carvedilol treatment to be associated with fewer myocardial infarctions (hazard ratio: 0.70; 95% confidence interval 0.52–0.97, p = 0.03) and

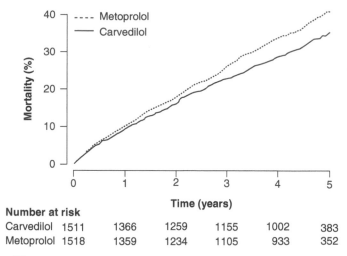

Number at risk

Carvedilol	1511	1366	1259	1155	1002	383
Metoprolol	1518	1359	1234	1105	933	352

Figure 18.2 All-cause mortality for patients enrolled in the Carvedilol Or Metoprolol European Trial (COMET) by type of beta-blocker. *Source*: From Ref. 30.

a lower composite endpoint of cardiovascular death or non-fatal myocardial infarction (hazard ratio: 0.81, 95% confidence interval 0.72–0.92, p = 0.0009) (31). Although this trial suggests that a nonselective third-generation beta blocker may be preferable to a β_1-selective agent, several methodological questions must be considered (32). One key question is whether the doses of the two agents were equivalent. The drug dosing in COMET aimed for a comparable reduction in resting heart rate between the two groups. While the resting heart rate reduction for patients who receive carvedilol was 13.3 beats per minute (identical to that achieved in the U.S. Carvedilol trials), the heart rate reduction in the metoprolol group was 11.7 beats per minute (compared with 15 beats per minute in the MDC trial) (9,30). Further, the preparation used in MERIT-HF was metoprolol succinate in a controlled release/extended release formulation (Metoprolol CR/XL). The mean dose of metoprolol tartrate was 159 mg daily in MERIT-HF compared with 85 mg daily of metoprolol succinate in COMET (9). Thus, the specific drug formulation, the lower average daily dose, and the more modest effects on resting heart rate confound comparison of the two drugs. Hence, it is difficult to be sure from COMET that metoprolol exerted a similar degree of β_1 blockade to carvedilol. At present, clinicians should consider initiating carvedilol as first-line therapy, given its broader antiadrenergic effects. For patients with marginal blood pressure in whom blockade may be deleterious, metoprolol XL/CR should be the initial drug of choice.

UNANSWERED QUESTIONS REGARDING BETA BLOCKER ADMINISTRATION
Asymptomatic Left Ventricular Dysfunction
Previous data indicate that beta blocker therapy should be used in patients after myocardial infarction, and in patients who undergo myocardial revascularization but have residual left ventricular dysfunction. The REVERT (Reversal of Vascular Remodeling with Toprol XL) trial randomized 149 patients with LVEF <40%, mild ventricular dilatation, and the absence of heart failure symptoms to metoprolol extended release or placebo (33). After 12 months, the metoprolol-treated patients had a 6 ± 1% increase in LVEF (p < 0.05) and a 14 ± 3 mL/m2 decrease in end-systolic volume compared with the placebo group. The study convincingly demonstrated that beta blocker treatment can improve left ventricular remodeling in asymptomatic patient with systolic dysfunction.

Current Heart Failure Society of America Practice Guidelines indicate that beta blocker therapy should be considered for patients with left ventricular systolic dysfunction (LVEF <40%) who are asymptomatic (NYHA class I), and are receiving ACE inhibitor therapy (34). Likewise, the 2009 American College of Cardiology/American Heart Association Practice Guidelines also recommend the use of beta blockers in Stage B (asymptomatic left ventricular dysfunction) (35).

Cardiac Pacemaker Implantation

Some physicians are now considering pacemaker implantation when symptomatic brady-cardia or heart block prevents the initiation of beta blocker therapy (36). Currently, no data exist to support this therapeutic approach. Further, the role of right ventricular pacing in worsening cardiac dyssynchrony and increasing the risk of heart failure hospitalization argues against a strategy that will promote predominant ventricular pacing, rather than utilize the patient's intrinsic ventricular activation sequence when QRS duration is <130 milliseconds. Beta blocker therapy should be considered following initiation of biventricu-lar pacing, if clinically indicated.

INITIATION OF THERAPY AND CONTRAINDICATION TO TREATMENT

Therapy should be initiated at the lowest possible dose and gradually uptitrated every two to four weeks as tolerated. A randomized trial suggested that the conventional sequence of drug initiation for new-onset heart failure with a vasodilator followed by a beta blocker should be reconsidered. Initiation of carvedilol before an ACE inhibitor resulted in a higher maintenance dose of the beta blocker, greater improvement in functional capacity, lower plasma N-terminal-pro-brain natriuretic peptide levels, and greater improvement in ventricular systolic function (Fig. 18.3) (37). Heart failure guidelines had previously recommended against routine initiation of beta blockers during a hospitalization for acute decompensated heart failure (ADHF). The IMPACT-HF trial prospectively randomized 363 ADHF patients to carvedilol initiation predischarge or post discharge at the discretion of the treating physician (38). At 60 days, 91% of patients randomized to predischarge beta blocker initiation were receiving the agent compared with only 73% of the postdischarge initiation group (38). Current guidelines now recommend that patients who have previously been receiving a beta blocker should continue it unless hemodynamic compromise exists and patients who are beta blocker naïve should initiate this therapy after establishment of a euvolemic state and prior to hospital discharge (35). Finally, continuation of beta blocker treatment during hospitalization for ADHF has been shown to be associated with lower in-hospital mortality and lower rehospitalization rates (39).

"Target" doses must be individualized. Beta blocker therapy has been shown to reduce mortality and hospitalizations independent of resting heart rate, treated heart rate, or change in heart rate (34). Therefore, practice guidelines do not recommend specific heart rate thresholds as surrogates for level of beta blockade. Instead, one simple rule applies: aim for the target dose validated in clinical trials (e.g., bisoprolol 10 mg daily, carvedilol 25 mg twice daily for weight less than 85 kg or 50 mg twice daily for weight more than 85 kg, or metoprolol succinate 200 mg daily) and strive for the highest tolerated dose in all heart failure patients (34,35).

Contraindications to beta blocker initiation include chronic obstructive pulmonary disease (COPD), diabetes mellitus, peripheral vascular disease, and low blood pressure (40). Despite legitimate concerns, the majority of patients with COPD can safely tolerate low-dose initiation and gradual uptitration of β_1-selective agents (40). However, even selective agents should not be used during acute exacerbations with bronchospasm or in severe forms of COPD or asthma. Similarly, beta blockers have been viewed by clinicians in the past as

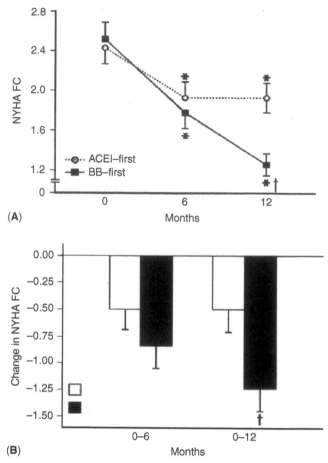

Figure 18.3 Effect of initiating carvedilol before perindopril [(beta-blocker, BB)-first group] compared with the effect of perindopril-first [angiotensin-converting enzyme inhibitor (ACEI)-first] group on New York Heart Association functional class (NYHA FC), *p < 0.05 versus baseline state, ⁺p < 0.05 versus absolute values and change from baseline in the ACEI-first group **(A)**; and plasma N-terminal-pro-brain natriuretic peptide concentrations, p < 0.005 versus baseline values + p < 0.01 versus absolute values and change from baseline in the ACEI-first group **(B)**. *Source*: From Ref. 37.

risky in diabetic patients because they may be associated with adverse effects on insulin sensitivity and could mask hypoglycemic symptoms. Diabetic heart failure patients have been shown to benefit from beta blockade; however, the absolute risk reduction is less than that observed for non-diabetic patients (40). Retrospective analysis of the COMET trial demonstrated a 22% reduction in new-onset diabetes mellitus among patients receiving carvedilol and fewer diabetic events (40). Proposed mechanisms of benefit remain unknown.

Despite theoretical concerns that beta blockers may worsen claudication or other symptoms of peripheral vascular disease due to unopposed α–mediated vasoconstriction, many studies (albeit few among documented heart failure patients) have failed to demonstrate an increase in symptoms during treatment with a selective or nonselective agent (40). Consideration should be given to avoiding beta blockade in patients with prominent vasospastic disorders, resting limb ischemia, or non-healing ulcers.

Patients with advanced heart failure have relatively low blood pressure and concerns exist that beta blockade may worsen hypotension and precipitate symptoms. Is should be noted that this group of patients also has the highest risk of death or hospitalizations regardless of treatment strategy. Retrospective analysis from the COPERNICUS trial demonstrated that among patients with a pretreatment systolic blood pressure of 85–95 mmHg, there was no evidence of an initial decline in blood pressure and many patients actually experienced a small increase in blood pressure compared with placebo (41). Nonetheless, the overall dose of beta blocker may need to be reduced and a small minority (<10%) of patients will be drug intolerant.

REFERENCES

1. Bristow MR. Beta-adrenergic receptor blockade in chronic heart failure. Circulation 2000; 101: 558–69.
2. Bristow MR. Mechanism of action of beta-blocking agents in heart failure. Am J Cardiol 1997; 80: 26L–40L.
3. Bristow MR, Gilbert EM, Abraham WT, et al. Carvedilol produces dose-related improvements in left ventricular function and survival in subjects with chronic heart failure. Circulation 1996; 94: 2807–16.
4. Waagstein F, Bristow MR, Swedberg K, et al. Beneficial effects of metoprolol in idiopathic dilated cardiomyopathy. Lancet 1993; 342: 1441–6.
5. Hall SA, Cigarroa CG, Marcoux L, et al. Time course of improvement in left ventricular function, mass, and geometry in patients with congestive heart failure treated with beta-adrenergic blockade. J Am Coll Cardiol 1995; 25: 1154–61.
6. Doughty RN, Whalley GA, Walsh HA, et al. Effect of carvedilol on left ventricular remodeling after acute myocardial infarction. the CAPRICORN substudy. Circulation 2004; 109: 201–6.
7. Satwani S, Dec GW, Narula J. Beta-adrenergic blockers in heart failure: review of mechanisms of action and clinical outcomes. J Cardiovasc Pharmacol Ther 2004; 9: 243–55.
8. Packer M, Bristow MR, Cohn JN, et al. For The Us CARVEDILOL Heart Failure Study Group. The effect of carvedilol on morbidity and mortality in patients with chronic heart failure. N Engl J Med 1996; 334: 1349–55.
9. MERIT-HF Study Group. Effect of metoprolol CR/XL in chronic heart failure: metoprolol CR/XL randomized intervention trial in congestive heart failure (MERIT-HF). Lancet 1999; 353: 2001–7.
10. Ghali JK, Dunselman P, Waagstein F, et al. Consistency of the beneficial effect of metoprolol succinate extended release across a wide range of doses of angiotensin-converting enzyme inhibitors and digitalis. J Card Fail 2004; 10: 452–9.
11. CIBIS Investigators and Committees. A randomized trial of beta-blockade in heart failure: THE Cardiac Insufficiency Bisoprolol Study (CIBIS). Circulation 1994; 90: 1765–73.
12. CIBIS II Investigators and Committees. The Cardiac insufficiency bisoprolol study II (CIBIS II): a randomized trial. Lancet 1999; 353: 9–13.
13. Bristow MR, Gilbert EM, Abraham WT, et al. For the MOCHA Investigators: Multicenter Oral Carvedilol Heart Failure Assessment (MOCHA): A six-month dose response evaluation in class II-IV patients. Circulation 1995; 92 (Suppl I): I142–6.
14. Packer M, Colucci WS, Sackner-Bernstein JD, et al. For The PRECISE Study Group. Double-blind, placebo-controlled study of the effects of carvedilol in patients with moderate to severe heart failure: the PRECISE trial. Circulation 1996; 94: 2793–9.
15. Colucci WS, Packer M. Bristow MR, et al for the US Carvedilol Study Group. Carvedilol inhibits clinical progression in patients with mild symptoms of heart failure. Circulation 1996; 94: 2800–6.
16. Australia-New Zealand Heart Failure Research Collaborative Group. Effects of carvedilol, a vasodilator-β-blocker, in patients with congestive heart failure due to ischemic heart disease. Circulation 1995; 92: 212–18.
17. Packer M, Coats AJ, Fowler MB, et al. Effect of carvedilol on survival in severe chronic heart failure. N Engl J Med 2001; 344: 1651–8.
18. Packer M, Fowler MB, Roecker EB, et al. Effect of carvedilol on the morbidity of patients with severe heart failure: results of the carvedilol prospective randomized cumulative survival (COPERNICUS) study. Circulation 2002; 106: 2194–9.
19. Krum H, Mohacsi P, Katus HA, et al. Are beta-blockers needed in patients receiving spironolactone for severe chronic heart failure? An analysis of the COPERNICUS study. Am Heart J 2006; 151: 55–61.

20. BEST Trial Investigators. A trial of the β-adrenergic blocker bucindolol in patients with advanced heart failure. N Engl J Med 2001; 344: 1659–67.

21. Ghali JK, Pina IL, Gottlieb SS, et al. Metoprolol CR/XL in female patients with heart failure. analysis of the experience in metoprolol extended-release randomized intervention trial in heart failure (MERIT-HF). Circulation 2002; 105: 1585–91.

22. Shekelle PG, Rich MW, Morton SC, et al. Efficacy of angiotensin-converting enzyme inhibitors and beta-blockers in the management of left ventricular systolic dysfunction according to race, gender, and diabetes status: a meta-analysis of major clinical trials. J Am Coll Cardiol 2003; 41: 1529–38.

23. Small KM, Wagoner LE, Levin AM, Kardia SLR, Liggett SB. Synergistic polymorphisms of the β1 and α2c-adrenergic receptors and the risk of congestive heart failure. N Engl J Med 2002; 347: 1135–42.

24. Bristow MR. Anti-adrenergic therapy of chronic heart failure: surprises and new opportunities. Circulation 2003; 107: 1100–2.

25. McNamara DM, Holubkov R, Janosko K, et al. Pharmacogenetic interactions between β-blocker therapy and the angiotensin-converting enzyme deletion polymporphism in patients with congestive heart failure. Circulation 2001; 103: 1644–8.

26. Di Lenarda A, Sabbadini G, Salvatore L, et al. The Heart-Muscle Disease Study Group. Long-term effects of carvedilol in idiopathic dilated cardiomyopathy with persistent left ventricular dysfunction despite chronic metoprolol. J Am Coll Cardiol 1999; 33: 1926–34.

27. Packer M, Antonopoulos GV, Berlin JA, et al. Comparative effects of carvedilol and metoprolol on left ventricular ejection fraction in heart failure: results of a meta-analysis. Am Heart J 2001; 141: 899–907.

28. Metra M, Giubbini R, Nodari S, et al. Differential effects of beta-blockers in patients with heart failure. a prospective, randomized, double-blind comparison of the long-term effects of metoprolol vs. carvedilol. Circulation 2000; 102: 546–51.

29. Kukin ML, Charney RH, Levy DK, et al. Prospective, randomized comparison of effect of long-term treatment with metoprolol or carvedilol on symptoms, exercise, ejection fraction, and oxidative stress in heart failure. Circulation 1999; 99: 2645–51.

30. Poole-Wilson PA, Swedberg K, Cleland JCF, et al. Comparison of carvedilol and metoprolol on clinical outcomes in patients with chronic heart failure in the Carvedilol Or Metoprolol European Trial (COMET): randomised controlled trial. Lancet 2003; 362: 7–13.

31. Remme WJ, Torp-Pedersen C, Cleland JGF, et al. Carvedilol protects better against vascular events than metoprolol in heart failure: results from COMET. J Am Coll Cardiol 2007; 49: 963–71.

32. Bristow MR, Feldman AM, Adams KF, Goldstein S. Selective versus non-selective beta-blockade for heart failure therapy. Are there lessons to be learned from the COMET trial? J Card Fail 2003; 9: 494–53.

33. Colucci WS, Katus TJ, Adams KF, et al. Metoprolol reverses left ventricular remodeling in patients with asymptomatic systolic dysfunction. The Reversal of Ventricular Remodeling with Toprol XL (REVERT) trial. Circulation 2007; 116: 49–56.

34. Adams KF, Lindenfeld JA, Arnold JM, et al. Heart Failure Society of America 2006 comprehensive heart failure practice guidelines. J Card Failure 2006; 12: 10–38.

35. Jessup M, Abraham WT, Casey DE, et al. 2009 Focused update: ACCF/AHA guidelines for the diagnsosis and management of heart failure in the adult. J Am Coll Cardiol 2009; 53: 1343–82.

36. Stecher EC, Fendrick AM, Knight BP, Aaronson KD. Prophylactic pacemaker use to allow beta blocker therapy in patients with chronic heart failure and bradycardia. Am Heart J 2006; 151: 20–8.

37. Sliwa K, Norton GR, Kone N, et al. Impact of initiating carvedilol before angiotensin-converting enzyme inhibitor therapy on cardiac function in newly diagnosed heart failure. J Am Coll Cardiol 2004; 44: 1825–30.

38. Gattis WA, O'Connor CM, Gallup DS, et al. Pre-discharge initiation of carvedilol in patients hospitalized in decompensated heart failure. results from the Initiation Management Pre-discharge process in assessment of carvedilol therapy in heart failure (IMPACT-HF) trial. J Am Coll Cardiol 2004; 43: 1534–41.

39. Butler J, Young JB, Abraham WT. Beta-blocker use and outcomes among hospitalized heart failure patients. J Am Coll Cardiol 2006; 47: 2452–9.

40. Naik SD, Freudenberger RS. Beta-blocker contraindications: are there patients or situations where use is inappropriate? Curr Heart Fail Rep 2007; 4: 93–8.

41. Rouleau JL, Roecker EB, Tendera M, et al. Influence of pretreatment systolic blood pressure on the effect of carvedilol in patients with severe chronic heart failure. J Am Coll Cardiol 2004; 43: 1423–9.

19

Angiotensin receptor blockers for heart failure

George V. Moukarbel

INTRODUCTION

Blockade of the renin-angiotensin-aldosterone system (RAAS) has become the corner-stone of heart failure therapy. A large number of clinical trials have provided evidence that the use of angiotensin-converting enzyme (ACE) inhibitors to inhibit the production of angiotensin II results in significantly improved clinical outcome in patients with heart failure and left ventricular (LV) systolic dysfunction (see chap. 17). These drugs work by inhibiting the enzyme responsible for the conversion of angiotensin I to angiotensin II (Fig. 19.1). Of the several angiotensin II receptor types identified so far, two are believed to mediate the majority of it its clinically relevant actions (1): (*i*) the angiotensin II type 1 (AT$_1$) receptor which is responsible for vasoconstriction, increased smooth muscle cell proliferation, increased matrix degradation, renal sodium and fluid retention, epinephrine release, and ventricular hypertrophy (2–4) and (*ii*) the angiotensin II type 2 (AT$_2$) receptor, which upon activation, leads to effects that seem to counteract those of the AT$_1$ receptor, particularly through vasodilation, reduction in cardiac fibrosis and hypertrophy, and increased apoptosis (1,3,4). Because of these "counter-balancing" effects of the angiotensin II receptors, selective AT$_1$ receptor blockers have emerged as an attractive alternative to ACE inhibitors for the blockade of the RAAS. These would impede the deleterious effects of the AT$_1$ receptors, while keeping angiotensin II available to stimulate the AT$_2$ receptors, therefore potentially deriving benefit from their activation. In addition, ACE inhibitors do not achieve complete and sustained suppression of angiotensin II production since evidence suggests that other pathways play an important role in its generation. These non-ACE-dependent pathways are mediated by serine proteases such as chymase, tonin, kallikrein, and cathepsin G, and may be responsible for the production of significant amounts of angiotensin II (5). In fact, clinical studies have shown that following long-term administration of ACE inhibitor, plasma levels of angiotensin II return to baseline levels (6,7), a phenomenon that was termed "ACE escape." Therefore, in comparison with ACE inhibitors, angiotensin receptor blockers (ARBs) can provide a more complete inhibition of the deleterious effects of angiotensin II.

The RAAS also interacts with the kinin-kallikrein system at the level of ACE, which is a kinase that breaks down bradykinin, which tends to accumulate with the use of an ACE inhibitor. Bradykinin causes nitric oxide–mediated vasodilation (8) and has been shown to contribute to the hemodynamic effects of ACE inhibitors. In patients with heart failure, the administration of a bradykinin receptor antagonist leads to the attenuation of the effects of

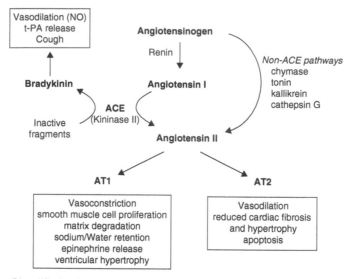

Figure 19.1 Simplified schematic diagram of the major pathways of angiotensin II production, action, and the link to the bradykinin system. *Abbreviations:* ACE, angiotensin-converting enzyme; NO, nitric oxide; t-PA, tissue plasminogen activator.

Table 19.1 The Effects of ACE Inhibitors, ARBs, and Their Combination on the Levels of Various Neurohormones and Receptor Activation

	ACE inhibitor	ARB	Combination
Renin	↑	↑	↑↑
Angiotensin II	↓ (↔ᵃ)	↑	↔ or ↑
Bradykinin	↑	↔	↑
AT₁ activation	↓	↓↓	↓↓
AT₂ activation	↓	↑↑	↑

ᵃACE escape.
Abbreviations: ACE, angiotensin-converting enzyme; ARBs, angiotensin receptor blockers; AT1 and AT2, Angiotensin II type 1 and 2; ↑, increases; ↓, decreases; ↔, no significant change.

an ACE inhibitor but not those of an ARB (9). Bradykinin also stimulates local tissue-type plasminogen activator release (10) which can contribute to the anti-ischemic effects seen with long-term ACE inhibitor therapy (11). On the other hand, accumulation of bradykinin is believed to participate in the genesis of side effects, mainly the nonproductive cough, seen in 5–35% of patients treated with ACE inhibitors (12). ARBs do not affect bradykinin degradation and are believed to have no significant impact on its levels. Table 19.1 summarizes the effects of ACE inhibitors, ARBs, and their combination on the levels of the main neurohormones and receptor activation of the RAAS.

In summary, these two classes of drugs act via distinct mechanisms: ACE inhibitors reduce the levels of angiotensin II, by blocking its production, and increase the levels of bradykinin, by blocking its degradation; while ARBs exert complete blockade of the AT₁ receptors and lead to increased stimulation of the AT₂ receptors. Because of this, the combined use of ACE inhibitor and ARB therapy has been suggested to have a "synergistic" effect. The ACE inhibitor will increase the levels of kinins, while the ARB blocks the adverse effects of angiotensin II that is generated via the ACE escape mechanism. In addition, combining both classes of drugs can effect a more complete inhibition of the RAAS in the face of the reactive increases in renin and consequently in angiotensin levels seen with either therapy alone (13).

CLINICAL STUDIES OF ARBS IN HEART FAILURE

Following the demonstration of potentially favorable hemodynamic and neurohormonal effects of ARBs in small cohorts of patients with heart failure (14,15), initial intermediate-scale randomized trials were conducted using ACE inhibitors with proven benefits in this patient population as active comparators. These trials examined the safety and tolerability profiles as well as the effects of ARBs on neurohormones, ventricular remodeling, and exercise tolerance.

The Evaluation of Losartan In The Elederly (ELITE) trial was among the first major studies to compare the effects of an ARB, losartan at 50 mg per day, to those of an ACE inhibitor, captopril at 50 mg three times per day, in patients with heart failure (16). The primary endpoint was an assessment of tolerability, as measured by the effect of therapy on serum creatinine. The trial enrolled 722 elderly patients in New York Heart Association (NYHA) class II–IV who had a left ventricular ejection fraction (LVEF) of ≤40% and were not treated with an ACE inhibitor. While the primary endpoint was not different in the two groups, death, which constituted one of the components of the secondary endpoint was reduced with losartan [risk reduction (RR) 46%; 95% confidence interval (CI) 5–69%; p = 0.035]; the overall number of events was, however, small. There was no difference in the rates of heart failure admissions in the two arms. In a similar group of 768 patients, the Randomized Evaluation of Strategies for Left Ventricular Dysfunction (RESOLVD) pilot study tested another ARB, candesartan against a proven ACE inhibitor, looking at functional capacity, left ventricular size and systolic function and neurohormonal levels over a period of 43 weeks. Though lacking the power to test for hard endpoints, a trend toward lower rates of death and heart failure hospitalization in the ACE inhibitor arm prompted early termination of the study. Endpoint analysis found nearly comparable effects between candesartan and enalapril. Their combination, however, appeared to be more effective at preventing left ventricular remodeling than either alone, and had favorable effects on the neurohormonal profile (7). Finally, in the Study of Patients Intolerant of Converting Enzyme Inhibitors (SPICE) trial, candesartan was well tolerated in patients with a history of ACE inhibitor intolerance (17). This 12-week randomized tolerability study with 270 participants enrolled provided evidence that ACE inhibitor–intolerant patients can be treated with an ARB.

Because of lack of power and appropriate design, firm conclusions regarding mortality and morbidity outcomes could not be drawn from the results of these studies (18). Conversely, the efficacy and safety of ARBs as an alternative therapy to, or in combination with, ACE inhibitors have been tested in several large, multicenter, randomized trials enrolling patients with heart failure and high-risk myocardial infarction. The following sections summarize the main findings of these studies, and highlight their similarities and differences with respect to patients' characteristics and clinical context. Table 19.2 provides an overview of the main characteristics of these trials.

TREATMENT OF PATIENTS WITH HEART FAILURE AND REDUCED LVEF
ARBs as Alternatives to ACE Inhibitors

The Evaluation of Losartan In The Elederly II (ELITE II) trial (19) was designed to be adequately powered to study the effects of losartan therapy on mortality and morbidity. The characteristics of the 3152 patients who were randomized were largely similar to those enrolled in the ELITE trial, as were the drug dosages. In contrast to the findings of the ELITE trial, losartan therapy in ELITE II was not superior to captopril in improving

Table 19.2 Characteristics of the Major Clinical Trials of ARBs in Patients with Heart Failure

Trial Name	ELITE II	HEAAL	CHARM-Alternative	Val-HeFT	CHARM-Added	CHARM-Preserved	I-PRESERVE	OPTIMAAL	VALIANT
No. of patients	3,152	3,846	2,028	5,010	2,548	3,023	4,128	5,477	14,703
Age ± SD (yrs)	71 ± 7	64 ± 12	67 ± 11	62 ± 11	64 ± 11	67 ± 11	72 ± 7	67 ± 10	65 ± 12
Women	31	30	32	20	21	39	60	29	31
African-Americans	2	1	4	7	5	5	2	<2	3
Diabetics	24	31	27	26	30	29	27	17	24
Ischemic etiology	79	64	68	58	62	56	25	100	100
NYHA/Killip class I	0	0	0	0	0	0	0	32	29
II	52	69	48	62	24	61	21	57	48
III	43	30	49	36	73	37	76	9	17
IV	5	1	3	2	3	2	3	2	6
Mean LVEF	31	32	30	27	28	54	59	NA	35
Use of neurohormonal blockers at baseline									
Beta-blockers	22	72	55	35	55	56	59	79	70
ACE Inhibitors	24 (prior)	0	0	93	100	20	25	0	41 (prior)
Aldo. Antagonists	<22	38	24	5	17	11	15	NA	<9
Treatment	Losartan vs. CPT	Losartan 150 mg vs. 50 mg	Candesartan vs. placebo	Valsartan vs. placebo	Candesartan vs. placebo	Candesartan vs. placebo	Irbesartan vs. placebo	Losartan vs. CPT	Valsartan vs. Valsartan + CPT vs. CPT
Follow up (months)	19	56	34	23	41	37	49	32	25
Effect of study drug vs. comparator on outcome									
Mortality	≈	≈	17% ↓	≈	≈	≈	≈	13% ↑ [p = 0.07]	≈
CV death	≈	≈	20% ↓	NA	17% ↓	≈	NA	17% ↑ [p = 0.03]	≈

									↓ with combination
HF Hosp.	≈	13% ↓	39% ↓	24% ↓	17% ↓	16% ↓ [p = 0.047]	≈	16% ↑ [p = 0.07]	
Adverse effects leading to discontinuation									
Hypotension	≈	1.0 vs. 0.8	3.7 vs. 0.9	1.3 vs. 0.8 †	4.5 vs. 3.1 †	2.4 vs. 1.1	3.0 vs. 3.0 †	1.7 vs. 2.2 †	1.4[a] vs. 1.9[a] vs. 0.8
Hyperkalemia	NA	0.5 vs. 0.2	1.9 vs. 0.3	NA	3.4 vs. 0.7	1.5 vs. 0.6	<1.0 vs. <1.0 †	NA	0.1 vs. 0.2 vs. 0.1 †
Renal dysfunction	NA	2.5 vs. 1.9	6.1 vs. 2.7	1.1 vs. 0.2	7.8 vs. 4.1	4.8 vs. 2.4	3.0 vs. 3.0 †	NA	1.1 vs. 1.3[a] vs. 0.8
Cough	0.3 vs. 2.7	NA	0.2 vs. 0.4 †	NA	NA	NA	NA	1.0 vs. 4.1	0.6[a] vs. 2.1 vs. 2.5
Any adverse event	9.7 vs. 14.7	7.7 vs. 7.0	21.5 vs. 19.3 †	9.9 vs. 7.2	24.2 vs. 18.3	17.8 vs. 13.5	16 vs. 14 †	7.0 vs. 14	5.8[a] vs. 9.0[a] vs. 7.7

Mean follow-up is provided for Val-HeFT, I-PRESERVE, and OPTIMAAL, and a median one for the other trials. Values are expressed as percentage, unless otherwise indicated. Covariate adjusted results are provided for the CHARM trials.

[a]Indicates significant difference from the CPT group.

Abbreviations: ACE, angiotensin-converting enzyme; Aldo, aldosterone; CPT, captopril; CV, cardiovascular; HF Hosp, heart failure hospitalization; LVEF, left ventricular ejection fraction; NA, not available; NYHA, New York Heart Association; SD, standard deviation; †, not significant; ≈, no difference; ↑, increase; ↓, decrease.

survival (hazard ratio 1.13; 95.7% CI 0.95–1.35; p = 0.16). There were no differences in the number of heart failure cases or any hospital admissions in the two groups. These disappointing findings were in part blamed on the low dose of losartan used in this trial compared with that of the ACE inhibitor. The issue of dosage was addressed in the Heart failure Evaluation with the Angiotensin receptor Antagonist Losartan (HEAAL) trial (20,21), which investigated whether high dose losartan (150 mg daily) is better than low dose (50 mg daily) in preventing death or hospitalization for heart failure (primary endpoint). The 3846 patients enrolled in this trial were ACE inhibitor intolerant and in NYHA class II–IV. After a median follow-up of 4.7 years, the primary endpoint was reduced in the high-dose losartan arm of the trial (hazard ratio 0.90; 95% CI 0.82–0.99; p = 0.027). This was mostly driven by a reduction in hospitalization for heart failure (hazard ratio 0.87; 95% CI 0.76–0.98; p = 0.025) at the expense of increased incidence of adverse effects (renal impairment, hypotension, and hyperkalemia). However, discontinuation of the study drug due to side effects was not significantly different in the two study arms. The results argue for the need to titrate therapy in this patient population, while closely monitoring for adverse effects. The Candesartan in Heart Failure Assessment of Reduction in Mortality and Morbidity (CHARM)-Alternative trial (22) randomly assigned a similar population of heart failure patients who were intolerant to ACE inhibitors to treatment with candesartan or placebo. Although it was not a direct comparison of ARB and ACE inhibitor, it provided evidence that in patients who cannot be maintained on ACE inhibitors, ARB therapy is feasible and is associated with improved clinical outcome (unadjusted risk reduction of 23% for the combined endpoint of cardiovascular death and heart failure hospitalization; p = 0.0004). This was comparable to the benefit seen in other large trials of ACE inhibitors (11).

ARBs in Combination with ACE Inhibitors

The Valsartan in Heart Failure Trial (Val-HeFT) randomly assigned 5010 patients with NYHA class II–IV heart failure and LVEF <40% to receive Valsartan or placebo (23). Although this was not required to be an add-on therapy to ACE inhibitors, about 93% of the patients enrolled were maintained on these drugs. An important point, however, is that unlike a planned combination therapy where dosage and titration of the two drugs are dictated by the study design, the choice and titration of the ACE inhibitor in Val-HeFT was dictated by the treating physician. After a mean follow-up of 23 months, there was no difference in the primary endpoint of mortality, but valsartan therapy was associated with a 13% significant (p = 0.009) reduction in the risk of the combined endpoint of mortality and morbidity, defined as the incidence of cardiac arrest with resuscitation, hospitalization for heart failure, or receipt of intravenous inotropic or vasodilator therapy for at least four hours. This reduction was, however, in a great part driven by a 24% reduction in the rate of heart failure hospitalization. An important finding when subgroups were analyzed was that in the 1610 patients who were taking both a beta blocker and an ACE inhibitor, valsartan was associated with a 42% significant (p = 0.009) increase in mortality. Despite the limitations inherent to subgroup analysis, this finding raised concerns about potential deleterious effects of excessive RAAS blockade; nevertheless, it was not substantiated in other trials.

The CHARM-Added trial (24) was designed to test whether the addition of an ARB to ACE inhibitor therapy could improve outcome in patients with NYHA class II–IV heart failure and reduced LVEF (≤40%). In this 2548–patient trial, the use of candesartan over a median follow-up of 41 months was associated with a 15% reduction in the combined endpoint of cardiovascular death and heart failure hospitalization (p = 0.011). More importantly, this benefit was consistent among all subgroups, including patients maintained on beta blockers (about 55% of the CHARM-Added population). This finding negated prior concerns regarding potential deleterious effects of "excessive" neurohormonal blockade.

TREATMENT OF PATIENTS WITH HEART FAILURE AND PRESERVED LVEF

There are only two completed major trials examining the role of ARB therapy in patients with heart failure and preserved LVEF: the CHARM-Preserved (25) and the Irbesartan in heart failure with PRESERVEd systolic function (I-PRESERVE) trials (26). In the CHARM-Preserved trial, patients who had an LVEF >40% were randomly assigned to candesartan or placebo, and were followed for a median of about 37 months. This trial had a high proportion of female patients and allowed for the use of other neurohormonal blockers (ACE inhibitors in 20% and beta blockers in 56% of the patients). The main finding was an overall 16% reduction in heart failure hospitalization with candesartan that was of borderline statistical significance (p = 0.047). The importance of this trial is that it provided the first evidence-based information regarding a potential therapy, although of modest benefit, in a large group of heart failure patients. The I-PRESERVE trial is the largest placebo-controlled trial in this patient population and it investigated the effects of the ARB irbesartan on morbidity and mortality in patients with heart failure and LVEF ≥45% (27). There were 4128 patients at least 60 years of age enrolled, whose mean LVEF was 59% and of whom almost 80% were in NYHA class III or IV. Patients were randomly assigned to receive 300 mg of irbesartan or placebo daily and were followed for a mean period of 49.5 months. It is important to note that background therapy at baseline included ACE inhibitors (25%), spironolactone (15%), and beta-blockers (59%) and that the use of these drugs increased during the course of the trial. Compared with the CHARM-Preserved, this trial enrolled slightly older patients and more women. Also, patients had more advanced symptoms and less ischemic etiology of their heart failure. The results showed a similar occurrence of the primary composite outcome of death and cardiovascular hospitalization in the two groups. There were also no differences in the occurrence of the various outcomes of death, myocardial infarction, stroke, heart failure, or their combinations. In particular, I-PRESERVE could not confirm any beneficial effect of the ARB in reducing heart failure hospitalization. Further analysis failed to identify specific subgroups of patients who might derive benefit from therapy. These data provide no support for the use of ARBs on top of standard therapy in patients with heart failure and preserved LVEF in the aim of improving mortality and morbidity. Their use in this patient population remains, however, important for other indications such as control of hypertension.

TREATMENT OF PATIENTS WITH POST-MYOCARDIAL INFARCTION HEART FAILURE

Two major trials studied the efficacy and safety of ARBs against an ACE inhibitor in high risk patients with recent myocardial infarction: The Optimal Therapy in Myocardial Infarction with the Angiotensin II Antagonist Losartan (OPTIMAAL) trial (28) and the VALsartan In Acute myocardial iNfarction Trial (VALIANT) (29). Both trials enrolled patients within 10 days of acute myocardial infarction who had evidence of either heart failure or left ventricular dysfunction (LVEF ≤35%), or both. The mean LVEF in VALIANT was 35%, while less than 14% of the OPTIMAAL patients had an LVEF <35%. All-cause mortality was the primary endpoint for the two trials. OPTIMAAL was a two-arm trial comparing losartan to captopril, while VALIANT compared the effects of valsartan as monotherapy and in combination with captopril to captopril monotherapy in a 1:1:1 randomized fashion. While there was a trend toward increased mortality in the losartan group in OPTIMAAL (relative risk 1.13; p = 0.07) that was consistent across different subgroups, valsartan was as effective as captopril in VALIANT. Furthermore, patients treated with the combination of the two drugs had similar outcomes, but showed a higher incidence of drug-related adverse events. Most importantly, a subgroup analysis in VALIANT did not reveal any adverse effects of the combination therapy in the patients maintained on beta-blockers. The finding of a trend toward a higher mortality rate and a significantly increased rate of cardio-vascular death with losartan therapy in OPTIMAAL may again be related to the underdos-age of the ARB, an issue that was avoided in VALIANT where valsartan was titrated to 160 mg twice daily. Also, differences in population characteristics might have caused the disparities in the outcomes seen in the two trials. Similar to the case of the heart failure population, losartan could not be considered comparable to captopril in the post-myocardial infarction patients.

ROLE OF ARBS IN ASYMPTOMATIC LV DYSFUNCTION

Unlike the case with ACE inhibitors (30,31), there is paucity of trial data that examine the role of ARBs in patients with asymptomatic LV dysfunction, with the goal of preventing the development of heart failure and reducing mortality. In the VALIANT trial (29), 4099 patients were in Killip class I at the time of randomization. Subgroup analysis revealed that the effects of the ARB and the combination therapy on mortality and the combined cardio-vascular endpoint were comparable to those of the ACE inhibitor. Combined with evidence of equivalent benefit seen in other heart failure trials, it can be inferred that ARBs might have a similar effect in patients with asymptomatic LV dysfunction. However, due to lack of direct trial evidence, their use in that setting should be reserved for patients who are intoler-ant of ACE inhibitors and their combined use with ACE inhibitors cannot be advocated.

ADVERSE EFFECTS OF ARB THERAPY

While clinical trials have shown benefit of ARBs in heart failure patients, as a standalone therapy or in combination with ACE inhibitors, they have raised safety concerns, especially regarding the combination. The overall incidence of side effects in those trials (Table 19.2) is likely to be an underestimate of the true incidence seen in clinical practice, as patients with a history of ACE inhibitor or ARB intolerance were excluded. However, it appears that the occurrence of cough with ARBs is significantly less than with ACE inhibitors. It is important to note that in CHARM-Alternative, cough was the cause of ACE inhibitor intol-erance in 72% of the patients. In this patient population, the frequency of cough during the course of the trial was similar in the candesartan and the placebo arms. Furthermore, only one patient out of the 39 patients in the candesartan arm who had a history of angioedema while treated with ACE inhibitors developed recurrence of symptoms (22). On the other hand, as is the case with ACE inhibitors, the main side effects encountered with ARB therapy included hypotension, hyperkalemia, and renal dysfunction. As shown in Table 19.2, their frequency is significantly increased in patients receiving the combination ther-apy. A meta-analysis (32) of the VALIANT, CHARM-Added, Val-HeFT, and RESOLVD trials found that compared with ACE inhibitor therapy, the use of combination ACE inhibi-tor/ARB was associated with a significantly increased relative risk of discontinuation because of adverse effects [1.28 (95% CI 1.17–1.40)], symptomatic hypotension [1.48 (95% CI 1.34–1.62)], and worsening renal function [1.76 (95% CI 1.49–2.09)]; there was also a nonsignificantly increased incidence of hyperkalemia defined as a serum potassium level >5.5 mEq/L [2.46 (95% CI (0.68–8.87)]. Despite the limitations inherent to pooled analysis, as well as the underrepresentation of real-world patients by clinical trials, these findings suggest that combination therapy is associated with increased risk and therefore should be reserved for appropriate patients and not adopted as routine practice. In addition, care should be taken to avoid combination therapy in patients maintained on aldosterone antagonists, as the risk of renal dysfunction and hyperkalemia would be substantially increased. Although a CHARM-Added subgroup analysis (33) suggested that ARBs could be used with an acceptable risk in patients taking spironolactone as well as an ACE inhibi-tor and a beta-blocker, such a strategy cannot be advocated at this time.

Table 19.3 Summary of the ACC/AHA, ESC, and HFSA Guideline Recommendations Pertinent to the Use of ARBs in Patients with Heart Failure

Indication	Class of Recommendation			Level of Evidence		
	ACC/AHA	ESC	HFSA	ACC/AHA	ESC	HFSA
Heart failure and reduced LVEF						
ACE Inhibitor intolerant	I	I	I	A	B	A
First-line alternatives to ACE inhibitors	IIa	IIa	IIb	A	B	B
Added to conventional therapy in persistently symptomatic patients	IIb	IIa (Mortality) / I (HF admission)	IIa	B	B / A	A
Routine combined use of ACE inhibitor/ARB/aldosterone antagonist	III		III	C		C
Heart failure and preserved LVEF						
Minimize symptoms and reduce hospitalizations	IIb	IIa	IIa	C	B	B
Post-myocardial infarction with heart failure or LV dysfunction						
As alternative to ACE inhibitors	I	I	IIb	A	B	A
Routine use in addition to ACE inhibitors and beta-blockers			III			A

Classification of Recommendations. I – Evidence and/or general agreement that a given procedure or treatment is beneficial, useful, and effective; II – Conflicting evidence and/or a divergence of opinion about the usefulness/efficacy of a procedure or treatment; IIa – Weight of evidence/opinion is in favor of usefulness/efficacy; IIb – Usefulness/efficacy is less well established by evidence/opinion; III – Evidence and/or general agreement that a procedure/treatment is not useful/effective and in some cases may be harmful. Level of Evidence. A – Data from multiple randomized clinical trials or meta-analyses. B – Data from a single randomized trial or nonrandomized studies. C – Only consensus opinion of experts, case studies, or standard-of-care.

Abbreviations: ACC, The American College of Cardiology; ACE, angiotensin-converting enzyme; AHA, American Heart Association; ARB, angiotensin receptor blockers; ESC, European Society of Cardiology; HFSA, Heart Failure Society of America; LVEF, left ventricular ejection fraction.

In 2010, concerns relating to an increased risk of developing cancer while on ARB therapy were raised after a meta-analysis of a few clinical trials showed that patients treated with ARBs had a modestly increased risk of incident cancer (34). This finding was not replicated in subsequent larger scale studies (35–37). The U.S. Food and Drug Administration (FDA) conducted a comprehensive analysis of about 156,000 patients enrolled in 31 clinical trials. This did not show evidence of increased risk of cancer with ARBs. The U.S. FDA concluded: treatment with ARBs does not increase the patient's risk of developing cancer (38).

CONCLUSIONS AND SUMMARY OF RECOMMENDATIONS

ARBs did not prove to be superior to ACE inhibitors in reducing adverse outcomes in patients with heart failure, as would have been theoretically expected on the basis of their mechanism of action. Possible reasons for this include insufficient doses used in trials (particularly with losartan), differences in activation and impact of other angiotensin II receptors, as well as the importance of the bradykinin system effects seen with ACE inhibition. It follows from the results of the above-mentioned trials that ARBs are an effective and valid therapy for heart failure patients who are intolerant of ACE inhibitors. In the post-myocardial infarction patients, they are equivalent to ACE inhibitors and can be used as first-line agents in this context. Also, it might be reasonable to use them instead of ACE inhibitors in chronic heart failure patients. Combined with ACE inhibitors, ARBs appear to have a beneficial effect of reducing morbidity, albeit at an increased risk for side effects. Therefore, patients on combination therapy should be closely monitored for the occurrence of hypotension, hyperkalemia, and renal insufficiency. Their use on top of triple therapy that includes an aldosterone antagonist is discouraged (39,40). Table 19.3 provides a comparative summary of the latest recommendations of the American College of Cardiology Foundation/American Heart Association (40), the European Society of Cardiology (39,41), and the Heart Failure Society of America (42) concerning the use of ARBs in patients with heart failure. When used, ARBs should be started at low doses and uptitrated to target doses proven in clinical trials (candesartan 32 mg once per day; valsartan 160 mg twice daily; losartan 150 mg once per day). Patients should be carefully monitored for side effects, especially in the early titration phases with particular attention to patients with borderline hemodynamics and renal function.

REFERENCES

1. Burnier M, Brunner HR. Angiotensin II receptor antagonists. Lancet 2000; 355: 637–45.
2. Ferrari R. Angiotensin-converting enzyme inhibition in cardiovascular disease: evidence with perindopril. Expert Rev Cardiovasc Ther 2005; 3: 15–29.
3. Unger T. The role of the renin-angiotensin system in the development of cardiovascular disease. Am J Cardiol 2002; 89: 3A–9A.
4. Goodfriend TL, Elliott ME, Catt KJ. Angiotensin receptors and their antagonists. N Engl J Med 1996; 334: 1649–54.
5. McConnaughey MM, McConnaughey JS, Ingenito AJ. Practical considerations of the pharmacology of angiotensin receptor blockers. J Clin Pharmacol 1999; 39: 547–59.
6. Biollaz J, Brunner HR, Gavras I, Waeber B, Gavras H. Antihypertensive therapy with MK 421: angiotensin II–renin relationships to evaluate efficacy of converting enzyme blockade. J Cardiovasc Pharmacol 1982; 4: 966–72.
7. McKelvie RS, Yusuf S, Pericak D, et al.; The RESOLVD Pilot Study Investigators. Comparison of candesartan, enalapril, and their combination in congestive heart failure: randomized evaluation of strategies for left ventricular dysfunction (RESOLVD) pilot study. Circulation 1999; 100: 1056–64.
8. Kuga T, Mohri M, Egashira K, et al. Bradykinin-induced vasodilation of human coronary arteries in vivo: role of nitric oxide and angiotensin-converting enzyme. J Am Coll Cardiol 1997; 30: 108–12.
9. Cruden NL, Witherow FN, Webb DJ, Fox KA, Newby DE. Bradykinin contributes to the systemic hemodynamic effects of chronic angiotensin-converting enzyme inhibition in patients with heart failure. Arterioscler Thromb Vasc Biol 2004; 24: 1043–8.

10. Witherow FN, Dawson P, Ludlam CA, Fox KA, Newby DE. Marked bradykinin-induced tissue plasminogen activator release in patients with heart failure maintained on long-term angiotensin-converting enzyme inhibitor therapy. J Am Coll Cardiol 2002; 40: 961–6.

11. Flather MD, Yusuf S, Kober L, et al. ACE-Inhibitor Myocardial Infarction Collaborative Group. Long-term ACE-inhibitor therapy in patients with heart failure or left-ventricular dysfunction: a systematic overview of data from individual patients. Lancet 2000; 355: 1575–81.

12. Dicpinigaitis PV. Angiotensin-converting enzyme inhibitor-induced cough: ACCP evidence-based clinical practice guidelines. Chest 2006; 129: 169S–73S.

13. Nussberger J, Wuerzner G, Jensen C, Brunner HR. Angiotensin II suppression in humans by the orally active renin inhibitor Aliskiren (SPP100): comparison with enalapril. Hypertension 2002; 39: E1–8.

14. Crozier I, Ikram H, Awan N, et al.; Losartan Hemodynamic Study Group. Losartan in heart failure. hemodynamic effects and tolerability. Circulation 1995; 91: 691–7.

15. Gottlieb SS, Dickstein K, Fleck E, et al. Hemodynamic and neurohormonal effects of the angiotensin II antagonist losartan in patients with congestive heart failure. Circulation 1993; 88: 1602–9.

16. Pitt B, Segal R, Martinez FA, et al. Randomised trial of losartan versus captopril in patients over 65 with heart failure (Evaluation of Losartan in the Elderly Study, ELITE). Lancet 1997; 349: 747–52.

17. Granger CB, Ertl G, Kuch J, et al. Randomized trial of candesartan cilexetil in the treatment of patients with congestive heart failure and a history of intolerance to angiotensin-converting enzyme inhibitors. Am Heart J 2000; 139: 609–17.

18. Greenberg BH. Role of angiotensin receptor blockers in heart failure: not yet resolvd. Circulation 1999; 100: 1032–4.

19. Pitt B, Poole-Wilson PA, Segal R, et al. Effect of losartan compared with captopril on mortality in patients with symptomatic heart failure: randomised trial--the Losartan heart failure survival study ELITE II. Lancet 2000; 355: 1582–7.

20. Konstam MA, Poole-Wilson PA, Dickstein K, et al. Design of the heart failure endpoint evaluation of AII-antagonist losartan (HEAAL) study in patients intolerant to ACE-inhibitor. Eur J Heart Fail 2008; 10: 899–906.

21. Konstam MA, Neaton JD, Dickstein K, et al. Effects of high-dose versus low-dose losartan on clinical outcomes in patients with heart failure (HEAAL study): a randomised, double-blind trial. Lancet 2009; 374: 1840–8.

22. Granger CB, McMurray JJ, Yusuf S, et al. Effects of candesartan in patients with chronic heart failure and reduced left-ventricular systolic function intolerant to angiotensin-converting-enzyme inhibitors: the CHARM-Alternative trial. Lancet 2003; 362: 772–6.

23. Cohn JN, Tognoni G. A randomized trial of the angiotensin-receptor blocker valsartan in chronic heart failure. N Engl J Med 2001; 345: 1667–75.

24. McMurray JJ, Ostergren J, Swedberg K, et al. Effects of candesartan in patients with chronic heart failure and reduced left-ventricular systolic function taking angiotensin-converting-enzyme inhibitors: the CHARM-added trial. Lancet 2003; 362: 767–71.

25. Yusuf S, Pfeffer MA, Swedberg K, et al. Effects of candesartan in patients with chronic heart failure and preserved left-ventricular ejection fraction: the CHARM-Preserved Trial. Lancet 2003; 362: 777–81.

26. Massie BM, Carson PE, McMurray JJ, et al. Irbesartan in Patients with heart failure and preserved ejection fraction. N Engl J Med 2008; 359: 2456–67.

27. McMurray JJ, Carson PE, Komajda M, et al. Heart failure with preserved ejection fraction: clinical characteristics of 4133 patients enrolled in the I-PRESERVE trial. Eur J Heart Fail 2008; 10: 149–56.

28. Dickstein K, Kjekshus J. Effects of losartan and captopril on mortality and morbidity in high-risk patients after acute myocardial infarction: the OPTIMAAL randomised trial. optimal trial in myocardial infarction with Angiotensin II Antagonist Losartan. Lancet 2002; 360: 752–60.

29. Pfeffer MA, McMurray JJ, Velazquez EJ, et al. Valsartan, captopril, or both in myocardial infarction complicated by heart failure, left ventricular dysfunction, or both. N Engl J Med 2003; 349: 1893–906.

30. Effect of enalapril on mortality and the development of heart failure in asymptomatic patients with reduced left ventricular ejection fractions. The SOLVD Investigattors. N Engl J Med 1992; 327: 685–91.

31. Pfeffer MA, Braunwald E, Moye LA, et al.; The SAVE Investigators. Effect of captopril on mortality and morbidity in patients with left ventricular dysfunction after myocardial infarction. results of the survival and ventricular enlargement trial. N Engl J Med 1992; 327: 669–77.

32. Phillips CO, Kashani A, Ko DK, Francis G, Krumholz HM. Adverse effects of combination angiotensin II receptor blockers plus angiotensin-converting enzyme inhibitors for left ventricular dysfunction: a quantitative review of data from randomized clinical trials. Arch Intern Med 2007; 167: 1930–6.

33. Weir RA, McMurray JJ, Puu M, et al. Efficacy and tolerability of adding an angiotensin receptor blocker in patients with heart failure already receiving an angiotensin-converting inhibitor plus aldosterone antagonist, with or without a beta blocker. Findings from the candesartan in heart failure: assessment of reduction in mortality and morbidity (charm)-added trial. Eur J Heart Fail 2008; 10: 157–63.

34. Sipahi I, Debanne SM, Rowland DY, Simon DI, Fang JC. Angiotensin-receptor blockade and risk of cancer: meta-analysis of randomised controlled trials. Lancet Oncol 2010; 11: 627–36.

35. ARB Trialists Collaboration. Effects of telmisartan, irbesartan, valsartan, candesartan, and losartan on cancers in 15 trials enrolling 138,769 individuals. J Hypertens 2011; 29: 623–35.

36. Bangalore S, Kumar S, Kjeldsen SE, et al. Antihypertensive drugs and risk of cancer: network meta-analyses and trial sequential analyses of 324,168 participants from randomised trials. Lancet Oncol 2011; 12: 65–82.

37. Pasternak B, Svanstrom H, Callreus T, Melbye M, Hviid A. Use of angiotensin receptor blockers and the risk of cancer. Circulation 2011; 123: 1729–36.

38. FDA Drug Safety Communication: No increase in risk of cancer with certain blood pressure drugs–Angiotensin Receptor Blockers (ARBs). 2011. [Available from: http://www.fda.gov/Drugs/DrugSafety/ucm257516.htm] (Accessed May 13, 2012)

39. Dickstein K, Cohen-Solal A, Filippatos G, et al. ESC Guidelines for the diagnosis and treatment of acute and chronic heart failure 2008: the Task Force for the Diagnosis and Treatment of Acute and Chronic Heart Failure 2008 of the European Society of Cardiology. Developed in collaboration with the Heart Failure Association of the ESC (HFA) and endorsed by the European Society of Intensive Care Medicine (ESICM). Eur Heart J 2008; 29: 2388–442.

40. Hunt SA, Abraham WT, Chin MH, et al. Focused update incorporated into the ACC/AHA 2005 guidelines for the diagnosis and management of heart failure in adults a report of the american college of cardiology foundation/american heart association task force on practice guidelines developed in collaboration with the international society for heart and lung transplantation. J Am Coll Cardiol 2009; 53: e1–e90.

41. Swedberg K, Cleland J, Dargie H, et al. Guidelines for the diagnosis and treatment of chronic heart failure: executive summary (update 2005): the task force for the diagnosis and treatment of chronic heart failure of the european society of cardiology. Eur Heart J 2005; 26: 1115–40.

42. Lindenfeld J, Albert NM, Boehmer JP, et al. HFSA 2010 comprehensive heart failure practice guideline. J Card Fail 2010; 16: e1–194.

20
Anticoagulation in systolic heart failure

Ronald S. Freudenberger

INTRODUCTION

Until the past decade, the risk of thromboembolic events (TEs), (stroke; pulmonary and peripheral thromboembolism), in patients with heart failure (HF) was poorly defined. The analyses that existed were from retrospective analyses of large HF treatment trials and from population based studies. Many of these studies enrolled patients with atrial fibrillation (AF) and flutter and did not specify thromboembolism as an endpoint. This is a particular problem since it has been shown that using precise scales to detect stroke significantly increases the detection of subtle neurological events (1). It is believed that HF in the absence of AF is associated with an increased risk of TE. This belief is based on several observations. First, many patients who present with stroke or TE have depressed left ventricular function (2–4). In the population-based Framingham Heart Study (5), the relative risk of stroke in individuals with HF was 4.1 for men and 2.8 for women, but many of these individuals had concurrent AF. In HF trials, annual stroke rates between 1.3% and 3.5% have been reported; however, almost all of these analyses included patients with AF. An analysis reported thromboembolic rates of only 1% per year in a population of patients in NYHA class II and III HF without AF (Table 20.1) (6). The Warfarin Aspirin Reduced Cardiac Ejection Fraction (WARCEF) study is the largest prospective, randomized, placebo controlled study that found an overall event rate (death, ischemic stroke, and intracerebral hemorrhage of 7.47 events/100 patient-years (7).

If we expand our definition of thrombotic related complications to include deaths from intracoronary thrombosis we greatly increase the true risk of thrombotic complications of HF (13). In one important study, nearly 50% of deaths adjudicated as sudden cardiac deaths were reclassified at autopsy as acute myocardial infarction or coronary thrombosis and 27% of deaths classified as progressive congestive heart failure were actually found to be due to coronary artery thrombosis (14).

This should be balanced against the fact that not all strokes in HF patients are thromboembolic. The majority of patients with HF have a history of diabetes, hypertension, and atherosclerosis. Some HF patients will have neurologic events and mesenteric ischemia due to low flow states, atherosclerotic disease, or a combination of the two. This suggests that perhaps the risks of anticoagulation will not be justified for primary prevention in patients with HF.

HEART FAILURE AS A PROTHROMBOTIC STATE

Heart failure has been described as a prothrombotic state as it relates to the concept of Virchow's triad: stasis of blood, abnormalities in the vessel wall, and abnormalities in blood constituents. Studies have shown that HF patients have higher levels of circulating

Table 20.1 Post Hoc Analyses of Heart Failure Trials

Trial	N	Follow-up (yrs)	AF(%)	CVA (% per yr)	Pulm. TE (% per yr)	Peripheral TE (% per yr)
V-HeFT-I (8)	632	2.3	15	1.8	0.3	0.3
Consensus (9)	253	0.5	50	4.6	NR	NR
V-HeFT-II (8)	804	2.6	15	1.8	0.3	0.08
SOLVD (10)	6797	3.3	6	1.2	0.3	0.3
CIBIS-II (11)	2647	1.3	1.4	NR	NR	NR
SCD-HEFT (12)	2114	4	0	2.64	0.3	0.3

Abbreviations: AF, atrial fibrillation; CVA, cardiovascular accident; Pulm TE, pulmonary thromboembolism; NR, not reported.

fibrinogen, antithrombin III, fibrinopeptide A and d-dimer (15,16). Neuroendocrine modulators may also increase the prothrombotic state by increasing angiotensin and endothelin which in turn increase levels of von Willebrand Factor (17). This, coupled with decreased levels of nitric oxide, has been shown to increase endothelial monocyte and platelet adhesion, potentially leading to *in situ* thrombosis (18,19). A study examining plasma markers of endothelial damage, dysfunction, and activation in patients with acute and chronic HF found that (12,18) levels of von Willebrand factor, soluble thrombomodulin (an index of endothelial damage/dysfunction), soluble E-selectin (an index of endothelial activation), and brain natiuretic peptide were all statistically significantly higher in acute and chronic HF compared with controls. Although this was a small study, it suggests a link between HF, inflammation, and thrombosis.

RISK FACTORS FOR THROMBOEMBOLISM IN PATIENTS WITH HF

Several analyses have attempted to identify potential risk factors for the development of stroke or thromboembolism. Other than ejection fraction (EF), a prior TE event and perhaps the presence of a pedunculated thrombus, these analyses have shed little light on potential risk factors and have provided results difficult to interpret. In a retrospective analysis of the Study of Left Ventricular Dysfunction (SOLVD) trials (10), after excluding patients with AF, the annual rate of TEs was 2.4% in women and 1.8% in men. Lower EF was associated with higher event rates in women but not in men. In addition, women were observed to have a higher proportion of pulmonary embolism. In an analysis of the Survival and Ventricular Enlargement (SAVE) Trial (20) the overall risk of stroke was 8.1% at 5 years and the only independent risk factors for stroke were LV function, older age, and non-use of aspirin or anticoagulants. The risk of stroke was found to be higher in patients with EF <28% versus EF >28% (twofold increase). Every decrease in EF by 5% was associated with an increase stroke risk by 18%. This analysis of ACEI versus placebo in patients post-myocardial infarction, did not exclude patients with AF and only looked at stroke events. This was in contrast to SOLVD which only showed an association with EF in women. An analysis of 2521 patients with moderately severe HF and an EF ≤35%, who participated in the Sudden Cardiac Death-Heart Failure Trial (SCD-HeFT) was performed. Patients with AF at the time of randomization were excluded in this analysis. The four-year rate of TEs was 3.5% with EF 30–35%, 3.6% with EF 20–30%, and 4.6% with EF <20% (extrapolated to 0.9%, 0.9% and 1.2% annual rate) (6). Hypertension at the time of randomization and EF were independent predictors. No other measured variables were significant in terms of outcome.

With regard to prior stroke, the Northern Manhattan Study (NOMAS) assessed 270 patients with first ischemic stroke and 288 age-, gender-, and race-matched controls for the incidence, risk factors, and clinical outcome of stroke patients hospitalized in one hospital. LV systolic function was measured and categorized as normal (>50%), mildly reduced (EF 41–50%), moderately reduced (31–40%), or severely decreased (≤30%). Decreased ejection fraction was found to be strongly associated with ischemic stroke even after adjusting for other stroke risk factors. Left ventricular dysfunction of any degree was more frequent in stroke patients (24.1% in stroke *vs.* 4.9% in controls p < 0.0001). Moderate/severe left ventricular dysfunction was also more common in stroke patients versus controls (13.3% *vs.* 2.4% p < 0.001). The adjusted odds ratio for mild left ventricular dysfunction was 3.96 and 3.88 for moderate/severe (adjusted for other stroke risk factors) (21). In another study, the rate of recurrent stroke following a first stroke was 9–10% per year in HF patients, suggesting that a previous event conferred a high risk of recurrence (22). In another study, the presence of intracardiac thrombus was identified in half of the cases of the patients with neurological events and patients with thrombus had a significantly higher rate of thromboembolism (5.3%/yr) (23). All of these studies taken together suggest a risk association with the presence and degree of systolic dysfunction.

WARFARIN USE FOR THE PREVENTION OF THROMBOEMBOLISM

Till some time back, there were no randomized controlled trials to help guide physicians in the use of warfarin for embolic prevention in HF patients. Unfortunately, the controlled trials that exist have suffered from poor recruitment and have been underpowered to make definitive conclusions. In retrospective analyses of large HF trials such as SAVE, SOLVD, and V-HeFT (Veterans Affairs Vasodilator-Heart Failure Trials) conflicting results have been found. In SOLVD and SAVE, there was a suggestion that warfarin was beneficial in HF patients. In SOLVD, anticoagulant treatment with warfarin was associated with a statistically significant decrease in mortality, death, or hospitalization for HF, but interestingly the benefit was not from the decreased risk of TEs. Warfarin had a 24% overall relative risk reduction for all-cause mortality. The SAVE trial demonstrated an 81% reduction in stroke risk in patients treated with anticoagulation.

On the other hand, other analyses of large HF studies have suggested that warfarin does not reduce rates of TEs in HF patients. In the analysis of the V-HeFT trial data (8), no significant difference in TEs was found when comparing patients treated with anticoagulation against those not treated. In the analysis of the SCD-HeFT data, warfarin use was not associated with reduced risk of TEs (6). Unfortunately, these findings are of limited value because anticoagulation use was not randomized or controlled, data were collected retrospectively, and endpoints were not predefined or standardized.

Three randomized controlled trials have been attempted to determine the optimal preventive therapy for TE in patients with a systolic HF. WASH (The Warfarin/Aspirin Study in Heart Failure) was a small pilot study designed to assess the feasibility of performing a larger outcome study to address the question of whether medical therapy with either aspirin or warfarin in HF patients could affect outcomes (24). The study included 279 patients with LV systolic dysfunction and EF <35%. It was an open label, randomized, placebo controlled study of warfarin (INR target 2.5) *vs.* 300 milligrams (mg) of aspirin *vs.* placebo. Patients with an absolute indication or contraindication to aspirin or warfarin were excluded. No difference in combined primary endpoints of all-cause mortality, non-fatal MI, and non-fatal stroke was found (26% *vs.* 32% *vs.* 26%, placebo *vs.* aspirin *vs.* warfarin, respectively). Patients on warfarin however did have fewer hospitalizations for congestive heart failure (freedom from hospitalization: 48% *vs.* 47% *vs.* 64% placebo *vs.* ASA *vs.* warfarin, respectively). It is important to note that this was a small pilot study designed to assess the feasibility of performing a larger outcome study and therefore not powered to make conclusive statements.

The WATCH study (The Warfarin and Antiplatelet Therapy in Chronic Heart Failure) randomized 1587 patients with HF and EF <30%. It was a randomized, blinded, non-placebo controlled study of warfarin (target INR 2.5) *vs.* aspirin *vs.* clopidogrel. Unfortunately, WATCH was terminated early because of poor recruitment and was therefore underpowered to make any definitive conclusions. Nevertheless, there was a strong trend favoring warfarin over aspirin in the incidence of non-fatal stroke (0.7% *vs.* 2.1%) and there was significantly less hospitalization in the warfarin group (16.1% *vs.* 22.2% *vs.* 18.3% for warfarin, aspirin, clopidogrel respectively). However, this was offset by a significantly higher bleeding rate in the warfarin group (5.5% *vs.* 3.6% *vs.* 2.5% warfarin, aspirin, clopidogrel respectively) (25).

A third multicenter randomized controlled trial, HELAS (efficacy of antithrombotic therapy in chronic HF) was reported (26). This was a double-blind placebo controlled trial of 197 patients with New York Heart Association (NYHA) class II–IV HF and EF ≤35%. Patients with known ischemic heart disease were randomized to aspirin 325 mg daily versus warfarin. Patients with idiopathic dilated cardiomyopathy were randomized to warfarin versus placebo. Patients with reversible ischemia, AF, mitral valve disease, hypertrophic cardiomyopathy, known LV thrombi, contraindication to aspirin or warfarin, and uncontrolled hypertension were excluded. Those who developed AF were withdrawn from the analysis. Primary endpoints were non-fatal stroke, peripheral or pulmonary embolism, myocardial infarction, re-hospitalization, and exacerbation of HF or death from any cause. Overall, the event rate was very low with an incidence of TEs of 2.2 per 100 patient-years. No difference was observed between aspirin and warfarin in the ischemic cardiomyopathy group, while there was a trend toward benefit of warfarin versus placebo in the non-ischemic cardiomyopathy group (8.9 events/100 patient-years in warfarin group *vs.* 14.8 events/100 patient-years in the placebo group). Unfortunately, this study also suffered from enrollment problems, yet again leaving the data to be underpowered to distinguish the differences in outcome between the treatment arms (Table 20.2).

When considering the option of anticoagulation, it is prudent to assess potential bleeding risks. Previous studies looking at risks of major hemorrhage in patients on long-term warfarin have reported ranges between two to three events per 100 patient-years. In the Stroke Prevention in Atrial Fibrillation Investigators trial (SPAF) the risk of major bleeding was 2.3% per 100 patientyears (27). A study was designed to assess the rates of thromboembolism and bleeding in an ambulatory cohort of patients with AF. Of 425

Table 20.2 Multicenter Trials of Anticoagulation and Antiplatlets

Trial	N	Intervention	Outcomes	Comment
Wash	279	Warfarin (INR 2.5) vs. ASA (300 mg)		Underpowered, signal of increased HF hospitalizations in ASA group
Watch	1587	Warfarin vs. ASA(162.5 mg) *vs.* clopidogrel (75 mg).		Underpowered, signal of increased HF hospitalizations in ASA group
Helas	197	Ischemic-ASA or warfarin Non-ischemic-warfarin or placebo	Stroke, embolization, infarction,hospitalization, exacerbation of heart failure, all-cause death	Underpowered

patients, 40% had concomitant HF and the overall event rate of major bleeding was 2.6% over two years (28). In another study of patients over 65 years with AF who were newly initiated on warfarin, the aggregate rate of major hemorrhage was 7.2% per 100 person years and significantly higher for those patients over 80 years old (13.08% vs. 4.75% for patients >80 years vs. less than 80 years). The higher than previously reported rate is probably a result of an older cohort and that only patients being initiated on warfarin were included. Given the aging population and the growing number of elderly patients with HF, this study underscores the importance of considering the potential risks of anticoagulation (29).

ASPIRIN USE FOR THE PREVENTION OF THROMBOEMBOLISM

Several studies have examined whether ASA may have a beneficial effect on thromboembolic event rates. In the SAVE trial, patients on aspirin was observed to have a 56% decreased risk of stroke following a myocardial infarction. In the SOLVD trial, aspirin also decreased the risk of thromboembolic events, but this association was only observed in women, where a 53% relative risk reduction was seen. V-HeFT-I showed a trend toward a reduction in thromboembolic events, whereas, V-HeFT-II did not show a benefit with aspirin. WASH and WATCH trials raised concern about the safety of aspirin use in the HF population as both showed an increase risk of HF hospitalization rates while no mortality benefit was seen. In WASH there was a trend toward a higher mortality rate in the aspirin group versus the warfarin and placebo groups. These studies and others have raised concern regarding the potential interaction between ACE inhibitors and ASA. Aspirin may attenuate the protective effects of ACE inhibitors by inhibiting prostaglandins and thus enhancing vasoconstriction. Given these data, it is difficult to be certain if aspirin provides a benefit in this population.

For these reasons the definitive study examining the use of warafrin or aspirin in patients with a low ejection fraction was conducted and published. The WARCEF trial randomized 2305 patients to either warfarin (target INR 2.0–3.5) or aspirin 325 mg. The patients were followed for up to 6 years (mean 3.5 years). The primary outcome was the time to the first event in a composite end point of ischemic stroke, intracerebral hemorrhage, or death from any cause.

The rates of the primary outcome were 7.47 events per 100 patient-years in the warfarin group and 7.93 in the aspirin group (hazard ratio with warfarin, 0.93; 95% CI, 0.79–1.10; P = 0.40). Thus, there was no significant overall difference between the two treatments. In a time-varying analysis, the hazard ratio changed over time, slightly favoring warfarin over aspirin by the fourth year of follow-up, but this finding was only marginally significant (P = 0.046). Warfarin, as compared with aspirin, was associated with a significant reduction in the rate of ischemic stroke throughout the follow-up period (0.72 events/100 patient-years vs. 1.36/100 patient-years; hazard ratio, 0.52; 95% CI, 0.33–0.82; P = 0.005). The rate of major hemorrhage was 1.78 events per 100 patient-years in the warfarin group as compared with 0.87 in the aspirin group (P < 0.001). The rates of intracerebral and intracranial hemorrhage did not differ significantly between the two treatment groups (0.27 events per 100 patient-years with warfarin and 0.22 with aspirin, P = 0.82). Further analysis of this study is currently underway. It may be possible to determine a subset of patients that will have an overall benefit of warfarin or aspirin (Fig. 20.1) (7).

SPECIAL POPULATIONS/MISCONCEPTIONS
Coronary Arterial Disease

In patients with coronary artery disease, platelet inhibitor therapy is generally prescribed. Although aspirin is the prophylactic antiplatelet drug of choice, it reduces the risk of

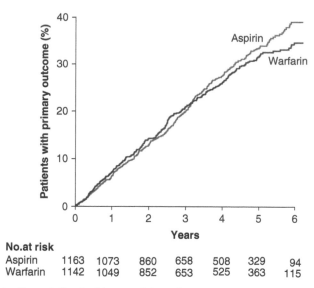

Figure 20.1   Cumulative incidence of the primary outcome. *Source*: From Ref. 7.

recurrent stroke, MI, and vascular death by only 13% (30). Clopidogrel was 8% better than aspirin in one large trial of patients with vascular disease and was associated with fewer gastrointestinal bleeding complications (31).

In trials reviewed by the Antithrombotic Trialists' Collaboration, (32), allocation of high-risk patients to antiplatelet therapy reduced the combined rates of serious vascular events by about a quarter, nonfatal myocardial infarction by a third, nonfatal stroke by a quarter, and vascular mortality by one-sixth. This meta-analysis has led to the broad recommendation to use antiplatelet agents for secondary prevention of myocardial infarction; however, the database included only two trials totaling 134 patients with HF. Despite the lack of data supporting the efficacy of aspirin, even in patients with ischemic cardiomyopathy, the recommendation has been generalized to patients with chronic HF, making some practitioners reluctant to allow inclusion of their patients in a trial comparing warfarin with aspirin for chronic HF. In fact, two studies—the Warfarin Re-Infarction Study (33) (WARIS) and the Anticoagulants in the Secondary Prevention of Events in Coronary Thrombosis (34) (ASPECT) trial—found warfarin effective for prevention of death (by 24%), myocardial infarction (by 34–53%) and stroke (by 40–55%) over 3 years in patients with ischemic heart disease. The beneficial effects were greater than those with aspirin, as found by meta-analysis, in which reductions in vascular-related death, myocardial infarction, and stroke were 15%, 31%, and 39%, respectively (35). A meta-analysis by Leor et al. found no difference between warfarin and aspirin with respect to these endpoints in patients with coronary disease (36).

Stents

Following coronary stent deployment several studies have addressed the use of dual antiplatelet therapy, with different endpoints. No studies have addressed optimal management beyond one year. "The Effects of pretreatment with clopidogrel and aspirin followed by long-term therapy in patients undergoing percutaneous coronary intervention: the PCI-CURE (37) trial" randomized 2658 patients with non-ST-elevation acute coronary syndrome undergoing PCI in double-blind treatment with clopidogrel (n = 1313) or placebo (n = 1345). Patients were pretreated with aspirin and study drug for a median of six days before PCI during the initial hospital admission, and for a median of 10 days overall. After PCI, most patients (>80%) in both groups received open-label thienopyridine for about four weeks, after which study drug was restarted for a mean of eight months. The primary endpoint was a composite of cardiovascular death, myocardial infarction, or urgent target-vessel revascularization within **30 days** of PCI. Fifty-nine (4·5%) patients in the clopidogrel group had the primary endpoint, compared with 86 (6·4%) in the placebo group (relative risk 0·70, 95% CI 0·50–0·97, P = 0·03). Long-term administration of clopidogrel after PCI (not a primary endpoint) was associated with a lower rate of cardiovascular death, myocardial infarction, or any revascularization (P = 0·03), and of cardiovascular death or myocardial infarction (P = 0·047). Overall (including events before and after PCI) there was a 31% reduction cardiovascular death or myocardial infarction (P = 0·002). At follow-up, there was no significant difference in major bleeding between the groups (P = 0·64).

The second trial was "The Clopidogrel for the Reduction of Events During Observation (CREDO) trial," a randomized, double-blind, placebo-controlled trial conducted among 2116 patients who were to undergo elective PCI or were deemed as having a high likelihood of undergoing PCI, enrolled at 99 centers in North America (38). Patients were randomly assigned to receive a 300-mg clopidogrel loading dose (n = 1053) or placebo (n = 1063) 3–24 hours before PCI. Thereafter, all patients received clopidogrel, 75 mg/d, through day 28. From day 29 through 12 months, patients in the loading-dose group received clopidogrel, 75 mg/d, and those in the control group received placebo. Both groups received aspirin throughout the study. At one year, long-term clopidogrel therapy was associated with a 26.9% relative reduction in the combined risk of death, MI, or stroke (95% CI, 3.9–44.4%; P = 0.02; absolute reduction, 3%). Clopidogrel pretreatment did not significantly reduce the combined risk of death, MI, or urgent target vessel revascularization at 28 days (reduction, 18.5%; 95% CI, -14.2% to 41.8%; P = 0.23). However, only 63% of patients in the clopidogrel group and 61% of patients in the control group completed the full one-year course of study drug. Patients treated with clopidogrel for one year experienced a trend toward an increase in major bleeding (8.8% clopidogrel vs. 6.7% placebo; P = 0.07).

The effects of warfarin alone on long-term restenosis and thrombosis are not adequately studied. In the *Stent Anticoagulation Restenosis Study Investigators* (39) dual antiplatelet therapy was found to be superior to aspirin plus warfarin in the first 30 days. Beyond this period, the effects of warfarin alone are not known. In the Full Anticoagulation versus Aspirin and Ticlopidine (FANTASTIC) study (40) there was 485 patients randomized to warfarin or aspirin plus ticlopidine. The primary endpoint was bleeding or peripheral vascular complications during the first six weeks after stent implantation. A primary endpoint occurred in 33 patients (13.5%) in the antiplatelet group and 48 patients (21%) in the anticoagulation group [odds ratio = 0.6 (95% CI 0.36 to 0.98), P = 0.03]. At six weeks and at six months there were no differences in major adverse cardiac events (a secondary endpoint) (Table 20.3).

Therefore, after stent deployment (studied mainly in bare metal stents, BMSs), short-term use of dual antiplatelet therapy with aspirin plus a thienopyridine is recommended based on studies demonstrating superiority compared with aspirin alone (37,40). However, given that these studies were not conducted in patients with ischemic cardiomyopathy and the event rate in both of these studies after the first several months of therapy was low, it is difficult to draw conclusions and apply them to long-term use after stent deployment in the cardiomyopathic population.

DRUG-ELUTING STENTS: SPECIAL CONSIDERATIONS

The cumulative incidence of target lesion revascularization is lower with drug-eluting stents (DESs) (1.9%/year) than with BMS (5%/year), with a majority of events occurring in the

Table 20.3   Major Cardiac Clinical Events Within a 6-Month Follow-Up in the FANTASTIC Study

	Antiplatelet Therapy, n (%)	Conventional Anticoagulation, n (%)	P
Death	2 (0.8)	5 (2.2)	0.21
Acute myocardial infarction	13 (5.4)	16 (7.1)	0.44
Q wave	3 (1.2)	7 (3.1)	0.16
Non–Q wave	10 (4.1)	9 (4.0)	0.93
Coronary artery bypass surgery	3 (1.2)	3 (1.3)	0.93
Repeat target lesion angioplasty	13 (5.4)	11 (4.9)	0.80
Total	31 (12.9)	35 (15.5)	0.40

first year with either type of stent (41). An apparently greater incidence of late stent thrombosis (1–12 months) in patients treated with DES is attributed to delayed re-endothelialization and higher complexity of coronary lesions (42,43). This has been associated with the interruption of clopidogrel and can be catastrophic, with mortality rates ranging from 20% to 45% (44). The incidence of stent thrombosis at three years is 2% (45). In a 478-patient registry of DES stent thrombosis, the majority of cases occurred after one year, and presented with MI (67% STEMI, 22% NSTEMI) (46). Nearly 30% of patients were taking dual-antiplatelet therapy (DAPT) at the time stent thrombosis occurred. By histological analysis in 127 patients who died >1 month after DES, localized strut hypersensitivity was seen with sirolimus eluting stents, whereas malapposition secondary to excessive fibrin deposition was seen with paclitaxel eluting stents (47). The best strategy for prevention of DES thrombosis beyond the first year is unknown.

Based on these data the ACC/AHA/SCAI advisory committee recommends treatment with dual antiplatelet therapy for one year in patients who receive DES who are not at high risk of bleeding, and for 3 months for BMS (44). The use of dual antiplatelet therapy versus warfarin following DES beyond the short term has not been studied.

Stroke

The landmark Warfarin and Aspirin for the Prevention of Recurrent Ischemic Stroke (WARSS) trial investigated whether warfarin was superior to aspirin in the prevention of recurrent ischemic stroke in patients with a prior noncardioembolic ischemic stroke (48). In this multicenter, double-blind, randomized trial, the effect of warfarin (at a dose adjusted to produce an international normalized ratio of 1.4–2.8) was compared with that of aspirin (325 mg per day) on the combined primary endpoint of recurrent ischemic stroke or death from any cause within two years. In the intention-to-treat analysis, no significant differences were found between the treatment groups in any of the outcomes measured. The primary endpoint of death or recurrent ischemic stroke was reached by 196 of 1103 patients assigned to warfarin (17.8 percent) and 176 of 1103 assigned to aspirin (16.0 percent; P = 0.25; hazard ratio comparing warfarin with aspirin, 1.13; 95% CI 0.92–1.38). The rates of major hemorrhage were low (2.22/100 patient-years in the warfarin group and 1.49/100 patient-years in the aspirin group). Also, there were no significant treatment-related differences in the frequency of or time to the primary end point or major hemorrhage according to the cause of the initial stroke (1237 patients had had previous small-vessel or lacunar infarcts, 576 had had cryptogenic infarcts, and 259 had had infarcts designated as due to severe stenosis or occlusion of a large artery). This study did not specifically examine patients with depressed

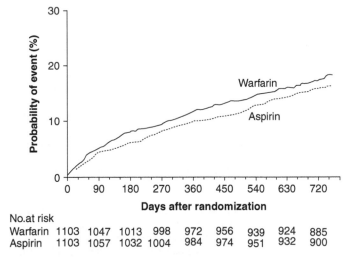

No.at risk

Warfarin	1103	1047	1013	998	972	956	939	924	885
Aspirin	1103	1057	1032	1004	984	974	951	932	900

Figure 20.2 Kaplan-Meier analyses of the time to recurrent ischemic stroke or death according to treatment assignment. *Source*: From Ref. 48.

left ventricular function, therefore an optimal approach for secondary prevention of stroke in patients with a depressed left ventricle is unknown (Fig. 20.2).

WHAT DO WE DO NOW?
The Guidelines
Current guidelines from the American Heart Association/American College of Cardiology do not support routine use of warfarin in dilated cardiomyopathy and stress the absence of randomized trial data (49). The American College of Chest Physicians guidelines (30) recognize the increased risk of stroke in patients with cardiomyopathy but does not advise warfarin treatment for stroke risk reduction in these patients. The Heart Failure Society of America guidelines suggest that "warfarin may be considered in patients with an EF <35%" (50). The European Society of Cardiology states that "there is little evidence to show that antithrombotic therapy modifies the risk of death or vascular events in patients with heart failure" (51). The European Stroke Initiative (52) has no specific recommendations for primary or secondary stroke prevention in patients with cardiomyopathy who are in sinus rhythm. Because there is no consensus in treatment guidelines, practitioners must individually apply a limited amount of data to each patient.

A Reasonable Approach
The WARCEF study found no significant overall difference between aspirin and warfarin with regard to the time to first event of death, ischemic stroke, and intracerebral hemorrhage. In the absence of definitive data we consider warfarin anticoagulation in patients with (*i*) an ejection fraction less than 20% (based on Freudenberger et al.), (*ii*) a prior stroke with reduced left ventricular function, based on NOMAS findings or the presence of a pedunculated thrombus in the left or right ventricle. This must be weighed carefully against the risk of bleeding in the patient based on age, and concomitant therapy. At present, we believe there is insufficient evidence to warrant treatment with dual antiplatelet therapy and warfarin in those who have undergone stent placement. We eagerly await further analysis of the WARCEF trial to help guide us in these important issues affecting a large number of patients and perhaps find subgroups where one drug may benefit from warfarin versus aspirin.

REFERENCES

1. Meschia JF. Management of acute ischemic stroke. what is the role of tPA and antithrombotic agents? Postgrad Med 2000; 107: 85–6; 89–93.
2. Samama MM. An epidemiologic study of risk factors for deep vein thrombosis in medical outpatients: the Sirius study. Arch Intern Med 2000; 160: 3415–20.
3. Anderson FA Jr, Wheeler HB, Goldberg RJ, et al. A population-based perspective of the hospital incidence and case-fatality rates of deep vein thrombosis and pulmonary embolism. the Worcester DVT study. Arch Intern Med 1991; 151: 933–8.
4. Isnard R, Komajda M. Thromboembolism in heart failure, old ideas and new challenges. Eur J Heart Fail 2001; 3: 265–9.
5. Kannel WB, Wolf PA, Verter J. Manifestations of coronary disease predisposing to stroke. The Framingham study. JAMA 1983; 250: 2942–6.
6. Freudenberger RS, Hellkamp AS, Halperin JL, et al. Risk of thromboembolism in heart failure: an analysis from the Sudden Cardiac Death in Heart Failure Trial (SCD-HeFT). Circulation 2007; 115: 2637–41.
7. Homma S, Thompson JLP, Pullicino PM, et al. Warfarin and aspirin in patients with heart failure and sinus rhythm. N Engl J Med 2012; 366: 1859–69.
8. Dunkman WB, Johnson GR, Carson PE, et al. Incidence of thromboembolic events in congestive heart failure. The V-HeFT VA cooperative studies group. Circulation 1993; 87: VI94–101.
9. The CONSENSUS Trial Study Group. Effects of enalapril on mortality in severe congestive heart failure. Results of the cooperative north scandinavian enalapril survival study (CONSENSUS). N Engl J Med 1987; 316: 1429–35.
10. Dries DL, Rosenberg YD, Waclawiw MA, et al. Ejection fraction and risk of thromboembolic events in patients with systolic dysfunction and sinus rhythm: evidence for gender differences in the studies of left ventricular dysfunction trials. J Am Coll Cardiol 1997; 29: 1074–80.
11. The Cardiac Insufficiency Bisoprolol Study II. CIBIS-II): a randomised trial. Lancet 1999; 353: 9–13.
12. Freudenberger RS, Hellkamp AS, Halperin JL, et al. The incidence of Thromboembolism in patients with NYHA class II and III heart failure: an analysis from the sudden cardiac death in heart failuretrial (SCD-HeFT). Circulation 2006; 115: 2637–41.
13. Roberts WC, Siegel RJ, McManus BM. Idiopathic dilated cardiomyopathy: analysis of 152 necropsy patients. Am J Cardiol 1987; 60: 1340–55.
14. Uretsky BF, Thygesen K, Armstrong PW, et al. Acute coronary findings at autopsy in heart failure patients with sudden death: results from the assessment of treatment with lisinopril and survival (ATLAS) trial. Circulation 2000; 102: 611–16.
15. Jafri SM, Ozawa T, Mammen E, et al. Platelet function, thrombin and fibrinolytic activity in patients with heart failure. Eur Heart J 1993; 14: 205–12.
16. Yamamoto K, Ikeda U, Furuhashi K, et al. The coagulation system is activated in idiopathic cardiomyopathy. J Am Coll Cardiol 1995; 25: 1634–40.
17. Sbarouni E, Bradshaw A, Andreotti F, et al. Relationship between hemostatic abnormalities and neuroendocrine activity in heart failure. Am Heart J 1994; 127: 607–12.
18. Chong AY, Freestone B, Patel J, et al. Endothelial activation, dysfunction, and damage in congestive heart failure and the relation to brain natriuretic peptide and outcomes. Am J Cardiol 2006; 97: 671–5.
19. Fischer D, Rossa S, Landmesser U, et al. Endothelial dysfunction in patients with chronic heart failure is independently associated with increased incidence of hospitalization, cardiac transplantation, or death. Eur Heart J 2005; 26: 65–9.
20. Loh E, Sutton MS, Wun CC, et al. Ventricular dysfunction and the risk of stroke after myocardial infarction. N Engl J Med 1997; 336: 251–7.
21. Hays AG, Sacco RL, Rundek T, et al. Left ventricular systolic dysfunction and the risk of ischemic stroke in a multiethnic population. Stroke 2006; 37: 1715–19.
22. Pullicino PM, Halperin JL, Thompson JL. Stroke in patients with heart failure and reduced left ventricular ejection fraction. Neurology 2000; 54: 288–94.
23. Katz SD, Marantz PR, Biasucci L, et al. Low incidence of stroke in ambulatory patients with heart failure: a prospective study. Am Heart J 1993; 126: 141–6.
24. Cleland JG, Findlay I, Jafri S, et al. The Warfarin/Aspirin Study in Heart failure (WASH): a randomized trial comparing antithrombotic strategies for patients with heart failure. Am Heart J 2004; 148: 157–64.
25. Cleland JG, Ghosh J, Freemantle N, et al. Clinical trials update and cumulative meta-analyses from the American College of Cardiology: WATCH, SCD-HeFT, DINAMIT, CASINO, INSPIRE, STRATUS-US, RIO-Lipids and cardiac resynchronisation therapy in heart failure. Eur J Heart Fail 2004; 6: 501–8.

26. Cokkinos DV, Haralabopoulos GC, Kostis JB, et al. Efficacy of antithrombotic therapy in chronic heart failure: the HELAS study. Eur J Heart Fail 2006; 8: 428–32.

27. Hart RG, Halperin JL, Pearce LA, et al. Lessons from the stroke prevention in atrial fibrillation trials. Ann Intern Med 2003; 138: 831–8.

28. Parkash R, Wee V, Gardner MJ, et al. The impact of warfarin use on clinical outcomes in atrial fibrillation: a population-based study. Can J Cardiol 2007; 23: 457–61.

29. Hylek EM, Evans-Molina C, Shea C, et al. Major hemorrhage and tolerability of warfarin in the first year of therapy among elderly patients with atrial fibrillation. Circulation 2007; 115: 2689–96.

30. Albers GW, Amarenco P, Easton JD, et al. Antithrombotic and thrombolytic therapy for ischemic stroke: the Seventh ACCP Conference on Antithrombotic and Thrombolytic Therapy. Chest 2004; 126: 483S–512S.

31. CAPRIE Steering Committee. A randomised, blinded, trial of clopidogrel versus aspirin in patients at risk of ischaemic events (CAPRIE). Lancet 1996; 348: 1329–39.

32. Antiplatelet Trialists' Collaboration. Collaborative overview of randomised trials of antiplatelet therapy–III: reduction in venous thrombosis and pulmonary embolism by antiplatelet prophylaxis among surgical and medical patients. BMJ 1994; 308: 235–46.

33. Hurlen M, Abdelnoor M, Smith P, et al. Warfarin, aspirin, or both after myocardial infarction. N Engl J Med 2002; 347: 969–74.

34. Anticoagulants in the Secondary Prevention of Events in Coronary Thrombosis (ASPECT) Research Group. Effect of long-term oral anticoagulant treatment on mortality and cardiovascular morbidity after myocardial infarction. Lancet 1994; 343: 499–503.

35. Al-Khadra AS, Salem DN, Rand WM, et al. Antiplatelet agents and survival: a cohort analysis from the Studies of Left Ventricular Dysfunction (SOLVD) trial. J Am Coll Cardiol 1998; 31: 419–25.

36. Leor J, Reicher-Reiss H, Goldbourt U, et al. Aspirin and mortality in patients treated with angiotensin-converting enzyme inhibitors: a cohort study of 11,575 patients with coronary artery disease. J Am Coll Cardiol 1999; 33: 1920–5.

37. Mehta SR, Yusuf S, Peters RJ, et al. Effects of pretreatment with clopidogrel and aspirin followed by long-term therapy in patients undergoing percutaneous coronary intervention: the PCI-CURE study. Lancet 2001; 358: 527–33.

38. Steinhubl SR, Berger PB, Mann JT, et al. Early and sustained dual oral antiplatelet therapy following percutaneous coronary intervention: a randomized controlled trial. JAMA 2002; 288: 2411–20.

39. Leon MB, Baim DS, Popma JJ, et al. A clinical trial comparing three antithrombotic-drug regimens after coronary-artery stenting. Stent Anticoagulation Restenosis Study Investigators. N Engl J Med 1998; 339: 1665–71.

40. Bertrand ME, Legrand V, Boland J, et al. Randomized multicenter comparison of conventional anticoagulation versus antiplatelet therapy in unplanned and elective coronary stenting. The full anticoagulation versus aspirin and ticlopidine (fantastic) study. Circulation 1998; 98: 1597–603.

41. Stettler C, Wandel S, Allemann S, et al. Outcomes associated with drug-eluting and bare-metal stents: a collaborative network meta-analysis. Lancet 2007; 370: 937–48.

42. Kuchulakanti PK, Chu WW, Torguson R, et al. Correlates and long-term outcomes of angiographically proven stent thrombosis with sirolimus- and paclitaxel-eluting stents. Circulation 2006; 113: 1108–13.

43. Cutlip DE, Baim DS, Ho KK, et al. Stent thrombosis in the modern era: a pooled analysis of multicenter coronary stent clinical trials. Circulation 2001; 103: 1967–71.

44. Grines CL, Bonow RO, Casey DE, et al. Prevention of premature discontinuation of dual antiplatelet therapy in patients with coronary artery stents: a science advisory from the American heart association, American college of cardiology, society for cardiovascular angiography and interventions, American college of surgeons, and American dental association, with representation from the american college of physicians. J Am Dent Assoc 2007; 138: 652–5.

45. de la Torre-Hernandez JM, Alfonso F, Hernandez F, et al. Drug-eluting stent thrombosis: results from the multicenter Spanish registry ESTROFA (Estudio ESpanol sobre TROmbosis de stents FArmaco-activos). J Am Coll Cardiol 2008; 51: 986–90.

46. Waksman R. The international FDA approved DES thrombosis registry (DESERT). Paper presented at: Annual Meeting of Transcatheter Cardiovascular Therapeutics. November 9, 2011. San Francisco, California, 2011.

47. Nakazawa G, Finn A, Vorpahl M, et al. Coronary responses and differential mechanisms of late stent thrombosis attributed to first generation sirolimus- and paclitaxel-eluting stents. J Am Coll Cardiol 2011; 57: 390–8.

48. Mohr JP, Thompson JL, Lazar RM, et al. A comparison of warfarin and aspirin for the prevention of recurrent ischemic stroke. N Engl J Med 2001; 345: 1444–51.

49. Hirsh J, Fuster V, Ansell J, et al. American Heart Association/American College of Cardiology Foundation guide to warfarin therapy. Circulation 2003; 107: 1692–711.

50. HFSA 2006 Guideline Executive Summary. Executive summary: HFSA 2006 Comprehensive Heart Failure Practice Guideline. J Card Fail 2006; 12: 10–38.

51. Swedberg K, Cleland J, Dargie H, et al. Guidelines for the diagnosis and treatment of chronic heart failure: executive summary (update 2005): the task force for the diagnosis and treatment of chronic heart failure of the european society of cardiology. Eur Heart J 2005; 26: 1115–40.

52. Hacke W, Kaste M, Olsen TS, et al. European stroke initiative: recommendations for stroke management. Organisation of stroke care. J Neurol 2000; 247: 732–48.

21

Role of mineralocorticoid receptor antagonists in patients with heart failure

Mara Giattina and Flora Sam

ALDOSTERONE PHYSIOLOGY

The renin angiotensin aldosterone system (RAAS) is an adaptation to maintain adequate salt and water balance and circulatory homeostasis during periods of deprivation. This sensitive regulation involves various sensors and has complex feedback mechanisms. In response to decreased renal perfusion, renin is secreted by the juxtaglomerular cells lining the renal afferent arterioles. Renin cleaves circulating angiotensinogen, forming angiotensin I, which is then further cleaved by angiotensin-converting enzyme (ACE) into the biologically active form angiotensin II. Angiotensin II acts to maintain circulatory homeostasis by potent renal and systemic vasoconstriction, proximal tubule sodium reabsorption, and signaling the adrenal cortex to secrete the steroid hormone, aldosterone. Aldosterone promotes the reabsorption of sodium, in exchange for potassium, in the distal nephron as well as the colon, salivary, and sweat glands. Aldosterone is also secreted directly in response to elevated potassium, causes potassium and magnesium urinary loss, therefore playing an integral role in electrolyte homeostasis. Because of its physiologic role in the regulation of sodium and potassium, it has been termed a mineralocorticoid (1).

The interplay of these hormones is complex. There is negative feedback loop once kidney perfusion and salt delivery are restored, but there is also evidence that aldosterone may amplify tissue ACE and angiotensin II responses and can increase the number of angiotensin receptors (2,3). Research has further elucidated angiotensin-independent stimuli for aldosterone secretion besides potassium, including corticotrophin, catecholamine, endothelins, and vasopressin (1). Aldosterone production is not confined to the adrenal cortex; it has now been discovered in the endothelium and smooth muscle cells of the heart and blood vessels, suggesting possible autocrine or paracrine local control mechanisms (4,5). In addition, mineralocorticoid receptor (MR) binding is not specific to aldosterone; it is also activated by normal circulating cortisol levels, suggesting activation besides those periods of salt and aldosterone excess (6).

The actions of aldosterone have been shown to be far more diverse than its classic role as a mineralocorticoid, with significant implications for patients with heart failure (HF). Along with angiotensin II, aldosterone plays an important role in cardiac and vascular remodeling. Downstream effects include cytokine production, inflammatory cell chemotaxis and adhesion, fibroblast growth, and collagen synthesis, culminating in an inflammatory and fibrotic reparative process. In animal models, aldosterone administration increases the media/lumen ratio in the vasculature and impairs the response to acetylcholine demonstrating endothelial dysfunction (7). Coagulation is another crucial response to tissue injury, and aldosterone and angiotensin II may contribute to its regulation by stimulating the production of plasminogen activator inhibitor-1 (PAI-1), an inhibitor of fibrinolysis (8). The expression of aldosterone in endothelium and smooth muscle cells of the heart and blood vessels suggests there could be a direct regulatory role in response to myocardial injury.

In summary, renin, angiotensin, and aldosterone work synergistically to preserve circulatory homeostasis including vasoconstriction, potentiation of sympathetic response, retention of salt and water, maintenance of electrolyte balance, and tissue reparative processes.

PATHOPHYSIOLOGY OF ALDOSTERONE IN HEART FAILURE

This normal physiologic role of these homeostatic controls goes awry in patients with HF (Fig. 21.1). Decreased cardiac output impairs renal perfusion and leads to increased sympathetic tone, activation of RAAS, widespread retention of sodium and water, and vasoconstriction. The resulting increased systemic resistance, volume overload, and increased cardiac demand can lead to further hemodynamic decompensation in cardiac function. Such is the progressively downward spiraling course of patients with HF. Aldosterone has also been shown to be produced by the failing heart and is markedly elevated in HF patients where it is inversely correlated with left ventricular (LV) ejection fraction (LVEF) and directly with LV end-diastolic pressure (LVEDP) (9). Levels are further elevated by decreased hepatic perfusion and clearance of aldosterone in the low flow state of HF (10).

Data suggest that aldosterone independently affects both the sympathetic and parasympathetic nervous system. Aldosterone blunts the normal baroreceptor heart rate response and potentiates norepinephrine action on the vasculature, further contributing to an elevation in blood pressure (11,12). It also prevents the normal uptake of norepinephrine in the myocardium, the process that enables normal cardiac tissue to avoid excessive adrenergic stimulation (13). Impaired cardiac norepinephrine uptake has been shown to be a strong adverse prognostic marker for overall mortality in congestive HF (CHF) secondary to both idiopathic dilated and ischemic cardiomyopathy (14).

As with the neurohormonal and downstream renal effects of the RAAS, the inflammatory and tissue reparative processes can have a vital role in homeostasis following injury,

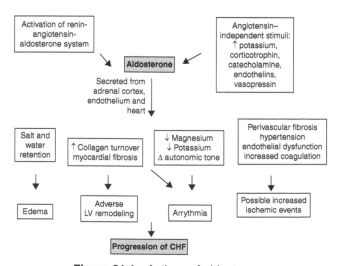

Figure 21.1 Actions of aldosterone.

but have a detrimental effect as an adaptive response to HF. Aldosterone may promote myocardial and vascular fibrosis independent of the hemodynamic effects (15,16). In rodent models, administration of sodium and aldosterone causes hypertension as well as an inflammatory reaction followed by the growth of fibroblasts, synthesis of collagen, and perivascular fibrosis of systemic small arteries and arterioles. Endothelial dysfunction, reduced vascular compliance, and poor vasodilatory reserve may result. Adverse cardiac remodeling also occurs with fibrosis of the myocardium and depressed mechanical function (17,18). This extracellular matrix turnover and adverse cardiac remodeling is a common endpoint in the pathology of hypertensive heart disease, dilated cardiomyopathy, and after myocardial infarction and may also be associated with proinflammatory changes as well as alterations in the fatty acid oxidation machinery (19). Cardiac fibrosis is also a major determinant of diastolic dysfunction and can provide a substrate for arrhythmogenicity and thus sudden death (20).

The relative contributions of the different hormones are difficult to tease out since the system works in concert; however, it seems clear that aldosterone plays a significant direct role. In a study on stroke-prone hypertensive rats, the beneficial stroke-reducing effect of treatment with an angiotensin-converting enzyme inhibitor (ACEI) was reduced when exogenous aldosterone was administered (21). In primary aldosteronism, patients exhibit vascular remodeling and reduced vascular response of small subcutaneous resistance arteries (22,23).

Renal Pathology

Similar to its effects on the heart and vessels, aldosterone has been shown to have salt-dependent effects on kidney morphology, causing nephrosclerosis and hypertrophy of distal collecting tubule cells, which can be prevented by mineralocorticoid receptor antagonism in animal models (24). This compromises kidney function in patients with HF who are already especially vulnerable to renal dysfunction because of their dependence on adequate cardiac output for normal kidney perfusion and function. This further impairs secretion of salt and water. As with the other effects of the RAAS system, aldosterone does not mediate these effects alone but functions in concert with the other hormones of the RAAS.

ALDOSTERONE "ESCAPE"

There are several reasons why direct inhibition of the mineralocorticoid receptor may be beneficial. As described above, the renin–angiotensin system involves a complex interplay of hormones, which are implicated in the exacerbation and progression of CHF. Thus there are several sites of potential treatment benefit. The best studied drugs to date are ACEI and angiotensin II receptor blockers (ARBs), which are an integral part of the standard of care for HF and are reviewed in detail elsewhere. Renin inhibitors have also been introduced. However, the system exhibits "aldosterone escape," a phenomenon whereby inhibition of upstream targets such as ACEI and ARB results in only transient lowering of aldosterone levels, followed by return to elevated levels in some patients (25,26). This is because aldosterone is also produced via angiotensin-independent mechanisms, including potassium, sympathetic activation, and perhaps also local vascular control mechanisms. This residual aldosterone may be clinically relevant as aldosterone is closely related to poor outcome and mortality in CHF (27). In a study of CHF patients, those 10% of patients who exhibited aldosterone escape while on ACEI had decreased exercise capacity compared with those with suppressed aldosterone levels (28). In addition, cortisol binds and activates the mineralocorticoid receptor and may be responsible for much of the downstream effects of receptor activation during normal volume loading conditions (6). Thus, direct MR antagonism has the potential to more completely ameliorate the adverse downstream effects of the RAAS, even in patients treated with ACEIs and/or ARBs despite the presence of "aldosterone escape."

Experimental data support this theory. In animal models, MR antagonism reduces inflammation, extracellular matrix production, and perivascular fibrosis, while improving endothelial dysfunction and attenuating platelet aggregation. There is a decreased incidence of cerebral and renal vascular lesions. Similar improvements were noted in cardiac tissue with decreased coronary inflammation, reduced interstitial fibrosis, regress of hypertrophy, and improved myocardial compliance. Mineralocorticoid receptor blockade also decreases sympathetic drive in rats through direct action on the brain (7,29).

CLINICAL APPLICATIONS OF MINERALOCORTICOID RECEPTOR INHIBITORS IN HEART FAILURE
Systolic Heart Failure (or Heart Failure Reduced Ejection Fraction)

The clinically available mineralocorticoid receptor antagonists, spironolactone, and eplerenone have each been evaluated in placebo-controlled double blind international trials with positive results. The Randomized Aldactone Evaluation Study (RALES) was the first large-scale clinical trial to evaluate outcome in HF (30). The study enrolled 1663 patients with chronic NYHA Class III–IV HF and LVEF <35%, who were randomized to receive spironolactone versus placebo. Patients with both ischemic and non-ischemic CHF were included. The initial dose of spironolactone was 25 mg daily, with titration to 50 mg daily if progressive HF symptoms developed. The trial was halted early after a mean follow-up of 24 months when it found treatment was associated with a 30% reduction in all-cause mortality and a 35% decrease in death from cardiac causes and CHF hospitalizations. Enrolled patients were on optimal CHF treatment for that time which included ACEI but not β-blockers. Following publication of these results, spironolactone prescribing increased significantly and is recommended guideline therapy for systolic HF (31).

The EPHESUS trial was the second large trial with mineralocorticoid receptor blockade and it demonstrated a mortality benefit in patients post myocardial infarction (MI) with LV dysfunction (32). Enrolled patients were 3–14 days post acute MI with clinical CHF or diabetes and LVEF <40%, and were randomized to eplerenone or placebo. This was in addition to standard medical therapy, including an ACEI or ARB in 87%, and β-blockade in 75%. Eplerenone was started at a dose of 25 mg, and then titrated to 50 mg if tolerated; mean dose was 43 mg. After a mean follow-up of 16 months, treatment conferred a significant 15% reduction in risk of all-cause mortality (Fig. 21.2). Death from cardiovascular causes and rate of hospitalization were also similarly significantly reduced. All causes of cardiovascular mortality (acute MI, HF, and sudden death) were reduced, though the reduction in sudden death was statistically significant with a relative risk of 79%.

These trials were robust evidence of the mortality and morbidity benefit of mineralocorticoid receptor antagonism. Several smaller studies have attempted to further delineate the underlying mechanisms of this treatment benefit and it appears to be multifactorial.

There has been support for the role of mineralocorticoid receptor antagonism in ameliorating the vascular changes and fibrosis associated with activation of RAAS. Myocardial fibrosis and collagen formation are of significant pathophysiological significance in HF, have prognostic implications, and have been shown to correlate with a marker of collagen turnover, procollagen type III amino terminal peptide (PIIINP) (11). A RALES substudy found that baseline levels of PIIINP correlated with an increased risk of death and hospitalization. Survival benefit in the group treated with spironolactone was associated with decreased level of this marker at six months. Interestingly, the spironolactone effect on outcome was significant only in patients with above-median baseline levels of PIIINP (Table 21.1) (20). Other studies corroborate this treatment effect on markers of fibrosis, including PIIINP and PAI-1, a mediator of fibrosis and inhibitor of fibrinolysis (8,11,33). Particularly during the critical post-MI period, studies have demonstrated reduced collagen

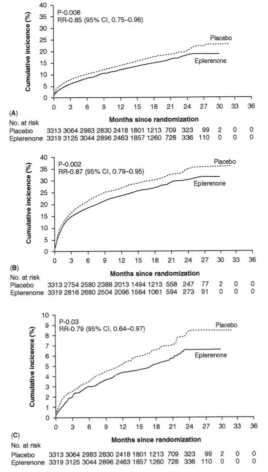

Figure 21.2 Treatment benefit conferred by Eplerenone in the EPHESUS Trial. *Source*: From Ref. 32.

Table 21.1 Adjusted Relative Risk of Death and of Death or Hospitalization (Spironolactone Vs. Placebo), According to Baseline Serum Level of PIIINP, a RALES Substudy

	PIIINP > Median		**PIIINP < Median**	
	RR (95% CI)	P	RR (95% CI)	P
Death	0.44 (0.26–0.75	0.002	1.11 (0.66–1.88)	0.7
Death or hospitalization	0.45 (0.29–71)	0.0004	0.85 (0.55–33)	0.48

PIIINP is procollagen type III amino-terminal peptide.
Source: From Ref. 20.

turnover, improved LV remodeling, a significantly higher LVEF, and smaller indexed LV end diastolic volume (LVEDV) (33–36). These treatment benefits were in addition to standard medical therapy including ACEI and/or ARB.

Endothelial dysfunction also improved with treatment. In a double-blinded, placebo controlled randomized study of 10 patients with chronic HF, one-month treatment with spironolactone improved endothelium-dependent vasodilation in the forearm microcirculation (3). Spironolactone also augmented an induced vasoconstrictive response. These patients did not have differences in BP to explain these findings. Studies have also demonstrated improved exercise capacity in patients with mild to moderate CHF treated with spironolactone, which could be related to the improvement in endothelial function and vasodilatory capacity. This is relevant as improving endothelial dysfunction has been suggested as a therapeutic target in CHF (3,35).

The autonomic effects of mineralocorticoid receptor antagonism have also been investigated. In a study of patients with NYHA class II–III CHF and severely depressed systolic function, treatment with spironolactone increased cardiac norepinephrine uptake as assessed by 123I-metaiodobenzylguanidine scintigraphy (123I-MIBG) (13). MR antagonism has been shown to improve QT dispersion and heart rate variability and blunt the early morning rise in HR, a time frame which correlates with the high frequency of MI and sudden death. These effects, together with decreased adrenergic tone and observed higher magnesium levels, may account for the reduction in ventricular ectopy observed with spironolactone treatment (12,13). These factors could contribute to the decrease in sudden death seen in RALES and EPHESUS.

In summary, several mechanisms could account for the observed benefits of mineralocorticoid receptor antagonism in HF patients with systolic dysfunction, including limitation of excessive extracellular matrix turnover, improvement in LV remodeling and LVEF, improved endothelial function, and changes in autonomic tone. All of these are of great importance in the pathology of HF.

Based on this data, the American College of Cardiology/American Heart Association (ACC/AHA) Guidelines give a class I recommendation for the addition of an aldosterone antagonist in carefully selected patients with moderate to severe CHF or a recent MI and a reduced LVEF who can be carefully monitored for preserved renal function and normal potassium concentration. Under conditions where monitoring for hyperkalemia or renal dysfunction is not anticipated to be feasible, the risks may outweigh the benefits of aldosterone antagonists (Table 21.2) (37).

Diastolic Heart Failure (or Heart Failure Preserved Ejection Fraction)

Almost half of patients with HF have a relatively normal ejection fraction yet, beyond symptom relief, there is no therapy that has been shown to reduce morbidity or mortality in these patients. The RAAS plays an important role in the pathophysiology because of its unique role in promoting fibrosis at a molecular level. LV hypertrophy (LVH) is one of the characteristic features of this disease process, confers an excess risk of cardiovascular events, and can be affected by RAAS blockade independent of BP lowering. Treatment with MR antagonists has been shown to reduce collagen turnover as assessed by PIIINP, which correlates with LV mass and diastolic dysfunction (38). In the 4E-LVH study, eplerenone was compared with enalapril and the combination of eplerenone/enalapril in patients with LVH and hypertension (39). Blood pressure reduction, LVH regression, and reduction in microalbuminuria occurred in all treatment arms, but were greatest in the combination arm. Investigators used alternate antihypertensive medications in all treatment arms to equalize diastolic BP, and found that BP lowering correlated poorly with LVH regression, suggesting that other factors besides BP lowering may be important in affecting LV mass. Studies in patients randomized to MR antagonists have demonstrated a reduction in LA volume and other significant improvements in diastolic filling patterns independent of BP lowering effects (35,40,41), however, other studies provide more mixed results (42,43).

Thus, conclusive evidence of clinical improvement in this subset of patients is lacking at this point. The randomized, placebo-controlled TOPCAT trial (Trial of Aldosterone

Table 21.2 Guidelines for Minimizing the Risk of Hyperkalemia in Patients Treated with Aldosterone Antagonists

1. Impaired renal function is a risk factor for hyperkalemia during treatment with aldosterone antagonists. The risk of hyperkalemia increases progressively when serum creatinine exceeds 1.6 mg/dl[a]. In elderly patients or others with low muscle mass in whom serum creatinine does not accurately reflect glomerular filtration rate, determination that glomerular filtration rate or creatinine clearance exceeds 30 ml/min is recommended.
2. Aldosterone antagonists should not be administered to patients with baseline serum potassium in excess of 5.0 mEq/l.
3. An initial dose of spironolactone 12.5 or eplerenone 25 mg is recommended, after which the dose may be increased to spironolactone 25 mg or eplerenone 50 mg if appropriate.
4. The risk of hyperkalemia is increased with concomitant use of higher doses of ACEIs (captopril ≥75 mg daily; enalapril or lisinopril ≥10 mg daily).
5. Nonsteroidal anti-inflammatory drugs and cyclo-oxygenase-2 inhibitors should be avoided.
6. Potassium supplements should be discontinued or reduced.
7. Close monitoring of serum potassium is required; potassium levels and renal function should be checked in 3 days and at 1 week after initiation of therapy and at least monthly for the first 3 months.
8. Diarrhea or other causes of dehydration should be addressed emergently.

[a]Although the entry criteria for the trials of aldosterone antagonists included creatinine >2.5 mg/dL, the majority of patients had a much lower creatinine.
Abbreviations: ACEIs, indicates angiotensin-converting enzyme inhibitors.
Source: From Ref. 37.

Antagonist Therapy in Adults with Preserved Ejection Fraction Congestive Heart) is currently underway to determine whether spironolactone will improve outcomes in patients with CHF and preserved systolic function.

Hypertension

Hypertension is a well-established major cardiovascular risk factor, and lowering of blood pressure has been shown to reduce cardiovascular morbidity and mortality. The pathology of hypertension and increased peripheral resistance results from vascular remodeling and endothelial dysfunction of small resistance arteries (44). ACEIs and ARBs are well-established drug classes in the treatment of hypertension. Along with angiotensin II, aldosterone is a mediator of these processes and is locally produced in the endothelium and vascular smooth muscle cells, thus aldosterone blockade is an obvious target for blood pressure lowering. This was evaluated in a randomized trial of eplerenone versus placebo, in addition to existing treatment regimen, in patients whose blood pressure was not adequately controlled on ACEI or ARB. Treatment was started at doses of 50 mg, with subsequent titration to 100 mg daily. Blood pressure was significantly reduced in recipients of eplerenone and side effects and incidence of hyperkalemia were few and comparable to placebo (45). Hence, there is some data that addition of MR antagonist to ACEI or ARB provides safe and effective BP reduction. The JNC7 lists aldosterone antagonists as recommended treatment for hypertension with the compelling indications of HF and post-myocardial infarction based on the RALES and EPHESUS trials (46).

Diabetes and Renal Disease

Diabetes, chronic kidney disease (CKD) and microalbuminuria are risk factors for cardiovascular disease. Blockade of the RAAS protects the kidney from target-organ damage caused by hypertension and diabetes. ACEI and ARB have well-defined roles in treating HTN, and are recommended as first-line agents in diabetics because of evidence that they slow progressive kidney damage and the worsening of albuminuria beyond their BP-lowering effects (46). High concentrations of aldosterone have been observed in obese, hypertensive, diabetic patients (47). Given the association of aldosterone with nephrosclerosis, mineralo-corticoid receptor antagonists may be a similarly effective tool in reducing the progression of diabetic and hypertensive renal disease. There is clinical evidence that the addition of MR antagonists decreases proteinuria, an ndependent predictor of mortality in patients with CKD (24). However, especially given the higher risk of hyperkalemia in those with CKD already on ACEI or ARB therapy, there are no sufficient long-term clinical data yet, regarding treatment benefit and acceptable safety profile to back their effectiveness in this population.

Experimental data demonstrated beneficial effects of MR inhibition on LVH regression and cardiac remodeling. LVH is common in chronic renal failure and its combination (renal failure and LVH) is associated with increased cardiovascular morbidity and mortality (48). Similarly impaired renal function is associated with increased morbidity and mortality in patients with chronic HF with both preserved and reduced LVEF (49). A clinical trial in dialysis patients using spironolactone was completed to evaluate the effect of MR antagonism on cardiac hypertrophy in the end-stage renal disease population and the results are still pending.

Combination Therapy with Other Agents

Though neurohormonal blockade has become the mainstay of treatment for CHF, there has been concern regarding negative results with overly aggressive neurohormonal blockade with multiple agents including BBs, ARBs, ACEIs, and mineralocorticoid receptor antagonists (50). However, combinations have been used safely in several trials to date (30,32,39,51). In EPHESUS, an MR antagonist was added to optimal CHF therapy including high rates of treatment with β-blocker and ACEI or ARB with significant mortality benefit and an acceptable safety profile. However vigilance to creatinine and potassium monitoring when using these drugs in combination cannot be overemphasized. What has not been studied adequately is the combination of triple RAAS blockade; the ACC/AHA Guidelines recommend against the routine concomitant use of an ACEI, ARB, and aldosterone antagonist for lack of sufficient safety data at this point (class III recommendation) (37).

AGENTS AND THEIR USE
Spironolactone

Spironolactone competitively antagonizes aldosterone binding, but may cause endocrine disturbances as a result of its nonselective binding affinity for progesterone and androgen receptors. Thus side effects of impotence, gynecomastia, breast pain, and menstrual irregularities occur in up to 10% of patients. In RALES, this was a reason for discontinuation in 2% of patients. Because it is generic, the cost is significantly less than eplerenone. Spironolactone should be initiated at a dose of 12.5 mg daily, with titration to 25 mg daily if appropriate (37).

Eplerenone

Eplerenone is a selective aldosterone blocker with much greater selectivity for the mineralocorticoid receptor relative to other steroid receptors. Though it is more expensive than generic spironolactone, the adverse sexual side effects are not an issue. Recommended dose range is from 25 mg to 50 mg daily (37).

PRECAUTIONS TO USE

The electrolyte consequences of MR blockade are significant. Along with other RAAS hormones, aldosterone has an integral role in potassium regulation. Especially in patients treated with concomitant ACEI and/or ARB or those with renal dysfunction, this crucial regulatory system is blocked and hyperkalemia can result in dire consequences. Severe hyperkalemia occurred in relatively few patients in the large clinical trials (less than 2% in RALES and 5.5% in EPHESUS); however, these trials used strict inclusion criteria and patients were very closely monitored. Trials excluded concomitant treatment with K-sparing diuretics, creatinine greater than 2.5 mg/dL, and potassium greater than 5.0 mmol/L. Potassium and creatinine were measured at 48 hours, one week, four weeks, then one week after any change in dose. If potassium levels were greater than 5.5 mmol/L, the study drug was reduced or temporarily discontinued. Though inclusion criteria required creatinine concentration less than 2.5 mg/dL, the mean creatinine was much lower, around 1.1 mg/dL. Among those with a creatinine clearance less than 50 mL/min, the rate of serious hyperkalemia rose to 10% (32).

The online publication of RALES led to a wider use of spironolactone and the subsequent incidence of hyperkalemia rose dramatically. A Canadian population-based study found that prescriptions for spironolactone increased up to five fold and rates of hospitalization for hyperkalemia and associated mortality tripled (Fig. 21.3) (31).

On the other hand, CHF patients are generally treated with diuretics and often have low potassium and magnesium levels, and electrolytes that can significantly affect ventricular ectopy. These electrolyte abnormalities can be offset by treatment with ACEI, ARB and/or MR antagonists. In EPHESUS, the rates of hypokalemia significantly decreased from 13.1% in placebo versus 8.4% with eplerenone (32). This can be viewed as a benefit of treatment in select patients as long as electrolytes and renal function are carefully monitored.

ACC/AHA CHF Guidelines specifically address precautions to reduce the incidence of hyperkalemia when using MR antagonists (Table 21.2).

FUTURE STUDIES

Mineralocorticoid inhibitors continue to have an evolving role in optimal treatment of CHF and treatment questions remain.

Though both clinically available agents spironolactone and eplerenone have treatment benefits based on available trial evidence, they have never been directly compared. Because of generic availability and significant cost savings, a reasonable strategy might be to initiate treatment with spironolactone and change to eplerenone should side effects develop.

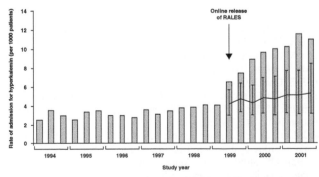

Figure 21.3 Incidence of hyperkalemia associated with online publication of RALES. *Source*: From Ref. 31.

The vast bulk of data available thus far pertains to those with moderate to severe CHF with LVEF <40%. Clinical data on those with less severe clinical CHF has recently been published (52). The EMPHASIS-HF trial showed a mortality benefit and reduction in hospitalization with eplerenone in patients with mild CHF (NYHA Class II and depressed LV systolic function). As mentioned, the TOPCAT trial is currently underway to evaluate those with preserved systolic function and diastolic heart failure.

There is biochemical evidence that treatment with MR antagonists affects inflammation and fibrinolysis and clinical evidence of mortality benefit post MI in patients with CHF; however, the direct effect of aldosterone on atherosclerosis has not been examined. Indirect evidence suggests the potential for an interaction since spironolactone decreases PAI-1 activity, a regulator of fibrosis that is expressed at high levels in atherosclerotic plaque and is a marker for increased risk of cardiovascular death in patients with unstable angina. This may be one of the mechanisms underlying the correlation between activation of RAAS and increased risk for ischemic cardiovascular events (8).

SUMMARY

Inappropriate activation of the RAAS is maladaptive in HF, leading to salt and water retention, autonomic changes, endothelial dysfunction, and adverse remodeling of the vasculature and myocardium. These changes contribute to the progressive nature of HF. The suppression of neurohormonal tone has a major impact on morbidity and mortality in HF patients and is a mainstay of current CHF therapy. Studies to date also emphasize the importance of inflammation, collagen turnover, and fibrosis in the pathogenesis of HF and suggest clinical improvement with its attenuation. Aldosterone appears to have a significant role in these pathological processes, and MR antagonists have been shown to reduce morbidity and mortality among patients with moderate to severe HF. The standard of care for patients with symptomatic CHF and LV systolic dysfunction should include an MR antagonist, given in combination with other proven therapies including β-blockade and ACEI or ARB. Careful regular monitoring of serum potassium and creatinine is an essential component to routine care of patients treated with these agents.

REFERENCES

1. Weber KT. Mechanisms of disease: aldosterone in congestive heart failure. N Engl J Med 2001; 345: 1689–97.
2. Robert V, Heymes C, Silvestre JS, et al. Angiotensin AT1 receptor subtype as a cardiac target of aldosterone: role in aldosterone-salt induced fibrosis. Hypertension 1999; 33: 981–6.
3. Farquharson CAJ, Struthers AD. Spironolactone increases nitric oxide bioactivity, improves endothelial vasodilator dysfunction, and suppresses vascular angiotensin I/angiotensin II conversion in patients with chronic heart failure. Circulation 2000; 101: 594–7.
4. Hatakeyama H, Miymori I, Fujita T, et al. Vascular aldosterone: biosynthesis and a link to angiotensin II- induced hypertrophy of vascular smooth muscle cells. J Biol Chem 1994; 289: 24316–20.
5. Struthers AD. Aldosterone-induced vasculopathy. Mol Cell Endocrin 2004; 217: 239–41.
6. Funder JW. RALES, EPHESUS and redox. J Steroid Biochemistry Mol Biol 2005; 93: 121–5.
7. Virdis A, Fritsch Neves M, Amiri F, et al. Spironolactone improves angiotensin-induced vascular changes and oxidative stress. Hypertension 2002; 40: 504–10.
8. Brown NJ, Kim K-S, Chen Y-Q, et al. Synergistic effect of adrenal steroids and angiotensin II on plasminogen activator inhibitor-1 production. J Clin Endocrinol Metab 2000; 85: 336–44.
9. Mizuno Y, Yoshimura M, Yasue H, et al. Aldosterone production is activated in failing ventricle in humans. Circulation 2001; 103: 72–7.
10. Tait JF, Bougas J, Little B, et al. Splanchnic extraction and clearance of aldosterone in subjects with minimal and marked cardiac dysfunction. J Clin Endocrinol Metab 1965; 25: 219–28.
11. MacFadyen RJ, Barr CS, Struthers AD. Aldosterone blockade reduces vascular collagen turnover, improves heart rate variability and reduces early morning rise in heart rate in heart failure patients. Cardiovasc Res 1997; 35: 30–4.

12. Yee K-M, Pringle SD, Struthers AD. Circadian variation in the effects of aldosterone blockade on heart rate variability and QT dispersion in congestive heart failure. J Am Coll Cardiol 2001; 37: 1800–7.

13. Barr CS, Lang CC, Hanson J, et al. Effects of adding spironolactone to an angiotensin-converting enzyme inhibitor in chronic congestive heart failure secondary to coronary artery disease. Am J Cardiol 1995; 76: 1259–65.

14. Merlet P, Valette H, Dubois-Rande J-L, et al. Prognostic value of cardiac metaiodobenzylguanidine imaging in patients with heart failure. J Nucl Med 1992; 33: 471–7.

15. Weber KT, Brilla CG. Pathological hypertrophy and cardiac interstitium: fibrosis and renin-angiotensin-aldosterone systome. Circulation 1991; 83: 1849–65.

16. Young M, Fullerton M, Dilley R, et al. Mineralocorticoids, hypertension and cardiac fibrosis. J Clin Invest 1994; 93: 2578–83.

17. Qin W, Rudolph AE, Bond BR, et al. Transgenic model of aldosterone-driven cardiac hypertrophy in heart failure. Circ Res 2003; 93: 69–76.

18. Zannad F, Dousset B, Alla F. Treatment of congestive heart failure: Interfering the aldosterone-cardiac extracellular matrix relationship. Hypertension 2001; 38: 1227–32.

19. Lebrasseur NK, Duhaney TS, De Silva D, et al. Myocardial effects of fenofibrate in aldosterone-induced hypertension. Hypertension 2007; 50:489–96.

20. Zannad F, Alla F, Dousset B, et al. Limitation of excessive extracellular matrix turnover may contribute to survival benefit of spironolactone therapy in patients with congestive heart failure: insights from the Randomized Aldactone Evaluation Study (RALES). Circulation 2000; 102: 2700–6.

21. MacLeod AB, Vasdev S, Smeda JS. The role of blood pressure and aldosterone in the production of hemorrhagic stroke in captopril-treated hypertensive rats. Stroke 1997; 28: 1821–9.

22. Rizzoni D, Porteri E, Castellano M, et al. Vascular hypertrophy and remodeling in secondary hypertension. Hypertension 1996; 28: 785–90.

23. Taddei S, Virdis A, Mattei P, et al. Vasodilation to acetylcholine in primary and secondary forms of human hypertension. Hypertension 1993; 21: 929–33.

24. Epstein M. Aldosterone blockade: An emerging strategy for abrogating progressive renal disease. Am J Med 2006; 119: 912–19.

25. McKelvie RS, Yusuf S, Pericak D, et al. Comparison of candesartan, enalapril and their combination in congestive heart failure: a randomized evaluation of strategies for left ventricular dysfunction (RESOLVD) pilot study. Circulation 1999; 100: 1056–64.

26. Pitt B. "Escape" of aldosterone production in patients with left ventricular dysfunction treated with an angiotensin converting enzyme inhibitor: implications for therapy. Cardiovasc Drugs Ther 1995; 9: 145–9.

27. Swedberg K, Eneroth P, Kjekshus J, et al. Hormones regulating cardiovascular function in patients with severe congestive heart failure and their relation to mortality. CONSENSUS trial study group. Circulation 1990; 82: 1730–6.

28. Cicoira M, Zanolla L, Franceschini L, et al. Relation of aldosterone "escape" despite angiotensin-converting enzyme inhibitor administration to impaired exercise capacity in chronic congestive heart failure secondary to ischemic or idiopathic dilated cardiomyopathy. Am J Cardiol 2002; 89: 403–7.

29. Brilla CG, Matsubara LS, Weber KT. Anti-aldosterone treatment and the prevention of myocardial fibrosis in primary and secondary hyperaldosteronism. J Mol Cell Cardiol 1993; 25: 563–75.

30. Pitt B, Zannad F, Remme WJ, et al. The effect of spironolactone on morbidity and mortality in patients with severe heart failure. N Engl J Med 1999; 341: 709–17.

31. Juurlink DN, Mamdani MM, Lee DS, et al. Rates of hyperkalemia after publication of the randomized aldactone evaluation study. N Engl J Med 2004; 351: 543–51.

32. Pitt B, Remme W, Zannad F, et al. Eplerenone, a selective aldosterone blocker, in patients with left ventricular dysfunction after myocardial infarction. N Engl J Med 2003; 348: 1309–21.

33. Hayashi M, Tsutamoto T, Wada A, et al. Immediate administration of mineralocorticoid receptor antagonist spironolactone prevents post-infarct left ventricular remodeling associated with supression of a marker of myocardial collagen synthesis in patients with first anterior acute myocardial infarction. Circulation 2003; 107: 2559–65.

34. Modena MG, Aveta P, Menozzi A, et al. Aldosterone inhibition limits collagen synthesis and progressive left ventricular enlargement after anterior myocardial infarction. Am Heart J 2001; 141: 41–6.

35. Cicoira M, Zanolla L, Rossi A, et al. Long-term, dose-dependent effects of spironolactone on left ventricular function and exercise tolerance in patients with chronic heart failure. J Am Coll Cardiol 2002; 40: 304–10.

36. Tsutamoto T, Wada A, Maeda K, et al. Effect of spironolactone on plasma brain natriuretic peptide and left ventricular remodeling in patients with congestive heart failure. J Am Coll Cardiol 2001; 37: 1228–33.

37. ACC/AHA 2005. Guideline update for the diagnosis and. management of chronic heart failure in the adult—Summary article. Circulation 2005; 112: 1825–52.

38. Bernal J, Pitta SR, Thatai D. Role of the renin-angiotensin-aldosterone system in diastolic heart failure. Am J Cardiovasc Drugs 2006; 6: 373–81.

39. Pitt B, Reichek N, Willenbrock R, et al. Effects of eplerenone, enalapril and eplerenone/enalapril in patients with essential hypertension and left ventricular hypertrophy: the 4E—Left Ventricular Hypertrophy study. Circulation 2003; 108: 1831–8.

40. Grandi AM, Imperiale D, Santillo R, et al. Aldosterone antagonist improves diastolic function in essential hypertension. Hypertension 2002; 40: 647–52.

41. Roongsritong C, Sutthiwan P, Bradley J, et al. Spironolactone improves diastolic function in the elderly. Clin Cardiol 2005; 28: 484–7.

42. Mottram PM, Haluska B, Leano R, et al. Effect of aldosterone antagonism on myocardial dysfunction in hypertensive patients with diastolic heart failure. Circulation 2004; 110: 558–65.

43. Sato A, Hayashi M, Saruta T. Relative long-term effects of spironolactone in conjunction with an angiotensin-converting enzyme inhibitor on left ventricular mass and diastolic function in patients with essential hypertension. Hypertens Res 2002; 25: 837–42.

44. Schiffrin EL. Reactivity of small blood vessel in hypertension: relation with structural changes. Hypertension 1992; 19: II-1–9.

45. Krum H, Nolly H, Workman D, et al. Efficacy of eplerenone added to renin-angiotensin blockade in hypertensive patients. Hypertension 2002; 40: 117–23.

46. The seventh report of the Joint National. Committee on Prevention, Detection, Evaluation, and Treatment of High Blood Pressure.

47. Goodfriend TL, Egan B, Stepniakowski K, et al. Relationships among plasma aldosterone, high-density lipoprotein cholesterol, and insulin in humans. Hypertension 1995; 25: 30–6.

48. Foley RN, Parfrey PS, Sarnak MJ. Epidemiology of cardiovascular disease in chronic renal disease. J Am Soc Nephrol 1998; 9: S16–23.

49. Heywood JT, Fonarow GC, Costanzo MR, et al. High prevalence of renal dysfunction and its impact on outcome in 118,465 patients hospitalized with acute decompensated heart failure: a report from the ADHERE database. J Card Fail 2007; 13: 422–30.

50. Cohn JN, Tognoni G. A randomized trial of the angiotensin-receptor blocker valsartan in chronic heart failure. N Engl J Med 2001; 345: 1667–75.

51. McMurray JJV, Ostergren J, Swedberg K, et al. Effects of candesartan in patients with chronic heart failure and reduced left ventricular systolic function taking angiotensin-converting-enzyme inhibitors: the CHARM-Added trial. Lancet 2003; 362: 767–71.

52. Zannad F, McMurray JJ, Krum H, et al. EMPHASIS-HF Study Eplerenone in patients with systolic heart failure and mild symptoms. N Engl J Med 2011; 364: 11–21.

22

Treatment of heart failure with preserved ejection fraction

Barry A. Borlaug

INTRODUCTION

Approximately half of all patients with chronic heart failure (HF) have a preserved ejection fraction (HFpEF) (1). Morbidity and mortality are high, and similar to patients with systolic heart failure (SHF) (2). In contrast to the wealth of data available from large-scale clinical trials in SHF, there is little evidence to guide treatment decisions in HFpEF (3). This relates to an incomplete pathophysiologic understanding, the lack of randomized trial data currently available, and the relatively equivocal findings noted in the studies published to date. Treatments with dramatic benefits in SHF have had less impressive effects in HFpEF (4,5). Fundamental disparities in ventriculoarterial mechanical properties in HFpEF produce different clinical responses to common drugs such as vasodilators and diuretics, and novel agents more specifically targeting these abnormalities may ultimately prove more effective (6). In this chapter, we shall first examine the pathophysiology of HFpEF to better predict and understand responses to various treatments. Data regarding specific medications, most of them commonly used in SHF, will be reviewed. Finally, future therapies that are or will soon be tested in clinical trials will be explored.

PATHOPHYSIOLOGY AND PUTATIVE THERAPEUTIC TARGETS
Diastolic Dysfunction

Abnormalities of diastolic function are commonly seen in patients with HFpEF and plausibly explain many of the commonly observed clinical findings, leading many to refer to this disease as "diastolic heart failure." Diastolic dysfunction can broadly be defined by abnormalities in pressure decay during isovolumic relaxation (often termed early or "active" relaxation) and changes in the distensibility of the left ventricle (often referred to as "passive" compliance, Fig. 22.1) (6). Basic studies have shown that these distinctions are largely artifactual, since both active (e.g., sarcoplasmic calcium handling) and passive processes (phosphorylation status of sarcomeric macromolecules such as titin) appear to be involved in each component of diastole (6). Although diastolic dysfunction has been considered for years to be a key player in the pathophysiology of HFpEF, there was lack of human data to support this.

In the first invasive pressure–volume study of HFpEF patients, Kawaguchi et al. found that the increase in cardiac filling pressures in HFpEF appeared more related to an increase in extrinsic restraint applied to the heart during diastole than to abnormal relaxation or compliance (7). Subsequently, Zile and colleagues measured left ventricular pressures and

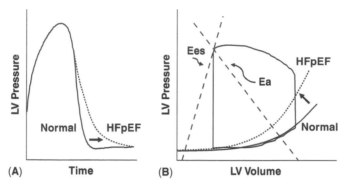

Figure 22.1 (**A**) Prolonged relaxation is common in heart failure preserved ejection fraction (HFpEF) (dotted line), reducing the atrioventricular filling gradient during early diastole. (**B**) Pressure–volume loop from a single beat. Bottom curve is the diastolic pressure–volume relationship or chamber compliance. This is shifted up and to the left with HFpEF (dotted line), such that LV pressure is higher at a given chamber volume. Dashed lines show ventricular end-systolic elastance (Ees), given by the slope of the end-systolic pressure–volume relationship, and arterial stiffness or elastance (Ea), the negative slope running through the end-diastolic and end-systolic coordinates.

echo-Doppler-derived volumes in 47 patients with HFpEF and compared them with those of 10 healthy controls (8), finding that ventricular filling pressures, diastolic relaxation velocity, and chamber stiffness were abnormal in HFpEF. However, diastolic dysfunction is also commonly seen in elderly patients with hypertension—yet these patients do not have clinical HF. To determine how specific diastolic dysfunction is to HFpEF, Lam et al. noninvasively compared diastolic parameters in HFpEF with both hypertensives and normal controls in a larger population-based study (9). Indeed, estimated chamber compliance, filling pressures, and relaxation rate were all impaired in hypertensives compared with healthy volunteers, but importantly, they were significantly more abnormal in HFpEF. These findings and others have led many to speculate that hypertensive heart disease exists on a continuum with HFpEF, meaning that early and aggressive treatment of the structural abnormalities seen with arterial hypertension (such as concentric remodeling) may be of benefit (3,6,9). Altering cardiac loading conditions may indirectly affect diastole (discussed below), but there are currently no agents available that can *directly* treat diastolic dysfunction.

Arterial Afterload and Ventricular-Vascular Stiffening
The vasculature becomes stiffer with aging (10), as does the left ventricle during both diastole and systole (11,12). This phenomenon, which is a key promoter of systolic hypertension in elderly adults, is exaggerated in many patients with HFpEF (13). Arterial hypertension is virtually universal in HFpEF (2,13,14), related largely to ventriculoarterial stiffening.

Kawaguchi et al. first showed that ventricular end-systolic elastance (Ees; Fig. 22.1) and arterial stiffness (effective arterial elastance, Ea) are markedly elevated in HFpEF (7), while Lam et al. found that these parameters were also elevated in many asymptomatic hypertensives (9). This should not be taken to mean that ventricular and arterial stiffening are not pathologic phenomena, because the dramatic pressure alterations seen are clearly deleterious in their effects on cardiovascular homeostasis (13). Indeed, Hundley and colleagues found that aortic stiffness was higher in patients with HFpEF than in old and young controls without HF, and in multivariate analysis, aortic distensibility best predicted aerobic exercise capacity (15).

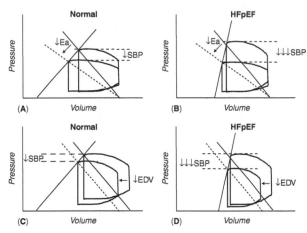

Figure 22.2 **(A–D)** Effects of elevated ventricular stiffness (Ees) on blood pressure regulation in heart failure preserved ejection fraction (HFpEF). An acute reduction in afterload (Ea) produces a much larger drop in blood pressure in the HFpEF patient **(B)** compared with a healthy control **(A)**. Similarly, the a given reduction in preload (end-diastolic volume, EDV) from diuresis or venodilation causes a much larger reduction in blood pressure in HFpEF **(D)** than normal **(C)**. Increases in preload and afterload would have similarly exaggerated effects in HFpEF, explaining the common occurrence of hypertensive crisis and acute pulmonary edema in HFpEF.

Figure 22.2 shows how ventricular systolic stiffening promotes exaggerated swings in blood pressure with minimal changes in preload and afterload. This has important repercussions in the care of patients with HFpEF, because a given amount of diuresis or vasodilator therapy will have much more potent effects in the stiffer "high gain" heart-artery system, increasing myocardial oxygen demand with stress, and decreasing cardiac efficiency (13). Therapies reducing vascular stiffening have been shown to improve exercise capacity in normal elderly patients (16) and those with diastolic dysfunction and a hypertensive response to exercise (17,18).

There is also important crosstalk between arterial afterload and diastolic function (13). Diastolic relaxation is inversely related to afterload in hypertensive and nonhypertensive subjects across a broad age-range (19). Loading sequence appears to be equally important, with increases in afterload during the late portion of systole (due to wave reflections—enhanced in the setting of vascular stiffening) being most strongly associated with abnormal relaxation (19). Blood pressure reduction improves diastolic relaxation velocity, although one drug has not emerged as being superior in this regard (20). Afterload reduction also allows the ventricle to contract down to a smaller end-systolic volume, improving diastolic recoil and "suction" effects during early diastole to augment filling. The reduction in preload allows the ventricle to operate in a more compliant range of the diastolic pressure–volume relationship (Fig. 22.3) (6).

Cardiovascular Reserve Function

Ventricular function may be normal at rest, but impaired under the duress of exercise, excessive afterload, or increases in central blood volume. Such abnormal cardiac reserve function is emerging as an important player in HFpEF. Kitzman and colleagues first compared hemodynamic and exercise responses in patients with HFpEF to normal volunteers. (21). They found marked exercise limitation, related to an inability to augment cardiac

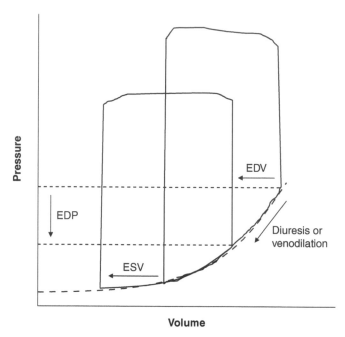

Figure 22.3 Reducing end-diastolic volume (EDV) with diuresis or venodilation moves the left ventricle from the steeper, stiffer portion of its diastolic pressure–volume relationship to a more favorable, compliant limb, with marked reduction in end-diastolic filling pressure (EDP). This, along with afterload reduction, allows the ventricle to contract down to a lower end-systolic volume (ESV), enhancing early diastolic recoil and "suction" to improve early diastolic filling.

output with exercise. This was related to impaired recruitment of ventricular preload volume, despite dramatically greater increases in filling pressures, leading the authors to conclude that exercise limitation in HFpEF was due to a failure of the Frank–Starling mechanism from diastolic dysfunction (21). In a later study comparing HFpEF to closely matched elderly hypertensive controls (22), patients with HFpEF displayed abnormal heart rate and cardiac output reserve responses, with impaired systemic vasodilation even during low level exercise. In contrast to the earlier study, there were no differences in preload reserve. Chronotropic incompetence has been observed by other groups in HFpEF (23), raising questions about the role of heart rate–slowing agents in this population (see the section "**Beta-Adrenergic Antagonists**"). We have shown that compared with hypertensive controls, HFpEF patients display markedly abnormal contractile responses and abnormal ventriculoarterial coupling with exercise, even at early, low workload, emphasizing the importance of limitations with systolic, diastolic, vascular and chronotropic reserve functions in HFpEF (24). HFpEF patients have impaired cellular ATP bioavailability, due to abnormalities in creatine shuttle kinetics (25), and this may contribute to abnormal reserve responses.

Systolic Dysfunction

By definition, one will assume that systolic function is normal in HFpEF, although a number of studies suggest this may not be the case. EF is a fairly nonspecific gauge of contractility, being potently affected by loading conditions and chamber remodeling. Several investigators have demonstrated abnormalities in regional systolic function in

HFpEF, predominantly reduced longitudinal shortening (26–29). Others have questioned the significance of these findings (30), because longitudinal shortening deficiencies may be compensated for by increases in radial shortening, particularly with concentric chamber remodeling (31), frequently seen in HFpEF—preserving global EF (14). Baicu et al. found that most chamber-level systolic parameters were similar in HFpEF patients to healthy controls, although they did find abnormalities in myocardial contractility (32). This finding has been corroborated by other groups (33,34), although the significance of this finding has been questioned, because it often is seen in the absence of HF as well (30). We have found that both chamber and myocardial level systolic function are indeed abnormal in a much larger, nonselected, population-based study of HFpEF (35). Intriguingly, systolic function was increased in the hypertensive controls compared with both healthy volunteers and HFpEF, suggesting this may serve as a chronic adaptation. Importantly, abnormal myocardial contractility was associated with increased mortality over long-term follow-up, emphasizing the clinical importance of this phenomenon.

Other Proposed Mechanisms

Maurer and colleagues have reported enlarged left ventricular chamber volumes in patients with HFpEF, associated with increases in extracellular fluid volume (36,37). Because pressure increases exponentially with increases in chamber filling (as the ventricle becomes stiffer at higher preloads; Fig. 22.3), it has been suggested that this may partly explain the elevated filling pressures seen in HFpEF. However, other groups have not replicated these findings (8,9,33), and one large study found that chamber volumes were if anything smaller in HFpEF (9). In addition to diastolic dysfunction and overfilling, ventricular filling pressures may also be increased when there are enhanced extrinsic restraining forces transmitted to the left ventricle, mediated via the pericardium and right heart (38). These forces become more operative when heart size increases, such that all four cardiac chambers similarly abut the rigid pericardium and become tightly coupled. Invasive human data support this hypothesis of enhanced restraint as a contributor (7), and Melenovsky et al. in their study have shown that while cavity size is normal, total heart volume is markedly enlarged in HFpEF (due to wall thickening and bi-atrial and right-sided enlargement), creating the substrate for enhanced restraining effects (33). Finally, pulmonary hypertension is extremely common in HFpEF (39), and many elderly patients with dyspnea and pulmonary hypertension on echo are eventually found to in fact have HFpEF (40). Increasing pulmonary artery pressures potently increase mortality in patients with HFpEF (39), and agents targeting pulmonary vascular function may be useful in the future.

ROLE OF SPECIFIC AGENTS
Angiotensin Receptor Antagonists and Converting Enzyme Inhibitors

The candesartan in heart failure-assessment of reduction in mortality (CHARM) trial was the first clinical trial published to date of a therapy for HFpEF, randomizing over 3000 subjects with NYHA class II–IV symptoms and EF >40% to candesartan or placebo (4). Over a median follow-up of three years, there was a nonsignificant 11% reduction in death or heart failure admission, driven exclusively by reduction in the latter. However, the population studied (male predominance, one-third with mild systolic dysfunction by EF, half with HF due to coronary disease) differed from the typical patient with HFpEF seen in most population-based studies (elderly, hypertensive women with absent or mild coronary disease, typically with EF >65%). Little and colleagues have shown in a number of elegant studies that losartan improves exercise capacity in association with a blunting of the hypertensive response to exercise, even in comparison with other antihypertensive that have similar effects on blood pressure (17,18). This is speculated to be related to attenuation of afterload-exacerbated diastolic dysfunction as discussed earlier. The valsartan in diastolic dysfunction (VALIDD) trial randomized 384 patients with hypertension and diastolic dysfunction to aggressive antihypertensive therapy based on valsartan or placebo (20). The investigators found that blood pressure reduction *per se* was associated with an improvement in diastolic relaxation velocity, but there was no difference between angiotensin antagonist-based therapy and placebo. This study population did not have HFpEF, and angiotensin blockers may have alternative effects independent of diastole. The irbesartan in heart failure with preserved systolic function (I-PRESERVE) trial of irbesartan for HFpEF is the largest trial to date in this population, showing no evidence of benefit from angiotensin antagonists overall or within any of the prespecified subgroups (41).

In contrast to the panoply of trial data regarding converting enzyme inhibitor in SHF, there is surprisingly little data available on HFpEF. In an early study, patients with prior myocardial infarction, HF, and EF >50% treated with enalapril derived improved functional status, exercise capacity, EF, ventricular mass, and diastolic filling (42). The perindopril in elderly people with chronic heart failure (PEP-CHF) trial randomized elderly patients with HFpEF to perindopril or placebo (5). Enrollment and event rates were lower than expected, reducing statistical power, and there was considerable crossover to open label perindopril therapy during the study. There was no reduction in the endpoint of death or HF admission at two years of follow-up, although there was a trend (p = 0.055) toward a reduction in the primary endpoint at one year, along with reduced HF hospitalizations, improved 6-minute walk distances and functional class, suggesting a benefit of this class of drugs in HFpEF.

Beta-Adrenergic Antagonists

Beta-blockers are frequently prescribed based on the premise that slowing the heart rate will allow more time for diastolic filling, improving preload volume and limiting pulmonary venous hypertension. While reducing the heart rate to less than 60–80 beats per minute does indeed increase the diastolic time period, this usually does not improve cardiac filling, because only diastasis (when transmitral flow is absent) is lengthened (43). Beta-blockers prolong relaxation, increase afterload and wave reflections, and can exacerbate chronotropic incompetence—all commonly seen and potentially problematic in HFpEF (22). Nonetheless, it is well known that beta blockers are effective *chronically* in SHF despite these negative acute effects (3) and the role of beta blockers in HFpEF remains controversial, with little trial data available. The SENIORS study randomized elderly patients with HF to the beta blocker nebivolol or placebo and found a 14% reduction in death or cardiovascular hospitalization with nebivolol (44). However, few patients had an EF >50%, and an echocardiographic substudy showed that the improvements in ventricular function and remodeling were confined to the group with systolic dysfunction (45).

Nitrates and Diuretics

Nitric oxide stimulates intracellular production of cyclic guanosine monophosphate, enhancing the rate of relaxation and improving diastolic compliance through phosphorylation of calcium handling and contractile proteins (6). Nitrates reduce afterload and potently reduce wave reflections (46), which may diminish afterload-induced diastolic dysfunction (19). Nitrate venodilation reduces central blood volume, moving the ventricle to lower operating volumes and a more compliant portion of the pressure–volume relationship (Fig. 22.3). Acute reductions in filling of the right heart with nitrates may decrease the amount of extrinsic pericardial restraining effects on left-sided filling, decreasing left heart pressures, and paradoxically increasing cardiac output (38,47). Diuretics have similar effects by decreasing circulating blood volume, affording relief of both pulmonary and systemic congestion. Caution must be used with both nitrates and diuretics because HFpEF patients tend to have more exaggerated changes in blood pressure and flow due to combined ventriculoarterial stiffening as described earlier (7,13). A recent small randomized trial (n = 44) testing the phophodiesterase 5 inhibitor sildenafil in HFpEF reported significant improvements in pulmonary artery pressures, resistance, cardiac filling pressures, quality of life, and measures of gas exchange (48).

Mineralocorticoid Antagonists

In addition to promoting volume retention, aldosterone is a potent pro-fibrotic hormone (49), suggesting that aldosterone antagonists may improve diastolic compliance in HFpEF (6). Ventricular hypertrophy is a key contributor to systolic and diastolic stiffening (6), and spironolactone is very effective for inducing hypertrophy regression (50). Aldosterone receptor blockade improves diastolic function in hypertensives (51), and the large NIH-sponsored TOPCAT study is currently underway to further evaluate the efficacy of spironolactone in HFpEF.

Calcium Channel Antagonists

Verapamil improves diastolic filling rates and exercise capacity in small studies of elderly subjects with systolic hypertension (16), hypertrophic cardiomyopathy (52) and HFpEF (53). Part of this effect may be related to acute reduction of ventriculoarterial stiffening (16) or changes in diastolic ventricular filling rates (52,53). However, as with beta-blockers, there may be exacerbation of chronotropic incompetence (22,23), and calcium channel blockers enhance filling rates at the cost of an acute increase in diastolic filling pressures and prolongation of relaxation (54).

Other Agents

Ancillary analysis from subjects with EF >45% from the Digitalis Investigation Group trial, known as DIG trial, showed that digoxin was associated with a trend toward reduction in HF hospitalizations over three years, but there was also a trend toward increased admissions for unstable angina (55). Overall, there was no effect on mortality or cardiovascular hospitalizations. Fukuta et al. followed a group of 137 patients with HFpEF over a median of 21 months and found a lower mortality in the group treated chronically with statins (56). Atrial systole may play an important role in maintaining normal ventricular filling volume and pressure in patients with HFpEF. Atrial fibrillation is extremely common in this disease, and restoration of sinus rhythm with antiarrhythmic drugs or ablative strategies may be useful, although this has not been studied specifically in HFpEF.

Nonpharmacologic Measures

Exercise training improves aerobic capacity in patients with SHF (57), and has been shown to attenuate age-related diastolic dysfunction in animal models (58). Vascular stiffening may be mitigated by exercise training, though diastolic properties seem to remain unchanged (59). Myocardial ischemia causes acute diastolic dysfunction (6), leading to the recommendation to strongly consider revascularization in such patients (3), although episodes of acute pulmonary edema tend to recur (60). Diabetes mellitus is associated with hypertrophic remodeling (61), ventriculoarterial stiffening (61), and diastolic dysfunction (62), suggesting that glucose control may be important. Obesity is a risk factor for HFpEF (63), and weight reduction should be recommended to appropriate patients. Just as in SHF, anemia is common in HFpEF and predicts increased mortality (64), although it again remains unknown whether direct treatment will affect outcome. Finally, sleep-disordered breathing is frequently seen in HFpEF, and worsening apnea–hypopnea indices are associated with more severe diastolic dysfunction (65), so early detection and treatment for sleep disordered breathing is likely of benefit in HFpEF.

FUTURE DIRECTIONS

Concentric chamber remodeling is a central component in HFpEF and is associated with systolic and diastolic dysfunction, so therapies directly targeting hypertrophy are appealing (6). ACE inhibitors, angiotensin antagonists, and aldosterone inhibitors have all been shown to be effective (50), but new drugs such as phosphodiesterase 5 and rho-kinase inhibitors that directly target hypertrophic signaling rather than hemodynamics may prove additionally useful (6). The PDE5 inhibitor sildenafil, which also targets ventriculoarterial stiffening and the pulmonary vasculature, is currently being tested as a treatment for HFpEF in the NIH-sponsored PhosphdiesteRasE-5 Inhibition to Improve CLinical Status and EXercise Capacity in Diastolic Heart Failure (RELAX) Trial. Novel agents targeting the quality or quantity of extracellular proteins, such as matrix metalloproteinases and advanced glycation endproduct breakers show promise (66,67), and a human HFpEF trial is of this agent is nearing completion. Some studies have demonstrated that a large part of the increase in diastolic stiffness of the myocyte is related to changes in the isoform and/or phosphorylation status of the sarcomeric macromolecule titin, thus novel small-molecule inhibitors or activators might be engineered to affect myocyte stiffness directly (6). The role of heart rate remains unresolved, with some studies showing that chronotropic incompetence is strongly associated with more severe exercise disability (22,23), while conventional wisdom states that heart rate should be slowed. The restoration of chronotropic competence in heart failure patients with normal ejection fraction (RESET) study trial was designed to test the effects of rate adaptive pacing in patients with HFpEF and chronotropic incompetence, but the study was prematurely discontinued by the sponsor because of slow enrollment. Mechanical systolic and diastolic dyssynchrony is common in HFpEF, even with a narrow QRS complex (68), but it remains unknown whether resynchronization therapy will ever be applicable to these patients, or if this form of dyssynchrony can effectively be resynchronized. Cardiac reserve function with exercise is clearly abnormal in HFpEF, and agents that either restore normal cellular milieu, by altering redox status (69) and maladaptive signaling (70), or that improve energy supply by affecting ATP flux (25), may ultimately provide more focused therapies. Recent small studies of exercise training in HFpEF have shown improvements in exercise capacity and diastolic function, and larger scale studies are needed in this regard (71). Exercise training improves exercise capacity and diastolic function in patients with heart failure with preserved ejection fraction: results of the Ex-DHF pilot study (72).

RECOMMENDATIONS

In contrast to the abundance of rigorously tested and well-established therapies for SHF, treatment guidelines for HFpEF are currently limited to expert consensus opinion (3). Revascularization for patients with documented ischemia and restoration of sinus rhythm may be useful in selected cases. Blood pressure control is central, as hypertension is the dominant risk factor and promoter of HFpEF—associated with ventriculoarterial stiffening, hypertrophic remodeling, and diastolic/systolic dysfunction. Based upon the encouraging results from the CHARM-Preserved and PEP-CHF trials, angiotensin antagonist or converting enzyme inhibitor–based therapy is generally considered first line. Diuretics and nitrates help maintain euvolemia and allow the ventricle to operate at lower chamber volumes, while minimizing pericardial restraining effects, avoiding marked elevations in cardiac filling pressures and attendant symptoms of dyspnea. Additional antihypertensives such as calcium channel blockers or beta blockers are often prescribed, particularly when blood pressure is not adequately controlled on the latter agents, although caution must be exercised because of the commonly coexistence of chronotropic incompetence. Antihypertensive therapies and diuretics may lead to much more dramatic fluctuations in blood pressure in HFpEF due to ventriculoarterial stiffening (13), and just as in SHF, a close outpatient follow-up and individualized care are essential in the management of patients with HFpEF.

REFERENCES

1. Owan TE, Hodge DO, Herges RM, et al. Trends in prevalence and outcome of heart failure with preserved ejection fraction. N Engl J Med 2006; 355: 251–9.
2. Bhatia RS, Tu JV, Lee DS, et al. Outcome of heart failure with preserved ejection fraction in a population-based study. N Engl J Med 2006; 355: 260–9.
3. Hunt SA, Abraham WT, Chin MH, et al. ACC/AHA 2005 Guideline update for the diagnosis and management of chronic heart failure in the adult: a report of the American College of Cardiology/American Heart Association task force on practice guidelines (writing committee to update the 2001 guidelines for the evaluation and management of heart failure): developed in collaboration with the american college of chest physicians and the international society for heart and lung transplantation: endorsed by the heart rhythm society. Circulation 2005; 112: e154–235.
4. Yusuf S, Pfeffer MA, Swedberg K, et al. Effects of candesartan in patients with chronic heart failure and preserved left-ventricular ejection fraction: the CHARM-Preserved trial. Lancet 2003; 362: 777–81.
5. Cleland JG, Tendera M, Adamus J, et al. The perindopril in elderly people with chronic heart failure (PEP-CHF) study. Eur Heart J 2006; 27: 2338–45.
6. Borlaug BA, Kass DA. Mechanisms of diastolic dysfunction in heart failure. Trends Cardiovasc Med 2006; 16: 273–9.
7. Kawaguchi M, Hay I, Fetics B, Kass DA. Combined ventricular systolic and arterial stiffening in patients with heart failure and preserved ejection fraction: implications for systolic and diastolic reserve limitations. Circulation 2003; 107: 714–20.
8. Zile MR, Baicu CF, Gaasch WH. Diastolic heart failure–abnormalities in active relaxation and passive stiffness of the left ventricle. N Engl J Med 2004; 350: 1953–9.
9. Lam CS, Roger VL, Rodeheffer RJ, et al. Cardiac structure and ventricular-vascular function in persons with heart failure and preserved ejection fraction from Olmsted County, Minnesota. Circulation 2007; 115: 1982–90.
10. Avolio AP, Chen SG, Wang RP, et al. Effects of aging on changing arterial compliance and left ventricular load in a northern Chinese urban community. Circulation 1983; 68: 50–8.
11. Chen CH, Nakayama M, Nevo E, et al. Coupled systolic-ventricular and vascular stiffening with age: implications for pressure regulation and cardiac reserve in the elderly. J Am Coll Cardiol 1998; 32: 1221–7.
12. Redfield MM, Jacobsen SJ, Borlaug BA, Rodeheffer RJ, Kass DA. Age- and gender-related ventricular-vascular stiffening: a community-based study. Circulation 2005; 112: 2254–62.
13. Borlaug BA, Kass DA. Ventricular-vascular interaction in heart failure. Heart Fail Clin 2008; 4: 23–36.
14. Klapholz M, Maurer M, Lowe AM, et al. Hospitalization for heart failure in the presence of a normal left ventricular ejection fraction: results of the New York Heart Failure Registry. J Am Coll Cardiol 2004; 43: 1432–8.
15. Hundley WG, Kitzman DW, Morgan TM, et al. Cardiac cycle-dependent changes in aortic area and distensibility are reduced in older patients with isolated diastolic heart failure and correlate with exercise intolerance. J Am Coll Cardiol 2001; 38: 796–802.
16. Chen CH, Nakayama M, Talbot M, et al. Verapamil acutely reduces ventricular-vascular stiffening and improves aerobic exercise performance in elderly individuals. J Am Coll Cardiol 1999; 33: 1602–9.
17. Warner JG Jr, Metzger DC, Kitzman DW, Wesley DJ, Little WC. Losartan improves exercise tolerance in patients with diastolic dysfunction and a hypertensive response to exercise. J Am Coll Cardiol 1999; 33: 1567–72.
18. Little WC, Zile MR, Klein A, et al. Effect of losartan and hydrochlorothiazide on exercise tolerance in exertional hypertension and left ventricular diastolic dysfunction. Am J Cardiol 2006; 98: 383–5.
19. Borlaug BA, Melenovsky V, Redfield MM, et al. Impact of arterial load and loading sequence on left ventricular tissue velocities in humans. J Am Coll Cardiol 2007; 50: 1570–7.
20. Solomon SD, Janardhanan R, Verma A, et al. Effect of angiotensin receptor blockade and antihypertensive drugs on diastolic function in patients with hypertension and diastolic dysfunction: a randomised trial. Lancet 2007; 369: 2079–87.
21. Kitzman DW, Higginbotham MB, Cobb FR, Sheikh KH, Sullivan MJ. Exercise intolerance in patients with heart failure and preserved left ventricular systolic function: failure of the Frank-Starling mechanism. J Am Coll Cardiol 1991; 17: 1065–72.

22. Borlaug BA, Melenovsky V, Russell SD, et al. Impaired chronotropic and vasodilator reserves limit exercise capacity in patients with heart failure and a preserved ejection fraction. Circulation 2006; 114: 2138–47.

23. Brubaker PH, Joo KC, Stewart KP, et al. Chronotropic incompetence and its contribution to exercise intolerance in older heart failure patients. J Cardiopulm Rehabil 2006; 26: 86–9.

24. Borlaug BA, Olson TP, Lam CSP, et al. Global cardiovascular reserve dysfunction in heart failure with preserved ejection fraction. J Am Coll Cardiol 2010; 56: 845–54.

25. Smith CS, Bottomley PA, Schulman SP, Gerstenblith G, Weiss RG. Altered creatine kinase adenosine triphosphate kinetics in failing hypertrophied human myocardium. Circulation 2006; 114: 1151–8.

26. Yip G, Wang M, Zhang Y, et al. Left ventricular long axis function in diastolic heart failure is reduced in both diastole and systole: time for a redefinition? Heart 2002; 87: 121–5.

27. Yu CM, Lin H, Yang H, et al. Progression of systolic abnormalities in patients with "isolated" diastolic heart failure and diastolic dysfunction. Circulation 2002; 105: 1195–201.

28. Brucks S, Little WC, Chao T, et al. Contribution of left ventricular diastolic dysfunction to heart failure regardless of ejection fraction. Am J Cardiol 2005; 95: 603–6.

29. Wang J, Khoury DS, Yue Y, Torre-Amione G, Nagueh SF. Preserved left ventricular twist and circumferential deformation, but depressed longitudinal and radial deformation in patients with diastolic heart failure. Eur Heart J 2008; 29: 1283–9.

30. Aurigemma GP, Zile MR, Gaasch WH. Contractile behavior of the left ventricle in diastolic heart failure: with emphasis on regional systolic function. Circulation 2006; 113: 296–304.

31. Aurigemma GP, Silver KH, Priest MA, Gaasch WH. Geometric changes allow normal ejection fraction despite depressed myocardial shortening in hypertensive left ventricular hypertrophy. J Am Coll Cardiol 1995; 26: 195–202.

32. Baicu CF, Zile MR, Aurigemma GP, Gaasch WH. Left ventricular systolic performance, function, and contractility in patients with diastolic heart failure. Circulation 2005; 111: 2306–12.

33. Melenovsky V, Borlaug BA, Rosen B, et al. Cardiovascular features of heart failure with preserved ejection fraction versus nonfailing hypertensive left ventricular hypertrophy in the urban Baltimore community: the role of atrial remodeling/dysfunction. J Am Coll Cardiol 2007; 49: 198–207.

34. Vinch CS, Aurigemma GP, Simon HU, et al. Analysis of left ventricular systolic function using midwall mechanics in patients >60 years of age with hypertensive heart disease and heart failure. Am J Cardiol 2005; 96: 1299–303.

35. Borlaug BA, Lam CSP, Roger VL, Rodeheffer RJ, Redfield MM. Contractility and ventricular systolic stiffening in hypertensive heart disease: insights in the pathogenesis of heart failure with preserved ejection fraction. J Am Coll Cardiol 2009; 54: 410–8.

36. Maurer MS, Burkhoff D, Fried LP, et al. Ventricular structure and function in hypertensive participants with heart failure and a normal ejection fraction: the Cardiovascular Health Study. J Am Coll Cardiol 2007; 49: 972–81.

37. Maurer MS, King DL, El-Khoury Rumbarger L, Packer M, Burkhoff D. Left heart failure with a normal ejection fraction: identification of different pathophysiologic mechanisms. J Card Fail 2005; 11: 177–87.

38. Dauterman K, Pak PH, Maughan WL, et al. Contribution of external forces to left ventricular diastolic pressure. Implications for the clinical use of the Starling law. Ann Intern Med 1995; 122: 737–42.

39. Lam CS, Roger VL, Rodeheffer RJ, et al. Pulmonary hypertension in heart failure with preserved ejection fraction: a community-based study. J Am Coll Cardiol 2009; 53: 1119–26.

40. Shapiro BP, McGoon MD, Redfield MM. Unexplained pulmonary hypertension in elderly patients. Chest 2007; 131: 94–100.

41. Massie BM, Carson PE, McMurray JJ, et al. I-PRESERVE Investigators. Irbesartan in patients with heart failure and preserved ejection fraction. N Engl J Med 2008; 359: 2456–67.

42. Aronow WS, Kronzon I. Effect of enalapril on congestive heart failure treated with diuretics in elderly patients with prior myocardial infarction and normal left ventricular ejection fraction. Am J Cardiol 1993; 71: 602–4.

43. Little WC, Brucks S. Therapy for diastolic heart failure. Prog Cardiovasc Dis 2005; 47: 380–8.

44. Flather MD, Shibata MC, Coats AJ, et al. Randomized trial to determine the effect of nebivolol on mortality and cardiovascular hospital admission in elderly patients with heart failure (SENIORS). Eur Heart J 2005; 26: 215–25.

45. Ghio S, Magrini G, Serio A, et al. Effects of nebivolol in elderly heart failure patients with or without systolic left ventricular dysfunction: results of the SENIORS echocardiographic substudy. Eur Heart J 2006; 27: 562–8.

46. Nichols WW, O'Rourke MF. McDonald's Blood Flow in Arteries, 3rd edn. Philadelphia, London: Lea and Febiger, 1990.

47. Frenneaux M, Williams L. Ventricular-arterial and ventricular-ventricular interactions and their relevance to diastolic filling. Prog Cardiovasc Dis 2007; 49: 252–62.
48. Guazzi M, Vicenzi M, Arena R, Guazzi MD. Pulmonary hypertension in heart failure with preserved ejection fraction: a target of phosphodiesterase-5 inhibition in a 1-year study. Circulation 2011; 124: 164–74.
49. Weber KT. Aldosterone in congestive heart failure. N Engl J Med 2001; 345: 1689–97.
50. Pitt B, Reichek N, Willenbrock R, et al. Effects of eplerenone, enalapril, and eplerenone/enalapril in patients with essential hypertension and left ventricular hypertrophy: the 4E-left ventricular hypertrophy study. Circulation 2003; 108: 1831–8.
51. Grandi AM, Imperiale D, Santillo R, et al. Aldosterone antagonist improves diastolic function in essential hypertension. Hypertension 2002; 40: 647–52.
52. Bonow RO, Dilsizian V, Rosing DR, et al. Verapamil-induced improvement in left ventricular diastolic filling and increased exercise tolerance in patients with hypertrophic cardiomyopathy: short- and long-term effects. Circulation 1985; 72: 853–64.
53. Setaro JF, Zaret BL, Schulman DS, Black HR, Soufer R. Usefulness of verapamil for congestive heart failure associated with abnormal left ventricular diastolic filling and normal left ventricular systolic performance. Am J Cardiol 1990; 66: 981–6.
54. Nishimura RA, Schwartz RS, Holmes DR, Jr., Tajik AJ. Failure of calcium channel blockers to improve ventricular relaxation in humans. J Am Coll Cardiol 1993; 21: 182–8.
55. Ahmed A, Rich MW, Fleg JL, et al. Effects of digoxin on morbidity and mortality in diastolic heart failure: the ancillary digitalis investigation group trial. Circulation 2006; 114: 397–403.
56. Fukuta H, Sane DC, Brucks S, Little WC. Statin therapy may be associated with lower mortality in patients with diastolic heart failure: a preliminary report. Circulation 2005; 112: 357–63.
57. Coats AJ, Adamopoulos S, Meyer TE, Conway J, Sleight P. Effects of physical training in chronic heart failure. Lancet 1990; 335: 63–6.
58. Brenner DA, Apstein CS, Saupe KW. Exercise training attenuates age-associated diastolic dysfunction in rats. Circulation 2001; 104: 221–6.
59. Gates PE, Tanaka H, Graves J, Seals DR. Left ventricular structure and diastolic function with human ageing. Relation to habitual exercise and arterial stiffness. Eur Heart J 2003; 24: 2213–20.
60. Kramer K, Kirkman P, Kitzman D, Little WC. Flash pulmonary edema: association with hypertension and reoccurrence despite coronary revascularization. Am Heart J 2000; 140: 451–5.
61. Devereux RB, Roman MJ, Paranicas M, et al. Impact of diabetes on cardiac structure and function: the strong heart study. Circulation 2000; 101: 2271–6.
62. Liu JE, Palmieri V, Roman MJ, et al. The impact of diabetes on left ventricular filling pattern in normotensive and hypertensive adults: the Strong Heart Study. J Am Coll Cardiol 2001; 37: 1943–9.
63. Kenchaiah S, Evans JC, Levy D, et al. Obesity and the risk of heart failure. N Engl J Med 2002; 347: 305–13.
64. Brucks S, Little WC, Chao T, et al. Relation of anemia to diastolic heart failure and the effect on outcome. Am J Cardiol 2004; 93: 1055–7.
65. Fung JW, Li TS, Choy DK, et al. Severe obstructive sleep apnea is associated with left ventricular diastolic dysfunction. Chest 2002; 121: 422–9.
66. Martos R, Baugh J, Ledwidge M, et al. Diastolic heart failure: evidence of increased myocardial collagen turnover linked to diastolic dysfunction. Circulation 2007; 115: 888–95.
67. Little WC, Zile MR, Kitzman DW, et al. The effect of alagebrium chloride (ALT-711), a novel glucose cross-link breaker, in the treatment of elderly patients with diastolic heart failure. J Card Fail 2005; 11: 191–5.
68. Nagueh SF. Mechanical dyssynchrony in congestive heart failure: diagnostic and therapeutic implications. J Am Coll Cardiol 2008; 51: 18–22.
69. Moens AL, Takimoto E, Tocchetti CG, et al. Reversal of cardiac hypertrophy and fibrosis from pressure overload by tetrahydrobiopterin: efficacy of recoupling nitric oxide synthase as a therapeutic strategy. Circulation 2008; 117: 2626–36.
70. Takimoto E, Champion HC, Li M, et al. Chronic inhibition of cyclic GMP phosphodiesterase 5A prevents and reverses cardiac hypertrophy. Nat Med 2005; 11: 214–22.
71. Kitzman DW, Brubaker PH, Morgan TM, Stewart KP, Little WC. Exercise training in older patients with heart failure and preserved ejection fraction: a randomized, controlled, single-blind trial. Circ Heart Fail 2010; 3: 659–67.
72. Edelmann F, Gelbrich G, Düngen HD, et al. Exercise training in Diastolic Heart Failure. J Am Coll Cardiol 2011; 58: 1780–91.

23

Cardiac resynchronization therapy

William T. Abraham

INTRODUCTION

Electrophysiological disturbances are common in the setting of chronic left ventricular dysfunction with or without heart failure. Approximately one-third of patients with systolic heart failure have a QRS duration greater than 120 msec, which is most commonly manifested as left bundle branch block (1,2). Such electrical disturbances result in left ventricular (i.e., *intra*ventricular) dyssynchrony with paradoxical septal wall motion, which further impairs the pumping ability of an already struggling heart (3–6). In particular, left ventricular dyssynchrony causes suboptimal ventricular filling, a prolonged duration of mitral regurgitation, and a reduction in left ventricular dP/dt. *Inter*ventricular dyssynchrony also occurs in the setting of a bundle branch block, adversely affecting the timing of left and right ventricular ejection. Ventricular dyssynchrony, defined electrocardiographically by a prolonged QRS duration, has been associated with increased mortality in heart failure patients (7–10).

Despite equivocal results from early attempts to use right-sided, dual chamber pacing to treat advanced systolic heart failure (11–16), atrial-synchronized biventricular pacing has proved useful in the management of certain patients with chronic systolic heart failure and ventricular dyssynchrony. This form of pacing therapy is now referred to as cardiac resynchronization therapy. The development of cardiac resynchronization therapy for the treatment of heart failure has progressed rapidly over the past several years. Early studies provided proof of concept, supporting the benefit of biventricular pacing in heart failure, via mechanistic, short-term, and longer-term observational studies (5,6,17–25). Cazeau et al. (17) performed the first application of atrial-synchronized biventricular pacing by using four chamber pacing in a 54-year-old man with New York Heart Association (NYHA) class IV heart failure and significant conduction disturbances (QRS duration of 200 msec, PR interval of 200 msec, and an inter-atrial conduction interval of 90 msec). After placing standard transvenous pacing leads in the right atrium and right ventricle, the left atrium was paced by a lead placed in the coronary sinus, while the left ventricle was paced by an epicardial lead located on the left ventricular free wall. After six weeks of pacing, the patient experienced a marked improvement in his clinical status with a weight loss of 17 kg and a disappearance of peripheral edema. His functional class improved to NYHA class II.

Such favorable anecdotal experiences led to small studies evaluating the acute hemodynamic effects of biventricular pacing. Positive results were achieved in studies by Foster and colleagues (18) and Saxon and associates (5), who evaluated the effects of temporary epicardial, atrial-synchronized biventricular pacing in postoperative cardiac surgery patients with reduced left ventricular function. Overall, patients demonstrated acute improvements in cardiac hemodynamic performance. The consequences of the acute and longer-term effects of biventricular pacing in heart failure were evaluated soon after and were equally encouraging, with patients showing consistent, often sustained, improvement in exercise tolerance, NYHA functional class, and cardiac output (19–25).

The first randomized controlled trials designed to evaluate the effects of cardiac resynchronization therapy on quality of life, functional status, and exercise capacity were begun in 1998–1999 (26–35). These trials affirmed that cardiac resynchronization therapy was safe and clinically effective in heart failure patients. In addition, cardiac resynchronization therapy was shown to improve left ventricular size and function. Finally, randomized controlled trials were initiated, starting in 2000, to assess the effects of cardiac resynchronization therapy on morbidity and mortality (36–38). The first of these trials reported demonstrated improved morbidity as well as reduced mortality for patients with moderate-to-severe heart failure (37). This study showed that the addition of defibrillation therapies in conjunction with cardiac resynchronization further improved patient outcomes. Also, additional trials have been initiated and some have been completed in an effort to expand the indication for cardiac resynchronization therapy to populations of heart failure patients other than those originally studied.

The mechanisms of action and proven clinical benefits of cardiac resynchronization therapy are reviewed in this chapter. In addition, recommendations for patient selection based on the results of randomized controlled trials are made, to encourage the evidence-based application of cardiac resynchronization in heart failure patients. Finally, future directions in resynchronization therapy are discussed with a focus on studies in patients with asymptomatic/mildly symptomatic heart failure and in patients with echocardiographic but not electrocardiographic dyssynchrony.

MECHANISMS OF ACTION OF CARDIAC RESYNCHRONIZATION THERAPY

Early studies of biventricular pacing provided important insight into the mechanisms of action of cardiac resynchronization therapy through electrocardiographic and echocardiographic data. The hemodynamic improvement seen with cardiac resynchronization therapy is related to its ability to increase left ventricular filling time, decrease septal dyskinesis, and reduce mitral regurgitation or the deleterious effects of ventricular dyssynchrony in the failing heart. Over time, these effects of resynchronization therapy result in improvements in ventricular geometry and function, compatible with reverse remodeling of the heart. Other mechanisms, as yet undetermined, may contribute to the clinical benefits of cardiac resynchronization therapy.

Increased Left Ventricular Filling Time

In the presence of a long AV delay and/or an interventricular conduction delay (IVCD), left ventricular activation is delayed, but atrial activation is not. Hence, both early passive left ventricular filling and the atrial "kick" may occur simultaneously, resulting in deceased total transmitral blood flow and diminished preloading of the left ventricle (39). These events are often seen as a fusion of the E and A waves on Doppler echocardiogram of transmitral blood flow. With atrial-synchronized biventricular pacing, both ventricles are activated simultaneously; thus, the left ventricle is able to complete contraction and begin relaxation earlier, which increases the filling time. The effect of cardiac resynchronization can be seen by the return of normal E and A wave separation on Doppler echocardiogram of transmitral blood flow.

Decreased Septal Dyskinesis

Although left ventricular activation and contraction are delayed in the presence of an IVCD, septal activation and contraction are not. This timing mismatch results in septal dyskinesis or paradoxical septal wall motion, as the septum moves away from the left ventricular free wall during systole. This paradoxical septal wall motion impairs mitral valve function thereby increasing mitral regurgitation and reducing the septum's contribution to left ventricular stroke volume (40). With cardiac resynchronization therapy, the ventricles are activated simultaneously, thus improving the ventricular contraction pattern by allowing left ventricular ejection to occur prior to relaxation of the septum, resulting in decreased mitral regurgitation and increased left ventricular stroke volume (27).

Reduced Mitral Regurgitation

In the presence of a long PR interval and/or an IVCD, mitral valve closure may not be complete, since atrial contraction is not followed by a properly timed ventricular systole. If the time lag is long enough, a ventricular-atrial pressure gradient may develop and cause diastolic mitral regurgitation (41). By resynchronizing AV activation and contraction, normal mitral valve timing is restored and regurgitation is potentially reduced or eliminated. In addition, the improvement in left ventricular contraction pattern also serves to minimize the regurgitant flow across the mitral valve, as noted above. Serial evaluations in large numbers of heart failure patients with ventricular dyssynchrony have confirmed a marked reduction in mitral regurgitant flow following initiation of cardiac resynchronization therapy (31).

Left Ventricular Reverse Remodeling

Numerous small mechanistic studies and the results of randomized controlled trials suggest a beneficial effect of cardiac resynchronization therapy on ventricular remodeling. Left ventricular end-systolic and end-diastolic dimensions have been shown to decrease and ejection fraction to increase modestly during chronic resynchronization therapy. Yu and colleagues (42) evaluated 25 NYHA class III or IV heart failure patients with baseline ejection fractions <40% and QRS durations >140 msec treated with biventricular pacing therapy. Subjects were assessed serially during 3 months of pacing and after pacing had been withheld for four weeks. During cardiac resynchronization therapy, there was a progressive improvement in ventricular structure and function. At three months, significant improvements were noted in ejection fraction, dP/dt, myocardial performance index, and mitral regurgitation. Left ventricular end-diastolic and end-systolic volumes were significantly reduced from 205 ± 68 to 168 ± 67 mL and from 162 ± 54 to 122 ± 42 mL, respectively. However, withholding pacing resulted in a progressive but not immediate loss of effect (i.e., pathophysiological adverse remodeling again ensued resulting in increased ventricular volumes and a reduction in ejection fraction).

Such observations have since been made in studies of hundreds of heart failure patients. In the Multicenter InSync Randomized Clinical Evaluation (MIRACLE), serial Doppler echocardiograms were obtained at baseline, three, and six months in 323 optimally treated NYHA class III and IV heart failure patients (31). Cardiac resynchronization therapy for six months was associated with reduced end-diastolic and end-systolic volumes (both p < 0.001), reduced left ventricular masses (p < 0.01), increased ejection fractions (p < 0.001), reduced mitral regurgitant blood flows (p < 0.001), and improved myocardial performance indices (p < 0.001) as compared with control (Fig. 23.1).

MAJOR CLINICAL TRIALS OF CARDIAC RESYNCHRONIZATION THERAPY

A number of observational as well as randomized controlled trials have been completed and others are currently underway to evaluate the safety, efficacy, and long-term effects of cardiac resynchronization therapy in the heart failure population. The weight of evidence supporting the beneficial effects of cardiac resynchronization therapy for the treatment of

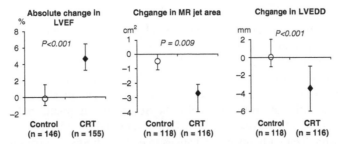

Figure 23.1 Effects of cardiac resynchronization therapy on measures of left ventricular structure and function. From left to right, paired median change from baseline at 6 months is shown for left ventricular ejection fraction (LVEF), mitral (MR) regurgitant jet area, and left ventricular end-diastolic dimension (LVEDD) determined echocardiographiclly. Baseline values for LVEF, MR jet area, and LVEDD were 22 ± 6%, 7.2 ± 4.9 cm², and 69 ± 10 mm, respectively, in the control group (open circles) and 22 ± 6%, 7.6 ± 6.4 cm², and 70 ± 10 mm, respectively, in the resynchronization group (solid diamonds). *Source*: From Ref. 31.

Table 23.1 Major Randomized Controlled Trials of Cardiac Resynchronization Therapy

Study (n random.)	NYHA	QRS	Sinus	ICD?
MIRACLE (524[a])	III, IV	≥130	Normal	No
MUSTIC SR 58	III	>150	Normal	No
MUSTIC AF (43)	III	>200[d]	AF	No
PATH CHF (42)	III, IV	≥120	Normal	No
CONTAK CD (581[c])	III–IV	≥120	Normal	Yes
MIRACLE ICD (362[b])	III-IV	≥130	Normal	Yes
PATH CHF II 89	III, IV	≥120	Normal	No
COMPANION 1520	III, IV	≥120	Normal	No
PACMAN 328	III	≥150	Normal	No
MIRACLE ICD II 186	II	≥130	Normal	Yes
VecToR 420	II–IV	≥140	Normal	No
CARE HF 813	III, IV	≥120[e]	Normal	No

LVEF ≤35% for all trials.
[a]Includes 71 patients enrolled in 3-month pilot study.
[b]Excludes class II patients.
[c]Includes 248 patients enrolled in a 3-month cross-over phase.
[d]RV paced QRS.
[e]Echo-based criteria for QRS <150 msec.
Abbreviations: AF, atrial fibrillation; ICD, implantable cardioverter-defibrillator; LVEF, left ventricular ejection fraction; NYHA, New York Heart Association.

heart failure is now quite substantial. To date, over 4000 patients have been evaluated in randomized single- or double-blinded controlled trials, and several hundred more patients have been assessed in uncontrolled or observational studies. Table 23.1 reviews the inclusion criteria and current status of completed and of some ongoing randomized controlled trials of cardiac resynchronization in heart failure. These studies include the Pacing Therapies in Congestive Heart Failure (PATH-CHF) trial (26–28), the Multisite Stimulation in Cardiomyopathy (MUSTIC) studies (29,34), the MIRACLE trial (31), MIRACLE ICD (35), the VENTAK CHF/CONTAK CD Trials (32), the Cardiac Resynchronization in Heart Failure (CARE HF) trial (38), and the Comparison of Medical Therapy, Pacing and Defibrillation in Heart Failure (COMPANION) trials (36,37).

PATH-CHF

The PATH-CHF study (26–28) was a single-blind, randomized, controlled cross-over trial designed to evaluate the effects of biventricular pacing on acute hemodynamic function and to assess any chronic clinical benefit in NYHA class III or IV heart failure patients with idiopathic or ischemic dilated cardiomyopathy. Primary endpoints were the effect of pacing on oxygen consumption at peak exercise and at anaerobic threshold during cardiopulmonary exercise testing and 6-minute hall walk. Secondary endpoints included changes in NYHA class, quality of life (assessed by the Minnesota Living with Heart Failure questionnaire), and hospitalization frequency. Changes in echocardiographic parameters, left ventricular ejection fraction (LVEF), cardiac output, and filling pattern were also assessed.

The PATH-CHF study consisted of four phases: (*i*) a preoperative patient evaluation phase, (*ii*) an intraoperative acute testing phase using a proprietary computer and software to guide the selection of an optimal AV delay and pacing site for the chronic pacing phase, (*iii*) a randomized cross-over protocol using two different pacing modes, each four weeks in duration with a four-week control phase in between, and (*iv*) a chronic pacing phase.

The study began in the summer of 1995 and enrolled 42 patients. An interim analysis assessing the differences in benefit between pacing and no pacing was performed in the spring of 1998, and the results were encouraging, with a trend toward improvement in all primary and secondary endpoints during pacing (28). However, the results were weakened by the small number of patients studied, the study's single-blind design, and the observation that functional endpoints did not return to baseline during the "pacing off" control or wash-out period.

MUSTIC

Begun in March 1998, the MUSTIC trial was designed to evaluate the safety and clinical efficacy of cardiac resynchronization in patients with severe heart failure of either an idiopathic or an ischemic origin (29,34). MUSTIC was really two studies. The first study involved 58 randomized patients with NYHA class III heart failure, normal sinus rhythm, and QRS duration of at least 150 msec. All patients were implanted with a device, and after a run-in period, patients were randomized in a single-blind fashion to receive either active pacing or to no pacing. After 12 weeks, patients were crossed-over and remained in the alternate study assignment for 12 weeks. After completing this second 12-week period, the device was programmed to the patient's preferred mode of therapy.

The second MUSTIC study involved few patients (only 37 completers) with atrial fibrillation and slow ventricular rates (either spontaneously or from radiofrequency ablation). A VVIR biventricular pacemaker and leads for each ventricle were implanted, and the same randomization procedure described above was applied. However, biventricular VVIR pacing versus single site right ventricular VVIR pacing, instead of no pacing, were compared in this group.

The primary endpoints for MUSTIC were exercise tolerance (assessed by measurement of peak VO_2 or the 6-minute hall walk test) and quality of life (assessed using the Minnesota Living with Heart Failure questionnaire). Secondary endpoints included rehospitalizations and/or drug therapy modifications for worsening heart failure. Results from the normal sinus rhythm arm of MUSTIC showed that during the active pacing phase, the mean distance walked in 6 minutes was 23% greater than that during the inactive pacing phase ($p < 0.001$) (29). Significant improvement was also seen in quality of life and NYHA class. Fewer hospitalizations occurred during active resynchronization therapy as well. Similar effects have been reported in the atrial fibrillation arm of MUSTIC (34), although the magnitude of benefit appeared to be somewhat less than that seen in patients in normal sinus rhythm.

MIRACLE

The early, positive results from observational studies and from single-blinded controlled trials led to the development of the MIRACLE trial (30). As the first prospective, randomized, double-blind, parallel-controlled clinical trial, MIRACLE was designed to validate the results from previous cardiac resynchronization studies and to further evaluate the therapeutic efficacy and identify mechanisms of potential benefit of cardiac resynchronization therapy. Primary endpoints were NYHA class, quality of life score (using the Minnesota Living with Heart Failure questionnaire), and 6-minute hall walk distance. Secondary endpoints included assessments of a composite clinical response, cardiopulmonary exercise performance, neurohormone and cytokine levels, QRS duration, cardiac structure and function, and a variety of measures of worsening the heart failure and combined morbidity and mortality.

The MIRACLE trial began in October 1998 and was completed late in 2000. Four hundred fifty-three patients with moderate to severe symptoms of heart failure associated with a LVEF <35% and a QRS duration >130 msec were randomized (double-blind) to either cardiac resynchronization (n = 228) or to a control group (n = 225) for six months, while conventional therapy for heart failure was maintained (31). Compared with the control group, patients randomized to cardiac resynchronization demonstrated a significant improvement in quality of life score (–18.0 vs. –9.0 points, p = 0.001), 6-minute walk distance (+39 vs. +10 m, p = 0.005), NYHA functional class ranking (–1.0 vs. 0.0 class, p < 0.001), treadmill exercise time (+81 vs. +19 sec, p = 0.001), peak VO_2 (+1.1 vs. 0.1 mL/kg/min, p < 0.01), and LVEF (+4.6% vs. –0.2%, p < 0.001). Cardiac resynchronization therapy patients demonstrated a highly significant improvement in the composite clinical heart failure response endpoint, as compared with control subjects, suggesting an overall improvement in the heart failure clinical status (Fig. 23.2). Further, fewer patients in the cardiac resynchronization group required hospitalization (8% vs. 15%) or intravenous medications (7% and 15%) for the treatment of worsening heart failure (both p < 0.05) when compared with the control group. This 50% reduction in hospitalization for the

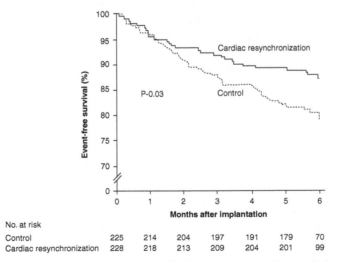

No. at risk

Control	225	214	204	197	191	179	70
Cardiac resynchronization	228	218	213	209	204	201	99

Figure 23.2 Effect of cardiac resynchronization on the composite endpoint of death or hospitalization for heart failure. Kaplan–Meier estimates of the time to death or hospitalization for worsening heart failure among patients randomized to the control group and those randomized to cardiac resynchronization. The risk of an event was 40% lower in the resynchronization group (95% CI, 4–63%; p = 0.03) *Source*: From Ref. 31.

cardiac resynchronization group was accompanied by a significant reduction in the length of stay, resulting in a 77% decrease in total days hospitalized over six months compared with the control group. Implantation of the device was successful in 92% of patients. The results of this trial led to the U.S. Food and Drug Administration approval of the InSync system in August 2001.

MIRACLE ICD

MIRACLE ICD was a prospective, multicenter, randomized, double-blind, parallel-controlled clinical trial intended to assess the safety and clinical efficacy of a combined implantable cardioverter-defibrillator (ICD) and cardiac resynchronization system in patients with dilated cardiomyopathy (LVEF ≤35%, LVEDD ≥55 mm), NYHA class III or IV heart failure (a cohort of class II patients was also enrolled), IVCD (QRS ≥130 msec), and an indication for an ICD. The MIRACLE ICD study was designed to be nearly identical to the MIRACLE trial. Primary and secondary efficacy measures were essentially the same as those evaluated in the MIRACLE trial, but measures of cardioverter-defibrillator function (including the efficacy of antitachycardia therapy with biventricular pacing) were also included.

Of 369 patients receiving devices and randomized, 182 were controls (cardioverter defibrillator activated, cardiac resynchronization OFF) and 187 were in the resynchronization group (cardioverter defibrillator activated, cardiac resynchronization ON) (35). At six months, patients assigned to cardiac resynchronization had a greater improvement in median quality of life score (–17.5 *vs.* –11.0, p = 0.02) and functional class (–1 *vs.* 0, p = 0.007) than controls, but were no different from controls in the change in distance walked in 6 minutes (55 m *vs.* 53 m, p = 0.36). Peak oxygen consumption increased by 1.1 mL/kg/min in the cardiac resynchronization group, versus 0.1 mL/kg/min in controls (p = 0.04), while treadmill exercise duration increased by 56 sec in the resynchronization group and decreased by 11 sec in controls (p = 0.0006). The magnitude of improvement was comparable to that seen in the MIRACLE trial (Figs. 23.3 and 23.4), suggesting that heart failure patients with an ICD indication benefit as much from cardiac resynchronization therapy as those patients without an indication for an ICD.

Of note in the MIRACLE ICD trial, the efficacy of biventricular antitachycardia pacing was significantly greater than that seen in right ventricular antitachycardia pacing. This observation suggests another potential benefit of an ICD combined with a resynchronization device in such patients. Finally, no pro-arrhythmia was observed and arrhythmia termination capabilities were not impaired by the addition of resynchronization therapy. This device was approved for use in NYHA class III and IV systolic heart failure patients with ventricular dyssynchrony and an ICD indication in June 2002.

CONTAK CD

The CONTAK CD trial enrolled 581 symptomatic heart failure patients with ventricular dyssynchrony and malignant ventricular tachyarrhythmias, who were all candidates for an ICD. Following unsuccessful implant attempts and withdrawals, 490 patients were available for analysis (32). The study did not meet its primary endpoint of a reduction in disease progression, defined by a composite endpoint of morbidity (heart failure hospitalization), mortality, and ventricular arrhythmia requiring defibrillator therapies, although the trends were in a direction favoring cardiac improved outcome with resynchronization therapy. However, the CONTAK CD trial did demonstrate statistically significant improvements in peak oxygen uptake and quality of life in the resynchronization group compared with control subjects, although quality of life was improved only in NYHA class III and IV patients without right bundle branch block. Left ventricular dimensions were also reduced, and

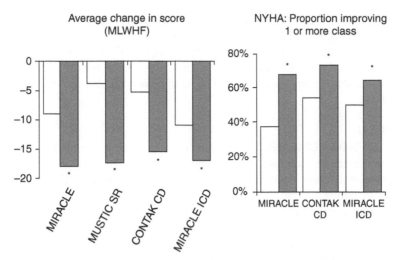

Figure 23.3 Effects of cardiac resynchronization therapy on quality of life and functional status. Left panel demonstrates the effect of resynchronization therapy on quality of life determined by the Minnesota Living with Heart Failure Questionnaire (MLWHF) while the right panel depicts the proportion of patients with an improvement in NYHA functional class ranking of at least one class. Data are taken from four independent randomized controlled trials of resynchronization therapy, as indicated in the figure. Improvements seen in patients actively treated with cardiac resynchronization (shaded bars) significantly exceed those observed in the control groups (white bars), with all p-values less than 0.05 as depicted by the asterisk. The consistency of effect is visible across the four studies.

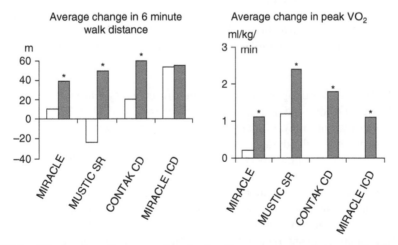

Figure 24.4 Effects of cardiac resynchronization therapy on exercise capacity. The effects of resynchronization therapy on the 6-minute hall walk distance and on peak oxygen consumption (VO$_2$) are shown on the right and left panels, respectively. Data are taken from four independent randomized controlled trials of resynchronization therapy, as indicated in the figure. Improvements seen in patients actively treated with cardiac resynchronization (shaded bars) significantly exceed those observed in the control groups (white bars), with all p-values less than 0.05 as depicted by the asterisk. As in Figure 24.3, the consistency of effect is visible across the four studies with the exception of the 6-minute hall walk finding observed in the case of MIRACLE ICD.

LVEFs increased, as seen in other trials of cardiac resynchronization therapy. Importantly, the improvement seen in peak VO_2 with cardiac resynchronization was again comparable to that observed in the MIRACLE trial. Improvements in NYHA functional class were not observed in this study. The CONTAK CD device was approved for use in NYHA class III and IV systolic heart failure patients with ventricular dyssynchrony and an ICD indication in May 2002.

COMPANION

Begun in early 2000, COMPANION was a multicenter, prospective, randomized, controlled clinical trial designed to compare drug therapy alone to drug therapy in combination with cardiac resynchronization in patients with dilated cardiomyopathy, an IVCD, NYHA class III or IV heart failure, and no indication for a device (36,37). COMPANION randomized 1520 patients into one of three treatment groups in a 1:2:2 allocation: Group 1 (308 patients) received optimal medical care only, Group II (617 patients) received optimal medical care and the Guidant CONTAK TR (biventricular pulse generator), and Group III (595 patients) received optimal medical care and the CONTAK CD (combined heart failure/bradycardia/tachycardia device). The primary endpoint of the COMPANION trial was a composite of all-cause mortality and all-cause hospitalization (measured as time to first event) beginning from time of randomization. Secondary endpoints included all-cause mortality and a variety of measures of cardiovascular morbidity. When compared with optimal medical therapy alone, the combined endpoint of mortality or heart failure hospitalization was reduced by 35% for patients receiving cardiac resynchronization therapy and 40% for patients receiving cardiac resynchronization plus defibrillator therapy (both p < 0.001). For the mortality endpoint alone, cardiac resynchronization therapy patients had a 24% risk reduction (p = 0.060) and cardiac resynchronization therapy plus defibrillator implanted patients experienced a risk reduction of 36% (p < 0.003), when compared with optimal medical therapy. COMPANION confirmed the results of earlier cardiac resynchronization therapy trials in improving symptoms, exercise tolerance, and quality of life for heart failure patients with ventricular dyssynchrony. In addition, COMPANION showed for the first time the impact of cardiac resynchronization plus defibrillator therapy in reducing all-cause mortality.

CARE HF

The CARE HF trial was designed to evaluate the effects of resynchronization therapy without an ICD on morbidity and mortality in patients with NYHA class III or IV heart failure and ventricular dyssynchrony. Eight hundred thirteen patients with LV ejection fractions of 35% or less and ventricular dyssynchrony defined as a QRS duration greater than or equal to 150 msec or a QRS duration between 120 msec and 150 msec with echocardiographic evidence of dyssynchrony were enrolled in this randomized, unblinded, controlled trial and followed for an average of 29.4 months (38). Four hundred four patients were assigned to receive optimal medical therapy alone and 409 patients were randomized to optimal medical therapy plus cardiac resynchronization therapy alone (i.e., without a combined defibrillator). The primary endpoint, risk of death from any cause or unplanned hospitalization for a major cardiac event, analyzed as time to first event, was significantly reduced by 37% in the treatment group compared with control subjects (hazard ratio, 0.63; 95% CI, 0.51–0.77; p < 0.001). In the resynchronization therapy group, 82 patients (20%) died during follow-up compared with 120 patients (30%) in the medical group, yielding a significant 36% reduction in all-cause mortality with resynchronization therapy (hazard ratio, 0.64; 95% CI, 0.48–0.85; p < 0.002). Resynchronization therapy also significantly reduced the risk of unplanned hospitalization for a major cardiac event by 39%, all-cause mortality plus heart failure hospitalization by 46%, and heart failure hospitalization by 52%.

LIMITATIONS OF CARDIAC RESYNCHRONIZATION THERAPY

The success rate for placement of a transvenous cardiac resynchronization system has ranged from about 88% to 92% in clinical trials. This means that 8–12% of patients undergoing an implant procedure will not attain a functioning system using this approach. Patients with failed implants must then settle for either another attempt at transvenous placement of the left ventricular lead or epicardial placement of the lead, or they must resign themselves to the absence of cardiac resynchronization therapy. Implant-related complications are similar to those seen with standard pacemaker and defibrillator technologies, with the additional risk of dissection or perforation of the coronary sinus during placement of the left ventricular lead. Although rare, this event may lead to substantial morbidity and even mortality in heart failure patients. Finally while many patients benefit from resynchronization therapy, about one-quarter to one-third of patients have no demonstrable benefit as measured in clinical trials. In such responders, the risk–benefit ratio for cardiac resynchronization is likely unfavorable. Unfortunately, there exist no reliable prospective predictors of responsiveness to resynchronization therapy at the present time.

CANDIDATES FOR CARDIAC RESYNCHRONIZATION THERAPY

The criteria for selecting patients for cardiac resynchronization therapy are primarily determined by the inclusion/exclusion criteria of the major randomized controlled trials, especially MIRACLE, MIRACLE ICD, CONTAK CD, COMPANION, and CARE-HF. The recommendations that follow are consistent with the 2009 update to the American College of Cardiology/American Heart Association clinical practice guideline for heart failure (43). Patients with chronic, moderate, or severe (NYHA class III-ambulatory class IV) heart failure despite optimal standard medical therapy, an LVEF ≤35%, left ventricular end diastolic diameter ≥55–0 mm, QRS duration ≥120 msec, and with or without an indication for an ICD should receive cardiac resynchronization therapy unless contraindicated.

It is worth emphasizing that ventricular dyssynchrony is currently defined by a prolonged QRS duration on a standard 12-lead electrocardiogram and not by the presence of mechanical dyssynchrony determined by an imaging study, such as an echocardiogram. While the use of mechanical dyssynchrony measures seems like an attractive alternative to the electrocardiogram, its value in predicting responsiveness to cardiac resynchronization has not been proven. To the contrary, the largest trial to date evaluating the predictive value of echocardiographic dyssynchrony demonstrated that imaging should not replace the electrocardiogram in selecting patients for resynchronization therapy (44). Thus, no patient meeting the guideline recommendation for cardiac resynchronization therapy should be denied therapy based on a negative echocardiographic dyssynchrony study.

FUTURE DIRECTIONS

Both completed and ongoing studies are evaluating various potential opportunities to benefit more patients with resynchronization therapy. Several studies have focused on patients with asymptomatic or mildly symptomatic (NYHA class I and II) heart failure. Following an encouraging pilot study in NYHA class II heart failure (45), the REsynchronization reVErses Remodeling in Systolic left vEntricular dysfunction (REVERSE) trial randomized 610 patients with NYHA functional class I or II heart failure with a QRS ≤120 msec and a LV ejection fraction ≤40% to active CRT (CRT-ON; n = 419) or an implanted control (CRT-OFF; n = 191) for 12 months. The primary endpoint was the heart failure clinical composite response, scoring patients as improved, unchanged, or worsened. The prospectively powered secondary endpoint was LV end-systolic volume index. Hospitalization for worsening heart failure was evaluated in a secondary endpoint. The heart failure clinical composite response endpoint, which compared only the percent worsened, indicated 16%

worsened in CRT-ON compared with 21% in CRT-OFF (p = 0.10). Patients assigned to CRT-ON experienced a greater improvement in LV end-systolic volume index (−18.4 ± 29.5 mL/m2 *vs.* −1.3 ± 23.4 mL/m2, p < 0.0001) and other measures of LV remodeling. Time-to-first heart failure hospitalization was significantly delayed in CRT-ON (hazard ratio: 0.47, p = 0.03). Thus, the REVERSE trial suggests that resynchronization therapy, in combination with optimal medical therapy, reduces the risk for heart failure hospitalization and improves ventricular structure and function in NYHA functional class I and II patients. Trials such as the MADIT CRT study are attempting to confirm these observations in larger groups of patients (47).

Another focus of ongoing resynchronization research attempts to expand the indication to patients with narrow QRS durations and mechanical dyssynchrony determined echocardiographically. Small studies performed to date have yielded mixed results (48). The ongoing Echocardiography-guided Cardiac Resynchronization Therapy (EchoCRT) trial should answer the question in a definitive way. Initiated in August 2008, EchoCRT will randomize more than 1250 patients with QRS durations <130 msec and echocardiographic evidence of dyssynchrony to resynchronization therapy or no therapy in a double-blind outcome study.

SUMMARY

Cardiac resynchronization therapy is an established therapeutic modality for patients with ventricular dyssynchrony and moderate-to-severe heart failure. Experience has shown it to be safe and effective, with patients demonstrating significant improvement in clinical symptoms, measures of functional status and exercise capacity, echocardiographic parameters, morbidity and mortality. Ongoing and future clinical trials should help to further define the ideal patient with systolic heart failure for cardiac resynchronization and may eventually expand the indication for resynchronization therapy to other patient subsets.

REFERENCES

1. Farwell D, Patel NR, Hall A, et al. How many people with heart failure are appropriate for biventricular resynchronization? Eur Heart J 2000; 21: 1246–50.
2. Aaronson KD, Schwartz JS, Chen TM, et al. Development and prospective validation of a clinical index to predict survival in ambulatory patients referred for cardiac transplant evaluation. Circulation 1997; 95: 2660–7.
3. Xiao HB, Brecker SJ, Gibson DG. Effects of abnormal activation on the time course of the left ventricular pressure pulse in dilated cardiomyopathy. Br Heart J 1992; 68: 403–7.
4. Littmann L, Symanski JD. Hemodynamic implications of left bundle branch block. J Electrocardiol 2000; 33(Suppl): 115–21.
5. Saxon LA, Kerwin WF, Cahalan MK, et al. Acute effects of intraoperative multisite ventricular pacing on left ventricular function and activation/contraction sequence in patients with depressed ventricular function. J Cardiovasc Electrophysiol 1998; 9: 13–21.
6. Kerwin WF, Botvinick EH, O'Connell JW, et al. Ventricular contraction abnormalities in dilated cardiomyopathy: effect of biventricular pacing to correct interventricular dyssynchrony. J Am Coll Cardiol 2000; 35: 1221–7.
7. Xaio HB, Roy C, Fujimoto S, et al. Natural history of abnormal conduction and its relation to prognosis in patients with dilated cardiomyopathy. Int J Cardiol 1996; 53: 163–70.
8. Unverferth DV, Magorien RD, Moeschberger ML, et al. Factors influencing the one-year mortality of dilated cardiomyopathy. Am J Cardiol 1984; 54: 147–52.
9. Shamim W, Francis DP, Yousufuddin M, et al. Intraventricular conduction delay: a prognostic marker in chronic heart failure. Int J Cardiol 1999; 70: 171–8.
10. Brophy JM, Deslauriers G, Rouleau JL. Long-term prognosis of patients presenting to the emergency room with decompensated congestive heart failure. Can J Cardiol 1994; 10: 543–7.
11. Hochleitner M, Hortnagl H, Ng CK, et al. Usefulness of physiologic dual-chamber pacing in drug-resistant idiopathic dilated cardiomyopathy. Am J Cardiol 1990; 66: 198–202.

12. Hochleitner M, Hortnagl H, Hortnagl H, et al. Long-term efficacy of physiologic dual-chamber pacing in the treatment of end-stage idiopathic dilated cardiomyopathy. Am J Cardiol 1992; 70: 1320–5.
13. Brecker SJ, Xiao HB, Sparrow J, et al. Effects of dual-chamber pacing with short atrioventricular delay in dilated cardiomyopathy. Lancet 1992; 340: 1308–12.
14. Innes D, Leitch JW, Fletcher PJ. VDD pacing at short atriventricular intervals does not improve cardiac output in patients with dilated heart failure. PACE 1994; 17: 959–65.
15. Linde C, Gadler F, Edner M, et al. Results of atrioventricular synchronous pacing with optimized delay in patients with severe congestive heart failure. Am J Cardiol 1995; 75: 919–23.
16. Gold MR, Feliciano Z, Gottlieb SS, Fisher ML. Dual-chamber pacing with a short atrioventricular delay in congestive heart failure: a randomized study. J Am Coll Cardiol 1995; 26: 967–73.
17. Cazeau S, Ritter P, Bakdach S, et al. Four chamber pacing in dilated cardiomyopathy. PACE 1994; 17: 1974–9.
18. Foster AH, Gold MR, McLaughlin JS. Acute hemodynamic effects of atrio-biventricular pacing in humans. Ann Thorac Surg 1995; 59: 294–300.
19. Bakker P, Meijburg H, de Vries J, et al. Biventricular pacing in end-stage heart failure improves functional capacity and left ventricular function. J Interv Card Electrophysiol 2000; 4: 395–404.
20. Cazeau S, Ritter P, Lazarus A, et al. Multisite pacing for end-stage heart failure: early experience. Pacing Clin Electrophysiol 1996; 19: 1748–57.
21. Blanc JJ, Etienne Y, Gilard M, et al. Evaluation of different ventricular pacing sites in patients with severe heart failure: results of an acute hemodynamic study. Circulation 1997; 96: 3273–7.
22. Leclercq C, Cazeau S, Le Breton H, et al. Acute hemodynamic effects of biventricular DDD pacing in patients with end-stage heart failure. J Am Coll Cardiol 1998; 32: 1825–31.
23. Kass DA, Chen CH, Curry C, et al. Improved left ventricular mechanics from acute VDD pacing in patients with dilated cardiomyopathy and ventricular conduction delay. Circulation 1999; 99: 1567–73.
24. Gras D, Mabo P, Tang T, et al. Multisite pacing as a supplemental treatment of congestive heart failure: preliminary results of the Medtronic Inc. InSync Study. Pacing Clin Electrophysiol 1998; 21: 2249–55.
25. Gras D, Leclercq C, Tang A, et al. Cardiac resynchronization therapy in advanced heart failure the multicenter InSync clinical study. Eur J Heart Fail 2002; 4: 311–20.
26. Auricchio A, Stellbrink C, Sack S, et al. The pacing therapies for congestive heart failure (path-chf) study: rationale, design, and endpoints of a prospective randomized multicenter study. Am J Cardiol 1999; 83: 130D–5D.
27. Auricchio A, Stellbrink C, Block M, et al.; For the Pacing Therapies for Congestive Heart Failure Study Group. Effect of pacing chamber and atrioventricular delay on acute systolic function of paced patients with congestive heart failure. Circulation 1999; 99: 2993–3001.
28. Auricchio A, Klein H, Spinelli J. Pacing for heart failure: selection of patients, techniques, and benefits. Eu J Heart Fail 1999; 1: 275–9.
29. Cazeau S, Leclercq C, Lavergne T, et al.; For the Multisite Stimulation in Cardiomyopathies (MUSTIC) Study Investigators. Effects of multisite biventricular pacing in patients with heart failure and intraventricular conduction delay. N Engl J Med 2001; 344: 873–880.
30. Abraham WT, On behalf of the Multicenter InSync Randomized Clinical Evaluation (MIRACLE) Investigators and Coordinators. Rationale and design of a randomized clinical trial to assess the safety and efficacy of cardiac resynchronization therapy in patients with advanced heart failure: the Multicenter InSync Randomized Clinical Evaluation (MIRACLE). J Card Fail 2000; 6: 369–80.
31. Abraham WT, Fisher WG, Smith AL, et al.; For the Multicenter InSync Randomized Clinical Evaluation (MIRACLE) Investigators and Coordinators. Double-blind, randomized controlled trial of cardiac resynchronization in chronic heart failure. N Engl J Med 2002; 346: 1845–53.
32. Higgins SL, Hummel JD, Niazi IK, et al. Cardiac resynchronization therapy for the treatment of heart failure in patients with intraventricular conduction delay and malignant ventricular tachyarrhythmias. J Am Coll Cardiol 2003; 42: 1454–9.
33. Linde C, Leclercq C, Rex S, et al.; On behalf of the MUltisite STimulation In Cardiomyopathies (MUSTIC) Study Group. Long-term benefits of biventricular pacing in congestive heart failure: results from the Multisite STimulation In Cardiomyopathy (MUSTIC) Study. J Am Coll Cardiol 2002; 40: 111–18.
34. Leclercq C, Walker S, Linde C, et al. Comparative effects of permanent biventricular and right-univentricular pacing in heart failure patients with chronic atrial fibrillation. Eur Heart J 2002; 23: 1780–7.
35. Young JB, Abraham WT, Smith AL, et al. Safety and efficacy of combined cardiac resynchronization therapy and implantable cardioversion defibrillation in patients with advanced chronic heart failure. The Multicenter InSync ICD Randomized Clinical Evaluation (MIRACLE ICD) trial. JAMA 2003; 289: 2685–94.

36. Bristow MR, Feldman AM, Saxon LA, For the COMPANION Steering Committee and COMPANION Clinical Investigators. Heart failure management using implantable devices for ventricular resynchronization: comparison of medical therapy, pacing, and defibrillation in chronic heart failure (COMPANION) trial. J Card Fail 2000; 6: 276–85.

37. Bristow MR, Saxon LA, Boehmer J, et al. Effect of cardiac resynchronization therapy with and without an implantable defibrillator on morbidity and mortality in advanced chronic heart failure: the COMPANION trial. N Engl J Med 2004; 43: 248–56.

38. Cleland JGF, Daubert J-C. Erdmann E, et al.; for the Cardiac Resynchronization — Heart Failure (CARE-HF) Study Investigators. The effect of cardiac resynchronization on morbidity and mortality in heart failure. N Engl J Med 2005; 352: 1539–49.

39. Nishimura RA, Hayes DL, Holmes DR Jr, et al. Mechanism of hemodynamic improvement by dual-chamber pacing for severe left ventricular dysfunction: an acute Doppler and catheterization hemodynamic study. J Am Coll Cardiol 1995; 25: 281–8.

40. Grines CL, Bashore TM, Boudoulas H, et al. Functional abnormalities in isolated left bundle branch block. The effect of interventricular asynchrony. Circulation 1989; 79: 845–53.

41. Panidis IP, Ross J, Munley B, et al. Diastolic mitral regurgitation in patients with atrioventricular conduction abnormalities: a common finding by Doppler echocardiography. J Am Coll Cardiol 1986; 7: 768–74.

42. Yu CM, Chau E, Sanderson JE, et al. Tissue doppler echocardiographic evidence of reverse remodeling and improved synchronicity by simultaneously delaying regional contraction after biventricular pacing therapy in heart failure. Circulation 2002; 105: 438–45.

43. Hunt SA, Abraham WT, Chin MH, et al. 2009 focused update incorporated into the ACC/AHA 2005 guidelines for the diagnosis and management of heart failure in adults: a report of the American College of Cardiology Foundation/American Heart Association Task Force on Practice Guidelines developed in collaboration with the International Society for Heart and Lung Transplantation. Circulation 2009; 119: e391–479.

44. Chung ES, Leon AR, Tavazzi L, et al. Results of the predictors of response to CRT (PROSPECT) trial. Circulation 2008; 117: 2608–16.

45. Abraham WT, Young JB, Leon AR, et al.; On behalf of the Multicenter InSync ICD II Study Group. Effects of cardiac resynchronization on disease progression in patients with left ventricular systolic dysfunction, an indication for an implantable cardioverter defibrillator, and mildly symptomatic chronic heart failure. Circulation 2004; 110: 2864–8.

46. Linde C, Abraham WT, Gold MR, REVERSE (REsynchronization reVErses Remodeling in Systolic left vEntricular dysfunction) Study Group. Randomized trial of cardiac resynchronization in mildly symptomatic heart failure patients and in asymptomatic patients with left ventricular dysfunction and previous heart failure symptoms. J Am Coll Cardiol 2008; 52: 1834–43.

47. Moss AJ, Brown MW, Cannom DS, et al. Multicenter Automatic Defibrillator Implantation Trial–Cardiac Resynchronization Therapy (MADIT-CRT): design and clinical protocol. Ann Noninvasive Electrocardiol 2005; 10(Suppl): 34–43.

48. Beshai JF, Grimm RA, Nagueh SF, et al.; RethinQ Study Investigators. Cardiac-resynchronization therapy in heart failure with narrow QRS complexes. N Engl J Med 2007; 357: 2461–71.

24

Management of atrial and ventricular arrhythmias in heart failure

Usha Tedrow and William G. Stevenson

In the heart failure patient population, cardiac arrhythmias frequently contribute to worsened symptoms, periodic decompensations, and increased mortality in the form of sudden death. Arrhythmia recognition and management is an important aspect of caring for these patients. Chronic heart failure predisposes to both supraventricular and ventricular arrhythmias. The etiologic diversity of patients with heart failure impacts on the incidence of arrhythmias and on diagnostic and therapeutic strategies. Arrhythmia prevention and management plans, taking into account the potential benefits and risks of implantable defibrillators, left ventricular pacing for cardiac resynchronization therapy, antiarrhythmic drugs, and ablation, often require careful integration with heart failure management.

ANTIARRHYTHMIC DRUGS

Antiarrhythmic drugs must be used cautiously with careful assessment of risks and benefits in patients with heart failure. The potential for drug toxicity is increased by diminished hepatic or renal excretion and drug interactions are common. In addition, depressed ventricular function is associated with a greater risk of drug-induced arrhythmia, such as polymorphic ventricular tachycardia (VT) (e.g., *torsade de pointes*) from drug-induced QT prolongation. Many drugs have negative inotropic effects that can aggravate heart failure.

Antiarrhythmic Effects of β-Adrenergic Blockers

β-adrenergic blockers are a first line therapy for many arrhythmias. These agents have antiarrhythmic effects and demonstrated efficacy for improving mortality and reducing sudden death in heart failure (1–3). β-adrenergic blockers can help control the ventricular response to atrial fibrillation and diminish symptoms of palpitations from supraventricular arrhythmias and premature ventricular contractions (4). Many ventricular arrhythmias are aggravated by sympathetic stimulation. β-adrenergic blockers are also effective in reducing many ventricular arrhythmias. In addition, sympathetic stimulation can blunt or reverse the electrophysiologic effects of amiodarone and other antiarrhythmic drugs. A combination of a β-adrenergic blocker with another antiarrhythmic drug can be useful. Aggravation of bradyarrhythmias is the major arrhythmia-related adverse effect.

Class I Sodium Channel Blocking Antiarrhythmic Drugs

The class I antiarrhythmic drugs are largely reserved for control of frequent symptomatic arrhythmias in patients who have an implantable defibrillator when amiodarone, dofetilide, or sotalol are less attractive options or ineffective. Class I sodium channel blocking drugs (mexiletine, tocainide, procainamide, quinidine, disopyramide, flecainide, and propafenone) have negative inotropic effects (with the possible exception of quinidine) (5,6). Blockade of sodium channels diminishes intracellular sodium and thereby may decrease intracellular calcium by its effect on the sodium calcium exchanger (the opposite effect of digitalis). Quinidine may lack negative inotropic effects because of vasodilation and QT interval prolongation, which allow additional time for calcium to enter during the plateau phase of the action potential, may offset the negative inotropic effects of the sodium channel blockade. In addition to a long-term risk of drug-induced systemic lupus erythematosis, procainamide is metabolized to N-acetylprocainamide (NAPA), which is a Class III antiarrhythmic drug that has QT prolonging effects of its own and accumulates in patients with renal insufficiency. Of note, procainamide is only currently available as an intravenous preparation in the United States.

Class I antiarrhythmic drugs also have a potential for proarrhythmia that is likely aggravated by the electrophysiologic changes of heart failure and hypertrophy (7,8). These adverse effects of Class I antiarrhythmic drugs likely explain the increases in mortality observed when these agents were administered to patients with prior myocardial infarction, to those with heart failure and atrial fibrillation, and to those who had been resuscitated from a cardiac arrest (2,7,9).

Amiodarone

Amiodarone is the major option for antiarrhythmic drug therapy in patients with heart failure, largely because it is a relatively safe from a cardiac standpoint (10–12). Amiodarone blocks cardiac sodium, potassium, and calcium currents and has sympatholytic effects. It has activity against both ventricular and supraventricular arrhythmias. Older trials and meta-analyses suggested mortality benefit, mainly limited to patients with concomitant β–blocker therapy. However, the randomized optimal medical therapy versus amiodarone portion of the Sudden Cardiac Death in Heart Failure Trial (SCD HeFT) showed no effect on mortality in patients with New York Heart Association Class II and III heart failure and ejection fraction <35% (10,11). In a subgroup analysis, those with the most severe heart failure (Class III) actually had worse outcomes when treated with amiodarone, while amiodarone did not have any effect in Class II heart failure (13). Noncardiac toxicities and drug-induced bradycardia are the major limitations (below).

Ventricular proarrhythmia is unusual. Amiodarone has been initiated in the outpatient setting without an increase in mortality (10,11,14). Bradyarrhythmias due to potent effects on the sinus and AV nodes are the major cardiac risk, occurring in 1–7% of patients in randomized trials, and in up to a third of patients in some case series (14,15).

In patients with compensated heart failure, amiodarone is well tolerated from a hemodynamic standpoint when administered at a loading dose of 600–800 mg daily for one to two weeks (10–12,15,16). In patients with advanced heart failure, administration of the loading dose and, in particular, large oral doses (e.g., >1200 mg daily) can exacerbate heart failure (17).

Noncardiac toxicities are a major problem. In randomized trials 41% of patients discontinue therapy by two years due to real or perceived side effects. The true incidence of side effects is lower, as indicated by the observation that placebo was discontinued in 27% of patients in these trials (14). However, it is often difficult to distinguish an amiodarone-induced side effect from symptoms of heart failure. Amiodarone-induced pulmonary toxicity occurs in approximately 1% of patients per year of therapy (18). Chronic therapy at doses exceeding 300 mg per day increases the risk. A chest radiograph should be obtained annually. Annual pulmonary function tests are recommended by some physicians, particularly for those patients taking a daily dose in excess of 300 mg.

A decrease in diffusing capacity can indicate development of pulmonary toxicity (19). When pulmonary toxicity is suspected, a right heart catheterization to assess the possibility of pulmonary vascular congestion, and a high-resolution chest computed tomography scan to assess interstitial fibrosis can be helpful in distinguishing pulmonary toxicity from heart failure (19,20).

Thyroid abnormalities occur in up to 18% of patients (21). Hypothyroidism is easily managed with thyroid replacement therapy and does not generally warrant discontinuation of amiodarone. Hyperthyroidism is a much more difficult problem, and can be refractory to management with antithyroid medications. Because the gland is saturated with iodine from the amiodarone, thyroid ablation with radioactive iodine is not possible. Discontinuation of the drug and medical therapy for hyperthyroidism in consultation with an endocrinologist is often required. Routine thyroid-stimulating hormone (TSH) assay every six months as well as an assessment of hepatic transaminases at those times for potential liver toxicity are reasonable.

Additionally, long-term use of amiodarone is associated with corneal and cutaneous deposits which are usually mainly cosmetic difficulties for the patient. In contrast, optic neuritis and peripheral neuropathy are also associated with use of amiodarone, and warrant discontinuation of the drug to prevent further neurologic deterioration.

Amiodarone increases the energy required for defibrillation and can render an implantable cardiac defibrillator (ICD) ineffective in some patients. It can also impair arrhythmia detection by slowing the rate of VT. These concerns warrant careful testing of ICD function and defibrillation after amiodarone therapy is initiated in patients with ICDs.

Dofetilide

Dofetilide is a Class III antiarrhythmic drug that is approved for therapy of atrial fibrillation. It blocks the repolarizing potassium current I_{Kr}, increasing action potential duration and the QT interval. Its major toxicity is proarrhythmia from *torsade de pointes*, which occurs in more than 3% of patients (22). It is primarily eliminated renally with a plasma half-life of 9.5 hours. It requires initiation with continuous electrocardiographic monitoring in-hospital for a minimum of 72 hours to detect the development of QT prolongation and *torsade de pointes*. It should not be administered to patients with significant renal insufficiency (creatinine clearance <20 mL/min). Taking these precautions and avoiding drug administration to patients with prolonged QT intervals, dofetilide can be administered safely to patients with heart failure. The Danish Investigations of Arrhythmia and Mortality on Dofetilide Study (DIAMOND) showed that, in patients with Class III–IV heart failure, during a median follow-up of 18 months, there was no difference in mortality between dofetilide-treated and placebo groups (22). Dofetilide-treated patients were less likely to be rehospitalized for exacerbation of heart failure (30% compared with 38%), possibly due to a reduction in atrial fibrillation.

Sotalol

Sotalol is a mixture of two stereoisomers. The *d* isomer has Class III effects similar to dofetilide, from blockade of the potassium current I_{Kr}. The *l* isomer is a potent nonselective β-adrenergic blocker. Sotalol has not been specifically evaluated in heart failure patients. In survivors of myocardial infarction who have depressed ventricular function, chronic therapy with the *d* isomer of sotalol increases mortality (23). Sotalol causes *torsade de pointes* with a similar incidence to that of dofetilide and can aggravate bradyarrhythmias and heart failure through its β-blocking effects. Therapy should be initiated in-hospital during continuous electrocardiographic monitoring. It also has a renal route of excretion and should be avoided in patients with renal insufficiency. Its antiarrhythmic efficacy for atrial fibrillation is less than that of amiodarone (24).

Dronedarone

Dronedarone is a relatively new antiarrhythmic drug with similar properties to amiodarone but the drug does not contain iodine. It was hoped this medication would retain the efficacy without typical amiodarone-associated toxicities. Earlier studies suggested increased mortality rates in heart failure patients (25). However, dronedarone diminishes renal creatinine excretion without diminishing glomerular filtration rate. Unfavorable changes in heart failure therapies may have been implemented based on dronedarone-induced increases in creatinine that did not actually indicate a deterioration in renal function. FDA approval in the United States includes a "black box" warning against use of dronedarone in patients with symptomatic heart failure. Dronedarone was then studied in atrial fibrillation and flutter (26). Patients with creatinine levels over 1.7 mg/dL and with NYHA class III or IV heart failure were excluded. Dronedarone appeared to decrease time to recurrence of atrial arrhythmia and seemed to improve rate control. Mortality was also improved although the trial was not powered to demonstrate a mortality benefit (hazard ratio, 0.73 p = 0.01). No evidence of thyroid or lung disease was seen as compared with placebo over the one-year follow-up. In January 2011, the FDA released reports of two patients who suffered significant hepatotoxicity thought related to the drug, and now monitoring of hepatic enzymes is recommended. In addition, the recent PALLAS (Permanent Atrial Fibrillation Outcome Study Using Dronedarone on top of Standard therapy) study which enrolled patients with permanent atrial fibrillation and no symptomatic heart failure was stopped early due to an increase in cardiovascular events including stroke, heart failure, cardiovascular death and arrhythmic death. Overall dronedarone is currently reserved for those with a structurally normal heart, few cardiovascular risk factors, who have failed standard therapies.

SUPRAVENTRICULAR TACHYCARDIAS

Atrial fibrillation and atrial flutter are the most common supraventricular arrhythmias encountered. Rarely, an incessant supraventricular tachycardia (SVT) from ectopic atrial tachycardia or atrioventricular re-entry from an accessory pathway causes a tachycardia-induced cardiomyopathy (27). Such SVTs typically have a rate greater than 120 beats per minute and despite depressed systolic function, marked ventricular dilation is often absent. Control of the arrhythmia can be followed by return of ventricular function to normal over weeks to several months. A persistently rapid response to atrial fibrillation can also cause a tachycardia-induced cardiomyopathy.

Atrial Fibrillation

The prevalence of atrial fibrillation increases with the severity of heart failure. Atrial fibrillation is found in 6% of patients with mild heart failure and more than 40% of patients with advanced heart failure (Fig. 24.1) (8,22,28–32). The potential adverse effects of atrial fibrillation include loss of A-V synchrony, rapid or slow ventricular rate responses that are no longer under optimal physiologic control, variable time for cardiac filling due to oscillations of R–R intervals and risk of thromboembolism (4,8,33–35). In some but not all studies, atrial fibrillation has been associated with increased mortality and more frequent hospitalizations (8,28,29,32,36).

Patients with atrial fibrillation and heart failure are at increased risk of stroke; anticoagulation with warfarin is warranted (37–39). Those who have had an episode of atrial fibrillation may experience asymptomatic episodes even when sinus rhythm is present on periodic examinations. During drug therapy or following ablation, despite apparent maintained sinus rhythm, patients appear to remain at risk for stroke. Therefore continued

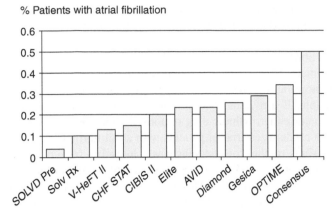

% Patients with atrial fibrillation

Figure 24.1   The incidence of atrial fibrillation in various heart failure and arrhythmia trials.

anticoagulation with warfarin is warranted, if not contraindicated by bleeding risks. Adequate control of heart rate is also extremely important.

Despite the potential adverse effects of atrial fibrillation, pharmacologic therapy to attempt to maintain sinus rhythm has not proven beneficial as compared with simple rate control and anticoagulation (4,40). Pharmacologic attempts to maintain sinus rhythm have been disappointing (41). The Atrial Fibrillation and Congestive Heart Failure Trial (AF-CHF) randomized 1376 patients with LV ejection fraction <0.35 (mean 0.27) and symptomatic heart failure (NYHA Class III or IV in 31% of patients) to rhythm control versus rate control strategy (41). Amiodarone was administered in 82% of the rhythm-control group during the first year, and over 80% of patients in the rhythm control group were in sinus rhythm during follow-up visits over the first two years. After a mean follow-up of 37 months cardiovascular mortality was similar in the two groups (27% *vs.* 25%) and there was no benefit in stroke (3% *vs.* 4%), or worsening heart failure (28% *vs.* 31%). The rhythm control group tended to be hospitalized more often (64% *vs.* 59%, p = 0.06) and have more bradyarrhythmias requiring hospitalization (6% *vs.* 3%, p = 0.02).

These findings are in concert with those of randomized trials in other patient populations. In the Atrial Fibrillation Follow-up Investigation of Rhythm Management (AFFIRM) trial most of the patients in AFFIRM had normal ejection fractions, 26% had low ejection fractions, and 939 (23%) had a history of congestive heart failure. Overall, there was a trend toward increased mortality for the strategy of administering antiarrhythmic drugs to attempt to maintain sinus rhythm (rhythm control group).

Rhythm Control with Medication

Although a routine strategy of antiarrhythmic drug therapy to maintain sinus rhythm can not be advocated with presently available agents, it should be recognized that patients who agree to randomization in these trials are willing to accept a rate control strategy and probably do not have substantial symptoms from their atrial fibrillation. In the congestive heart failure survival trial of antiarrhythmic therapy (CHF-STAT) trial, AFFIRM, and dofetilide trials, patients who maintained sinus rhythm had better outcomes as compared with those with persistent atrial fibrillation (22,30). Patients treated with dofetilide who achieved sinus rhythm had fewer hospitalizations for heart failure exacerbations (22). It remains unclear whether atrial fibrillation has adverse effects that increase mortality, or is simply a marker of more severe heart failure. It is also possible that the adverse effects of available drug therapy offset any benefit of sinus rhythm in the broad heart failure population. Thus, it is reasonable to individualize the approach in this patient population.

We favor an attempt to maintain sinus rhythm for heart failure patients with a first episode of atrial fibrillation, when rate control is difficult to achieve, and when atrial fibrillation is symptomatic or its onset is associated with deterioration in heart failure. In the absence of symptoms and evidence of hemodynamic impairment, maintaining rate control alone is reasonable. If a rhythm control strategy is chosen, amiodarone, dofetilide, and sotalol are the major antiarrhythmic drug options. Amiodarone is most likely to be effective (15,42). In a randomized trial of patients with atrial fibrillation without heart failure, maintenance of sinus rhythm for one year was achieved in 69% of patients treated with amiodarone as compared with 39% of those treated with sotalol or the Class I antiarrhythmic drug propafenone (24). In the DIAMOND trial, 12% of patients who had atrial fibrillation on entry into the study converted to sinus rhythm by one month when treated with dofetilide; only 1% of atrial fibrillation patients in the placebo group converted to sinus rhythm. Dofetilide also reduced the risk of recurrent atrial fibrillation once sinus rhythm had been restored (hazard ratio 0.35) (22). Amiodarone and dofetilide have not been directly compared.

Catheter Ablation of Atrial Fibrillation

More controversial is the possibility of catheter ablation for rhythm control of atrial fibrillation in heart failure. Catheter ablation of AF involves extensive left atrial ablation around the antral regions of the pulmonary veins and often other regions (Fig. 24.2) (43). Efficacy ranges from less than 50% to greater than 80% depending on whether a single or multiple procedures are considered, whether atrial fibrillation is persistent versus paroxysmal, and whether severe underlying heart disease is present. The incidence of major complications in a large survey was 6% including cardiac tamponade, stroke, phrenic nerve injury, fatal esophageal–atrial fistulae and serious pulmonary vein stenosis. In single-center reports from experienced centers the incidence of major complications is in the range of 1–2% (44,45).

In patients with heart failure, lower success rates and greater risk would be anticipated, although in selected patients who are referred to experienced centers, ablation can have a favorable outcome. Hsu and coworkers performed catheter ablation in 58 patients (mean age of 56 years) with symptomatic heart failure and LV ejection fraction <0.45 (mean 0.35) who had atrial fibrillation (persistent in 91%) with heart failure who were referred to their center (46). Two ablation procedures were required in half of the patients. Sinus rhythm was maintained in 78% of patients during a mean follow-up of one year. One patient experienced pericardial tamponade during the procedure and one patient died of worsening heart failure during follow-up. Left ventricular function, exercise capacity, and quality of life improved. The outcomes compared favorably to those of a matched control group without heart failure.

A small randomized study compared pulmonary vein isolation to AV junction ablation and biventricular pacing in 81 patients with symptomatic heart failure (LV ejection fraction of <0.40, mean 0.28; mean age 60 years) and atrial fibrillation which was persistent in approximately half of the patients (47). At 6 months of follow-up, 8 of the 41 patients randomized to pulmonary vein isolation underwent a second ablation procedure; 71% were in sinus rhythm without antiarrhythmic medications. At 6 months the composite endpoint of 6-minute walk distance, LV ejection fraction, and quality of life favored the pulmonary vein isolation group. There were no dangerous complications in either group.

Whether a rhythm control strategy with catheter ablation will avoid drug toxicities and improve outcomes compared with rate control alone is not known. It is important to

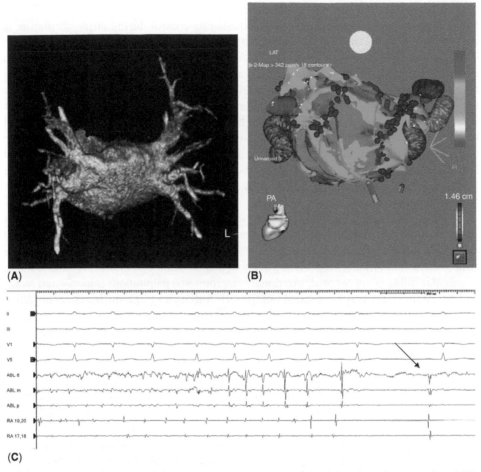

Figure 24.2 (**A**) Shown is a chamber reconstruction of the left atrium from cardiac MRI, seen in a posterior view. The pulmonary veins are seen to enter the left atrium with a common trunk on the left, and with three main branches on the right. The right inferior vein also has a proximal ramification. (**B**) An electroanatomic map of the left atrium with merged MRI information, intracardiac ultrasound, and information from catheter position during mapping. Integrated imaging is critical to the safe performance of atrial fibrillation ablation. The maroon dots encircling the veins indicate radiofrequency ablation sites, placed in sequence in the atrial antrum to electrically isolate the veins from the rest of the atrium. This is the usual plan for ablation of patients with paroxysmal atrial fibrillation and pulmonary vein triggers. (**C**) Termination of atrial fibrillation to sinus rhythm during radiofrequency ablation. The top five tracings are surface ECG, with QRS complexes visible. Signals from the ablation catheter are seen in the next three rows, with rapid fractionated activity near a pulmonary vein. The activity slows down and organizes as the AF terminates. A sinus beat is seen at the end of the tracing, (arrow).

recognize that patients in the small studies available are selected by referral to experienced centers, and are generally younger than the larger population of patients with atrial fibrillation and heart failure. As techniques and success rates for AF ablation improve, catheter ablation may be more commonly used. For patients with heart failure undergoing valve surgery or coronary artery bypass grafting, a surgical MAZE procedure also could be considered to control atrial arrhythmias.

Rate Control and AV Junctional Ablation

When sinus rhythm is not maintained, adequate rate control during atrial fibrillation is of paramount importance (12,27,33,39,48,49). A poorly controlled ventricular rate can exacerbate heart failure and contribute to further deterioration in ventricular function. A resting heart rate below 80–90 beats/min and remaining below 100/min with comfortable ambulation is a reasonable goal. β-adrenergic blockers and digoxin are the first-line options for rate control (39). Digoxin is less effective when sympathetic tone is elevated, but useful because it lacks adverse hemodynamic effects. The calcium channel blockers, diltiazem and verapamil, slow down the heart rate but should be avoided in patients with advanced heart failure due to their negative inotropic effects and potential for increasing mortality in patients with heart failure due to coronary artery disease (50). Amiodarone is an effective drug for rate control but other agents are preferable due to its toxicities.

When adequate rate control cannot be achieved with pharmacologic means, catheter ablation of the AV junction with implantation of a permanent pacemaker should be consi dered. AV junction ablation achieves rate control and regularizes the heart rhythm. The atria continue to fibrillate, necessitating anticoagulation. Although the atrial contribution to ventricular filling is not restored, exertional symptoms and palpitations improve and recurrent hospitalizations may be reduced (49,51–57). Although symptoms improve, objective demonstration of improvement in exercise time or oxygen uptake are not usually observed (33,52). In some patients left ventricular ejection fraction improves, which may be a consequence of the decrease in rate, or better ability to measure ejection fraction once the heart rate is regularized (58).

Two problems are of concern with this procedure. Occasional patients experience deterioration in heart failure after this procedure (59,60). A change in ventricular activation sequence produced by right ventricular pacing might be responsible (as discussed in Part IV, Chapter 23 (23). First, patients at the greatest risk for hemodynamic deterioration have severely depressed ventricular function and functional mitral regurgitation. Biventricular pacing, also known as cardiac resynchronization (left ventricular and right ventricular pacing) reduces this risk. Second, sudden death due to *torsade de pointes* occurs after ablation, potentially the result of electrophysiologic changes produced by the sudden reduction in heart rate. Pacing at 90 beats per minute for the initial one to three months after ablation appears to reduce this risk (61).

If a heart failure patient with atrial fibrillation is being considered for cardiac surgery to correct a valvular lesion or to revascularize, left atrial appendage removal or ligation has been suggested, in the hope of reducing the risk thrombus formation and embolism. This is the subject of several ongoing devices under investigation (62).

Atrial Flutter

As for atrial fibrillation, rate control and anticoagulation are important (39,63–65). Although some studies suggest less risk of left atrial thrombus formation in patients with atrial flutter than that observed in patients with atrial fibrillation, others suggest a similar risk in these two groups (63–67). Chronic anticoagulation with warfarin is prudent. Recurrent atrial flutter responds poorly to pharmacologic therapy and rate control is often more difficult to achieve than for atrial fibrillation (68). Antiarrhythmic drugs that slow down the rate of atrial flutter without blocking AV nodal conduction, such as Class I antiarrhythmic drugs, can lead to life-threatening 1:1 AV conduction .

The most common form of atrial flutter is due to circulation of a single reentry wavefront around the tricuspid annulus. Radiofrequency catheter ablation of the isthmus between the tricuspid annulus and inferior vena cava is an excellent option, and is more effective than antiarrhythmic drug therapy (69,70), abolishing atrial flutter in >95% of patients. Procedural risk is minimal. Less commonly an apparent atrial flutter is due to reentry involving an area of scar in the right or left atrium. Ablation of these types of flutter is more difficult, with somewhat lower efficacy. Ablation of flutter in the left atrium is associated with a risk of arterial embolism from left atrial catheter manipulation.

Despite effective ablation of atrial flutter, these patients are susceptible to atrial fibrillation which occurs in 20–40% of patients within the following two to five years (70). When atrial flutter develops during chronic drug therapy of atrial fibrillation, ablation of flutter may allow maintenance of sinus rhythm, but drug therapy for prevention of atrial fibrillation is still likely to be required (71).

VENTRICULAR ARRHYTHMIAS AND SUDDEN CARDIAC DEATH

Sudden cardiac death accounts for 20–50% of the mortality in patients with heart failure (72). Ventricular arrhythmias are a major etiology, and implantable defibrillators (ICDs) are warranted for many high-risk patients. Other mechanisms of sudden death also occur (73–76).

Bradyarrhythmias caused 41% of in-hospital unexpected cardiac arrests in one series (76). Conduction disease associated with heart failure, myocardial ischemia, antiarrhythmic and β-adrenergic blocking drugs, and hyperkalemia are important potential etiologies. Bradyarrhythmias and pulseless electrical rhythm may be a more common presentation of cardiac arrest in nonischemic cardiomyopathies (NICMs) as compared with ischemic cardiomyopathies (ICMs). Similarly, compared with stable outpatients, patients hospitalized with advanced heart failure may have a higher incidence of electromechanical dissociation as a cause of sudden death (73,77). Unexpected and unrecognized acute myocardial infarction, pulmonary embolism, stroke, and ruptured aortic aneurysms also cause some of these deaths.

In chronic dilated heart failure, the incidence of sudden death increases with the severity of heart failure (31,78–86). In patients with minimal to modest symptoms of heart failure, the annual risk of sudden death ranges from 2% to 6% per year. Those with more advanced symptoms, New York Heart Association functional class III–IV, have a risk of 5–12% per year. As the severity of heart failure increases, deaths due to pump failure increase to a greater extent than sudden deaths. Thus the proportion of sudden deaths decreases from 50–80% for mild to moderate heart failure, to 5–30% for severe heart failure. The risk of sudden death is approximately similar for a given severity of ventricular dysfunction regardless of whether heart failure is due to ICM as compared with NICM (74,87,88).

ICDs provide effective therapy for most episodes of VT or fibrillation (Fig. 24.3A) and are warranted for many high risk patients. The superiority of ICDs to therapy with amiodarone has been convincingly demonstrated for patients who have been resuscitated from a cardiac arrest (9,16,89–91). In the Antiarrhythmics Versus Implantable Defibrillator (AVID) trial, total mortality at three years was reduced from 36% to 25%; an 11% absolute reduction in mortality and a 31% relative reduction in mortality compared with antiarrhythmic drug therapy (amiodarone in over 95% of patients). Two smaller trials also show similar trends (9,89,90). The arrhythmia history, etiology of heart failure, severity of ventricular dysfunction, and, in advanced heart failure, the candidacy for cardiac transplantation or destination left ventricular assist device therapy are important considerations in selecting patients for ICDs. Whether the patient may benefit from LV pacing for cardiac resynchronization is also an important consideration Part IV, Chapter 23.

Monomorphic Ventricular Tachycardia

Patients with ICM typically have large areas of infarction (Fig. 24.4A). Surviving myocyte bundles present within the infarction create channels for conduction set up reentry circuits (92,93). The VT that results is typically monomorphic, with each QRS complex resembling

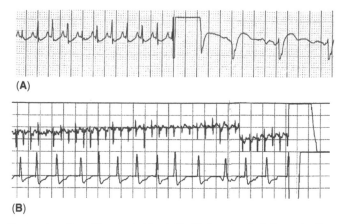

(A)

(B)

Figure 24.3 Two examples of implantable defibrillator shock delivery. In the upper (**A**) tracing, a ventricular electrogram (EGM) is shown. Rapid ventricular tachycardia is terminated by a shock from the device. In the lower (**B**) tracing, simultaneous atrial and ventricular EGMs are shown. The atrial EGM shows very rapid irregular signals consistent with atrial fibrillation, and the irregular response on the ventricular channel is also consistent with atrial fibrillation. In this case, an inappropriate shock occurred due to atrial fibrillation with rapid ventricular response.

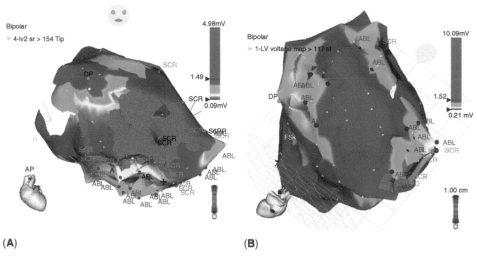

(A)   (B)

Figure 24.4 Left ventricular electroanatomic maps from two patients with VT due to of ischemic (**A**) and nonischemic (**B**) cardiomyopathy. Maps were created during LV mapping by moving a catheter from point to point on the ventricle. Points on the map are color coded for voltage in millivolts (mV). Areas in purple represent normal myocardium. Low voltage yellow, green, and red regions (<1.5 mV) are abnormal scars or infarcts and areas of gray represent unexcitable scar. Notably the ischemic cardiomyopathy has a large area of low voltage anteroapical scar, whereas the nonischemic cardiomyopathy has patchy low voltage disease.

the preceding and following QRS complex (Fig. 24.5). Because the arrhythmia substrate is relatively fixed and stable, VT is usually inducible with programmed stimulation, allowing electrophysiologic testing to be used to detect these reentry circuits, thereby identifying

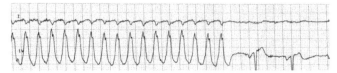

Figure 24.5 An episode of spontaneously terminating monomorphic ventricular tachycardia in a patient with ischemic cardiomyopathy.

patients at risk of spontaneous episodes. Although, in general, absence of inducible VT at electrophysiologic testing indicates a reasonably low risk of sudden arrhythmic death after myocardial infarction, in patients with poor ventricular function, absence of inducible VT does not necessarily convey a low sudden death risk (94,95).

In patients with idiopathic NICM, large areas of scar or infarction are usually absent (Fig. 24.4B) and programmed stimulation rarely induces sustained monomorphic VT if it has not occurred spontaneously (96,97). A negative electrophysiology study has little prognostic value (98–102). Interestingly, of the occasional NICM patients who develop sustained monomorphic VT, most have areas of ventricular scar that can be intramural or epicardial in location as the substrate for reentry circuits (103,104). The scar may be a consequence of replacement fibrosis from the myopathic process itself or due to infarcts from embolism of left ventricular or atrial thrombus to a coronary artery. Scars causing VT in the absence of coronary artery disease should prompt consideration of sarcoidosis, Chagas' disease, and arrhythmogenic right ventricular dysplasia (105–112). Approximately 5 to 10% of NICM patients with monomorphic VT have reentry through the bundle branches causing their VT (103,113,114). This tachycardia is also inducible by programmed stimulation, and is amenable to cure by catheter ablation of the right bundle branch.

Chronic Therapy for Sustained Monomorphic VT

Following restoration of sinus rhythm, potential precipitating and aggravating factors should be sought and corrected. However, it should be recognized that sustained monomorphic VT is associated with an underlying structural abnormality in the vast majority of cases and that the risk of recurrence during long-term follow-up likely exceeds 20% regardless of antiarrhythmic drug therapy or correction of myocardial ischemia or other potential aggravating factors. When monomorphic VT occurs with elevated serum cardiac enzymes indicating infarction, the risk of recurrent VT remains high despite treatment for ischemia (115). The major role of electrophysiologic testing is to confirm the diagnosis when SVT with aberrancy is a consideration, and guiding ablation therapy, if needed.

If VT is incessant, it should be suppressed with an antiarrhythmic drug therapy or catheter ablation (116). The possibility of idiopathic VT causing tachycardia-induced cardiomyopathy should be considered. Implantation of an ICD is recommended for most of the patients with sustained VT as discussed below. The device can often terminate the arrhythmia by painless, antitachycardia pacing. If VT recurs causing symptomatic ICD therapies, antiarrhythmic drugs or catheter ablation can be considered at that time. Episodes of VT are a marker for increased risk of death and heart failure, even when promptly terminated by an ICD (see below) (117).

Sustained Polymorphic Ventricular Tachycardia

Polymorphic VT has a continually changing QRS complex. It is often caused by potentially reversible conditions. Acute myocardial ischemia or infarction is a common etiology and

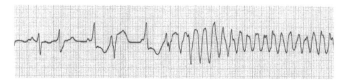

Figure 24.6   Shown is an episode of *torsade de pointes* initiated by a long-short RR interval.

warrants evaluation. *Torsade de pointes* associated with QT interval prolongation is the other major form of polymorphic VT. Less commonly, polymorphic VT is associated with cardiomyopathy or prior infarction without clear precipitating triggers.

Torsade de Pointes

Polymorphic VT associated with QT interval prolongation is referred to as *torsade de pointes* (118). Any cause of QT interval prolongation can cause *torsade de pointes* (119–122). Hypokalemia, bradycardia, drugs such as sotalol, dofetilide, ibutilide, quinidine, n-acetylprocainamide, haloperidol, and erythromycin are relatively common causes. (A more extensive list is available at the www.QTdrugs.org web site maintained by the university of Arizona.) Electrophysiologic changes that accompany ventricular hypertrophy in chronic heart failure may increase susceptibility to *torsade de pointes*.

   Torsade de pointes is often "bradycardia-dependent" or "pause dependent," with a characteristic initiating sequence (Fig. 24.6). A sudden increase in R–R interval as may occur following a premature beat, creates a pause. The QT interval of the beat terminating the pause is prolonged. The first beat of the tachycardia interrupts the T-wave of that beat. Interventions that increase heart and shorten refractoriness are protective. Emergent treatment is intravenous administration of 1 to 2 g of magnesium sulfate. If episodes continue, therapy directed at accelerating the heart rate with intravenous administration of isoproterenol and/or transvenous pacing is warranted.

   Patients who have had *torsade de pointes* should avoid all drugs that prolong the QT interval. Although amiodarone prolongs the QT interval, it rarely causes *torsade de pointes*, possibly because it also blocks ionic currents that also cause the arrhythmia. Patients with heart failure are particularly susceptible to *torsade de pointes* and therapy with amiodarone is not protective (123,124). Treatment with an ICD is reasonable. ICDs also provide pacing to prevent bradycardia and suppress pauses following premature beats that may help prevent polymorphic VT (125).

Syncope

There are a variety of causes of syncope and determining the etiology is often challenging. Among 491 consecutive patients with advanced heart failure, Middlekauff and coworkers found that 12% had a history of syncope (126). In 45% of patients, syncope was attributed to a cardiac arrhythmia, orthostatic hypotension, or a noncardiac cause was identified in 25%, and no clear cause was identified in 30% of patients. The rate of sudden death during the following year was 45%. The sudden death risk was similar for patients with identifiable cardiac causes and presumptively identified noncardiac causes of syncope, suggesting that even when an apparently benign explanation is found, patients with heart failure and syncope remain at high risk for sudden death.

   In patients with NICM and syncope, a negative electrophysiologic study does not indicate a low risk. Knight and coworkers placed ICDs in 14 patients with NICM, unexplained syncope, and a negative electrophysiology study. During an average follow-up of 2 years, half of the patients received therapy from the ICD for VT or ventricular fibrillation (127). Of 639 consecutive patients with non-ischemic cardiomyopathy referred for heart transplantation reported by Fonarow and coworkers, 147 (23%) had a history of syncope (128). Twenty-five of these patients received an ICD; 40% received an appropriate shock for VT and none died suddenly during a mean follow-up of 22 months. Of the 122 patients who had a history of syncope but did not receive an ICD, 15% died suddenly during follow-up. Actuarial survival at 2 years was 84.9% with an ICD therapy and 66.9% with conventional therapy.

Based on the above data, implantation of an ICD is a reasonable consideration for most patients with heart failure and unexplained syncope (127–129).

PRIMARY PREVENTION OF SUDDEN DEATH IN HEART FAILURE

The single most useful risk factor that has been used to select patients for ICD therapy is the left ventricular ejection fraction (Table 24.1). The Sudden Cardiac Death in Heart Failure Trial (SCD-HeFT) randomized 2521 patients with NYHA class II or III heart failure and LV ejection fraction of 0.35 or less to a single-chamber ICD, amiodarone, or placebo (13). Heart failure was due to ischemic cardiomyopathy in 52% of patients. After a median follow-up of 46 months mortality was reduced by 7% (from 29% in the control group to 22%) for the ICD group, a relative risk reduction of 23%. Amiodarone was of no benefit, with a mortality of 28%. Benefit was similar for patients with ischemic and nonischemic cardiomyopathy. Benefit was greatest for patients with mild heart failure (functional class II). The smaller number of patients with functional class III heart failure did not have a mortality benefit, consistent with the notion that as heart failure progresses, progressive pump failure becomes a more important cause of death, such that the survival benefit from an ICD is limited.

Other randomized trials have evaluated the use of ICDs for primary prevention of sudden death. In patients with prior myocardial infarction and depressed ventricular function most of whom had functional class 1 or II symptoms, ICDs also reduced mortality (130,131). In a study of patients with nonischemic dilated cardiomyopathy, LV ejection fraction <35% and nonsustained VT or premature ventricular contraction frequency >10 per hour, there was a favorable trend for mortality reduction (132). Based on these studies present guidelines recommend ICD implantation for patients with reasonable expectation for one year of survival who have significantly depressed ventricular function and acceptable functional class (Table 24.2) (133).

Risk Stratification

ICDs treat rapid VT in approximately only 20% patients treated for primary prevention, and inappropriate ICD therapies occur with a similar frequency in some trials (117). Better identification of patients who will benefit from an ICD is the focus of much research (134). For a marker of risk to be useful clinically it requires the following: (i) the marker identifies a high risk group and (ii) specific therapy directed at the high risk group improves survival. Several noninvasive markers of potential electrical instability, including ambient ventricular ectopy, nonsustained VT, signal-averaged ECG, measures of heart rate variability, and T-wave alternans have a physiologic basis for predicting arrhythmia risk. However, in most cases, the prevalence of abnormal markers increases in parallel to the severity of heart failure and disappointingly, have not been found to be sufficiently specific for arrhythmia risk to guide selection of ICD therapy (135). T-wave alternans assesses a measure of repolarization variability that has been linked to susceptibility to ventricular fibrillation in animal models, and to inducible arrhythmias in humans, but has not proven clinically useful (136,137). Programmed electrical stimulation to detect inducible VT does identify patients with scars that can support reentry and is associated with increased

Table 24.1 ICD Primary Prevention Trials

	MADIT I	CABG-Patch	MUSTT	MADIT II	DEFINITE	SCD HeFT
Target population	Post-myocardial infarction	Post-coronary artery bypass grafting	Nonsustained VT	Post-myocardial infarction	Nonischemic Cardiomyopathy, ventricular ectopy	NYHA Class II and III heart failure and EF <35%
Treatment	ICD vs. best-available drug therapy	ICD vs. control	ICD vs. EPS-guided drug therapy or no therapy	ICD vs. best available therapy	ICD vs. best available therapy	ICD vs. amiodarone versus best medical therapy
Patients enrolled	196	900	704	1232	458	2521
Arrhythmia qualifier	Spontaneous NSVT + inducible, nonsuppressible VT/VF	None (abnormal signal averaged ECG)	Spontaneous NSVT + inducible VT/VF	None	PVCs > 10/hr or NSVT	None
LVEF (%) qualifier	≤35	<36	None	≤30	<35%	<35%
CHF qualifier	None	None	None	None	None	Class II or III
NYHA IV (%)	Excluded	Excluded	Excluded	5	Excluded	Excluded
Mean LVEF (%)	26	27	30	23	21	25
Outcome	Survival advantage in ICD group	No difference in survival	Survival advantage in ICD group	Survival advantage in ICD group	Trend to survival advantage in ICD group	Survival advantage in ICD group
Total mortality rate	16% ICD vs. 34% drug @ 1 yr	27% ICD vs. 24% control @ 4 yrs	24% ICD vs. 48% no treatment vs. 55% drug treatment @ 5 yrs[a]	14.2% ICD vs. 19.8% control at 20 months	7.9 % ICD vs. 14.1% at 2 yrs, p = 0.08	28.9% ICD vs. 36.1% placebo at 5 yrs
Comments	Drug therapy: 80% amiodarone, 11% Class IA, 9% no antiarrhythmic drug at discharge	EFs for inclusion are pre-revascularization due to study design where patients received ICDs surgically at the time of CABG	Most patients randomized to drug therapy were taking Class IA agents which could have enhanced mortality in drug group	1. Survival curves diverge at 9 months rather than soon after implant. 2. Survival advantage balanced by worsened heart failure in ICD arm	Possibly nonsignificant result due to lower numbers and a shorter followup than SCD HeFT	1. Survival curves diverge at 18 months rather than soon after implant 2. No survival advantage to amiodarone

[a]EP study guided drug therapy + ICD, EP study guided drug therapy without ICD, No antiarrhythmic therapy, respectively.

Abbreviations: CABG, coronary artery bypass graft; ICD, implantable cardiac defibrillator; LVEF, left ventricular ejection fraction; NSVT, nonsustained ventricular tachycardia; NYHA, New York Heart Association; PVC, premature ventricular contraction, VF, ventricular fibrillation; VT, ventricular tachycardia.

Table 24.2 Use of Implantable Defibrillators for Primary Prevention in Patients with Heart Failure[a]

Ischemic Cardiomypathy:
LVEF <35% due to prior myocardial infarction and
At least 40 days after acute MI and NYHA functional class II or III
(Class I recommendation, Level of Evidence: A)
LVEF <30% due to prior myocardial infarction and
One month after MI or three months after surgical revascularization and
NYHA functional class I
(Class I recommendation, Level of Evidence: A)
LVEF <40% and
Nonsustained VT and inducible VF or sustained VT at EP study
(Class I recommendation, Level of Evidence: B)
Nonischemic Cardiomypathy:
LVEF less than or equal to 35% and NYHA functional Class II or III.
(Class I recommendation, Level of Evidence: B)
LVEF of less than or equal to 35% and NYHA functional Class I.
(Class IIB recommendation, Level of Evidence: C)
Familial cardiomyopathy associated with sudden death.
  (Class IIB recommendation, Level of Evidence: C)
Both Ischemic and Nonischemic Cardiomyopathy:
Non-hospitalized patients awaiting cardiac transplantation
(Class IIA recommendation, Level of Evidence: C)
Syncope and advanced structural heart disease where thorough invasive and noninvasive
  investigations have failed to define a cause
(Class IIA recommendation, Level of Evidence: C)

[a]"Recommendations for consideration of ICD therapy, particularly those for primary prevention, apply only to patients who are receiving optimal medical therapy and have a reasonable expectation of survival with a good functional status for more than 1 year." *Source*: From Ref. 133, Epstein, AE *et alia*.
Abbreviations: ICD, implantable cardiac defibrillator; LVEF, left ventricular ejection fraction; MI, myocardial infarction, NYHA, New York Heart Association; VF, ventricular fibrillation; VT, ventricular tachycardia.

risk in patients with prior myocardial infarction (138). Electrophysiologic testing can be useful in selected patients.

Ventricular Ectopy and Nonsustained VT

Ventricular ectopic activity and nonsustained VT of three or more consecutive beats are common in heart failure patients; 34–79% of patients have one or more runs of nonsustained VT on 24-hour ambulatory recordings (87,139,140). These are typically short; only 30% of patients have runs >5 beats in duration (87). Fast, long runs of nonsustained VT and polymorphic VT should prompt a careful search for possible myocardial ischemia and possible causes of *torsade de pointes*. Occasionally ventricular ectopic activity is due to an aggravating factor that requires treatment, or is a marker for hemodynamic deterioration. Hyper or hypokalemia, hypoxemia, apneic periods during sleep and myocardial ischemia are potential causes that deserve evaluation when a marked change in the frequency of ectopic activity occurs (141–144).

Frequent ventricular ectopy and nonsustained VT are markers for increased mortality and sudden death, but appear to reflect the severity of underlying heart failure and ventricular dysfunction, rather than a specific arrhythmia risk (87,139,140). Furthermore, suppression of nonsustained VT, such as by amiodarone, does not necessarily improve survival. Asymptomatic arrhythmias should, in general, not receive specific antiarrhythmic therapy.

Ventricular Ectopy Causing Ventricular Dysfunction

It has been recognized that very frequent ventricular ectopy can cause or contribute to ventricular dysfunction, which improves following successful ablation, similar to tachycardia-induced cardiomyopathy (145,146). These patients typically have more than 6000 ectopic beats per 24 hours and often more than 20,000 or >15% of total beats are ectopic beats. In some cases, determination of whether the arrhythmia is contributing to ventricular dysfunction or is secondary to a myopathic process can be determined only by suppressing the arrhythmia with amiodarone or ablation.

Heart Failure Severity and ICDs

The severity of heart failure is an important consideration in assessing whether an ICD is warranted (Table 24.2) (133,147). Successful termination of VT or ventricular fibrillation meaningfully extends survival when the patient has well-compensated heart failure and returns to the pre-arrhythmia functional state. Extension of survival is limited when deteriorating heart failure or associated complications lead to death from pump failure soon after an episode of VT. Patients with severely decompensated heart failure are less likely to benefit from an ICD and are at an increased risk for harm from the implantation and testing procedure. Present guidelines stipulate that recommendations for primary prevention ICDs "apply only to patients who are receiving optimal medical therapy and only to patients who are receiving optimal medical therapy and have a reasonable expectation of survival with a good functional status for more than 1 year" (133,148).

The risk–benefit balance of ICDs is difficult to assess for patients with advanced heart failure. In post-hoc subgroup analyses of the SCD-HeFT trial ICDs conferred benefit for patients with functional Class II, but not Class III heart failure patients (13). Similarly, a post-hoc analysis of subgroups in the AVID trial there was a survival benefit demonstrable for patients with ejection fractions between 0.20 and 0.34, but patients with worse left ventricular function (ejection fraction <0.20) did not have a statistically significant improvement in survival (149). In a post-hoc analysis of the Canadian Implantable Defibrillator Study (CIDS), the study population was divided into quartiles of risk based on age, ejection fraction, and functional class. ICD therapy was associated with a 50% reduction in death in the highest risk quartile, but conferred no benefit in the three lower risk quartiles (90).

Thus, the benefit of ICD therapy as reflected by an extension of survival appears to follow a bell-shaped curve. Patients with mild heart failure generally have a lower risk of arrhythmia events and as a population receive less benefit during initial follow-up. With increasing severity of heart failure the incidence of arrhythmic events (VT and ventricular fibrillation) increase so that the benefit of the ICD increases, until, mortality from pump failure increases to the extent that effective arrhythmia termination minimally extends survival (150). In some cases, heart failure symptoms become intolerable and patients seek to have the tachyarrhythmia therapies of the device turned off to avoid painful shocks as death approaches. Extrapolating data from trials to an individual patient is often difficult.

In general, patients with compensated heart failure are candidates for ICD implantation when they have an indication for an ICD. Some patients with decompensated heart failure should not receive an ICD, even through the risk of ventricular arrhythmias is high. For some of these patients, amiodarone may be a better option. However, some patients with transient class IV symptoms survive for years after resuscitation from a cardiac arrhythmia (151).

The possibility for cardiac transplantation and left ventricular assist devices as home destination therapy also impacts on the potential benefit of an ICD. Most patients who are accepted onto elective transplantation waiting lists are sufficiently compensated to wait at home for a donor heart to become available. Sudden death is a significant risk for these patients. Of 434 patients accepted onto the elective transplantation list between 1984 and 1997, at one center 25% received a donor heart, 26% of patients died, and 72% of these deaths were sudden (82). Even for patients who have very poor functional capacity, a dramatic extension of survival occurs when successful defibrillation allows a patient to receive a transplant. Protection from sudden arrhythmic death with an ICD allows some patients with advanced heart failure to await cardiac transplantation at home, avoiding or delaying in-patient waiting until hemodynamic deterioration necessitates inotropic support. Implantation of an ICD is reasonable in these patients even though progressive hemodynamic deterioration is anticipated (82,152,153).

Bradycardia Pacing with ICDs

All ICDs incorporate pacing for bradycardia. Dual chamber (atrioventricular) pacing, activity responsiveness, and mode switching for atrial arrhythmias are available. Approximately, 50% of patients who require ICD therapy have indications for or subsequently evolve the need for permanent pacing for bradyarrhythmia. Use of the ICD for bradycardia pacing is preferable to placement of a separate pacemaker, thereby avoiding adverse interactions between the devices and minimizing the number of leads implanted. If sinus rhythm rather than atrial fibrillation is present, maintenance of AV synchrony is generally preferred. This is achieved with a dual chamber defibrillator that requires placement of an atrial lead as well as the ventricular lead (154).

Although dual chamber is generally preferred to ventricular pacing alone for patients with bradycardia, the consequences of AV pacing warrant careful consideration due to the potential for adverse hemodynamic effects of right ventricular apical pacing (RVAP). As discussed in chapter 18, RVAP produces QRS prolongation similar to left bundle branch block, and is associated with worse ventricular performance than ventricular activation over the normal His-Purkinje system which produces a shorter QRS duration (155–157). The Dual Chamber Pacing or Ventricular Backup Pacing in patients with an Implantable Defibrillator (DAVID) trial randomized 506 ICD patients with ejection fractions less than 40% to dual chamber pacing at a base rate of 70 beats per minute versus ventricular backup pacing at a rate of 40 beats per minute (158). It was expected that dual chamber pacing would allow better medical management of heart failure and lower incidence of atrial fibrillation. However, the trial was stopped early for increased hospitalizations for heart failure in the group receiving dual chamber pacing, opposite to the original hypothesis. The adverse effect was attributed to a 60% rate of RVAP in the dual chamber pacing group versus a 1% rate of RVAP in patients with ventricular backup pacing. It is therefore desirable to avoid RVAP when there is normal ventricular activation (i.e., narrow QRS duration). In some patients, back-up ventricular pacing below the intrinsic heart rate, which results in supraventricular conduction and rare ventricular pacing, might be preferable to chronic RVAP in the dual chamber mode. The implementation of left ventricular pacing leads (discussed in chap. 18) may obviate this concern, but further investigation is required.

ICD Implantation Considerations

The ICD implantation procedure usually includes initiation of ventricular fibrillation and testing of defibrillation from the ICD to make certain that the lead configuration and energy available will effectively defibrillate. Induced ventricular fibrillation is associated with mild, transient ventricular dysfunction, which is well tolerated in the majority of patients (159). In patients with advanced heart failure defibrillation threshold testing occasionally precipitates a hemodynamic deterioration (153). In one series, 3 of 59 patients (5%) who were being evaluated for cardiac transplantation developed electromechanical dissociation after successful defibrillation. In decompensated patients ICD implantation should be deferred until medical therapy has been optimized and heart failure improved. In general, the mortality from defibrillation implantation is less than 1%, but this has not been specifically assessed in heart failure populations.

Continuing Care

Patients with ICDs should be followed in a specialized clinic. Routine device interrogations assessing sensing and pacing function, remaining battery life, and arrhythmias detected by the ICD are generally performed every three to four months. Follow-up can be periodically in the office, or intermittently via telephone-based home monitoring, where the physician caring for the patient can look at device downloads on a secure Internet website.

Up to 40% of patients receive inappropriate therapies from the ICD at some point during follow-up. Heart rate is the major criterion for arrhythmia detection. A rate exceeding the programmed detection threshold will trigger therapy with either antitachy-cardia pacing (ATP) or high voltage shocks. Thus sinus tachycardia or a rapid supraventricular tachycardia can lead to painful shocks. Inappropriate therapy, as for rapid atrial fibrillation or flutter can often be recognized and managed with reprogramming of the ICD. Occasionally inappropriate therapy is due to oversensing of diaphragmatic activity or T-waves. Electrical noise indicating a lead fracture or loose connection of the lead in the pulse generator header can also cause inappropriate shocks. Following the first symptomatic therapy from the ICD after implantation, patient assessment with interrogation of the device is usually warranted to confirm appropriate function of the ICD and assess the possibility that therapy was inappropriate, triggered by a supraventricular arrhythmia. If the patient receives more than one shock in a short period of time or has symptoms of arrhythmia or a change in symptoms that persists following an ICD shock, urgent evaluation is required. Failure of ICD therapy to terminate the arrhythmia, persistence of a ventricular tachycardia at a rate that is slower than the programmed detection criteria, and persistence of a supraventricular arrhythmia, such as atrial fibrillation, are possible causes. Occurrence of ventricular tachycardia or ventricular fibrillation is a marker for greater mortality, heart failure hospitalizations, and decreased quality of life and warrants assessment (160–164).

Even inappropriate shocks, most commonly due to atrial fibrillation, were predictors of increased mortality in one study (165). Myocardial ischemia, electrolyte disturbances, and intercurrent illness are important potential causes of arrhythmia exacerbations that should be considered. Recurrent symptomatic episodes warrant antiarrhythmic drug therapy or catheter ablation (166).

Occasionally it is necessary to temporarily disable an ICD to prevent incessant shocks or antitachycardia pacing such as may be triggered by an "electrical storm" of recurrent VT or atrial fibrillation with a rapid ventricular response (Fig. 24.3B) in a patient in the intensive care unit (167). Application of a magnet over the ICD pulse generator suspends arrhythmia detection as long as the magnet is in place, allowing time for implementation of other therapy. While the magnet is in place the patient must be closely monitored and external cardioversion used as appropriate to treat arrhythmias.

Antiarrhythmic Drug Interactions with ICDs

Many patients with ICDs require antiarrhythmic drug therapy to control supraventricular arrhythmias (most commonly atrial fibrillation and flutter) or reduce episodes of VT. In the presence of an ICD, the potential for fatal drug-induced proarrhythmia is low. The ICD will terminate *torsade de pointes* and provide pacing for bradyarrhythmias. Antiarrhythmic drugs can impede effective ICD termination of arrhythmias and should be used cautiously.

Some antiarrhythmic drugs may increase the energy required for defibrillation. At the time of ICD implantation, defibrillation testing is performed by inducing ventricular fibrillation and observing that an ICD shock will terminate fibrillation, though the utility of routine defibrillator testing is an area of increasing controversy (168). Most ICDs are capable of providing a 30–42 Joule shock. A 10-Joule safety margin is recommended and confirmed by demonstrating that ventricular fibrillation is terminated by a shock 10 Joules below the maximum energy available from the ICD. Amiodarone therapy can increase the energy required for defibrillation; however, the size of the effect is typically small relative to the available output from modern ICD systems. If the defibrillation threshold is close to the maximal energy of the ICD, antiarrhythmic drug therapy could increase it such that maximal energy shocks from the ICD are no longer effective. Class III antiarrhythmic drugs that block potassium channels, sotalol and dofetilide, may decrease the defibrillation threshold, though this is controversial. In general, repeat defibrillation testing should be considered when a possibly ineffective shock occurs, when the device is reprogrammed beyond the sensitivity of prior testing, or when therapy with amiodarone is initiated in patient with known high defibrillation threshold (169).

Psychological Support

The presence of an ICD "safety-net" is greatly reassuring for most patients. Those who have experienced repeated, painful ICD shocks, however, often live in fear of an arrhythmia recurrence (170–174). Some patients needlessly restrict activities and suffer significant depression and anxiety. Patient support groups and counseling are often beneficial. Some patients require therapy with anxiolytics and antidepressant medications, particularly those who have suffered multiple repetitive shocks.

CONCLUSION

Managing atrial and ventricular arrhythmias and their risks is an important component of caring for patients with heart failure. Antiarrhythmic drugs and catheter ablation are important therapies. ICDs provide effective and reliable treatment of sustained VT and fibrillation and decrease the risk of arrhythmic death. The degree to which this benefit translates to an improvement in survival depends on the severity of pump dysfunction, which is an important consideration. Many ICD recipients need active arrhythmia management to prevent symptoms and adverse consequences of ventricular and atrial arrhythmias.

REFERENCES

1. Exner DV, Dries DL, Waclawiw MA, et al. β-adrenergic blocking agent use and mortality in patients with asymptomatic and symptomatic left ventricular systolic dysfunction: a post hoc analysis of the studies of left ventricular dysfunction. J Am Coll Cardiol 1999; 33: 916–23.
2. Kennedy HL, Brooks MM, Barker AH, et al. β-blocker therapy in the Cardiac Arrhythmia Suppression Trial. CAST Investigators. Am J Cardiol 1994; 74: 674–80.
3. Exner DV, Reiffel JA, Epstein AE, et al. β-blocker use and survival in patients with ventricular fibrillation or symptomatic ventricular tachycardia: the Antiarrhythmics Versus Implantable Defibrillators (AVID) trial. J Am Coll Cardiol 1999; 34: 325–33.
4. Khand AU, Rankin AC, Kaye GC, et al. Systematic review of the management of atrial fibrillation in patients with heart failure. Eur Heart J 2000; 21: 614–32.
5. Ravid S, Podrid PJ, Lampert S, et al. Congestive heart failure induced by six of the newer antiarrhythmic drugs. J Am Coll Cardiol 1989; 14: 1326–30.
6. Stevenson WG. Mechanisms and management of arrhythmias in heart failure. Curr Opin Cardiol 1995; 10: 274–81.
7. Flaker GC, Blackshear JL, McBride R, et al. Antiarrhythmic drug therapy and cardiac mortality in atrial fibrillation. The Stroke Prevention in Atrial Fibrillation Investigators. J Am Coll Cardiol 1992; 20: 527–32.
8. Stevenson WG, Stevenson LW, Middlekauff HR, et al. Improving survival for patients with atrial fibrillation and advanced heart failure. J Am Coll Cardiol 1996; 28: 1458–63. [Erratum appears in J Am Coll Cardiol 1997; 30: 1902].

9. Kuck KH, Cappato R, Siebels J, et al. Randomized comparison of antiarrhythmic drug therapy with implantable defibrillators in patients resuscitated from cardiac arrest: the Cardiac Arrest Study Hamburg (CASH). Circulation 2000; 102: 748–54.

10. Nul DR, Doval HC, Grancelli HO, et al. Heart rate is a marker of amiodarone mortality reduction in severe heart failure. The GESICA-GEMA Investigators. Grupo de Estudio de la Sobrevida en la Insuficiencia Cardiaca en Argentina-Grupo de Estudios Multicentricos en Argentina. J Am Coll Cardiol 1997; 29: 1199–205.

11. Singh SN, Fletcher RD, Fisher SG, et al. Amiodarone in patients with congestive heart failure and asymptomatic ventricular arrhythmia. Survival Trial of Antiarrhythmic Therapy in Congestive Heart Failure. N Engl J Med 1995; 333: 77–82.

12. Massie BM, Shah NB, Pitt B, et al. Importance of assessing changes in ventricular response to atrial fibrillation during evaluation of new heart failure therapies: experience from trials of flosequinan. Am Heart J 1996; 132: 130–6.

13. Bardy GH, Lee KL, Mark DB, et al. Amiodarone or an implantable cardioverter-defibrillator for congestive heart failure. N Engl J Med 2005; 352: 225–37.

14. Anonymous. Effect of prophylactic amiodarone on mortality after acute myocardial infarction and in congestive heart failure: meta-analysis of individual data from 6500 patients in randomised trials. Amiodarone Trials Meta-Analysis Investigators. Lancet 1997; 350: 1417–24.

15. Weinfeld MS, Drazner MH, Stevenson WG, et al. Early outcome of initiating amiodarone for atrial fibrillation in advanced heart failure. J Heart Lung Transplant 2000; 19: 638–43.

16. Anonymous. A comparison of antiarrhythmic-drug therapy with implantable defibrillators in patients resuscitated from near-fatal ventricular arrhythmias. The Antiarrhythmics versus Implantable Defibrillators (AVID) Investigators. N Engl J Med 1997; 337: 1576–83.

17. Gottlieb SS, Riggio DW, Lauria S, et al. High dose oral amiodarone loading exerts important hemodynamic actions in patients with congestive heart failure. J Am Coll Cardiol 1994; 23: 560–4.

18. Dusman RE, Stanton MS, Miles WM, et al. Clinical features of amiodarone-induced pulmonary toxicity. Circulation 1990; 82: 51–9.

19. Singh SN, Fisher SG, Deedwania PC, et al. Pulmonary effect of amiodarone in patients with heart failure. the congestive heart failure-survival trial of antiarrhythmic therapy (CHF-STAT) investigators (veterans affairs cooperative study no. 320). J Am Coll Cardiol 1997; 30: 514–17.

20. Siniakowicz RM, Narula D, Suster B, et al. Diagnosis of amiodarone pulmonary toxicity with high-resolution computerized tomographic scan. J Cardiovasc Electrophysiol 2001; 12: 431–6.

21. Loh KC. Amiodarone-induced thyroid disorders: a clinical review. Postgrad Med J 2000; 76: 133–40.

22. Torp-Pedersen C, Møller M, Bloch-Thomsen PE, et al. Dofetilide in patients with congestive heart failure and left ventricular dysfunction. Danish Investigations of Arrhythmia and mortality on dofetilide study group. N Engl J Med 1999; 341: 857–65.

23. Pratt CM, Camm AJ, Cooper W, et al. Mortality in the Survival With ORal D-sotalol (SWORD) trial: why did patients die? Am J Cardiol 1998; 81: 869–76.

24. Roy D, Talajic M, Dorian P, et al. Amiodarone to prevent recurrence of atrial fibrillation. Canadian Trial of Atrial Fibrillation Investigators. N Engl J Med 2000; 342: 913–20.

25. Kober L, Torp-Pedersen C, McMurray JJ, et al. Increased mortality after dronedarone therapy for severe heart failure. N Engl J Med 2008; 358: 2678–87.

26. Singh BN, Connolly SJ, Crijns HJ, et al. Dronedarone for maintenance of sinus rhythm in atrial fibrillation or flutter. N Engl J Med 2007; 357: 987–99.

27. Shinbane JS, Wood MA, Jensen DN, et al. Tachycardia-induced cardiomyopathy: a review of animal models and clinical studies. J Am Coll Cardiol 1997; 29: 709–15.

28. Mahoney P, Kimmel S, DeNofrio D, et al. Prognostic significance of atrial fibrillation in patients at a tertiary medical center referred for heart transplantation because of severe heart failure. Am J Cardiol 1999; 83: 1544–7.

29. Dries DL, Exner DV, Gersh BJ, et al. Atrial fibrillation is associated with an increased risk for mortality and heart failure progression in patients with asymptomatic and symptomatic left ventricular systolic dysfunction: a retrospective analysis of the SOLVD trials. Studies of Left Ventricular Dysfunction. J Am Coll Cardiol 1998; 32: 695–703.

30. Deedwania PC, Singh BN, Ellenbogen K, et al. Spontaneous conversion and maintenance of sinus rhythm by amiodarone in patients with heart failure and atrial fibrillation: observations from the veterans affairs congestive heart failure survival trial of antiarrhythmic therapy (CHF-STAT). the department of veterans affairs CHF-STAT investigators. Circulation 1998; 98: 2574–9.

31. anonymous. Effects of enalapril on mortality in severe congestive heart failure. Results of the Cooperative North Scandinavian Enalapril Survival Study (CONSENSUS). The CONSENSUS trial study group. N Engl J Med 1987; 316: 1429–35.

32. Crijns HJ, Tjeerdsma G, de Kam PJ, et al. Prognostic value of the presence and development of atrial fibrillation in patients with advanced chronic heart failure. Eur Heart J 2000; 21: 1238–45.

33. Kay GN, Ellenbogen KA, Giudici M, et al. The Ablate and Pace Trial: a prospective study of catheter ablation of the AV conduction system and permanent pacemaker implantation for treatment of atrial fibrillation. APT Investigators. J Interv Card Electrophysiol 1998; 2: 121–35.

34. Pardaens K, Van Cleemput J, Vanhaecke J, et al. Atrial fibrillation is associated with a lower exercise capacity in male chronic heart failure patients. Heart 1997; 78: 564–8.

35. Verma A, Newman D, Geist M, et al. Effects of rhythm regularization and rate control in improving left ventricular function in atrial fibrillation patients undergoing atrioventricular nodal ablation. Canadian J Cardiol 2001; 17: 437–45.

36. Carson PE, Johnson GR, Dunkman Wb, et al. The influence of atrial fibrillation on prognosis in mild to moderate heart failure. The V-HeFT Studies. The V-HeFT VA Cooperative Studies Group. Circulation 1993; 87:VI102–10.

37. Dries DL, Domanski MJ, Waclawiw MA, et al. Effect of antithrombotic therapy on risk of sudden coronary death in patients with congestive heart failure. Am J Cardiol 1997; 79: 909–13.

38. Anonymous. Predictors of thromboembolism in atrial fibrillation: I. Clinical features of patients at risk. The Stroke Prevention in Atrial Fibrillation Investigators.[comment]. Ann Intern Med 1992; 116: 1–5.

39. Fuster V, Ryden LE, Asinger RW, et al. ACC/AHA/ESC guidelines for the management of patients with atrial fibrillation: executive summary. a report of the american college of cardiology/american heart association task force on practice guidelines and the European Society of Cardiology Committee for Practice Guidelines and Policy Conferences (Committee to Develop Guidelines for the Management of Patients With Atrial Fibrillation): Developed in Collaboration With the North American Society of Pacing and Electrophysiology. J Am Coll Cardiol 2001; 38: 1231–66.

40. Tuinenburg AE, Van Gelder IC, Van Den Berg MP, et al. Lack of prevention of heart failure by serial electrical cardioversion in patients with persistent atrial fibrillation. Heart 1999; 82: 486–93.

41. Roy D, Talajic M, Nattel S, et al. Rhythm control versus rate control for atrial fibrillation and heart failure. N Engl J Med 2008; 358: 2667–77.

42. Roy D, Talajic M, Dorian P, et al. Amiodarone to prevent recurrence of atrial fibrillation. Canadian Trial of Atrial Fibrillation Investigators. N Engl J Med 2000; 342: 913–20.

43. Calkins H, Bruqada J, Packer DL, et al. HRS/EHRA/ECAS expert consensus statement on catheter and surgical ablation of atrial fibrillation: recommendations for personnel, policy, procedures and follow-up. a report of the heart rhythm society (HRS) task force on catheter and surgical ablation of atrial fibrillation developed in partnership with the european heart rhythm association (EHRA) and the European Cardiac Arrhythmia Society (ECAS); in collaboration with the American College of Cardiology (ACC), American Heart Association (AHA), and the Society of Thoracic Surgeons (STS). Endorsed and approved by the governing bodies of the American College of Cardiology, the American Heart Association, the European Cardiac Arrhythmia Society, the European Heart Rhythm Association, the Society of Thoracic Surgeons, and the Heart Rhythm Society. Europace 2007; 9: 335–79.

44. Pappone C, Rosanio S, Augello G, et al. Mortality, morbidity, and quality of life after circumferential pulmonary vein ablation for atrial fibrillation: outcomes from a controlled nonrandomized long-term study. J Am Coll Cardiol 2003; 42: 185–97.

45. Pappone C. Pulmonary vein stenosis after catheter ablation for atrial fibrillation. J Cardiovasc Electrophysiol 2003; 14: 165–7.

46. Hsu LF, Jais P, Sanders P, et al. Catheter ablation for atrial fibrillation in congestive heart failure. N Engl J Med 2004; 351: 2373–83.

47. Khan MN, Jais P, Cummings J, et al. Pulmonary-vein isolation for atrial fibrillation in patients with heart failure. N Engl J Med 2008; 359: 1778–85.

48. Grogan M, Smith HC, Gersh BJ, et al. Left ventricular dysfunction due to atrial fibrillation in patients initially believed to have idiopathic dilated cardiomyopathy. Am J Cardiol 1992; 69: 1570–3.

49. Ueng KC, Tsai TP, Tsai CF, et al. Acute and long-term effects of atrioventricular junction ablation and VVIR pacemaker in symptomatic patients with chronic lone atrial fibrillation and normal ventricular response. J Cardiovasc Electrophysiol 2001; 12: 303–9.

50. Heywood JT. Calcium channel blockers for heart rate control in atrial fibrillation complicated by congestive heart failure. Canadian J Cardiol 1995; 11: 823–6.

51. Brown CS, Mills RM, Conti JB, et al. Clinical improvement after atrioventricular nodal ablation for atrial fibrillation does not correlate with improved ejection fraction. Am J Cardiol 1997; 80: 1090–1.

52. Brignole M, Menozzi C, Gianfranchi L, et al. Assessment of atrioventricular junction ablation and VVIR pacemaker versus pharmacological treatment in patients with heart failure and chronic atrial fibrillation: a randomized, controlled study. Circulation 1998; 98: 953–60.

53. Proclemer A, Della Bella P, Tondo C, et al. Radiofrequency ablation of atrioventricular junction and pacemaker implantation versus modulation of atrioventricular conduction in drug refractory atrial fibrillation. Am J Cardiol 1999; 83: 1437–42.

54. Fitzpatrick AP, Kourouyan HD, Siu A, et al. Quality of life and outcomes after radiofrequency His-bundle catheter ablation and permanent pacemaker implantation: impact of treatment in paroxysmal and established atrial fibrillation. Am Heart J 1996; 131: 499–507.

55. Manolis AG, Katsivas AG, Lazaris EE, et al. Ventricular performance and quality of life in patients who underwent radiofrequency AV junction ablation and permanent pacemaker implantation due to medically refractory atrial tachyarrhythmias. J Interv Card Electrophysiol 1998; 2: 71–6.

56. Levy T, Walker S, Mason M, et al. Importance of rate control or rate regulation for improving exercise capacity and quality of life in patients with permanent atrial fibrillation and normal left ventricular function: a randomised controlled study. Heart 2001; 85: 171–8.

57. Falk RH. Atrial fibrillation. N Engl J Med 2001; 344: 1067–78. [Erratum appears in N Engl J Med 2001; 344: 1876].

58. Edner M, Kim Y, Hansen KN, et al. Prospective study of left ventricular function after radiofrequency ablation of atrioventricular junction in patients with atrial fibrillation. Br Heart J 1995; 74: 261–7.

59. Twidale N, Manda V, Holliday R, et al. Mitral regurgitation after atrioventricular node catheter ablation for atrial fibrillation and heart failure: acute hemodynamic features. Am Heart J 1999; 138: 1166–75.

60. Vanderheyden M, Goethals M, Anguera I, et al. Hemodynamic deterioration following radiofrequency ablation of the atrioventricular conduction system. Pacing Clin Electrophysiol 1997; 20: 2422–8.

61. Geelen P, Brugada J, Andries E, et al. Ventricular fibrillation and sudden death after radiofrequency catheter ablation of the atrioventricular junction. Pacing Clin Electrophysiol 1997; 20: 343–8.

62. Crystal E, Lamy A, Connolly SJ, et al. Left Atrial Appendage Occlusion Study (LAAOS): a randomized clinical trial of left atrial appendage occlusion during routine coronary artery bypass graft surgery for long-term stroke prevention. Am Heart J 2003; 145: 174–8.

63. Corrado G, Sgalambro A, Mantero A, et al. Thromboembolic risk in atrial flutter. The FLASIEC (FLutter Atriale Societa Italiana di Ecografia Cardiovascolare) multicentre study. Eur Heart J 2001; 22: 1042–51.

64. Lanzarotti CJ, Olshansky B. Thromboembolism in chronic atrial flutter: is the risk underestimated? J Am Coll Cardiol 1997; 30: 1506–11.

65. Schmidt H, von der Recke G, Illien S, et al. Prevalence of left atrial chamber and appendage thrombi in patients with atrial flutter and its clinical significance. J Am Coll Cardiol 2001; 38: 778–84.

66. Seidl K, Hauer B, Schwick NG, et al. Risk of thromboembolic events in patients with atrial flutter. Am J Cardiol 1998; 82: 580–3.

67. Wood KA, Eisenberg SJ, Kalman JM, et al. Risk of thromboembolism in chronic atrial flutter. Am J Cardiol 1997; 79: 1043–7.

68. Crijns HJ, Van Gelder IC, Tieleman RG, et al. Long-term outcome of electrical cardioversion in patients with chronic atrial flutter. Heart 1997; 77: 56–61.

69. Natale A, Newby KH, Pisano E, et al. Prospective randomized comparison of antiarrhythmic therapy versus first-line radiofrequency ablation in patients with atrial flutter. J Am Coll Cardiol 2000; 35: 1898–904.

70. Paydak H, Kall JG, Burke MC, et al. Atrial fibrillation after radiofrequency ablation of type I atrial flutter: time to onset, determinants, and clinical course. Circulation 1998; 98: 315–22.

71. Huang DT, Monahan KM, Zimetbaum P, et al. Hybrid pharmacologic and ablative therapy: a novel and effective approach for the management of atrial fibrillation. J Cardiovasc Electrophysiol 1998; 9: 462–9.

72. Solomon SD, Anavekar N, Skali H, et al. Influence of ejection fraction on cardiovascular outcomes in a broad spectrum of heart failure patients. Circulation 2005; 112: 3738–44.

73. Pratt CM, Greenway PS, Schoenfeld MH, et al. Exploration of the precision of classifying sudden cardiac death. Implications for the interpretation of clinical trials. Circulation 1996; 93: 519–24.

74. Uretsky BF, Thygesen K, Armstrong PW, et al. Acute coronary findings at autopsy in heart failure patients with sudden death: results from the assessment of treatment with lisinopril and survival (ATLAS) trial. Circulation 2000; 102: 611–16.

75. Stevenson WG, Sweeney MO. Arrhythmias and sudden death in heart failure. Jpn Circ J 1997; 61: 727–40.

76. Faggiano P, d'Aloia A, Gualeni A, et al. Mechanisms and immediate outcome of in-hospital cardiac arrest in patients with advanced heart failure secondary to ischemic or idiopathic dilated cardiomyopathy. Am J Cardiol 2001; 87: 655–7.

77. Grubman EM, Pavri BB, Shipman T, et al. Cardiac death and stored electrograms in patients with third-generation implantable cardioverter-defibrillators. J Am Coll Cardiol 1998; 32: 1056–62.

78. anonymous. Effect of enalapril on survival in patients with reduced left ventricular ejection fractions and congestive heart failure. The SOLVD Investigators. N Engl J Med 1991; 325: 293–302.

79. anonymous. Effect of metoprolol CR/XL in chronic heart failure: Metoprolol CR/XL Randomised Intervention Trial in Congestive Heart Failure (MERIT-HF). Lancet 1999; 353: 2001–7.

80. Cohn JN, Johnson GR, Shabetai R, et al. Ejection fraction, peak exercise oxygen consumption, cardiothoracic ratio, ventricular arrhythmias, and plasma norepinephrine as determinants of prognosis in heart failure. The V-HeFT VA Cooperative Studies Group. Circulation 1993; 87(6 Suppl): VI5–16.

81. Anonymous. The Cardiac Insufficiency Bisoprolol Study II (CIBIS-II): a randomised trial. Lancet 1999; 353: 9–13.

82. Nagele H, Rodiger W. Sudden death and tailored medical therapy in elective candidates for heart transplantation. J Heart Lung Transplant 1999; 18: 869–76.

83. Uretsky BF, Sheahan RG. Primary prevention of sudden cardiac death in heart failure: will the solution be shocking? J Am Coll Cardiol 1997; 30: 1589–97.

84. Cohn JN, Goldstein SO, Greenberg BH, et al. A dose-dependent increase in mortality with vesnarinone among patients with severe heart failure. Vesnarinone Trial Investigators. N Engl J Med 1998; 339: 1810–16.

85. Pitt B, Poole-Wilson PA, Segal R, et al. Effect of losartan compared with captopril on mortality in patients with symptomatic heart failure: randomised trial–the Losartan Heart Failure Survival Study ELITE II. Lancet 2000; 355: 1582–7.

86. Pitt B, Zannad F, Remme WJ, et al. The effect of spironolactone on morbidity and mortality in patients with severe heart failure. Randomized Aldactone Evaluation Study Investigators. N Engl J Med 1999; 341: 709–17.

87. Teerlink JR, Jalaluddin M, Anderson S, et al. Ambulatory ventricular arrhythmias in patients with heart failure do not specifically predict an increased risk of sudden death. PROMISE (Prospective Randomized Milrinone Survival Evaluation) Investigators. Circulation 2000; 101: 40–6.

88. Stevenson WG, Stevenson LW, Middlekauff HR, et al. Sudden death prevention in patients with advanced ventricular dysfunction. Circulation 1993; 88: 2953–61.

89. Connolly SJ, Gent M, Roberts RS, et al. Canadian implantable defibrillator study (CIDS) : a randomized trial of the implantable cardioverter defibrillator against amiodarone. Circulation 2000; 101: 1297–302.

90. Sheldon R, Connolly S, Krahn A, et al. Identification of patients most likely to benefit from implantable cardioverter-defibrillator therapy: the Canadian Implantable Defibrillator Study. Circulation 2000; 101: 1660–4.

91. Connolly SJ, Hallstrom AP, Cappato R, et al. Meta-analysis of the implantable cardioverter defibrillator secondary prevention trials. AVID, CASH and CIDS studies. Antiarrhythmics vs Implantable Defibrillator study. Cardiac Arrest Study Hamburg. Canadian Implantable Defibrillator Study. Eur Heart J 2000; 21: 2071–8.

92. de Bakker JM, van Capelle FJ, Janse MJ, et al. Slow conduction in the infarcted human heart. 'Zigzag' course of activation. Circulation 1993; 88: 915–26.

93. Stevenson WG, Friedman PL, Sager PT, et al. Exploring postinfarction reentrant ventricular tachycardia with entrainment mapping. J Am Coll Cardiol 1997; 29: 1180–9.

94. Buxton AE, Lee KL, DiCarlo L, et al. A randomized study of the prevention of sudden death in patients with coronary artery disease. Multicenter Unsustained Tachycardia Trial Investigators. N Engl J Med 1999; 341(25): 1882–90. [Erratum appears in N Engl J Med 2000; 342(17): 1300].

95. Moss AJ, Hall WJ, Cannom DS, et al. Improved survival with an implanted defibrillator in patients with coronary disease at high risk for ventricular arrhythmia. Multicenter Automatic Defibrillator Implantation Trial Investigators. N Engl J Med 1996; 335: 1933–40.

96. Stevenson WG, Stevenson LW, Weiss J, et al. Inducible ventricular arrhythmias and sudden death during vasodilator therapy of severe heart failure. Am Heart J 1988; 116: 1447–54.

97. Turitto G, Ahuja RK, Caref EB, et al. Risk stratification for arrhythmic events in patients with nonischemic dilated cardiomyopathy and nonsustained ventricular tachycardia: role of programmed ventricular stimulation and the signal-averaged electrocardiogram. J Am Coll Cardiol 1994; 24: 1523–8.

98. Hammill SC, Trusty JM, Wood DL, et al. Influence of ventricular function and presence or absence of coronary artery disease on results of electrophysiologic testing for asymptomatic nonsustained ventricular tachycardia. Am J Cardiol 1990; 65: 722–8.

99. Lindsay BD, Osborn JL, Schechtman KB, et al. Prospective detection of vulnerability to sustained ventricular tachycardia in patients awaiting cardiac transplantation. Am J Cardiol 1992; 69: 619–24.

100. Das SK, Morady F, DiCarlo L, et al. Prognostic usefulness of programmed ventricular stimulation in idiopathic dilated cardiomyopathy without symptomatic ventricular arrhythmias. Am J Cardiol 1986; 58: 998–1000.

101. Meinertz T, Treese N, Kasper W, et al. Determinants of prognosis in idiopathic dilated cardiomyopathy as determined by programmed electrical stimulation. Am J Cardiol 1985; 56: 337–41.

102. Poll DS, Marchlinski FE, Buxton AE, et al. Usefulness of programmed stimulation in idiopathic dilated cardiomyopathy. Am J Cardiol 1986; 58: 992–7.

103. Delacretaz E, Stevenson WG, Ellison KE, et al. Mapping and radiofrequency catheter ablation of the three types of sustained monomorphic ventricular tachycardia in nonischemic heart disease. J Cardiovasc Electrophysiol 2000; 11: 11–17.

104. Nazarian S, Bluemke DA, Lardo AC, et al. Magnetic resonance assessment of the substrate for inducible ventricular tachycardia in nonischemic cardiomyopathy. Circulation 2005; 112: 2821–5.

105. Ellison KE, Friedman PL, Ganz LI, et al. Entrainment mapping and radiofrequency catheter ablation of ventricular tachycardia in right ventricular dysplasia. J Am Coll Cardiol 1998; 32: 724–8.

106. Pinski SL. The right ventricular tachycardias. J Electrocardiol 2000; 33(Suppl): 103–14.

107. Corrado D, Basso C, Thiene G, et al. Spectrum of clinicopathologic manifestations of arrhythmogenic right ventricular cardiomyopathy/dysplasia: a multicenter study. J Am Coll Cardiol 1997; 30: 1512–20.

108. Anonymous. Case records of the Massachusetts General Hospital. Weekly clinicopathological exercises. Case 20-2000. A 61-year-old man with a wide-complex tachycardia. N EnglJ Med 2000; 342: 1979–87.

109. Marcus FI, Fontaine G. Arrhythmogenic right ventricular dysplasia/cardiomyopathy: a review. Pacing Clin Electrophysiol 1995; 18: 1298–314.

110. Fontaine G, Fontaliran F, Hebert JL, et al. Arrhythmogenic right ventricular dysplasia. Annu Rev Med 1999; 50: 17–35.

111. Inoue S, Shinohara F, Sakai T, et al. Myocarditis and arrhythmia: a clinico-pathological study of conduction system based on serial section in 65 cases. Jpn Circ J 1989; 53: 49–57.

112. Delacretaz E, Stevenson WG, Winters GL, et al. Ablation of ventricular tachycardia with a saline-cooled radiofrequency catheter: anatomic and histologic characteristics of the lesions in humans. J Cardiovasc Electrophysiol 1999; 10: 860–5.

113. de Bakker JM, van Capelle FJ, Janse MJ, et al. Fractionated electrograms in dilated cardiomyopathy: origin and relation to abnormal conduction. J Am Coll Cardiol 1996; 27: 1071–8.

114. Lopera G, Stevenson WG, Soejima K, et al. Identification and ablation of three types of ventricular tachycardia involving the his-purkinje system in patients with heart disease. J Cardiovasc Electrophysiol 2004; 15:52–8.

115. Woelfel A, Wohns DH, Foster JR. Implications of sustained monomorphic ventricular tachycardia associated with myocardial injury. Ann Intern Med 1990; 112: 141–3.

116. Soejima K, Suzuki M, Maisel WH, et al. Catheter ablation in patients with multiple and unstable ventricular tachycardias after myocardial infarction: short ablation lines guided by reentry circuit isthmuses and sinus rhythm mapping. Circulation 2001; 104: 664–9.

117. Poole JE, Johnson GW, Hellkamp AS, et al. Prognostic importance of defibrillator shocks in patients with heart failure. N Engl J Med 2008; 359: 1009–17.

118. Passman R, Kadish A. Polymorphic ventricular tachycardia, long Q-T syndrome, and torsades de pointes. Med Clin North America 2001; 85: 321–41.

119. Torp-Pedersen C, Møller M, Bloch-Thomsen PE, et al. Dofetilide in patients with congestive heart failure and left ventricular dysfunction. Danish Investigations of Arrhythmia and Mortality on Dofetilide Study Group. N Engl J Med 1999; 341: 857–65.

120. Kowey PR, VanderLugt JT, Luderer JR. Safety and risk/benefit analysis of ibutilide for acute conversion of atrial fibrillation/flutter. Am J Cardiol 1996; 78: 46–52.

121. Mazur A, Anderson ME, Bonney S, et al. Pause-dependent polymorphic ventricular tachycardia during long-term treatment with dofetilide: a placebo-controlled, implantable cardioverter-defibrillator-based evaluation. J Am Coll Cardiol 2001; 37: 1100–5.

122. Maor N, Weiss D, Lorber A. Torsade de pointes complicating atrioventricular block: report of two cases. Int J Cardiol 1987; 14: 235–8.

123. Tomaselli GF, Rose J. Molecular aspects of arrhythmias associated with cardiomyopathies. Curr Opin Cardiol 2000; 15: 202–8.

124. Middlekauff HR, Stevenson WG, Saxon LA, et al. Amiodarone and torsades de pointes in patients with advanced heart failure. Am J Cardiol 1995; 76: 499–502.

125. Viskin S. Cardiac pacing in the long QT syndrome: review of available data and practical recommendations. J Cardiovasc Electrophysiol 2000; 11: 593–600.

126. Middlekauff HR, Stevenson WG, Stevenson LW, et al. Syncope in advanced heart failure: high risk of sudden death regardless of origin of syncope. J Am Coll Cardiol 1993; 21: 110–16.

127. Knight BP, Goyal R, Pelosi F, et al. Outcome of patients with nonischemic dilated cardiomyopathy and unexplained syncope treated with an implantable defibrillator. J Am Coll Cardiol 1999; 33: 1964–70.

128. Fonarow GC, Feliciano Z, Boyle NG, et al. Improved survival in patients with nonischemic advanced heart failure and syncope treated with an implantable cardioverter-defibrillator. Am J Cardiol 2000; 85: 981–5.

129. Fruhwald FM, Eber B, Schumacher M, et al. Syncope in dilated cardiomyopathy is a predictor of sudden cardiac death. Cardiology 1996; 87: 177–80.

130. Moss AJ, Hall WJ, Cannom DS, et al. Improved survival with an implanted defibrillator in patients with coronary disease at high risk for ventricular arrhythmia. Multicenter Automatic Defibrillator Implantation Trial Investigators. N Engl J Med 1996; 335: 1933–40.

131. Buxton AE, Lee KL, Fisher JD, et al. A randomized study of the prevention of sudden death in patients with coronary artery disease. Multicenter Unsustained Tachycardia Trial Investigators. N Engl J Med 1999; 341: 1882–90.

132. Kadish A, Dyer A, Daubert JP, et al. Prophylactic defibrillator implantation in patients with nonischemic dilated cardiomyopathy. N Engl J Med 2004; 350: 2151–8.

133. Epstein AE, DiMarco JP, Ellenbogen KA, et al. ACC/AHA/HRS 2008 Guidelines for Device-Based Therapy of Cardiac Rhythm Abnormalities: a report of the American College of Cardiology/American Heart Association Task Force on Practice Guidelines (Writing Committee to Revise the ACC/AHA/NASPE 2002 Guideline Update for Implantation of Cardiac Pacemakers and Antiarrhythmia Devices): developed in collaboration with the American Association for Thoracic Surgery and Society of Thoracic Surgeons. Circulation 2008; 117: e350–408.

134. Goldberger JJ, Cain ME, Hohnloser SH, et al. American Heart Association/American College of Cardiology Foundation/Heart Rhythm Society scientific statement on noninvasive risk stratification techniques for identifying patients at risk for sudden cardiac death: a scientific statement from the American Heart Association Council on Clinical Cardiology Committee on Electrocardiography and Arrhythmias and Council on Epidemiology and Prevention. Circulation 2008; 118: 1497–518.

135. Moss AJ. MADIT-II and implications for noninvasive electrophysiologic testing. Ann Noninvasive Electrocardiol 2002; 7: 179–80.

136. Chow T, Joshi D. Microvolt T-wave alternans testing for ventricular arrhythmia risk stratification. Expert Rev Cardiovasc Ther 2008; 6: 833–42.

137. Gold MR, Ip JH, Costantini O, et al. Role of microvolt T-wave alternans in assessment of arrhythmia vulnerability among patients with heart failure and systolic dysfunction: primary results from the T-wave alternans sudden cardiac death in heart failure trial substudy. Circulation 2008; 118: 2022–8.

138. Buxton AE, Lee KL, Hafley GE, et al. Limitations of ejection fraction for prediction of sudden death risk in patients with coronary artery disease: lessons from the MUSTT study. J Am Coll Cardiol 2007; 50: 1150–7.

139. Singh SN, Fisher SG, Carson PE, et al. Prevalence and significance of nonsustained ventricular tachycardia in patients with premature ventricular contractions and heart failure treated with vasodilator therapy. Department of Veterans Affairs CHF STAT Investigators. J Am Coll Cardiol 1998; 32: 942–7.

140. Doval HC, Nul DR, Grancelli HO, et al. Nonsustained ventricular tachycardia in severe heart failure. Independent marker of increased mortality due to sudden death. GESICA-GEMA Investigators. Circulation 1996; 94: 3198–203.

141. Davies SW, John LM, Wedzicha JA, et al. Overnight studies in severe chronic left heart failure: arrhythmias and oxygen desaturation. Br Heart J 1991; 65: 77–83.

142. Javaheri S. Effects of continuous positive airway pressure on sleep apnea and ventricular irritability in patients with heart failure. Circulation 2000; 101: 392–7.

143. Javaheri S, Corbett WS. Association of low PaCO2 with central sleep apnea and ventricular arrhythmias in ambulatory patients with stable heart failure. Ann Intern Med 1998; 128: 204–7.

144. Javaheri S, Parker TJ, Liming JD, et al. Sleep apnea in 81 ambulatory male patients with stable heart failure. Types and their prevalences, consequences, and presentations. Circulation 1998; 97:2 154–9.

145. Yarlagadda RK, Iwai S, Stein KM, et al. Reversal of cardiomyopathy in patients with repetitive monomorphic ventricular ectopy originating from the right ventricular outflow tract. Circulation 2005; 112: 1092–7.

146. Bogun F, Crawford T, Reich S, et al. Radiofrequency ablation of frequent, idiopathic premature ventricular complexes: comparison with a control group without intervention. Heart Rhythm 2007; 4: 863–7.

147. Gregoratos G, Abrams J, Epstein AE, et al. ACC/AHA/NASPE 2002 guideline update for implantation of cardiac pacemakers and antiarrhythmia devices: summary article: a report of the American College of Cardiology/American Heart Association Task Force on Practice Guidelines (ACC/AHA/NASPE Committee to Update the 1998 Pacemaker Guidelines). Circulation 2002; 106: 2145–61.

148. Goldenberg I, Moss AJ, Hall WJ, et al. Causes and consequences of heart failure after prophylactic implantation of a defibrillator in the multicenter automatic defibrillator implantation trial II. Circulation 2006; 113:2810–17.

149. Causes of death in the Antiarrhythmics Versus Implantable Defibrillators (AVID) Trial. J Am Coll Cardiol 1999; 34: 1552–9.

150. Bocker D, Bansch D, Heinecke A, et al. Potential benefit from implantable cardioverter-defibrillator therapy in patients with and without heart failure. Circulation 1998; 98: 1636–43.

151. Mecca A, Barakat T, Guo H, et al. Implantable cardioverter defibrillator therapy for patients with life- threatening ventricular arrhythmias and severe heart failure. Am J Cardiol 2000; 86: 875–7.

152. Saxon LA, Wiener I, DeLurqio DB, et al. Implantable defibrillators for high-risk patients with heart failure who are awaiting cardiac transplantation. Am Heart J 1995; 130: 501–6.

153. Sweeney MO, Ruskin JN, Garan H, et al. Influence of the implantable cardioverter/defibrillator on sudden death and total mortality in patients evaluated for cardiac transplantation. Circulation 1995; 92: 3273–81.

154. Best PJ, Hayes DL, Stanton MS. The potential usage of dual chamber pacing in patients with implantable cardioverter defibrillators. Pacing Clin Electrophysiol 1999; 22: 79–85.

155. Grines CL, Bashore TM, Boudoulas H, et al. Functional abnormalities in isolated left bundle branch block. The effect of interventricular asynchrony. Circulation 1989; 79: 845–53.

156. Nielsen JC, Bøttcher M, Nielsen TT, et al. Regional myocardial blood flow in patients with sick sinus syndrome randomized to long-term single chamber atrial or dual chamber pacing–effect of pacing mode and rate. J Am Coll Cardiol 2000; 35: 1453–61.

157. Tse HF, Lau CP. Long-term effect of right ventricular pacing on myocardial perfusion and function. J Am Coll Cardiol 1997; 29: 744–9.

158. Wilkoff BL, Cook JR, Epstein AE, et al. Dual-chamber pacing or ventricular backup pacing in patients with an implantable defibrillator: the Dual Chamber and VVI Implantable Defibrillator (DAVID) Trial. JAMA 2002; 288: 3115–23.

159. Spotnitz HM. Does ventricular fibrillation cause myocardial stunning during defibrillator implantation? J Card Surg 1993; 8: 249–56.

160. Pires LA, Lehmann MH, Steinman RT, et al. Sudden death in implantable cardioverter-defibrillator recipients: clinical context, arrhythmic events and device responses. J Am Coll Cardiol 1999; 33: 24–32.

161. Villacastin J, Almendral J, Arenal A, et al. Incidence and clinical significance of multiple consecutive, appropriate, high-energy discharges in patients with implanted cardioverter-defibrillators. Circulation 1996; 93: 753–62.

162. Exner DV, Pinski SL, Wyse DG, et al. Electrical Storm Presages Nonsudden Death: The Antiarrhythmics Versus Implantable Defibrillators (AVID) Trial. Circulation 2001; 103: 2066–71.

163. Mark DB, Anstrom KJ, Sun JL, et al. Quality of life with defibrillator therapy or amiodarone in heart failure. N Engl J Med 2008; 359: 999–1008.

164. Moss AJ, Greenberg H, Case RB, et al. Long-term clinical course of patients after termination of ventricular tachyarrhythmia by an implanted defibrillator. Circulation 2004; 110: 3760–5.

165. Daubert JP, Zareba W, Cannom DS, et al. Inappropriate implantable cardioverter-defibrillator shocks in MADIT II: frequency, mechanisms, predictors, and survival impact. J Am Coll Cardiol 2008; 51: 1357–65.

166. Stevenson WG, Soejima K. Catheter ablation for ventricular tachycardia. Circulation 2007; 115: 2750–60.

167. Hohnloser SH, Al-Khalidi HR, Pratt CM, et al. Electrical storm in patients with an implantable defibrillator: incidence, features, and preventive therapy: insights from a randomized trial. Eur Heart J 2006; 27:3027–32.

168. Exner DV, Pinski SL, Wyse DG, et al. Electrical storm presages nonsudden death: the antiarrhythmics versus implantable defibrillators (AVID) trial. Circulation 2001; 103: 2066–71.

169. Hohnloser SH, Dorian P, Roberts R, et al. Effect of amiodarone and sotalol on ventricular defibrillation threshold: the optimal pharmacological therapy in cardioverter defibrillator patients (OPTIC) trial. Circulation 2006; 114: 104–9.

170. Thomas SA, Friedmann E, Kelley FJ. Living with an implantable cardioverter-defibrillator: a review of the current literature related to psychosocial factors. AACN Clin Issues 2001; 12: 156–63.

171. Sears SF, Todaro JF, Urizar G, et al. Assessing the psychosocial impact of the ICD: a national survey of implantable cardioverter defibrillator health care providers. Pacing Clin Electrophysiol 2000; 23: 939–45.

172. Dunbar SB, Kimble LP, Jenkins LS, et al. Association of mood disturbance and arrhythmia events in patients after cardioverter defibrillator implantation. Depression Anxiety 1999; 9: 163–8.

173. Heller SS, Ormont MA, Lidagoster L, et al. Psychosocial outcome after ICD implantation: a current perspective. Pacing Clin Electrophysiol 1998; 21: 1207–15.

174. Fricchione GL, Vlay LC, Vlay SC. Cardiac psychiatry and the management of malignant ventricular arrhythmias with the internal cardioverter-defibrillator. Am Heart J 1994; 128: 1050–9.

25

Ultrafiltration for the management of volume overload

Bradley A. Bart

INTRODUCTION
Most of the signs and symptoms of heart failure are attributable to fluid overload. Patients with persistent congestion remain symptomatic and are at increased risk for prolonged hospitalization, rehospitalization, and death. Therefore, effective volume reduction therapies are needed to address the morbidity and mortality of heart failure. Diuretics relieve symptoms in the majority of heart failure patients, yet they are difficult to use and rarely result in complete clinical decongestion. Ultrafiltration, the mechanical removal of fluid directly from the vasculature, has been used in heart failure patients for over 30 years. Originally reserved only for patients with refractory heart failure, ultrafiltration is increasingly being used in a less sick population as an early therapy in for decompensated heart failure. This chapter reviews ultrafiltration for the management of fluid overload in heart failure.

CONGESTION IS THE PRIMARY THERAPEUTIC TARGET IN DECOMPENSATED HEART FAILURE
The majority of patients hospitalized for heart failure have symptoms of congestion attributable to fluid overload (1). Their hospital admission is often preceded by increases in weight indicating progressive fluid overload (2). Persistent congestion in the hospital and after discharge is associated with increased morbidity and mortality (3–7). Failure to achieve complete clinical decongestion may be one of the most important reasons why the rate of death or rehospitalization is as high as it is (30–60% within 60 days from a heart failure admission) (8). For these reasons, relief of congestion is perhaps the most important therapeutic goal for patients hospitalized with decompensated heart failure. Effective volume removal strategies could substantially reduce the morbidity and mortality of decompensated heart failure and decrease the $47 billion cost associated with caring for patients with this condition (9).

Most hospitalized patients with heart failure (up to 90%) receive diuretics in an attempt to reduce congestion; however, nearly half of these patients experience little or no weight loss at the time of hospital discharge (10). Therefore, health care providers need better ways of managing fluid overload in hospitalized patients with heart failure.

TREATMENT OF CONGESTION
Traditional Approaches to Fluid Overload
Purgatives, cathartics, leeches, and fluid restriction have been used effectively to relieve symptoms of fluid overload for millennia (11,12). Oral loop diuretics were introduced in

the middle of the 20th century and have been the mainstay of therapy for fluid overload ever since (13–15). Unfortunately, diuretics are often difficult to use due to significant dose variability, electrolyte depletion, and the frequent development of diuretic resistance (14,16–19). However, in the absence of other effective approaches to treating fluid overload, these limitations have been accepted by generations of healthcare providers (Table 25.1). There is a strong and consistent association between higher doses of diuretics and increased mortality (16,20–22). Whether this is due to indication bias is unclear. However, diuretics directly stimulate the sympathetic nervous system, decrease renal blood flow, contribute to functional and structural remodeling of nephron architecture (23) and may contribute to the development of left ventricular dysfunction (24). These physiologic responses could partially explain poor outcomes in patients receiving high doses of diuretics.

Ultrafiltration for Treatment of Congestion in Heart Failure

Ultrafiltration is the mechanical removal of fluid from the vasculature. Plasma water is separated from blood by convective solute transport (Fig. 25.1). Hydrostatic pressure is applied to blood across a semi-permeable membrane to create plasma water that is iso-osmotic with blood (23,25,26). Ultrafiltration differs from dialysis and hemofiltration. In dialysis, the movement of solutes and fluid is driven by a concentration gradient rather than a hydrostatic gradient resulting in significant shifting of solutes, particularly sodium and potassium. Hemofiltration is similar to ultrafiltration except that fluid and solutes are replaced during hemofiltration (26). The direct removal of fluid and solute from the vasculature during ultrafiltration allows for large amounts of fluid to be removed

Table 25.1   Limitations to the Use of Loop Diuretics for Decompensated Heart Failure

Variable dose response
Acquired resistance
Electrolyte depletion
Neurohormonal activation
Reduced glomerular filtration rate
Association with increased mortality

Abbreviation: GFR, glomerular filtration rate.

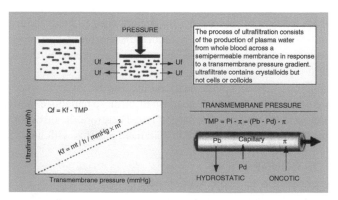

Figure 25.1   Convective solute transport occurs during ultrafiltration when blood is exposed to a semipermeable membrane under hydrostatic forces. Plasma water removed is iso-osmotic with blood. *Source*: From Ref. 26.

at the discretion of the treating physician—in contrast to the unpredictable urine output following treatment with diuretics. In addition, because plasma water removed during ultrafiltration is iso-osmotic with blood, there is no change in the serum concentration of electrolytes or other solutes. Ultrafiltration does not directly stimulate the sympathetic nervous system and may have beneficial effects on symptoms, progression of disease, and prognosis (Table 25.2).

CLINICAL EXPERIENCE WITH ULTRAFILTRATION
Case Series

The technique of ultrafiltration was first reported by Silverstein in 1974 (27). Since then, numerous uncontrolled case series have been published (28–33). In addition to removing large volumes of iso-osmotic fluid, ultrafiltration relieves symptoms of congestion and improves exercise capacity (34–37). Symptomatic relief may be related to improved cardiac filling pressures (30,31,34,35,38,39) and favorable effects on pulmonary function and ventilatory efficiency (35–37,40). In contrast to diuretics, ultrafiltration increases renal perfusion (41), increases diuretic responsiveness (31,42–45), and improves plasma neurohormone levels including norepinephrine, renin, and aldosterone (Table 25.3) (41,43,45).

Controlled Trials in Chronic Heart Failure

Seven randomized controlled trials of ultrafiltration have been published (Table 25.4). The first two trials randomized stable patients with mild heart failure to ultrafiltration or continued medical care (35,37). All patients were stabilized in a clinical research unit prior to randomization. Patients randomized to ultrafiltration experienced fluid removal at a rate of 500 cc/hour until right atrial pressure decreased 50% from baseline (usually 1–2 liters over 2–4 hours). Compared with control, patients treated with ultrafiltration experienced improvements in hemodynamics, neurohormonal responsiveness, pulmonary function, diastolic filling patterns, and exercise capacity. These changes were apparent immediately following ultrafiltration and persisted for up to six months (35,37).

The same investigative team subsequently performed a similar trial with an active control arm (34). Sixteen patients with stable, mild heart failure were randomized to fluid removal with ultrafiltration or IV furosemide given as a bolus followed by a continuous infusion. Both treatment groups were treated until there was a 50% decrease in right atrial pressure. The average volume removed in the ultrafiltration and furosemide groups were 1710 mL and 1460 mL, respectively; the average dose of furosemide received by patients in the active control arm was 248 mg. Acutely, there were significant decreases in right atrial pressure and pulmonary capillary wedge pressure in both treatment groups. However, filling pressures rapidly returned to baseline in the furosemide group while they remained decreased in the ultrafiltration group. In addition, patients in the ultrafiltration group had a significant and sustained improvement in exercise capacity, measured by peak oxygen

Table 25.2 Potential Advantages to Ultrafiltration for Decompensated Heart Failure

Predictable amount and rate of fluid removal
No electrolyte depletion
No direct stimulation of the sympathetic nervous system
Improved diuresis, natriuresis, and diuretic responsiveness
Improved outcomes

Table 25.3 Clinical Experience with Ultrafiltration for Heart Failure-Case Studies

Study	n	Population	Type of Therapy	UF Fluid Removal	Clinical Effects
Silverstein 1974 (27)	5	HF and end-stage renal failure	CAVH	3.6 L removed in a single session	Hypotension, leg cramps, and headaches occurred at UF rates of 400–500 mL/hr and were reversible with decreasing the UF rate.
Asaba H 1978 (32)	9	Volume overload state with diuretic resistance (3 pts with HF)	CVVUF	5.5 L removed in a single session	Improved symptoms, transient fall in blood pressure
Simpson 1986 (28)	9	Class IV HF with diuretic resistance	CVVUF	12.7 L removed during 2.9 sessions/patient, UF continued until muscle cramps or hypotension occurred	Sustained weight loss, improved diuretic response, transient hypotension, stable creatinine, stable hemodynamics, no change in PCWP, transient decrease in RA pressure.
Fauchald, 1986 (30)	6	Class IV HF refractory to medical therapy	CVVUF with hypertonic saline replacement	7.75 L removed during two sessions over 2 days	Reduced plasma volume, transient decrease in filling pressures, and transient increase in SVR; stable hemodynamics
Simpson, 1987 (29)	13	Class IV HF with diuretic resistance	CVVUF	3.7–23 L removed in 1–2 sessions	Transient decrease in RA pressure, stable hemodynamics, symptomatic improvement.
DiLeo M 1988 (33)	19	Acute and chronic HF refractory to medical therapy	CVVUF (2 peritoneal dialysis)	1.68–3.5 L removed per session over an average of 125 sessions/patient	Improved symptoms, restored diuretic responsiveness
Rimondini, 1987 (31)	11	Class IV HF refractory to medical therapy	CVVUF	2–3 L removed in a single session	Increased urine output and diuretic responsiveness, decreased filling pressures, stable hemodynamics.
Cipolla 1990 (43)	23	Class III–IV HF	CVVUF	2.98 L removed in single session with a goal of reducing RAP to 4–8 or causing an increase in HCT	Stable hemodynamics, decreased filling pressures, increased diuresis and natriuresis, stable renal function, decreased PNE
Canaud 1991 (42)	35	Class IV HF, refractory to medically therapy	CVVUF	4.3 L removed per day for 3 days	Improved diuresis and natriuresis, transient increase in creatinine, improved shortening index and ejection fraction

Study	N	Population	Technique	Fluid removed	Outcomes
Forslund 1992 (44)	5	Class IV HF, <6 month anticipated survival, on transplant list	CVVUF with hypertonic saline replacement	3.31 L removed in a single session	Transient improvement in hemodynamics, transient increase in PRA and ADH, no change in ANP or aldosterone
Marenzi 1993 (41)	32	Class II–IV HF with fluid overload	CVVUF	UF performed until RAP reached 50% of baseline	Variable responses in hemodynamics, neurohormones, diuresis, and renal function depending on baseline volume status
Guazzi 1994 (45)	22	Class III–IV HF with fluid overload	CVVUF	3.1 L removed in a single session	Transient decrease in hemodynamics, decreased filling pressures, decreased neurohormones, increased diuresis and natriuresis
Agostoni 1995 (36)	21	Stable class II–III HF	CVVUF	1.77 L removed in a single session	Improved exercise capacity, dynamic lung compliance, and hemodynamics
Wei 1995 (101)	7	HF with diuretic resistance and impaired renal function	CVVUF	2.19 L removed per session	Stable hemodynamics
Ramos 1996 (102)	30	HF refractory to medical therapy and renal failure	CVVUF	9.6 L removed from responders, 3.2 L from nonresponders during 2.4 treatments	Improved renal function, decreased filling pressures, transient hypotension, otherwise stable hemodynamics
Dormans 1996 (88)	12	Severe chronic HF refractory to medical therapy	Hemofiltration in 10, hemodialysis in 2	8.5 kg weight loss during 38 sessions/patients (1–113)	Poor outcomes, median survival 24 days
Agostoni, 2000 (40)	28	Stable chronic HF	CVVUF	3.97 L removed in a single session	Improved pulmonary volumes and mechanics, lower filling pressures, stable hemodynamics, improved symptoms
Marenzi 2001 (39)	24	Class IV HF refractory to medical therapy	CVVUF	4.88 L removed in a single session	Improved symptoms, improved diuresis, and diuretic responsiveness, stable hemodynamics, decreased filling pressures

(continued)

Table 25.3 (cont.) Clinical Experience with Ultrafiltration for Heart Failure-Case Studies

Study	n	Population	Type of Therapy	UF Fluid Removal	Clinical Effects
Jaski, 2003 (48)	21	Fluid overload and history of cardiovascular disease	CVVUF[a]	2.6 L removed in a single session	Stable hemodynamics and renal function
Sheppard 2004 (100)	19	Outpatients with refractory HF and diuretic resistance	Peritoneal dialysis in 5, hemofiltration in 14	Details not available	Improved symptoms, decreased use of inotropes, 7 deaths over 1 year, survivors had fewer hospitalizations
Costanzo, 2005 (103)	20	Hospitalized decompensated HF with renal insufficieny or diuretic resistance	CVVUF[a]	8.65 L removed over 3.7 days	Improved symptoms, stable hemodynamics and renal function, reduced neurohormones, reduced hospitalizations
Dahle, 2006 (87)	9	Hospitalized decompensated HF	CVVUF[a]	7 L removed over 33 hrs	Clinical improvement, stable renal function
Liang 2006 (89)	11	Hospitalized decompensated HF with diuretic resistance	CVVUF[a]	Goal of 4 L over 8 hrs for 1–5 days	Stable hemodynamics and creatinine, high morbidity and mortality
Jaski 2008 (104)	100	Hospitalized with HF as primary or secondary diagnosis	CVVUF[a]	7.0 L removed in 2.2 days	Significant weight loss, stable renal function, no device-related complications

Hemodynamics refers to heart rate, mean arterial pressure, and cardiac output; Filling pressure refers to right atrial, pulmonary artery, and pulmonary capillary wedge pressure.
[a]Ultrafiltration performed using Aquedex System 100 (CHF Solutions, Minneapolis, Minnesota, USA).
Abbreviations: ADH, antidiuretic hormone; ANP, atrionatriuretic peptide; CAVH, continuous arteriovenous hemofiltration; CVVUF, continuous venovenous ultrafiltration; HF, heart failure; PCWP, pulmonary capillary wedge pressure; PNE, plasma norepinephrine; PRA, plasma; renin activity; RA, right atrial; SVR, systemic vascular resistance; UF, ultrafiltration.

Table 25.4 Clinical Experience with Ultrafiltration for Heart Failure-Randomized Controlled Trials

Study	n	Population	Type of Therapy	Weight loss and Volume Effects	Laboratory and Clinical Effects
Pepi 1993 (37)	24	Stable HF	CVVUF at 600 mL/hr until RA pressure reached 50% of baseline vs. control	1.93 L removed in a single session from UF group	Increased peak oxygen consumption and exercise capacity, stable hemodynamics, decreased filling pressures, change in diastolic filling pattern, decreased radiographic lung congestion
Agostoni, 1993 (35)	36	Stable class II–III HF	CVVUF at 600 mL/hr until RA pressure reached 50% of baseline vs. control	1.88 L removed in single session from UF group	Increased peak oxygen consumption and exercise capacity, decreased neurohormones, decreased radiographic lung congestion
Agostoni, 1994 (34)	16	Stable class II–III HF	CVVUF at 500 mL/hr until RA pressure reached 50% of baseline vs. IV furosemide to achieve a similar fall in RA pressure	1.71 L removed in single UF session vs. 1.46 L with IV furosemide	Sustained improvements in filling pressures, exercise capacity, weight loss in ultrafiltration group vs. IV furosemide
Bart, 2005 (RAPID) (46)	40	Hospitalized patients with decompensated HF	CVVUF[a] vs. Standard care with diuretics	4.65 L (total) removed over 24 hours in UF group vs. 2.84 L removed in standard care group	Decreased dyspnea, HF symptoms and a trend toward greater weight loss in UF group vs. standard care, renal function and hemodynamics were stable in both groups
Costanzo 2007 (UNLOAD) (47)	200	Hospitalized patients with decompensated HF	CVVUF[a] vs. Standard care with diuretics	4.6 L (net) fluid removed over 48 hrs in UF group vs. 3.3 L removed in standard care group	Greater volume removal and weight loss, few rehospitalizations in UF group vs. standard care, renal function and hemodynamics were stable in both groups
Giglioli 2011 (49)	30	Hospitalized patients with decompensated HF	CVVUF vs. continuous infusion of IV furosemide	7.3% weight loss at end of treatment in UF group vs. 6.7% in IV furosemide group (NS)	Improved signs and symptoms, decreased plasma aldosterone and NT-proBNP levels, improved stroke volume, cardiac index in UF group vs IV furosemide

(continued)

Table 25.4 (cont.) Clinical Experience with Ultrafiltration for Heart Failure-Randomized Controlled Trials

Study	n	Population	Type of Therapy	Weight loss and Volume Effects	Laboratory and Clinical Effects
Mazen 2012 (105)	36	Hospitalized patients with decompensated HF admitted for hemodynamic monitoring	CVVUF vs. standard care with diuretics	5.2 L (total) fluid removed in UF group vs. 2.2 L removed in standard care group	Greater volume removal and a shorter time to discharge in UF group vs. standard care, no difference in renal function, hemodynamics, or rehospitalizations between both groups
CARRESS-HF Trial 2012 (74)	188	Hospitalized patients with HF and worsening renal function	CVVUF[a] vs. stepped pharmacologic care	Results not available at time of publishing	Results not available at time of publishing

[a]Ultrafiltration performed using Aquedex System 100 (CHF Solutions, Minneapolis Minnesota, USA).

Abbreviations: CVVUF, continuous venovenous ultrafiltration; IV, intravenous HF, heart failure; RA, right atrial; SCUF, slow continuous ultrafiltration.

consumption, whereas no such sustained improvement was observed in the furosemide group (Fig. 25.2). The authors state in their discussion that the clinical benefit following ultrafiltration does not appear to be solely related to the amount of fluid removed. Rather, the method of fluid removal or the content of the fluid removed may be more important. The lack of sustained benefit in the furosemide group may be explained, in part, by enhanced sodium retention following diuresis (14).

Controlled Trials in Decompensated Heart Failure

Ultrafiltration is safe and effective when used as an early treatment strategy for hospitalized patients with decompensated heart failure (46,47). In an early feasibility study, 40 patients

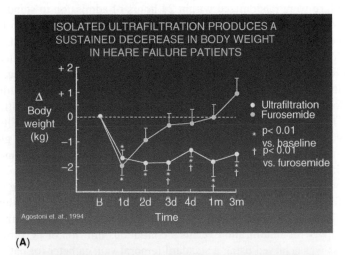

(A)

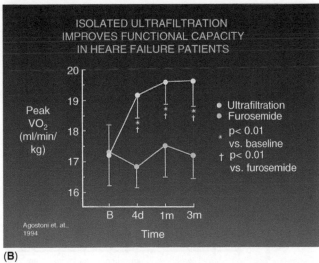

(B)

Figure 25.2 Changes in body weight and peak oxygen consumption in heart failure patients undergoing ultrafiltration or diuresis to achieve a 50% reduction in right atrial pressure (34). 16 patients with stable heart failure for at least 6 months, class II or III heart failure symptoms and no overt evidence of volume overload. Basal assessments were made in an ultrafiltration or IV Lasix was given. Ultrafiltration was performed at a rate of 500 mL per hour and continued until class I was a 50% drop in mean right intro pressure-the average food removal was 1710 mL. Furosemide was given as an intravenous bolus of 160 mg followed by continuous infusion until the same hemodynamic endpoint was met.

admitted for decompensated heart failure were randomized within 24 hours of admission to usual care with IV diuretics versus early ultrafiltration. Patients in the ultrafiltration group had all diuretics stopped at the time of randomization and underwent a single, eight-hour ultrafiltration session using a minimally invasive device and peripheral IV access (46,48). Compared with standard care with diuretics, ultrafiltration resulted in greater weight loss (NS), total fluid removal, and symptom relief at 24 and 48 hours (46). There were no significant changes in creatinine, heart rate, or blood pressure between the treatment groups.

Based on these promising results, a larger trial (Ultrafiltration versus Intravenous Diuretics for Patients Hospitalized for Acute Decompensated Heart Failure—the UNLOAD trial) was performed (47). In this trial, patients hospitalized with decompensated heart failure were randomized within 24 hours of admission to standard care with IV diuretics versus ultrafiltration. The fluid status of patients in the ultrafiltration group was managed exclusively by ultrafiltration (all diuretics were discontinued) for 48 hours (47). Weight loss at 48 hours, the primary endpoint of the study, was significantly greater for the ultrafiltration group compared with standard care (5.0 vs. 3.1 kg, p = 0.001). Importantly, the prespecified secondary endpoint of rehospitalizations within 90 days of the index hospitalization was significantly improved in the ultrafiltration group (Fig. 25.3). There was a slight increase in serum creatinine in the ultrafiltration group (NS); there were no significant differences in self-reported symptoms, in global assessment and Minnesota Living with Heart Failure scores, 6-minute walk distance, BNP levels, or mortality.

In another study, the acute hemodynamic effects of ultrafiltration were studied using arterial waveform analysis. In this randomized, single-center study, 30 patients hospitalized for acute heart failure with evidence of volume overload were randomized to volume reduction therapy with ultrafiltration versus a continuous infusion of IV furosemide (49). Vascular access was achieved using a standard femoral vein catheter for patients randomized to ultrafiltration. The fluid removal rate ranged from 100 to 300 mL per hour and was adjusted according to systolic blood pressure and clinical score (determined by the presence of signs and symptoms). Patients randomized to receive a continuous infusion of IV furosemide were treated with an initial dose of 250 mg/24 hrs. Furosemide doses were adjusted thereafter with the goal of achieving a negative fluid balance of at least 2000 mL per day. The treatment endpoint for both ultrafiltration and IV furosemide patients was based on a clinical score rating the degree of congestion.

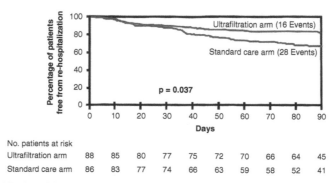

Figure 25.3 Kaplan–Meier survival curve for heart failure rehospitalizations within 90 days of discharge from index hospitalization in heart failure patients randomized to early ultrafiltration versus standard care with intravenous diuretics (47).

At the end of the active treatment period, ultrafiltration and IV furosemide patients achieved similar reductions in weight. However, patients in the ultrafiltration group significantly increased their stroke volume index, cardiac index, and cardiac power output and decreased their systemic vascular resistance, NTpro-BNP, aldosterone, and creatinine compared with patients receiving IV furosemide (Fig. 25.4). This study suggests that the acute hemodynamic and neurohormonal responses to volume reduction therapy differ according to the method of volume removal and that ultrafiltration results in more favorable responses compared with IV furosemide.

POSSIBLE MECHANISMS OF BENEFIT
Effective Fluid Removal

Ultrafiltration may result in more complete volume removal compared with loop diuretics because ultrafiltration allows the physician to precisely control the amount and rate of fluid removal. More complete fluid removal with ultrafiltration may increase the likelihood of favorable clinical outcomes based on decreased myocardial edema; decreased myocardial oxygen requirements due to decreased ventricular size and wall stress; improved coronary artery perfusion; reduced interventricular dependence; reduced mitral regurgitation; increased transrenal perfusion pressure; and decreased passive congestion of other organs including the liver and gut due to decreased intra-abdominal pressure (6,7,50–53).

Diuretic Sparing

Another possible explanation for improved outcomes following ultrafiltration is a diuretic sparing effect or "diuretic holiday." Diuretics are associated with adverse physiologic consequences such as activation of the sympathetic nervous system, decreased renal perfusion/function and electrolyte depletion (17,18,24,54,55). Furthermore, the use of loop diuretics is associated with increased mortality (16,20,22,56). Therefore, it is possible that reduced

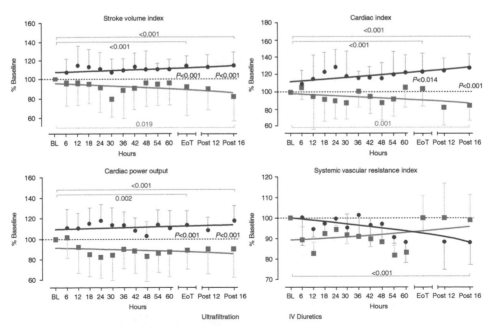

Figure 25.4 Trends over time in hemodynamic variables for patients treated with ultrafiltration and intravenous diuretics (49).

exposure to diuretics during and following ultrafiltration contributes to improved outcomes. This decrease in exposure to loop diuretics is attributable to the common practice of with-holding these drugs during ultrafiltration. This usually occurs at a time when patients would otherwise be receiving large doses of intravenous diuretics. In addition, ultrafiltration restores responsiveness to diuretics possibly decreasing chronic diuretic requirements after acute treatment (33,57).

Effective Sodium Removal

The removal of fluid in the form of hypotonic urine is an inefficient way to address fluid over-load and is an important disadvantage of loop diuretics (23). Moreover, the loss of hypotonic fluid can stimulate osmotic receptors and thirst, resulting in sodium retention and increased consumption of fluid (58–60). Volume reduction therapy with vasopressin antagonists is achieved by removal of free water with very little sodium excretion. These drugs produce minor changes in hemodynamics and a significant weight loss in heart failure patients (58,61). However, these changes are not associated with improved clinical outcomes (58).

In contrast to loop diuretics, ultrafiltration removes fluid that is iso-osmotic with plasma (23,26,27,42,62). Thus, the total sodium content in a given amount of fluid removed during volume reduction therapy in heart failure is substantially higher with ultrafiltration compared with loop diuretics. This enhanced sodium removal during ultrafiltration may result in greater reductions in extracellular fluid volume and improved outcomes (23,34,63,64).

Removal of Inflammatory Cytokines

Another possible mechanism of benefit for ultrafiltration is the removal of inflammatory cytokines. Inflammatory mediators have been implicated in the progression of heart failure (65–67) and are present in the ultrafiltrate of patients with heart failure and acute renal injury due to sepsis (68–73). In addition, ultrafiltrate obtained from pigs with endotoxin-mediated shock decreases cardiac function and other hemodynamic parameters when injected into healthy pigs (71).

PRESCRIPTION OF ULTRAFILTRATION
Patient Selection

There are many unresolved questions relating to the prescription of ultrafiltration for heart failure. Patient selection continues to be one of the most difficult issues. It seems intuitive that patients with significant volume overload and diuretic resistance may be the best candi-dates for ultrafiltration; however, this approach is untested. The Study of Heart Failure Hos-pitalizations After Aquapheresis Therapy Compared to Intravenous Diuretic Treatment (AVOID-HF) will attempt to address this issue in a multicenter, randomized, controlled trial comparing ultrafiltration to IV diuretics in patients hospitalized for heart failure and diuretic resistance. The trial is statistically powered for a primary endpoint of time to first heart fail-ure event (rehospitalization or unscheduled outpatient or emergency room treatment for HF) within 90 days after discharge from the index heart failure hospitalization (NCT01474200).

Worsening Renal Function

Significant renal insufficiency or worsening renal function following intravenous diuretics may also identify patients who will benefit from ultrafiltration. The Cardiorenal Rescue Study in Acute Decompensated Heart Failure (CARESS HF) will compare ultrafiltration to stepped pharmacologic care in patients hospitalized with heart failure who develop wors-ening renal function in the setting of persistent congestion (74). The results of this trial will inform clinicians concerning the most appropriate treatment options for patients with wors-ening renal function.

Treatment Termination Conditions

Plasma water withdrawal rates during ultrafiltration can range anywhere from 0 to 500 cc per hour with the new portable devices and the duration of a single ultrafiltration session can range anywhere from several hours to a week or more if multiple circuits are used. The optimal rate of fluid removal should not exceed the plasma refill rate, otherwise patients may experience transient intravascular volume depletion. This, in turn, could result in hemodynamic instability, activation of the sympathetic nervous system, and renal failure (39). Intravascular hemoconcentration may occur when fluid removal rates exceed the plasma refill rate and this could potentially be assessed with serial or continuous measurements of hematocrit, albumin, or total protein (75–77). These measurements could be used to guide the rate of volume reduction therapy during ultrafiltration. However, this approach has not been tested and there are potential barriers to the success of this strategy including the variability of repeated measurements, postural changes in blood components, and sympathetic control of the splanchnic circulation which could rapidly and dramatically change the circulating blood volume in the venous fluid compartment (77–80).

Commonly used clinical parameters to assess intravascular or extracellular fluid volume are insensitive and nonspecific (81,82). Symptoms and physical examination findings are poorly correlated with volume status; therefore, other parameters must be identified to optimally define treatment termination conditions for ultrafiltration.

Invasive hemodynamic monitoring has produced mixed results with respect to improving clinical outcomes (4,83). Other approaches for identifying optimal fluid removal/acute treatment termination conditions include the use of bioimpedance (84), neurohormone levels, and other biomarkers (81); and imaging of the inferior vena cava to assess collapsibility (85).

RISKS OF ULTRAFILTRATION

The risks of ultrafiltration are primarily related to vascular access, systemic anticoagulation, and intravascular volume depletion (86). Traditional ultrafiltration is performed using a relatively large catheter placed in a central vein. Transient discomfort at the vascular access site and catheter-related infections have been reported (28,46,47). Risks associated with vascular access are decreased through the use of peripheral venovenous ultrafiltration which, in some circumstances, can be performed through an 18 gauge IV (87). Rapid volume removal can result in leg cramps and orthostatic hypotension (27). Excessive fluid removal can result in intravascular volume depletion, hypotension, endorgan ischemia, and activation of the sympathetic nervous system (86). These risks are not unique to ultrafiltration and can occur in the setting of excessive diuresis with oral or intravenous diuretics. Transient hypotension can also occur when the rate of fluid removal exceeds the plasma refill rate which dictates the movement of fluid from the extravascular to intravascular space (39). Indeed, rapid fluid withdrawal during ultrafiltration has a differential effect on renal hemodynamics and catecholamine levels based on the extent of fluid retention at baseline. Patients without evidence of significant volume overload experience decreased renal perfusion and increased catecholamine levels following ultrafiltration compared with patients with massive fluid overload (41). In several small, uncontrolled case series involving moribund patients, there was a high incidence of dialysis and/or death in patients treated with ultrafiltration; however, without control groups, the poor clinical outcomes cannot be attributed directly to ultrafiltration (38,88,89). Patients in controlled trials were not as sick; however, ultrafiltration was tolerated well. In UNLOAD, 90-day mortality was 9.6% in the ultrafiltration group and 11.6% in the standard care group (47).

COST EFFECTIVENESS OF ULTRAFILTRATION

The cost of ultrafiltration must be considered in a broad context that includes downstream effects. So far, no prospective analyses have been performed. The added cost of ultrafiltration compared with the use of intravenous diuretics may be justified if ultrafiltration improves quality of life, decreases length of hospital stay, or prevents recurrent hospitalizations for heart failure. Results from the UNLOAD trial demonstrating decreased hospitalizations at 90 days are promising but not definitive with respect to cost effectiveness (47,90).

OTHER STRATEGIES OF FLUID REMOVAL IN HEART FAILURE

Strategies to relieve congestion continue to evolve. Changes in the dose or delivery of intravenous diuretics may result in better outcomes than current approaches (91–94). However, a randomized, double-blind, double dummy study showed no significant difference between high or low-dose, intermittent IV bolus, or continuous infusion dosing of furosemide in patients hospitalized with acute decompensated heart failure (95). The role of other agents such as vasopressin antagonists, adenosine receptor antagonists, and natriuretic peptides in the management of congestion is evolving and has yet to be defined (58,96–98).

FUTURE DIRECTIONS

Much has yet to be learned about the proper role of ultrafiltration in treating patients with heart failure. Ongoing research in this area will help clarify questions related to patient selection, clinical indications, and termination of treatment conditions. Fundamental questions remain concerning the mechanism of ultrafiltration therapy and how it may differ from IV diuretics. The advantages (and disadvantages) of ultrafiltration compared with standard treatment with IV diuretics need to be more clearly defined, especially as they relate to patient outcomes. In addition, the cost effectiveness of ultrafiltration will need to be closely studied. Ultrafiltration performed in ambulatory care setting may be very cost effective if it prevents unnecessary hospitalizations. Ultrafiltration has been performed in the ambulatory setting (99) and the development of portable devices may make ultrafiltration more attractive for some patients and providers (48,100). Patients with diuretic resistance may prefer one or more outpatient ultrafiltration sessions when the alternative is admission to an acute care hospital. Most hospitals and some ambulatory care centers are equipped with infusion clinics to deliver chemotherapy or to perform blood transfusions or plasmapheresis. These clinics could facilitate the use of outpatient ultrafiltration. Outpatient ultrafiltration is a promising approach that should be rigorously studied.

SUMMARY

Ultrafiltration is a safe and effective treatment for patients with heart failure and fluid overload. The amount and rate of fluid removed during ultrafiltration is determined by the provider and ultrafiltration, in contrast to diuretics, does not directly stimulate the sympathetic nervous system or deplete important electrolytes such as potassium and magnesium. Effective sodium removal may be one of the most attractive features of ultrafiltration possibly contributing to improved outcomes. More research is necessary to identify patients most likely to benefit from ultrafiltration and to determine the ideal prescription and therapeutic endpoints for this form of fluid removal.

REFERENCES

1. Adams KF Jr, Fonarow GC, Emerman CL, et al. Characteristics and outcomes of patients hospitalized for heart failure in the United States: rationale, design, and preliminary observations from the first 100,000 cases in the Acute Decompensated Heart Failure National Registry (ADHERE). Am Heart J 2005; 149: 209–16.

2. Chaudhry SI, Wang Y, Concato J, Gill TM, Krumholz HM. Patterns of weight change preceding hospitalization for heart failure. Circulation 2007; 116: 1549–54.

3. Nohria A, Tsang SW, Fang JC, et al. Clinical assessment identifies hemodynamic profiles that predict outcomes in patients admitted with heart failure. J Am Coll Cardiol 2003; 41: 1797–804.

4. Binanay C, Califf RM, Hasselblad V, et al. Evaluation study of congestive heart failure and pulmonary artery catheterization effectiveness: the ESCAPE trial. JAMA 2005; 294: 1625–33.

5. Gheorghiade M, Gattis WA, O'connor CM, et al. Effects of tolvaptan, a vasopressin antagonist, in patients hospitalized with worsening heart failure: a randomized controlled trial. JAMA 2004; 291: 1963–71.

6. Lucas C, Johnson W, Hamilton MA, et al. Freedom from congestion predicts good survival despite previous class IV symptoms of heart failure. Am Heart J 2000; 140: 840–7.

7. Rogers JG, Hellkamp AS, Young J, et al. Low congestion score 1-month after hospitalization predicts better function and survival. J Am Coll Cardiol 2007; 49: 47A.

8. Fonarow GC. Epidemiology and risk stratification in acute heart failure. Am Heart J 2008; 155: 200–7.

9. Gheorghiade M, Zannad F, Sopko G, et al. Acute heart failure syndromes: current state and framework for future research. Circulation 2005; 112: 3958–68.

10. Adhere - Acute Decompensated Heart Failure National Registry: Q1 2004 National Benchmark Report. 2004 Report No.: P0305403.

11. Saba MM, Ventura HO, Saleh M, Mehra MR. Ancient Egyptian medicine and the concept of heart failure. J Card Fail 2006; 12: 416–21.

12. Ventura HO, Mehra MR. Bloodletting as a cure for dropsy: heart failure down the ages. J Card Fail 2005; 11: 247–52.

13. Ventura HO, Mehra MR, Young JB. Treatment of heart failure according to William Stokes: the enchanted mercury. J Card Fail 2001; 7: 277–82.

14. Ellison DH. Diuretic therapy and resistance in congestive heart failure. Cardiology 2001; 96: 132–43.

15. Heart Failure Society Of America. HFSA 2006 Comprehensive Heart Failure Practice Guideline. J Card Fail 2006; 12: e1–e122.

16. Domanski M, Norman J, Pitt B, et al. Diuretic use, progressive heart failure, and death in patients in the Studies Of Left Ventricular Dysfunction (SOLVD). J Am Coll Cardiol 2003; 42: 705–8.

17. Weber KT. Furosemide in the long-term management of heart failure: the good, the bad, and the uncertain. J Am Coll Cardiol 2004; 44: 1308–10.

18. Francis GS, Siegel RM, Goldsmith SR, et al. Acute vasoconstrictor response to intravenous furosemide in patients with chronic congestive heart failure. activation of the neurohumoral axis. Ann Intern Med 1985; 103: 1–6.

19. Sackner-Bernstein JD, Obeleniene R. How should diuretic-refractory, volume-overloaded heart failure patients be managed? J Invasive Cardiol 2003; 15: 585–90.

20. Cooper HA, Dries DL, Davis CE, Shen YL, Domanski MJ. Diuretics and risk of arrhythmic death in patients with left ventricular dysfunction. Circulation 1999; 100: 1311–5.

21. Neuberg GW, Miller AB, O'connor CM, et al. Diuretic resistance predicts mortality in patients with advanced heart failure. Am Heart J 2002; 144: 31–8.

22. Ahmed A, Husain A, Love TE, et al. Heart failure, chronic diuretic use, and increase in mortality and hospitalization: an observational study using propensity score methods. Eur Heart J 2006; 27: 1431–9.

23. Schrier RW. Role of diminished renal function in cardiovascular mortality: marker or pathogenetic factor? J Am Coll Cardiol 2006; 47: 1–8.

24. McCurley JM, Hanlon SU, Wei SK, et al. Furosemide and the progression of left ventricular dysfunction in experimental heart failure. J Am Coll Cardiol 2004; 44: 1301–7.

25. Sharma A, Hermann DD, Mehta RL. Clinical benefit and approach of ultrafiltration in acute heart failure. Cardiology 2001; 96: 144–54.

26. Ronco C, Ricci Z, Bellomo R, Bedogni F. Extracorporeal ultrafiltration for the treatment of overhydration and congestive heart failure. Cardiology 2001; 96: 155–68.

27. Silverstein ME, Ford CA, Lysaght MJ, Henderson LW. Treatment of severe fluid overload by ultrafiltration. N Engl J Med 1974; 291: 747–51.

28. Simpson IA, Rae AP, Simpson K, et al. Ultrafiltration in the management of refractory congestive heart failure. Br Heart J 1986; 55: 344–7.

29. Simpson IA, Hutton I. Diuretics or ultrafiltration in the treatment of congestive cardiac failure? Br J Hosp Med 1987; 37: 144–5; 148.

30. Fauchald P, Forfang K, Amlie J. An evaluation of ultrafiltration as treatment of therapy-resistant cardiac edema. Acta Med Scand 1986; 219: 47–52.

31. Rimondini A, Cipolla C, Della Bella P, et al. Hemofiltration as short-term treatment for refractory congestive heart failure. Am J Med 1987; 83: 43–8.

32. Asaba H, Bergstrom J, Furst P, Shaldon S, Wiklund S. Treatment of diuretic-resistant fluid retention with ultrafiltration. Acta Med Scand 1978; 204: 145–9.

33. DiLeo M, Pacitti A, Bergerone S, et al. Ultrafiltration in the treatment of refractory congestive heart failure. Clin Cardiol 1988; 11: 449–52.

34. Agostoni P, Marenzi G, Lauri G, et al. Sustained improvement in functional capacity after removal of body fluid with isolated ultrafiltration in chronic cardiac insufficiency: failure of furosemide to provide the same result. Am J Med 1994; 96: 191–9.

35. Agostoni PG, Marenzi GC, Pepi M, et al. Isolated ultrafiltration in moderate congestive heart failure. J Am Coll Cardiol 1993; 21: 424–31.

36. Agostoni PG, Marenzi GC, Sganzerla P, et al. Lung-heart interaction as a substrate for the improvement in exercise capacity after body fluid volume depletion in moderate congestive heart failure. Am J Cardiol 1995; 76: 793–8.

37. Pepi M, Marenzi GC, Agostoni PG, et al. Sustained cardiac diastolic changes elicited by ultrafiltration in patients with moderate congestive heart failure: pathophysiological correlates. Br Heart J 1993; 70: 135–40.

38. Inoue T, Sakai Y, Morooka S, et al. Hemofiltration as treatment for patients with refractory heart failure. Clin Cardiol 1992; 15: 514–18.

39. Marenzi G, Lauri G, Grazi M, et al. Circulatory response to fluid overload removal by extracorporeal ultrafiltration in refractory congestive heart failure. J Am Coll Cardiol 2001; 38: 963–8.

40. Agostoni PG, Guazzi M, Bussotti M, et al. Lack of improvement of lung diffusing capacity following fluid withdrawal by ultrafiltration in chronic heart failure. J Am Coll Cardiol 2000; 36: 1600–4.

41. Marenzi G, Grazi S, Giraldi F, et al. Interrelation of humoral factors, hemodynamics, and fluid and salt metabolism in congestive heart failure: effects of extracorporeal ultrafiltration. Am J Med 1993; 94: 49–56.

42. Canaud B, Cristol JP, Klouche K, et al. Slow continuous ultrafiltration: a means of unmasking myocardial functional reserve in end-stage cardiac disease. Contrib Nephrol 1991; 93: 79–85.

43. Cipolla CM, Grazi S, Rimondini A, et al. Changes in circulating norepinephrine with hemofiltration in advanced congestive heart failure. Am J Cardiol 1990; 66: 987–94.

44. Forslund T, Riddervold F, Fauchald P, et al. Hormonal changes in patients with severe chronic congestive heart failure treated by ultrafiltration. Nephrol Dial Transplant 1992; 7: 306–10.

45. Guazzi MD, Agostoni P, Perego B, et al. Apparent paradox of neurohumoral axis inhibition after body fluid volume depletion in patients with chronic congestive heart failure and water retention. Br Heart J 1994; 72: 534–9.

46. Bart BA, Boyle A, Bank AJ, et al. Ultrafiltration versus usual care for hospitalized patients with heart failure: the relief for acutely fluid-overloaded patients with decompensated congestive heart failure (RAPID-CHF) trial. J Am Coll Cardiol 2005; 46: 2043–6.

47. Costanzo MR, Guglin ME, Saltzberg MT, et al. Ultrafiltration versus intravenous diuretics for patients hospitalized for acute decompensated heart failure. J Am Coll Cardiol 2007; 49: 675–83.

48. Jaski BE, Ha J, Denys BG, et al. Peripherally inserted veno-venous ultrafiltration for rapid treatment of volume overloaded patients. J Card Fail 2003; 9: 227–31.

49. Giglioli C, Landi D, Cecchi E, et al. Effects of ULTRAfiltration vs. DIureticS on clinical, biohumoral and haemodynamic variables in patients with deCOmpensated heart failure: the ULTRADISCO study. Eur J Heart Fail 2011; 13: 337–46.

50. Boyle A, Maurer MS, Sobotka PA. Myocellular and interstitial edema and circulating volume expansion as a cause of morbidity and mortality in heart failure. J Card Fail 2007; 13: 133–6.

51. Firth JD, Raine AE, Ledingham JG. Raised venous pressure: a direct cause of renal sodium retention in oedema? Lancet 1988; 1: 1033–5.

52. Mullens W, Abrahams Z, Skouri HN, et al. Elevated intra-abdominal pressure in acute decompensated heart failure: a potential contributor to worsening renal function? J Am Coll Cardiol 2008; 51: 300–6.

53. Rubboli A, Sobotka PA, Euler DE. Effect of acute edema on left ventricular function and coronary vascular resistance in the isolated rat heart. Am J Physiol 1994; 267: H1054–61.

54. Butler J, Forman DE, Abraham WT, et al. Relationship between heart failure treatment and development of worsening renal function among hospitalized patients. Am Heart J 2004; 147: 331–8.

55. Ikram H, Chan W, Espiner E, et al. Haemodynamic and hormone responses to acute and chronic frusemide therapy in congestive heart failure. Clin Sci 1980; 59: 443–9.

56. Domanski M, Tian X, Haigney M, Pitt B. Diuretic use, progressive heart failure, and death in patients in the DIG study. J Card Fail 2006; 12: 327–32.

57. Libetta C, Sepe V, Zucchi M, Campana C, Dal CA. Standard hemodiafiltration improves diuretic responsiveness in advanced congestive heart failure. Cardiology 2006; 105: 122–3.

58. Konstam MA, Gheorghiade M, Burnett JC Jr, et al. Effects of oral tolvaptan in patients hospitalized for worsening heart failure: the EVEREST outcome trial. JAMA 2007; 297: 1319–31.
59. De Smet HR, Menadue MF, Oliver JR, Phillips PA. Increased thirst and vasopressin secretion after myocardial infarction in rats. Am J Physiol Regul Integr Comp Physiol 2003; 285: R1203–11.
60. Fitzsimons JT. Angiotensin, thirst, and sodium appetite. Physiol Rev 1998; 78: 583–686.
61. Mehra MR, Rockman HA, Greenberg BH. Highlights of the 2007 scientific meeting of the heart failure society of America: Washington, DC, September 16–19, 2007. J Am Coll Cardiol 2008; 51: 320–7.
62. Ali SS, Olinger CC, Sobotka P, et al. Enhanced sodium extraction with ultrafiltration compared to intravenous diuretics. J Card Fail 2006; 12: S114.
63. Bart BA. Treatment of congestion in congestive heart failure: ultrafiltration is the only rational initial treatment of volume overload in decompensated heart failure. Circ Heart Fail 2009; 2: 499–504.
64. Bart BA, Insel J, Goldstein MM, et al. The improved outcomes following ultrafiltration versus intravenous diuretics in UNLOAD are not solely due to increased weight loss in the Ultrafiltration group. J Card Fail 2007; 13(6 Suppl 2): 188.
65. Braunwald E. Biomarkers in heart failure. N Engl J Med 2008; 358: 2148–59.
66. Mann DL, Young JB. Basic mechanisms in congestive heart failure. Recognizing the role of proinflammatory cytokines. Chest 1994; 105: 897–904.
67. Torre-Amione G, Kapadia S, Benedict C, et al. Proinflammatory cytokine levels in patients with depressed left ventricular ejection fraction: a report from the Studies of Left Ventricular Dysfunction (SOLVD). J Am Coll Cardiol 1996; 27: 1201–6.
68. Bellomo R, Tipping P, Boyce N. Interleukin-6 and interleukin-8 extraction during continuous venovenous hemodiafiltration in septic acute renal failure. Ren Fail 1995; 17: 457–66.
69. Blake P, Hasegawa Y, Khosla MC, et al. Isolation of "myocardial depressant factor(s)" from the ultrafiltrate of heart failure patients with acute renal failure. ASAIO J 1996; 42: M911–15.
70. De Vriese AS, Colardyn FA, Philippe JJ, et al. Cytokine removal during continuous hemofiltration in septic patients. J Am Soc Nephrol 1999; 10: 846–53.
71. Grootendorst AF, van Bommel EF, van Leengoed LA, et al. Infusion of ultrafiltrate from endotoxemic pigs depresses myocardial performance in normal pigs. J Crit Care 1993; 8: 161–9.
72. Ronco C, Tetta C, Lupi A, et al. Removal of platelet-activating factor in experimental continuous arteriovenous hemofiltration. Crit Care Med 1995; 23: 99–107.
73. Sander A, Armbruster W, Sander B, et al. Hemofiltration increases IL-6 clearance in early systemic inflammatory response syndrome but does not alter IL-6 and TNF alpha plasma concentrations. Intensive Care Med 1997; 23: 878–84.
74. Bart BA, Goldsmith SR, Lee KL, et al. Cardiorenal rescue study in acute decompensated heart failure: rationale and design of CARRESS-HF, for the heart failure clinical research network. J Card Fail 2012; 18: 176–82.
75. van BW. Evaluation of hemoconcentration from hematocrit measurements. J Appl Physiol 1972; 32: 712–13.
76. Boyle A, Sobotka PA. Redefining the therapeutic objective in decompensated heart failure: hemoconcentration as a surrogate for plasma refill rate. J Card Fail 2006; 12: 247–9.
77. Testani JM, Chen J, McCauley BD, Kimmel SE, Shannon RP. Potential effects of aggressive decongestion during the treatment of decompensated heart failure on renal function and survival. Circulation 2010; 122: 265–72.
78. Jacob G, Raj SR, Ketch T, et al. Postural pseudoanemia: posture-dependent change in hematocrit. Mayo Clin Proc 2005; 80: 611–14.
79. Fallick C, Sobotka PA, Dunlap ME. Sympathetically mediated changes in capacitance: redistribution of the venous reservoir as a cause of decompensation. Circ Heart Fail 2011; 4: 669–75.
80. Katz SD. The plot thickens: hemoconcentration, renal function, and survival in heart failure. Circulation 2010; 122: 233–5.
81. Nohria A, Mielniczuk LM, Stevenson LW. Evaluation and monitoring of patients with acute heart failure syndromes. Am J Cardiol 2005; 96: 32G–40G.
82. Androne AS, Hryniewicz K, Hudaihed A, et al. Relation of unrecognized hypervolemia in chronic heart failure to clinical status, hemodynamics, and patient outcomes. Am J Cardiol 2004; 93: 1254–9.
83. Abraham WT, Adamson PB, Bourge RC, et al. Wireless pulmonary artery haemodynamic monitoring in chronic heart failure: a randomised controlled trial. Lancet 2011; 377: 658–66.
84. Tang WH, Tong W. Measuring impedance in congestive heart failure: current options and clinical applications. Am Heart J 2009; 157: 402–11.
85. Guiotto G, Masarone M, Paladino F, et al. Inferior vena cava collapsibility to guide fluid removal in slow continuous ultrafiltration: a pilot study. Intensive Care Med 2010; 36: 692–6.

86. Kazory A, Ross EA. Contemporary trends in the pharmacological and extracorporeal management of heart failure: a nephrologic perspective. Circulation 2008; 117: 975–83.

87. Dahle TG, Blake D, Ali SS, et al. Large volume ultrafiltration for acute decompensated heart failure using standard peripheral intravenous catheters. J Card Fail 2006; 12: 349–52.

88. Dormans TP, Huige RM, Gerlag PG. Chronic intermittent haemofiltration and haemodialysis in end stage chronic heart failure with oedema refractory to high dose frusemide. Heart 1996; 75: 349–51.

89. Liang KV, Hiniker AR, Williams AW, et al. Use of a novel ultrafiltration device as a treatment strategy for diuretic resistant, refractory heart failure: initial clinical experience in a single center. J Card Fail 2006; 12: 707–14.

90. Colechin ES, Bower L, Sims AJ. Ultrafiltration Therapy for Fluid Overload in Heart Failure. NHS Centre for Evidence-based Purchasing, 2007: report #CEP07016.

91. Licata G, Di Pasquale P, Parrinello G, et al. Effects of high-dose furosemide and small-volume hypertonic saline solution infusion in comparison with a high dose of furosemide as bolus in refractory congestive heart failure: long-term effects. Am Heart J 2003; 145: 459–66.

92. Lahav M, Regev A, Ra'anani P, Theodor E. Intermittent administration of furosemide vs continuous infusion preceded by a loading dose for congestive heart failure. Chest 1992; 102: 725–31.

93. Dormans TP, van Meyel JJ, Gerlag PG, et al. Diuretic efficacy of high dose furosemide in severe heart failure: bolus injection versus continuous infusion. J Am Coll Cardiol 1996; 28: 376–82.

94. Aaser E, Gullestad L, Tollofsrud S, et al. Effect of bolus injection versus continuous infusion of furosemide on diuresis and neurohormonal activation in patients with severe congestive heart failure. Scand J Clin Lab Invest 1997; 57: 361–7.

95. Felker GM, Lee KL, Bull DA, et al. Diuretic strategies in patients with acute decompensated heart failure. N Engl J Med 2011; 364: 797–805.

96. O'connor CM, Starling RC, Hernandez AF, et al. Effect of nesiritide in patients with acute decompensated heart failure. N Engl J Med 2011; 365: 32–43.

97. Voors AA, Dittrich HC, Massie BM, et al. Effects of the adenosine A1 receptor antagonist rolofylline on renal function in patients with acute heart failure and renal dysfunction: results from PROTECT (placebo-controlled randomized study of the selective adenosine a1 receptor antagonist rolofylline for patients hospitalized with acute decompensated heart failure and volume overload to assess treatment effect on congestion and renal function). J Am Coll Cardiol 2011; 57: 1899–907.

98. Zakeri R, Burnett JC. Designer natriuretic peptides: a vision for the future of heart failure therapeutics. Can J Physiol Pharmacol 2011; 89: 593–601.

99. Sheppard R, Panyon J, Pohwani AL, et al. Intermittent outpatient ultrafiltration for the treatment of severe refractory congestive heart failure. J Card Fail 2004; 10: 380–3.

100. Peacock WF. Future options for management of heart failure in an emergency department observation unit. Crit Pathw Cardiol 2005; 4: 177–81.

101. Wei SS, Lee WT, Woo KT. Slow continuous ultrafiltration (SCUF)–the safe and efficient treatment for patients with cardiac failure and fluid overload. Singapore Med J 1995; 36: 276–7.

102. Ramos R, Salem BI, DePawlikowski MP, et al. Outcome predictors of ultrafiltration in patients with refractory congestive heart failure and renal failure. Angiology 1996; 47: 447–54.

103. Costanzo MR, Saltzberg M, O'Sullivan J, Sobotka P. Early ultrafiltration in patients with decompensated heart failure and diuretic resistance. J Am Coll Cardiol 2005; 46: 2047–51.

104. Jaski BE, Romeo A, Ortiz B, et al. Outcomes of volume-overloaded cardiovascular patients treated with ultrafiltration. J Card Fail 2008; 14: 515–20.

105. Hanna MA, Tang WH, Teo BW, et al. Extracorporeal ultrafiltration *vs.* conventional diuretic therapy in advanced decompensated heart failure. Congest Heart Fail 2012; 18: 54–63.

26
Heart failure and palliative care

Joshua M. Hauser and Robert O. Bonow

INTRODUCTION
Palliative Care and Hospice

Palliative care is care that aims to treat suffering and to improve the quality of life of patients and their families with serious illnesses. It involves an interdisciplinary team of physicians, nurses, social workers, chaplains, pharmacists, and volunteers and is appropriate at any stage of illness (1). Palliative care is a broader approach than hospice care, which typically occurs only for patients with an estimated prognosis of six months or less and for whom efforts at disease-modifying therapy are not being undertaken.

Palliative care can occur in both inpatient and outpatient settings, with increasing number of hospitals having dedicated palliative care units and consultation services (2). Hospice care, by contrast, generally occurs at home or in long-term care facilities with a smaller number of free-standing hospice facilities. The last decades have seen a dramatic rise in the number of patients cared for in hospice, such that in 2008, 963,000 patients died under hospice care, which represented almost 40% of deaths in the United States (3). Since 1987, hospice has been a Medicare benefit, and as such is also paid for by most major insurance companies. This has resulted in reliable data about its delivery. Since *palliative care* is a broader term and not a specific Medicare benefit, data about its use is less comprehensive. As a specialty, palliative care is now certified by the American Board of Medical Specialties and sponsoring boards include internal medicine, family medicine, emergency medicine, psychiatry, neurology, and others (4).

This chapter discusses the epidemiology of heart failure with an emphasis on palliative care, the prevalence, and treatment of common symptoms in patients with advanced heart failure and ends with a consideration of some issues unique to heart failure and palliative care.

Epidemiology and Mortality

In 2006, cardiovascular disease was the leading cause of death in the United States, the last year for which full figures from the Centers for Disease Control (CDC) are available: It accounted for 631,636 deaths or 26.0% of all deaths (5). In the same year, cancer accounted for 559,888 deaths or 23.0% of all deaths. Although heart disease is the leading cause of death in the United States, it represents a significant minority of patients in hospice programs. By contrast, in 2008, 11.7% of patients enrolled in hospice had a primary diagnosis of heart disease and 38.3% had a diagnosis of cancer (6). Given this relatively low number of patients with heart failure who use hospice, it is likely that many patients who might benefit from palliative care are not receiving it.

From an economic standpoint, the direct cost of care for patients with heart failure was estimated to be as high as $58 billion a year in 2000 (7). The indirect costs in terms of lost wages and family caregiving are likely significantly higher.

Newly diagnosed heart failure in the community carries a mortality of 24%, 37%, and 75% at one, two, and six years. For patients with advanced (New York Heart Association (NYHA) Class IV or Stage D) heart failure, the rate of rehospitalization or death is 81% at one year. In patients with a left ventricular ejection fraction of less than 25% and Stage D symptoms (such as dyspnea and angina at rest) for more than 90 days, oxygen consumption of 12 mL/kg or inotropic dependence, mortality is 50% at six months. For patients on continuous inotropic support, mortality is 75% at six months (8).

How is Heart Failure Different From Cancer?

Both cancer and heart failure are increasingly viewed as chronic illnesses, with an emphasis on survivorship, rehabilitation, and quality of life. This view of heart failure recognizes that there may not be a discrete point at which it is considered a "terminal illness." Rather, there are multiple stages during which a combination of disease-modifying and symptom-directed or palliative therapies are appropriate. This combination of approaches can make the decision to start hospice challenging for clinicians, patients, and families, especially if hospice is equated with giving up certain therapies.

For many years, the palliative care movement has conceived of the trajectory of many chronic as one in which there are multiple opportunities for disease-modifying and for palliative therapies. Data from Lunney and colleagues has provided empirical evidence to the stuttering trajectory of symptoms and care that heart failure patients experience in the last year of life (9). This trajectory may involve multiple exacerbations of symptoms, medication changes and management strategies and multiple emergency department visits and hospitalizations.

Although a patient's specific diagnosis will determine how he or she is treated medically, the experience of illness among patients with cancer and heart failure may be similar: A study that surveyed patients and their caregivers from England found that symptom burden, emotional wellbeing, and quality of life among a cohort of 50 advanced cancer and 50 advanced heart failure patients to be "indistinguishable" (10). What this study suggests is that although the pathophysiology of the illnesses these patients were experiencing was no doubt diverse, their experiences of illness were remarkably similar by these subjective measures.

Despite the fact that the patient's experience may be remarkably similar, there is evidence for differing perceptions of cancer and heart disease among physicians. These differences in disease perception have implications for how physicians care for patients with heart failure. As one example, McKinley and colleagues compared care delivered by general practitioners in the last year of life to people who died with cancer and with cardiovascular and respiratory disease (11). They found that when compared with people who died with cardiovascular and respiratory disease, those died with cancer were more likely to have had a "terminal phase" of their illness identified by their health care providers and to have received more palliative medications.

The transition to palliative care or hospice for patients with heart failure is often considered only after the most aggressive treatments have been tried. For many patients and their families, this represents a sudden shift in care and goals, despite the fact that they have experienced a long period of chronic illness. Based on overall studies of palliative care, it is likely that palliative care principles of symptom management, attention to goals for care, and support for patients and their families may have the greatest impact on quality of life when introduced as early as possible in a patient's management (12). This will not mean abandoning traditional care and management of heart failure, but rather an augmentation of these.

Guidelines

For patients with cancer, the National Comprehensive Cancer Network (NCCN) has specific guidelines for symptom management as well as for the integration of palliative care into the care of specific cancers (13). In cardiology and pulmonary medicine, guidelines issued by both the American College of Chest Physicians (14) and the American College of Cardiology/American Heart Association (ACC/AHA) (15) have addressed palliative strategies within their overall management guidelines. ACC/AHA guidelines include a section on "end-of-life considerations in the setting of heart failure." Among the recommendations for patients with end-stage heart failure are areas such as ongoing education for patients and their families concerning prognosis, functional capacity, the role of palliative care, implanted cardiac defibrillators (ICDs) deactivation, coordination of care, and the use of opioids for symptomatic relief.

The ACC/AHA guidelines also advise withholding of resuscitative measures in some patients with advanced heart failure in whom the benefit is likely to be small and that "aggressive procedures, including intubation and automated implanted cardiac defibrillators (AICDs), within the final days are not appropriate." Although identifying the "final days" presents a challenge to our recognized inaccuracies of prognostication (16), there are generally agreed upon criteria that include significantly decreased responsiveness, severely compromised functional status, and decreased urine output that palliative care physicians use to assess the last days of life.

Overall, ACC/AHA guidelines for palliative care and heart failure recognize that there is limited empirical data for many interventions for palliative care for patients with heart failure. For many of the recommendations in the ACC/AHA guidelines concerning disease-specific treatments, such as the use of angiotensin-converting enzyme (ACE) inhibitors and beta-blockers, evidence reaches the level of "Class A" (data derived from multiple randomized clinical trials or meta-analyses). For all of the recommendations concerning palliative care, however, the level of evidence is "Class C" (only consensus, case studies and standard of care as opposed to data from clinical trials). This suggests that the field may be early in its integration of palliative care. At the same time, it is likely that the types of evidence needed to support some of the palliative interventions may differ from traditional clinical trials for disease-modifying medications.

Another set of guidelines specifically concerning palliative care and heart failure has been issued by a group of cardiologists and palliative care physicians (17). These guidelines were issued from a consensus conference on "Palliative and Supportive Care in Advanced Heart Failure." They identified the need for research on symptom clusters, prognostication, and coordination of care approaches to heart failure as priorities as the fields of palliative care and heart failure become more tightly linked and move forward.

Symptom Prevalence Among Patients with Heart Failure

Symptoms that patients with heart failure experience include dyspnea, pain, fatigue, and depression. One of the largest trials that examined symptoms for patients near the end-of-life is the Study to Understand Prognoses and Preferences for Outcomes and Risks of Treatments (SUPPORT) trial (18). This study assessed symptoms of patients facing the end of life with multiple medical illnesses and included a cohort of patients with heart failure.

In one analysis of the SUPPORT trial that examined elderly patients with heart failure, Levenson and colleagues reported that 60% of patients had dyspnea and 78% had pain at some point during their illness. These symptoms persisted through the final days of life: Patient surrogates reported that 41% of patients were in severe pain and 63% were severely short of breath at some point during the final three days before death (19). Psychological symptoms, including depression, anxiety, and confusion were all between 10% and 20% in this sample from SUPPORT.

Smaller studies of the prevalence of symptoms in patients with heart failure have reported similar results. In the Cardiovascular Health Study, a longitudinal study of more than 5500 patients that began in 1989, investigators found a prevalence of dyspnea of 79%, chest pain of 28%, and fatigue of 82% among incident cases of heart failure (20).

Psychological symptoms also have a high prevalence in patients with heart failure. The prevalence of depression ranges from 24% to 42% in patients with heart failure (21). Predictors of depression in patients with heart failure include living alone, alcohol abuse, perception of medical care being a substantial economic burden, and overall poor health status (22). Its presence is associated with increased mortality in patients with heart failure (23). It is often overlooked in the treatment of heart failure—up to 50% of patients with depression had it go undetected in one study (24).

In a study on hospitalized patients with heart failure, Jiang and colleagues found that 35% of patients screened positively on the Beck Depression Inventory and 14% of patients had a diagnosable major depressive disorder. These numbers have prognostic implications for patients: Jiang's study found that untreated depression in the setting of heart failure is a risk factor for increased mortality (25).

Multiple symptoms may co-exist and influence each other. A smaller study of Veterans with heart failure identified the prevalence of pain and also looked at contributing factors to pain (26). In this study, 55% of heart failure patients reported pain, with a majority rating their pain as moderate to severe. Pain was reported more frequently than was dyspnea for this sample. In addition, depression, anxiety, and spiritual and social stress all correlated with pain severity. The authors suggest that the association of physical, psychological, social, and spiritual domains with pain suggests that multidisciplinary interventions are needed to address the complex nature of pain in heart failure.

The high symptom burden on patients with heart failure is not just for those who are hospitalized: A study of patients with heart failure in a community-based hospice found a prevalence of pain in 25%, dyspnea in 60%, and confusion in 48% (27). If anything, these numbers may underestimate the numbers in a general population of home-bound patients with heart failure, as it is likely that these patients were receiving symptomatic care through their hospice program.

TREATMENT OF SYMPTOMS
Standard Treatment for Heart Failure

Heart failure is unlike some illnesses in palliative care and hospice, because a number of its treatments have quality-of-life benefits as well as disease-modifying effects. This contrasts with many types of cancer in which the disease-modifying treatments whose goal is to increase length of life may have deleterious effects on quality of life. For example, two of the cornerstones of treatment for heart failure, laid out in the ACC/AHA guidelines (28) and multiple other sources (29,30) include the use of ACE inhibitors or angiotensin receptor blockers (ARBs), and beta-blockers. Both of these classes of medications have been shown to improve survival and decrease repeated hospitalizations. Since they have both quality-of-life and mortality benefits, these medicines should be continued in palliative care.

Two other medications for heart failure, diuretics and digoxin, also have effects on quality of life. In the setting of fluid overload from heart failure, furosemide can improve dyspnea. Its effects can be potentiated by spironolactone which, when added to a loop diuretic such as furosemide, has been shown to have both mortality and symptomatic benefits and also result in reduced hospitalizations in the setting of heart failure (31). Although digoxin has been shown not to improve mortality (32), it can have symptomatic benefits in terms of decreased dyspnea and result in fewer repeat hospitalizations. Therefore, these medications should be continued as well.

Intravenous inotropic medications (such as dobutamine or milrinone) represent a dilemma for many patients, families, and providers. Although these medications have been shown to result in excess mortality in randomized trials, they have also been shown in some settings to decrease hospitalizations and symptoms among patients with end-stage heart failure (33). Recommendations concerning these medications in advanced heart failure management generally includes their use as a "bridge" to cardiac transplantation and as a palliative measure in patients with end-stage heart failure whose symptoms are refractory to other treatments (34). For patients in hospice, the use of intravenous inotropes may represent a challenge to the philosophy of care (is this "aggressive care" or "palliative care"?), education ("do we have the resources among our nurses and/or physicians to administer these safely in the home or nursing home setting?") and finances ("in the face of capitated reimbursement which is how hospices are reimbursed, are we able to afford this medication?"). Although there are no clear guidelines at this point in time for the use of these medications in the palliative care or hospice context, there are case studies of patients benefiting from their use (35). As the number of patients with heart failure who elect to be cared for by hospices increases, more and more individual programs and physicians will face this dilemma (36).

Symptomatic Treatment

The treatments above directed at the underlying pathophysiology heart failure itself will frequently have symptomatic benefits. However, in addition to such "disease-modifying" treatments, additional symptomatic treatment is part of palliative care for patients with heart failure. Generally, evidence for these treatments is based on the experience of symptomatic treatment in the setting of cancer: A systematic review of palliative care interventions found moderate-to-strong evidence to support pharmacologic treatment of pain, dyspnea, and depression in the setting of advanced cancer, but limited evidence for these symptoms in the setting of heart failure (37).

Dyspnea

The key medications for the medical treatment of dyspnea in the setting of heart failure include diuretics and opioids. Wherever possible, treatment directed at the underlying etiology of dyspnea will help to avoid potential side effects of opioids.

Low-dose opioids have been shown to be safe and effective at relieving dyspnea in small studies (38,39). For patients who have not received opioids before, a dose of 2–4 mg of oral morphine every two to three hours, titrated to the comfort of breathing can help a clinician determine a standing dose of long-acting morphine. Patients with dyspnea only after specific activities often benefit from taking oral morphine before engaging in that activity, much the same way that patients might take an inhaler before any triggers of asthma or nitroglycerin before triggers of angina.

For dyspnea due to pulmonary edema, furosemide or another loop diuretic may be effective; and for dyspnea due to a pleural effusion, drainage by thoracentesis may be effective temporarily, but these effusions frequently recur. When dyspnea is due to cardiac ischemia (angina), a nitrate should be used. This can include immediate release sublingual nitroglycerin and extended oral or transdermal nitrates when the angina is recurrent and predictable. Patients who get anginal symptoms and dyspnea with a predictable amount of exertion can be counseled to take a nitrate before activity. When dyspnea is due to rapid atrial fibrillation, rate control with digoxin, a beta-blocker, or other agent is appropriate to decrease cardiac workload.

Clinicians also need to be alert to comorbid noncardiac conditions in patients with heart failure before ascribing all symptoms to their primary diagnosis. When dyspnea is due to co-existing asthma or chronic obstructive pulmonary disease (COPD), an appropriate symptomatic approach includes inhaled beta-agonists, inhaled steroids, or inhaled anticholinergic medications as well as oral steroids.

Sleep apnea has been shown to be associated to heart failure, and its treatment may help to improve symptoms of fatigue and dyspnea (40). The formal diagnosis of sleep apnea requires an overnight sleep study in a sleep laboratory. In patients who are home-bound, overnight pulse oximetry in the home can sometimes be an alternative. The standard treatment for sleep apnea is the use of night time continuous positive airway pressure (CPAP). A randomized trial has shown some efficacy using acetazolamide as treatment for sleep apnea (41). Although the use of CPAP may initially be difficult for many patients, it is frequently something that they can adapt to and tolerate after continued use.

Although oxygen is commonly used in hospice and hospital contexts, a review found limited data to support its use in relieving dyspnea secondary to heart failure (42), especially when used as the sole treatment for dyspnea. Oxygen may hold symbolic value as an example of continued care and attention for the patient and family and therefore, its use, including the possibility that it may contribute to prolonging life, can be discussed openly with patient and family. Some may feel that it is a requirement when they are in the hospital and not be aware that like any other intervention, its use can be considered in terms of overall goals for care for a given patient. Conversely, patients and families may perceive discontinuing oxygen as a sign that the physicians or other providers are "giving up" on a patient.

Along with the administration of oxygen, patients in the hospital context as well as those being discharged, may be accustomed to having their pulse oximetry measured at regular intervals and oxygen titrated accordingly. As the patient's clinical condition and goals for care change and as symptom relief becomes the primary focus for patients, both the administration of oxygen and the monitoring of it should be re-addressed with patients and their families.

Pain

Pain is common in patients with heart failure. Most of the pain in this population is likely noncardiac in origin and stems from co-existing arthritic or musculoskeletal disease (43). When it is cardiac in origin, anginal pain should be treated with nitrates. This may help to reduce the amount of opioids that patients might require. When cardiac pain is not relieved by nitrates or there is other prevalent pain in patients with heart failure, this can be treated with standard doses of opioids according to World Health Organization (WHO) criteria (44). This includes the use of nonsteroidal anti-inflammatory drugs (NSAIDs) and acetaminophen as step 1, mild opioids (such as hydrocodone) as step 2, and string opioids (such as morphine, oxycodone, and hydromorphone) as step 3.

Since renal insufficiency is common in patients with advanced heart failure, a few considerations apply. First, NSAIDs can worsen renal insufficiency. Second, both morphine and hydromorphone (Dilaudid) have metabolites that can accumulate and lead to adverse neuroexcitatory effects, including tremors, myoclonus, and more rarely, seizures. Fentanyl, delivered transdermally or submucosally or intravenously, is safer in the setting of renal failure. Generally, doses should start low and be increased slowly, especially in elderly patients. When neuroexcitatory side effects do occur, one can reduce the opioid dose, rotate opioids, or add a low dose of a benzodiazepine, such as clonazepam or lorazepam. This last approach should be reserved for cases when opioid dose reduction or opioid rotation are unsuccessful.

When pain has a neuropathic component, treatment with an adjuvant medication, such as a tricyclic antidepressant (e.g., nortriptyline, which has fewer anticholinergic side-effects than amitriptyline) or an anticonvulsant (e.g., gabapentin or pregabalin) are both effective. In general, gabapentin and pregabalin have fewer side effects than do the tricyclic antidepressants.

Depression

An approach to the treatment of depression includes counseling interventions and the use of selective serotonin reuptake inhibitors. Tricyclic antidepressants are often avoided due to potential cardiotoxic effects. The data concerning counseling and psychological interventions are mixed. A Cochrane review of depression in the setting of heart failure found that, although there is randomized clinical trial evidence for the effectiveness of counseling in the setting of depression after myocardial infarction, there is no such evidence for patients with heart failure. They did identify three observational trials suggesting some benefit to counseling (45).

Communication in Palliative Care

Careful attention to communication and clear goal setting is a cornerstone of palliative care. Investigators have found that patients and their families are able to articulate goals of care (46). These may include life prolongation but may also include a focus on specific symptoms, family support, and the ability to be home, even when very ill and near the end of life. The task of eliciting goals of care involves careful exploration of a patient's understanding, values, and preferences. One framework for this is a basic model of communication skills that focuses on six steps summarized by the acronym SPIKES: S is for setting, P is for perception, I is for invitation, K is for knowledge, E is for emotion, and S is for summary and planning. Although initially designed for "breaking bad news," (47) it can appropriately be applied to many serious conversations in medicine, such as new test results, prognosis, and overall goals of care. It has also been subjected to empirical validation among patients (48).

Do-not-Resuscitate Orders

For many hospitalized patients, discussion of resuscitation, discussion of do-not-resuscitate (DNR) orders is a frequent conversational task. As such, it can be considered a prototype for discussions about goals of care. Discussions about goals of care will generally include many more elements than simple resuscitation status. But resuscitation status, since it is frequently tracked in the medical record can give us some insight into the frequency with which palliative care goals are discussed with patients with heart failure.

Some years ago, Wachter and colleagues found that DNR orders were instituted for 5% of patients with heart failure, 47% of patients with unresectable malignancy, and 52% of patients with AIDS (49) despite similar prognoses. In a trial that analyzed data from the SUPPORT study, Krumholz and colleagues found a low level of preferences for DNR orders and a low level of discussions of resuscitation among patients with heart failure: 23% and 25%, respectively (50). A study of homebound elderly patients with end-stage heart failure and dementia, found higher rates than the hospitalized samples in Wachter and Krumholz's studies. These investigators found that patients with heart failure were less likely to have a DNR order (62% vs 91%) (51).

Overall, these studies reveal that patients with heart failure have a lower prevalence of DNR orders compared with other patients. Although these studies do not address the question of what is the "correct" number of patients who "should" have DNR orders, the lack of DNR orders may be a marker for a lack of discussion about goals of care and prognosis with these patients and their families.

Automated Implantable Cardiac Defibrillators

By definition, patients with heart failure have more frequent indications for AICDs than do patients with other diagnoses. Patients with these devices represent a specific population in whom the discussion of goals of care and of resuscitation is paramount because of (*i*) their severity of illness and (*ii*) the expanding numbers of patients who will be receiving AICDs as indications for these devices grow and as the population grows older (52). Conceptual literature concerning ethical issues in AICDs (53) is beginning to develop and includes issues of when these "should" be deactivated and models for how we discuss these decisions with patients. There are clearly parallels with overall advanced care planning discussions and discussions about general DNR orders.

In one empirical study in this area, Goldstein and colleagues examined family members' views on the management of AICDs in end-of-life care (54). They surveyed 100 family members of patients who died with AICDs in place and found that these family members reported discussions of possible deactivation in only 27 of 100 cases and often only in the last few days of life.

Hospice Criteria for Heart Failure

Hospice predicates an average prognosis of six months to qualify for the benefit. The main professional organization for hospices and palliative care organizations, The National Hospice and Palliative Care Organization (NHPCO), has published criteria for determining prognosis in the setting of heart failure and other noncancer diseases. Although the last update of these criteria was in 1996, they do provide a framework for prognostication for patients with heart failure. The criteria include "symptoms of recurrent heart failure at rest (including an ejection fraction of 20%)," "optimal treatment" with medications directed at heart failure, and a number of comorbidities include documented arrhythmias, syncope, previous cardiac arrest, and co-existing cerebrovascular disease (55).

A study by Fox and colleagues examined the performance of these criteria in a population from the SUPPORT trial and found deficiencies in their prognostic accuracy for chronic medical illnesses in general (56). These investigators tested the performance of three levels of the criteria (broad, intermediate, and narrow) in determining six-month prognosis. "Broad" inclusion criteria identified the most patients eligible for hospice care, of whom 70% survived longer than six months. Intermediate inclusion criteria identified only one third as many patients, of whom 65% survived longer than six months. "Narrow" inclusion criteria identified only 19 patients for inclusion, of whom 53% survived longer than six months. They concluded that for seriously ill hospitalized patients with advanced COPD, heart failure, or end-stage liver disease, recommended clinical prediction criteria from NHPCO are not effective in identifying a population with a survival prognosis of six months or less. Another analysis of SUPPORT data cited by Albert and colleagues demonstrated similar difficulties in our ability to prognosticate: Among those with a predicted survival of 10% at six months, 38% were alive six months later (57).

Investigators have developed more sensitive and better validated models of prognosis than for inpatients with heart failure. Fonarow and colleagues used admission blood urea nitrogen (>43 mg/dL), creatinine (<2.75 mg/dL) (58), and systolic blood pressure (<115 mmHg) to identify inhospital mortality of 20% when all the three criteria were met. Criteria identified by Lee and colleagues associated with high mortality included older age, lower systolic blood pressure, higher respiratory rate, higher urea nitrogen level, and hypo-natremia. They developed a scale that predicted one-year mortality of 1–10% for lowest risk heart failure patients and 50–75% for highest risk patients (59).

Overall, however, there is a paucity of scales to assist clinicians in applying palliative care principles to heart failure. A systematic review of 11 prognostic scales for nonmalig-nant illnesses, found evidence lacking for disease-specific prognostic scales in heart failure (60). Although there is evidence for short hospice survival among patients with heart failure, the most comprehensive trial of overall prognosis for patients enrolled in hospice that used national Medicare survival data, showed the hospice length of stay among heart failure patients to be slightly *greater* than among all hospice patients, regardless of diagno-sis: 43.5 days versus 36.0 days (61). In the absence of consistent predictors of a six-month prognosis, the goal of integrating palliative care into heart failure outside of a formal hospice referral is crucial.

Disease Management Programs

Disease management programs for patients with heart failure have shown marked success in reducing re-hospitalization and improving quality of life. They have been not only clini-cally successful, but also cost-effective as well (62). A review by Lorenz and colleagues of effective palliative interventions, which found a paucity of strong evidence for many symptomatic treatments in the setting of heart failure, did identify these disease manage-ment programs as effective (63).

Although these programs have generally been distinct from hospice programs, they share care processes and goals with hospice: They consist of an interdisciplinary team that proactively manages patients at home with the goal of (*i*) improved coordination and continuity of care and (*ii*) prevention of inappropriate hospitalization or emergency depart-ment use. They generally consist of phone calls or electronic contact with patients on a weekly or more frequent basis to inquire about symptoms such as dyspnea or chest pain and signs such as weight gain or edema and adjust medications (principally diuretics) and clinician visits accordingly. In addition to reductions in hospitalizations and costs for patients and increased patient satisfaction, some of these programs have shown mortality benefits (64–67). As palliative care and hospice continues to integrate into the care of patients with heart failure, integrating the management techniques of these programs will be a crucial.

CONCLUSION

Hospice and palliative care are now a clear part of guidelines not only from palliative care organizations, but also from the ACC and AHA. At the same time, increasing numbers of clinicians in cardiology and palliative care are advocating for early integration of symp-tomatic care in the management of patients with heart (68). Because many of the symptom-atic therapies for heart failure have disease-modifying aspects to them, this integration is all the more crucial and makes the distinction between "normal" care and "palliative care" blurry. Excellent care for heart failure should include the tenets of excellent palliative care throughout: Consistent symptom management, support for patients and their families, and discussion of overall and specific goals of care throughout.

The sentiment that palliative care is a dramatic, and often unwelcome, alternative to cure or "normal" care is not isolated to heart failure. For patients with heart failure and their families as well as their health care team, the instinct to "fight" may be vital, especially in the face of expanding technologies and treatments. A thoughtful approach to palliative care should not advocate giving these up. Rather, it should offer two accompanying elements: First, the integration of palliative care principles from diagnosis one and two, the recognition of when a patient might be helped by re-focusing the goals from "victory" in the form of a "cure" to "victory" in the form of the best possible quality of life and support we can offer.

REFERENCES

1. WHO def of palliative care. [Available from: http://www.who.int/cancer/palliative/definition/en/].
2. Morrison RS, Maroney-Galin C, Kralovec PD, Meier DE. The growth of palliative care programs in united states hospitals. J Palliat Med 2005; 8: 1127–34.
3. [Available from: www.nhpco.org].
4. [Available from: http://www.nhpco.org/i4a/pages/index.cfm?pageid=5072].
5. [Available from: http://www.cdc.gov/nchs/FASTATS/lcod.htm].
6. National Hospice and Palliative Care Organization, Hospice Care in America, 2009 Edition. [Available from: http://www.nhpco.org/files/public/Statistics_Research/NHPCO_facts_and_figures.pdf].
7. O'Connell JB. The economic burden of heart failure. Clin Cardiol 2000; 23: III-6–III-10.
8. Hauptman PJ, Havranek EP. Integrating palliative care into heart failure care. Arch Intern Med 2005; 165: 374–8.
9. Lunney JR, Lynn J, Foley DJ, et al. Patterns of functional decline at the end of life. JAMA 2003; 289: 2387–92.
10. O'Leary N, Murphy NF, O'Loughlin C, Tiernan E, McDonald K. A comparative study of the palliative care needs of heart failure and cancer patients. Eur J Heart Fail 2009; 11: 406–12.
11. McKinley RK, Stokes T, Exley C, et al. Care of people dying with malignant and cardiorespiratory disease in general practice. Br J Gen Pract 2004; 54: 909–13.
12. Zimmermann C, Riechelmann R, Krzyzanowska M, Rodin G, Tannock I. Effectiveness of specialized palliative care: a Systematic Review. JAMA 2008; 299: 1698–709.
13. NCCN guidelines. [Available from: www.nccn.org].
14. Selecky PA, Eliasson CA, Hall RI, et al. American college of chest physicians. Palliative and end-of-life care for patients with cardiopulmonary diseases: american college of chest physicians position statement. Chest 2005; 128: 3599–610.
15. Hunt SA, Abraham WT, Chin MH, et al. ACC/AHA 2005 Guideline update for the diagnosis and management of chronic heart failure in the adult – summary article. Circulation 2005; 112: 1–28.
16. Christakis NA, Lamont EB. Extent and determinants of error in doctors' prognoses in terminally ill patients: prospective cohort study. BMJ 2000; 320: 469–72.
17. Goodlin SJ, Hauptman PJ, Arnold R, et al. Consensus statement: palliative and supportive care in advanced heart failure. J Card Fail 2004; 10: 200–9.
18. SUPPORT Investigators. A controlled trial to improve care for seriously ill hospitalized patients. JAMA 1995; 274: 1591–8.
19. Levenson JW, McCarthy EP, Lynn J, Davis RB, Phillips RS. The last six months of life for patients with congestive heart failure. J Am Geriatr Soc 2000; 48: S101–9.
20. Sullivan MD, O'Meara ES. Heart failure at the end of life: symptoms, function, and medical care in the Cardiovascular Health Study. Am J Geriatr Cardiol 2006; 15: 217–25.
21. Guck TP, Elsasser GN, Kavan MG, et al. Depression in congestive heart failure. Congest Heart Fail 2003; 9: 163–9.
22. Havranek EP, Spertus JA, Masoudi FA, Jones PG, Rumsfeld JS. Predictors of the onset of depressive symptoms in patients with heart failure. J Am Coll Cardiol 2004; 44: 2333–8.
23. Rumsfeld JS, Jones PG, Whooley MA, et al. Depression predicts mortality and hospitalization in patients with myocardial infarction complicated by heart failure. Am Heart J 2005; 150: 961–7.
24. Koenig HG. Depression outcome in inpatients with congestive heart failure. Arch Intern Med 2006; 166: 991–6.
25. Jiang W, Alexander J, Christopher E, et al. Relationship of depression to increased risk of mortality and rehospitalization in patients with congestive heart failure. Arch Intern Med 2001; 161: 1849–56.
26. Goebel JR, Doering LV, Shugarman LR, et al. Heart failure: the hidden problem of pain. J Pain Symptom Manage 2009; 38: 698–707.
27. Zambroski CH, Moser DK, Roser LP, Heo S, Chung ML. Patients with Heart Failure who die in Hospice, Am Heart J 2005; 149: 558–64.
28. ACC guidelines.
29. Nohria A, Lewis E, Stevenson LW. Medical management of advanced heart failure. JAMA 2002; 287: 628–40.
30. Jessup M, Brozena S. Heart failure. N Engl J Med 2003; 348: 2007–18.

31. Pitt B, Zannad F, Remme WJ, et al. The effect of spironolactone on morbidity and mortality in patients with severe heart failure. Randomized Aldactone Evaluation Study Investigators. N Engl J Med 1999; 341: 709–17.

32. The Digitalis Investigation Group. The effect of digoxin on mortality and morbidity in patients with heart failure. N Engl J Med 1997; 336: 525–33.

33. Felker GM, O'Connor CM. Inotropic therapy for heart failure: an evidence-based approach. Am Heart J 2001; 142: 393–401.

34. Felker GM, O'tConnor CM. Inotropic therapy for heart failure: an evidence-based approach. Am Heart J 2001; 142: 393–401.

35. Rich MW, Shore BL. Dobutamine for patients with end-stage heart failure in a hospice program? J Palliat Med 2003; 6: 93–7.

36. Nauman DJ, Ray E, Hershberger RE. The use of positive inotropes in end-of-life heart failure care. Curr Heart Fail Rep 2007; 4: 158–63.

37. Lorenz KA, Lynn J, Dy SM, et al. Evidence for improving palliative care at the end of life: a systematic review. Ann Intern Med 2008; 1482: 147–59.

38. Williams SG, Wright DJ, Marshall P, et al. Safety and potential benefits of low dose diamorphine during exercise in patients with chronic heart failure. Heart 2003; 89: 1085–6.

39. Johnson MJ, McDonagh TA, Harkness A, McKay SE, Dargie HJ. Morphine for the relief of breathlessness in patients with chronic heart failure–a pilot study. Eur J Heart Fail 2002; 4: 753–6.

40. Kaneko Y, Floras JS, Usui K, et al. Cardiovascular effects of continuous positive airway pressure in patients with heart failure and obstructive sleep apnea. N Engl J Med 2003; 348: 1233–41.

41. Javaheri S. Acetazolamide improves central sleep apnea in heart failure: a double-blind, prospective study. Am J Respir Crit Care Med 2006; 173: 234–7.

42. Booth S, Wade R, Johnson M, Expert Working Group of the Scientific Committee of the Association of Palliative Medicine. The use of oxygen in the palliation of breathlessness. A report of the expert working group of the Scientific Committee of the Association of Palliative Medicine. Respir Med 2004; 98: 66–77.

43. [Available from: http://www.who.int/cancer/palliative/painladder/en/].

44. Lane DA, Chong AY, Lip GYH. Psychological interventions for depression in heart failure. Cochrane Database Syst Rev 2006; 25: CD003329.

45. Kaldjian LC, Curtis AE, Shinkunas LA, Cannon KT. Goals of care toward the end of life: a structured literature review. Am J Hosp Palliat Care 2009; 25: 501–11.

46. Baile WF, Buckman R, Lenzi R, et al. SPIKES: a six-step protocol for delivering bad news: application to the patient with cancer. Oncologist 2000; 5: 302–11.

47. Weiner JS, Arnold RM, Curtis JR, et al. Manualized communication interventions to enhance palliative care research and training: rigorous, testable approaches. J Palliat Med 2006; 9: 371–81.

48. Wachter RM, Luce JM, Hearst N, Lo B. Decisions about resuscitation: inequities among patients with different diseases but similar prognoses. Ann Intern Med 1989; 111: 525–32.

49. Krumholz HM, Phillips RS, Hamel MB, et al. Resuscitation preferences among patients with severe congestive heart failure: results from the SUPPORT Project. Circulation 1998; 98: 648–55.

50. Haydar ZR, Lowe AJ, Kahveci KL, Weatherford W, Finucane T. Differences in end-of-life preferences between congestive heart failure and dementia in a medical house calls program. J Am Geriatr Soc 2004; 52: 736–40.

51. McClellan MB, Tunis SR. Medicare coverage of ICDs. N Engl J Med 2005; 352: 222–4.

52. Berger JT. The ethics of deactivating implanted cardioverter defibrillators. Ann Intern Med 2005; 142: 631–4.

53. Goldstein NE, Lampert R, Bradley E, Lynn J, Krumholz HM. Management of implantable cardioverter defibrillators in end-of-life care. Ann Intern Med 2004; 141: 835–8.

54. National Hospice Organization. Medical Guidelines for Determining Prognosis in Selected Non-Cancer Diseases. Arlington, VA: National Hospice Organization, 1996.

55. Fox E, Landrum-McNiff K, Zhong Z, et al. Evaluation of prognostic criteria for determining hospice eligibility in patients with advanced lung, heart, or liver disease. SUPPORT Investigators. Study to understand prognoses and preferences for outcomes and risks of treatments. JAMA 1999; 282: 1638–45.

56. Albert NM, Davis M, Young J. Improving care of patients dying of heart failure. Cleve Clin J Med 2002; 69: 321–8.

57. Fonarow GC, Adams KF, Abraham WT, et al. Risk stratification for in-hospital mortality in acutely decompensated heart failure. JAMA 2005; 293: 572–80.

58. Lee DS, Austin PC, Rouleau JL, et al. Predicting mortality among patients hospitalized for heart failure: derivation and validation of a clinical model. JAMA 2003; 290: 2581–7.

59. Coventry PA, Grande GE, Richards DA, Todd CJ. Prediction of appropriate timing of palliative care for older adults with non-malignant life-threatening disease: a systematic review. Age Ageing 2005; 34: 218–27.
60. Christakis N, Escarce J. Survival of medicare patients after enrollment in hospice programs. NEJM 1996; 335: 172–8.
61. Chan DC, Heidenreich PA, Weinstein MC, Fonarow GC. Heart failure disease management programs: a cost-effectiveness analysis. Am Heart J 2008; 155: 332–8.
62. Lorenz KA, Lynn J, Dy SM, et al. Evidence for improving palliative care at the end of life: a systematic review. Ann Inter Med 2008; 148: 147–59.
63. Hebert KA, Horswell RL, Dy S, et al. Mortality benefit of a comprehensive heart failure disease management program in indigent patients. Am Heart J 2006; 151: 478–83.
64. Shah MR, Flavell CM, Weintraub JR, et al. Intensity and focus of heart failure disease management after hospital discharge. Am Heart J 2005; 149: 715–21.
65. Rich MW. Multidisciplinary heart failure clinics: are they effective in Canada? CMAJ 2005; 173: 53–4.
66. Akosah KO, Shaper AM, Haus LM, et al. Improving outcomes in heart failure in the community: long-term survival benefit of a disease-management program. Chest 2005; 127: 2042–8.
67. Goodlin SJ, Hauptman PJ, Arnold R, et al. Consensus statement: palliative and supportive care in advanced heart failure. J Card Fail 2004; 10: 200–9.

27
Gene therapy for heart failure

Stefan P. Janssens

INTRODUCTION

Although originally mainly envisioned for the treatment of monogenetic diseases, gene therapy has become a promising therapeutic approach for selected polygenetic cardiac disorders. During the past decades, the pathophysiology of a variety of cardiac diseases is better understood, which has paved the way for targeted gene-based interventions directed at key processes in the pathogenesis of myocardial dysfunction and advanced heart failure (HF). Myocardial ischemia is most often due to obstructive coronary disease and percutaneous coronary intervention or coronary artery bypass grafting to restore perfusion together with state-of-the-art medical treatment is the first-line therapy. A significant number of patients, however, will remain symptomatic despite these conventional interventions (referred to as no-option patients) or have severe and diffuse coronary artery damage, not amenable to routine interventions. These no-option patients might benefit from gene therapy aimed at enhancing neovascularization by either angiogenesis or vasculogenesis. Neovascularization is a physiologic endogenous process in response to ischemia, but when insufficient to resolve ischemia, proangiogenic therapies might prove useful.

Preclinical gene therapy studies have mainly focused on angiogenic gene transfer using either vascular endothelial growth factor (VEGF) isoforms VEGF121 and VEGF165 or fibroblast growth factor (FGF), mainly FGF-4 and FGF-5 isoforms. Intramyocardial delivery of a replication-deficient adenovirus carrying VEGF165 in Yucatan minipigs enhanced BrdU incorporation in cardiomyocytes four weeks after myocardial ischemia-reperfusion injury without concomitant reduction in infarct size or increase in global LV function (1). In contrast, intramyocardial adenoviral delivery of FGF-4 and FGF-5 in a porcine model of myocardial ischemia has been shown to increase both collateral vessel formation and left ventricular (LV) function (2,3). Despite promising results of some of these preclinical angiogenic gene transfer studies, translation in patients with ischemic cardiomyopathy has been rather disappointing, as discussed in the section Update on Human Gene Therapy for Cardiac Disease.

This review, therefore, will more specifically address gene-based strategies to enhance myocardial performance by increasing systolic or diastolic function in advanced HF. Heart transplantation currently remains the only long-term treatment option for these patients despite state-of-the-art medical and device therapy, but donor organ shortage remains a critical limitation. Hence, innovative gene-based strategies aimed at either improving cardiac function or slowing down disease progression constitute a valuable and particularly timely alternative in view of the growing incidence of advanced HF in a rapidly aging population.

Major gene-based strategies in established HF have focused on improved contraction, via enhanced β-adrenergic signaling, or on reversal of diastolic dysfunction, via enhanced intracellular calcium handling and sarcoplasmic reticulum (SR) calcium ATPase (SERCA) gene function. Intracoronary adenoviral delivery of genes encoding β2-adrenergic receptors resulted in enhanced β-adrenergic signaling and increased contraction (4). Likewise, overexpression of SERCA by adeno-associated viral transfer improved systolic and diastolic HF and mitigated disease progression (5).

But equally important may be gene-based efforts to prevent rather than reverse development of HF. Progression toward HF is often initiated by myocardial damage leading to cardiomyocyte death and adverse remodeling. Thus, minimizing cardiac damage or preventing myocyte death are potentially interesting gene therapy targets to halt or prevent progression toward HF. Experiments in animal models of ischemia-reperfusion have shown improved cardiac function after transfer of genes encoding the antiapoptotic factor bcl-2 (6) or cardioprotective NOS3 or AKt genes (7–9). These are promising strategies that need further validation.

GENE THERAPY MODALITIES FOR THE FAILING HEART
Targeted Gene Therapy

Irrespective of the delivery route used for gene delivery, there is always some systemic leakage of the vector leading to unwanted transduction of extracardiac tissues. In most cases, this minimal leakage will not have any tangible adverse effects, but side effects can occur in case of significant expression in nontarget tissues. In order to improve the safety profile, efforts have been made to develop targeted gene therapy strategies in which transgene expression is confined to the myocardium with minimal or ideally no ectopic expression. Theoretically, the optimal targeting strategy should allow systemic administration of therapeutic vectors and so far, two different targeting strategies have been explored to achieve this goal: transductional and transcriptional targeting.

Transductional Targeting

The goal of transductional targeting is to increase the cardiac tropism of different viral vectors and decrease the affinity for ectopic tissues. Most viral vectors have an intrinsic tropism for specific tissues such as the commonly used serotype-5 adenoviral vector, which predominantly transduces liver tissue after IV delivery. Transductional targeting with adenoviral vectors has not been explored extensively in cardiac gene therapy. In contrast, myocardial targeting with adeno-associated viral (AAV) vectors is more frequently applied because some AAV serotypes exhibit a natural tropism for striated muscles, such as AAV-1, AAV-6, and AAV-8 and -9 (10–12). The AAV-2 serotype is the most widespread vector used for gene therapy and modifications of the capsid proteins lead to a significant reduction of liver infection, resulting in an increased heart-to-liver ratio (13). Further attempts to achieve even greater cardiospecificity by packaging the genome of the AAV-2 serotype into the viral capsids of serotypes with high natural tropism for muscle have been successful (14). Even though a significant cardiac tropism has been achieved by these modifications, most viral vectors will still transduce ectopic tissues to some extent. Currently, transductional targeting is not routinely employed for cardiac gene therapy.

Transcriptional Targeting

In contrast to transductional targeting in which the virus's tropism for the heart is enhanced, the goal of transcriptional targeting is to minimize the expression of the therapeutic gene in nontarget tissues transduced with the viral vector. The latter can be achieved by using a cardiac-specific promoter that drives the therapeutic gene of interest. The ideal cardiac-specific promoter will only direct transgene expression in the myocardium and not in other tissues. For cardiac applications, three specific promoters have extensively been studied: myosin light chain-2 ventricular isoform (MLC-2v), alpha-myosin heavy chain (αMHC), and cardiac troponin T (cTnT) (15,16). These promoters for cardiac gene delivery have been shown to significantly limit ectopic expression in lungs and liver, two organs that are easily transduced following systemic leakage of viral vectors after intramyocardial delivery.

However, transcriptional targeting has been very difficult to achieve *in vivo* due to the weakness of most cardiac-specific promoters even at the target site. Different amplification strategies, such as adding a viral enhancer sequence to or multimerizing a cardiac-specific promoter (16,17) confer minimal amplification or suffer from limited cardiac specificity. A more robust two-step transcriptional amplification system, reported by Ray et al., may circumvent these limitations without compromising cardiac specificity but needs further validation before clinically applicable (18).

Therapeutic Delivery Routes for Gene Therapy

The ideal route for gene or vector delivery to the myocardium aims for maximal efficacy with minimal diffusion or leakage to extra-cardiac tissues. More specifically, three different routes are under investigation for this purpose: intravenous (IV), intramyocardial and intracoronary delivery and each has distinct advantages and disadvantages.

Intravenous Delivery

IV delivery is the easiest, most accessible and least invasive way for gene transfer but most constructs will disseminate to the whole body and result in off-target transduction. Larger constructs may be temporarily trapped in the precapillary network of the lungs and only very few will home to the myocardium. Similarly, systemic injection of radioactively labeled bone marrow cells only showed background signal in the myocardium after ischemia (19,20). The amount of cells accumulating in the myocardium is highly dependent on homing signals, but most cells will be trapped in the reticuloendothelial system of liver and spleen in case of mononuclear cell transfer. Systemic delivery is also irrelevant for naked DNA, because of its instability in serum and its very short half-life due to the presence of serum nucleases (21).

Intramyocardial Delivery

Direct injection into the myocardial wall has been the preferred delivery route in most preclinical small animal studies of cell and gene therapy. It has been proved to be a very efficient route for both viral and nonviral vectors as well as for cell delivery (22). Although this route traditionally required surgical exposure of the heart, dedicated small animal ultrasound imaging systems enable image-guided minimally invasive percutaneous cell or gene delivery (23). In contrast to small animal models, fluoroscopy-guided catheter-based endocardial delivery is feasible in large animals and patients and a valuable percutaneous alternative for intramyocardial injection. Independent of the technique used, direct injection usually leads to a more focal and patchy pattern in the myocardium and inevitably causes some diffusion into the circulation.

Intracoronary Delivery

Intracoronary injection is a very relevant method for cell or vector delivery but not for naked DNA due to its poor stability in serum. In contrast to intramyocardial injection, intracoronary infusion theoretically enables a more widespread distribution pattern covering the entire perfusion territory supplied by the respective artery. Although this is a

Table 27.1   Gene Transfer Vector Systems

	Nonviral	Adenovirus	Adeno-associated Virus	Retrovirus	Lentivirus
Vector genome	Naked DNA-ipoplexes	ds-DNA (serotype 5)	ss-DNA (serotype 2 parvovirus)	ss-RNA	ss-RNA
Transfer efficiency	Low in vivo More effective in vitro (lipoplexes)	High Quiescent and dividing cells	High Quiescent and dividing cells	Low Only dividing cells	Low Quiescent cells
Duration gene expression	Transient	Weeks	Long term	Long term	Long term
Toxicity	—	Local inflammatory response; Limited insertional mutagenesis	WT vector nonpathogenic in humans	Nonspecific integration	Nonspecific integration
Immune response	—	Dose-dependent; Pre-existing NAbs against Ad5	Moderate; Pre-existing NAbs against AAV2	Low	Low
Systemic delivery	No (serum nucleases)	No selective targeting	Serotype-specific tropism (AAV1–6 skeletal muscle; AAV8–9 myocardium)	Limited tropism	Limited tropism
Gene insert packaging capacity	—	8 kb (E1E3-deleted); 30 kb (gutless)	4.5 kb	7.5 kb	>8 kb
Upscaling	Easy	Easy in high titers	Difficult production	Difficult production	Difficult production

Abbreviation: AAV, adeno-associated virus.

straightforward and commonly used method for cell delivery, its success for gene delivery highly depends on viral vector type and titer. Transduction efficacy for adenoviral vectors following intracoronary delivery, for example, is superior to adeno-associated viral vectors, the preferred vector system for cardiac applications due to its intrinsic cardiac tropism (24,25). Delivery through the coronary arteries involves catheter-based techniques and is therefore mainly applicable in large animals and humans. Nevertheless, challenging surgical procedures have been developed to achieve coronary gene delivery in smaller animal models. The latter is achieved by positioning a small catheter into the left ventricular cavity or aortic root while cross clamping both the aorta and pulmonary artery (26).

Vectors for Gene Transfer
Transfer of genetic material to cells can be obtained by either viral or nonviral delivery methods (Table 27.1). The main goal of these vectors is protecting the DNA from serum nucleases and delivering the DNA across the membrane into the cell and its nucleus. Again, the different approaches all have distinct advantages and disadvantages.

Nonviral Vectors

Nonviral delivery of genetic material in the cell can be achieved by physical or chemical methods. Physical approaches are based on transient defects in the cell membrane, induced by physical forces, including injection of naked DNA, hydrodynamic injection, electroporation, and ultrasound.

Local injection of naked DNA can lead to transgene expression in tissues, such as muscle and liver, but generally results in very poor, and tissue-dependent transfer efficacy. This method does not induce any toxicity and elicits only a minimal immune response. The major drawback of naked DNA injection is rapid degradation by nucleases. Hydrodynamic injection is a more efficient method for gene transfer, as very fast injection of a large volume causes retrograde flow and increased pressure leading to transient membrane defects and DNA entry into the cell. This method has shown promise for liver-directed gene transfer, but cardiac applications are uncertain.

Electroporation and ultrasound transiently increase the permeability of the cell membrane by applying an external electrical field or sound waves, respectively. This transient membrane disruption allows diffusion of DNA in the cell with greater transfer efficacy than naked DNA and stable gene expression for over one year after electroporation.

The other nonviral delivery method is based on a chemical approach in which DNA is packed into particles composed of cationic polymers or lipids. After complex formation, these particles mainly enter the cell through endocytosis and release the DNA into the cytoplasm. Cationic lipid-based methods are generally used for *in vitro* transfection procedures with good transfer efficacy. When DNA and cationic lipids are brought together, small particles known as lipoplexes are formed, which efficiently transfect cultured cells in the absence of serum. However, interaction with negatively charged serum proteins *in vivo* causes large aggregates and precludes clinical use thus far. Cationic polymers are an alternative and polyethylenimine has been shown to yield similar results as cationic lipids. However, polymer toxicity and uncertainties on biodegradability remain major drawbacks for clinical translation. Despite the progress, nonviral methods generally result in transient expression and lower transfer efficacy as compared with viral methods and their use will likely remain limited to *in vitro* and preclinical studies.

Viral Vectors

During evolution, viruses have co-evolved with their hosts, and have undergone continuous selection to overcome significant barriers for infectivity and replication of genetic material in somatic cells. In the development of viral vectors for gene transfer purposes, the replication potential of the parental virus has been suppressed by removal of both disease-causing genes and genes required for replication. A gene of interest, which, in turn, will be expressed in host cells, can then replace the deleted gene sequences. There are currently four main types of viral vector systems available for gene therapy: adenoviral (Ad), adeno-associated virus (AAV), retroviral, and lentiviral vectors (Table 27.1). These vector systems all have their strengths and disadvantages, and the choice for any particular viral vector depends on the required duration of gene expression in the host, the size of the transgene, the target tissue, and biosafety issues. The main limitations of retroviruses, for example, are their low-titer stocks, risk of insertional mutagenesis, and their inability to efficiently transfect nondividing or slowly dividing cells, including cardiomyocytes or vascular endothelial cells. In contrast, lentiviral vectors are capable of transducing mitotically quiescent cells by genomic integration and have been successfully used in preclinical models of familial hypercholesterolemia (27). The most commonly used lentiviral vector system was based on the human immunodeficiency virus type 1 (HIV-1) (28). Because of biosafety concerns regarding pathogenicity of the parental virus, significant bioengineering efforts are ongoing to reduce the risk of producing replication-competent virus through recombination and to render the proviral 5'-long terminal repeats of the HIV transcriptionally inactive. More later additional modifications to the vector backbone have enhanced nuclear import and mRNA translation in target cells, and offer novel prospects for enhanced in vivo transduction efficiency in adult cardiomyocytes (29). While waiting for these emerging novel developments, Ad and AAV vectors have been favored in current clinical cardiac gene therapy protocols, and will be briefly described.

Adenoviral Vectors

Adenoviruses are nonenveloped double-stranded DNA viruses with a genome size of 36 kb. There are more than 50 different serotypes, which can readily infect tissues of the respiratory, urinary, and gastrointestinal tract as well as the liver and the conjunctivae. Most adenoviral vectors are derived from serotype 2 and 5 from species C, which are endemic and cause upper respiratory tract infection. The first-generation vectors are made replication-defective by deletion of the E1 gene and newer generations also contain additional deletions of the E3 gene. The combined E1 and E3 deletions leave a relatively large packaging capacity of 8 kb. In the laboratory, these viruses are easy to produce in high titers and can efficiently infect both dividing and nondividing cells. Ad vectors infect the target cell through interaction with the coxsackie-adenovirus receptor (CAR) followed by internalization through the interaction between the viral capsid and cellular integrins (30). These vectors can yield very high transgene expression even if there are only few CARs present on the target cells. The first- and second-generation vectors can trigger an immune response after IV delivery, but this effect is dose dependent (31) and the latest generation of Ad vectors in which almost the entire viral genome has been deleted can drastically reduce this immune reaction. The latter so-called gutless vectors, that lack all viral DNA except for the packaging sequence and replication-initiation sequences, are superior because of very high payload, packaging capability of 30 kb, and reduced immunogenicity further extending duration of transgene expression (32). However, they can still elicit an inflammatory reaction because of the presence of viral capsid proteins.

The major drawback of Ad vectors is the induction of a host immune response because almost 50% of the population carries antibodies against serotypes 1, 2, and 5. This immune response limits the duration of transgene expression and further limits potential re-administration of the vector (9). Another factor limiting the duration of transgene expression is inherent to Ad vectors because the adenoviral genome does not integrate into the host genome but is maintained episomally. This will result in dilution of the DNA with subsequent cell divisions but on the other hand will also limit the risk for insertional mutagenesis.

Adeno-Associated Viral Vectors

AAVs are single-stranded DNA viruses belonging to the parvoviruses, which are not pathogenic in humans. To date, 11 subtypes of the virus have been reported for which humans are the primary host and up to 80% of the population are seropositive for the most prevalent serotype 2. AAV vectors have mainly been based on serotype 2 and have been shown to efficiently transduce liver, muscle, and brain tissue. AAV vectors can transduce both dividing and nondividing cells but their efficacy is greatly enhanced during the S phase of the cell cycle. In contrast to Ad vectors, AAV vectors have only a limited packaging size of 4.5 kb even after removal of most of the viral genome. The viral infectivity highly depends on the presence or absence of a heparin sulfate-binding domain and the natural tropism of the serotype, such as the liver tropism of AAV6 and the cardiac tropism of AAV9. The latter was reported in rodents but does not fully translate in large animals and has not been studied in patients. Efficient gene transfer in the myocardium has been achieved by substituting the viral capsid from the AAV vectors with the capsid of a virus with intrinsic high myocardial tropism (13). Long-term transgene expression has been achieved and is mainly due to the existence of nonintegrated, extrachromosomal AAV genomes. There is only a very small fraction of AAV vectors that integrates into the host genome and these integrations occur mainly at transcription start sites or in transcribed genes (33). The kinetics of transgene expression are somewhat slower than with Ad vectors.

The major hurdles for clinical use of AAV vectors are the limited packaging size and the high incidence of pre-existing neutralizing antibodies not only against the AAV serotype 2 but also against serotype 1, which has been used in clinical heart failure trials (34). Modifications of the viral capsid or use of viral capsids from other serotypes may overcome this hurdle and are currently under investigation (32).

GENE THERAPY TARGETS IN HEART FAILURE

With rapid advancements in our understanding of the molecular basis of myocardial dysfunction, an increasing number of molecular targets is being pursued in various models of gene therapy for HF. Because an exhaustive review of all possible targets is beyond the scope of this chapter, we will summarize the most representative approaches with a particular focus on those that have been introduced in ongoing early clinical trials (Fig. 27.1).

Common molecular hallmarks of HF are the alterations in β-AR signaling and intracellular calcium signaling, which fundamentally govern contraction and relaxation in cardiomyocytes. Briefly, under normal circumstances, cardiac cell membrane depolarization triggers Ca^{2+} influx through the L-type calcium channels (LTCC) followed by a calcium-induced calcium release from the SR through the ryanodine receptors (RyRs). Increased catecholamine levels activate β-ARs and enhance contraction via enhanced transmembrane calcium influx, increased velocity and amplitude of SR Ca^{2+} release, and facilitated SERCA pump activity. The increased cytosolic Ca^{2+} in turn binds to the thin filament troponin C and activates contraction. As SR Ca^{2+} content is being depleted during contraction and RyRs are being inactivated, the cardiomyocyte switches from its systolic to its diastolic mode and cytosolic free Ca^{2+} is being sequestered again in the SR for the next contraction cycle via the SERCA2a ATPase pump [a process, negatively regulated on a beat-to-beat basis by a small inhibitory peptide, phospholamban (PLN)] or pumped out of the cell via the sodium Ca^{2+} exchanger.

It has been well accepted for decades that β-AR density is reduced as well as the responsiveness to β-agonists in the myocardium of HF patients. Yet the complex interplay between the different β-AR subtypes (type 1, 2, and 3), their downstream signaling

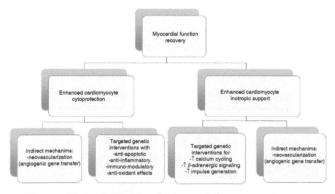

Figure 27.1 Strategies for heart failure gene therapy.

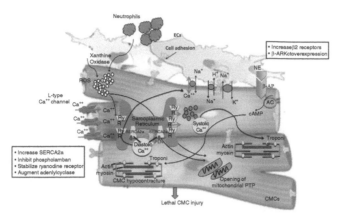

Figure 27.2 Pathophysiologic mechanisms resulting in loss of contractile force and targets for heart failure gene therapy. *Abbreviations*: cAMP, cyclic adenosine monophosphate; CMC, cardiac myocyte; ECs, endothelial cells; NE, norepinephrine; PTP, permeability transition pore; ROS, reactive oxygen species; SERCA, sarcoplasmic reticulum calcium ATPase.

components, including heterotrimeric G proteins, adenylate cyclase, and cyclic adenosine monophosphate (cAMP)-dependent and -independent effectors do not allow for a simplified and "one fits all" approach to improve cardiac function by β-AR gene transfer strategies. Similarly, the amplitude and velocity of intracellular calcium transients in cardiomyocytes is regulated by phosphorylation of two major kinases, namely, protein kinase A (PKA) and Ca^{2+}/calmodulin-dependent protein kinase II (CaMKII). These two important regulators in turn phosphorylate at least three distinct key Ca^{2+} regulators, namely, the LTCC, the RyRs, and PLN. To maintain cardiomyocyte homeostasis and proper excitation–contraction coupling, these phosphorylated proteins require dynamic and balanced active dephosphorylation by a series of phosphatases, the regulation and function of which is much less understood in HF.

By and large, important transporters and proteins that have been targeted in preclinical models using gene transfer can be grouped into those involved in (*i*) the β-adrenergic signaling cascade, (*ii*) calcium cycling regulation, (*iii*) cardiomyocyte cytoprotection, and (*iv*) impulse generation and conduction in the myocardium. For each, specific gene-based strategies vary depending on the underlying pathophysiologic mechanism in the experimental model. The goal is to correct a missing gene or a gene mutation, overexpress a deficient target molecule, administer genetically modified progenitor cells, or introduce loss of function approaches using dominant negative strategies (Fig. 27.2 and Table 27.2).

β-Adrenergic Signaling Cascade

As stated above, the paramount clinical observations of improved survival in severe HF patients following β-adrenergic receptor blocker administration, is somewhat paradoxic in view of many preclinical reports showing benefit of enhanced β-AR signaling in animal models of HF. Part of this is related to species-specific expression and regulation of β-AR subtypes, which generate significantly different cAMP levels and elicit different myocyte contractile responses. In addition, a tightly regulated interaction between β-ARs and downstream G-proteins reduces β-AR activity via a family of G-protein coupled receptor kinases (GRKs) in a process termed agonist-dependent desensitization (homologous desensitization) (35).

Table 27.2 β-AR and Ca^{2+} Cycling Targets for Heart Failure Gene Therapy: Preclinical Studies

Molecular Target Class	Mechanisms of Action	Experimental Model	Clinical Translation	References
β-AR signaling				
β-ARKct	Targeted inhibition of GRK2	Transgenic mice and somatic gene transfer	Controversy on gene transfer to augment β-AR	(38,76–78)
Ca++ cycling regulators				
SERCAa	PKA–CaMKII inhibition*	Gene transfer to augment SERCA2a rat, porcine model; mouse isoproterenol-induced cardiomyopathy*	Ongoing phase II trial with AAV1-SERCA2a	(48–50,79,80)
PLN	Pseudophosphorylated mutant (S16E)	Gene transfer to inhibit PLN (antisense and dominant–negative approaches): rat MI, sheep rapid pacing, CMP hamsters	Doubtful—different phenotype in human, loss of function mutations	(41–43,80,81)
RyR	Stabilization of channel by chemical compound JTV519	Canine pacing HF model	Uncertain	(47)
S100A1	Ca^{2+}-binding protein in SR and on sarcomere—independent of β-AR	Knockout and transgenic mice; isolated rat cardiomyocytes and post-MI	Uncertain in absence of large animalmodels or human cells	(82,83)
Parvalbumin	Ca^{2+} sequestering protein, Correction of prolonged diastolic Ca^{2+} decay	Rat isolated cardiomyocytes, transgenic mice, dogs (TAC)	Uncertain	(84)
Protein phosphatase 1	Dephosphorylation b PP1 (inhibits Ca-regulators and β-AR response)	—	—	—
Inhibitor protein-1	Inhibits PP1 and augments β-AR response	Transgenic PP1-mice dilated cardiomyopathy	Uncertain—preliminary in human isolated CMC	(81)
AC Type 6	Specific subtype overexpression	Variety of large and small animal models	Isoform-specific effects; clinical trials considered with AC6	(39,85,86)

Abbreviations: AAV, adeno-associated virus; CaMKII, Ca^{2+}/calmodulin-dependent protein kinase II; CMC, cardiac myocyte; CMP, cardiomyopathic; HF, heart failure; MI, myocardial infarction; PLN, phospholamban; RyR, ryanodine receptors; SR, sarcoplasmic reticulum; SERCA, sarcoplasmic reticulum calcium ATPase.

Importantly, the observations that GRK2 levels are increased in failing myocardium with uncoupling, downregulation of β1- and β2-AR and subsequent loss of inotropic reserve have led to strategies aimed at inhibiting activation of GRK2 (also known as β-ARK1) (35,36). These strategies have been successfully tested in transgenic mouse models or in adenoviral-mediated gene transfer studies (37), which from a clinical point of view are less representative. Intracardiac administration of β-ARKct peptide, a caboxy-terminal fragment of β-ARK, which inhibits endogenous kinase activity, using recombinant AAV vectors (serotype 6) in failing rat hearts has demonstrated sustained, sufficient expression levels of the peptide without significant toxicity, and significantly improved cardiac contractiltiy and reversed LV remodeling (38). Of note, these effects seemed to be synergistic to the benefit obtained with chronic β-blockade, but need validation and confirmation in larger animal models and in the clinical setting.

Calcium Cycling Regulation

Whereas pharmacologic therapies lack sufficient target selectivity and proper temporospatial distribution to reverse or correct specific calcium cycling defects, genetic correction of abnormalities in cardiac phosphorylation and to a lesser extent dephosphorylation cascades may become a promising target for HF treatment. Several experimental studies involving transgenic or gene transfer approaches to correct defective Ca^{2+} cycling have shown marked benefit in small and large animal models. They include overexpression of subtypes of adenylyl cyclase to boost cardiac cAMP production (39,40), modulation of PLN phosphorylation using phosphomimetic mutant forms (e.g., S16E, which promotes SERCA2a activity) (41–43), overexpression of SERCA2a using direct intramyocardial adenoviral gene transfer in rats with pressure overload-induced HF (44) or AAV-directed intracoronary gene transfer in pigs with volume overload-induced HF (45), correction of abnormal phosphatase PP1 regulation (46), stabilization of leaky RyR channel, and other SR Ca^{2+} releasing channels via CaMKII inhibition and subsequent restoration of phosphoregulation of RyR (47,48).

A common denominator of these strategies is the ultimate amelioration of SR Ca^{2+} uptake activity, which enhances the speed of Ca^{2+} removal during relaxation (and hence diastolic function) but by the same token increases the SR Ca^{2+} content, and therefore the amount of Ca^{2+} available for the subsequent contraction (enhanced systolic function). It should therefore not come as a surprise that the concept of SERCA2a gene therapy to replace the lost activity was among the first to be tested in preclinical models (26), isolated failing human cardiomyocytes (49) and in early phase clinical trials (50). Despite the early enthusiasm in rodents with pressure overload-induced myocardial dysfunction and in pigs with volume overload-induced LV failure (45), transgenic rats with cardiac SERCA2a overexpression failed to show a sustained benefit in LV performance at long-term follow-up after myocardial infarction and were prone to enhanced ventricular arrhythmogenicity (51). Moreover, SERCA2a gene transfer in isolated failing canine cardiomyocytes only conferred partial benefit characterized by improved diastolic function but loss of inotropic support and β-AR responsiveness (52). The reasons for these discrepancies are unclear but likely relate to species differences in calcium cycling and its tightly regulated phosphorylation and dephosphorylation cascades and to intricacies of experimental conditions (lifelong gain of function in transgenic rodents with likelihood of adaptive/compensatory changes versus acute gain of function following gene transfer without such chronic adaptation). However, the observation of deficient SR Ca^{2+} uptake in cardiomyocytes from failing human hearts, associated with reduced SR Ca^{2+}-ATPase gene function, has facilitated phase 2 SERCA gene transfer studies in selected HF patients.

Cardiomyocyte Protection

A variety of anti-inflammatory, antioxidant, antiapoptotic, angiogenic, and immunomodulatory gene-based interventions have been tested successfully in preclinical models of myocardial injury leading to cardiac dysfunction and negative LV remodeling. Most notably, genetic interference via decoy oligonucleotides against the NF-κB transcription factor, which acts as a masterswitch controlling expression of several downstream genes involved in inflammation has reduced infarct size in small and large animal models, and proved beneficial in experimental viral myocarditis and cardiac allografting (53). Similarly, gene transfer of antioxidant enzymes, including manganese superoxide dismutase (54) and heme oxygenase-1 can confer myocardial protection (55) and preserve LV function in rodents up to one year after ischemia-reperfusion injury (21,56) or after cardiac allografting (57). Finally, the recognition that apoptotic cardiomyocyte cell death contributes to LV dysfunction in both experimental and clinical HF has led many laboratories to pursue a variety of molecular targets within the intrinsic and extrinsic effector pathways for apoptosis. Adenoviral-mediated overexpression of antiapoptotic (Bcl-2, soluble Fas, NOS3, caspase-3 inhibitor p35) (6,58–60), angiogenic (hepatocyte growth factor) (61), or prosurvival genes (PI3-kinase and Akt) (62,63) has conferred marked cardioprotection against ischemic cell death both in small and large animal models.

Impulse Generation and Conduction

Genetic manipulations of processes involved in cardiac impulse generation, propagation, and repolarization are still in its infancy. Although efforts to create biologic pacemakers using adenovirus-mediated HCN gene transfer have shown proof of principle, the resulting pacemaker *If* current does not yet approximate the physiology of endogenous impulse-generating and -conducting cells (64–66). It remains therefore uncertain whether or not these strategies will be incorporated in future gene transfer strategies for HF treatment.

UPDATE ON HUMAN GENE THERAPY FOR CARDIAC DISEASE
Gene Therapy Studies

Similar to cell transfer studies, promising results in preclinical gene therapy studies have accelerated the start of clinical trials. Several randomized controlled phase 2 angiogenic gene delivery trials for coronary artery disease (CAD), have been completed. With several hundreds of patients having received active gene treatment, all studies have thus far documented a reassuring safety profile. Primary endpoints included myocardial perfusion or exercise tolerance and all but one of the five published and peer reviewed studies have reported either enhanced perfusion or exercise capacity (Table 27.3) (67–71).

Of the unpublished trials, some were prematurely stopped because of futility. Several factors are likely responsible for the variable outcome, including the type and dose of vector used, patient selection (unknown expression profile of growth factor receptors), choice of primary endpoint, and treatment of the control group. Moreover, therapeutic gene delivery efficacy and expression cannot always be easily assessed in CAD patients and little is known about vector biodistribution after intracoronary or intramyocardial delivery in patients, kinetics of transgene expression, or risk of inadvertent ectopic gene expression. Amidst some disappointment because of lack of successful translation from encouraging preclinical studies in CAD patients, these limitations emphasize the need for better vectors, dosing and delivery protocols, and importantly, for an optimized clinical trial design.

To limit inadvertent systemic expression of gene therapy products, and maintain long-term myocardial expression, several pseudotypes of AAVs have been introduced over the past 5 years in gene therapy studies in HF patients (34,50,72). In two phase 1 and phase 2 trials, patients with advanced HF of ischemic and nonischemic origin (CUPID study program) are

Table 27.3 Published Open-Label, Randomized, Controlled Gene Therapy Trials for Coronary Artery Disease

Trial	Patient Number	Gene of Interest	Study Design	Route of Delivery	Primary Endpoint and Result
KAT (68)	103	AdVEGF$_{165}$ or plasmid/ liposome VEGF$_{165}$ vs Ringer's lactate	Randomized, double-blind, placebo-controlled	Intracoronary infusion (injection at site of angioplasty)	Myocardial perfusion at 6 mo: positive, only in virus group
REVASC (70)	67	AdVEGF$_{121}$ vs best medical treatment	Randomized, controlled	Intramyocardial via thoracotomy	Exercise tolerance at 26 wk: positive
Euroinject One (69)	74	Naked VEGF$_{165}$ plasmid vs placebo plasmid	Randomized, double-blind, placebo-controlled	Percutaneous intramyocardial injection	Myocardial perfusion at 6 mo: negative
AGENT-2 (67)	52	AdFGF-4 vs vehicle	Randomized, double-blind, placebo-controlled	Intracoronary infusion	Myocardial perfusion (SPECT) at 8 wk: positive
CUPID (50) (Phase 1)	9	AAV1-SERCA2a	Open label	Intracoronary infusion	Safety acceptable – efficacy pending in Phase
VIF-CAD (71)	52	VEGFA165/bFGF plasmid vs placebo plasmid	Randomized, double-blind, placebo-controlled	Percutaneous intramyocardial injection	Myocardial perfusion (SPECT) at 5 mo: negative
CUPID (34) (Phase 2)	39	AAV1-SERCA2a	Randomized, double-blind, placebo-controlled, parallel-group, dose-ranging	Intracoronary infusion	Safety acceptable – benefit with highest dose in 7 efficacy parameters
VIF-CAD (71)	52	VEGFA165/bFGF plasmid vs placebo plasmid	Randomized, double-blind, placebo-controlled	Percutaneous intramyocardial injection	Myocardial perfusion (SPECT) at 5 mo: negative
CUPID (34) (Phase 2)	39	AAV1-SERCA2a	Randomized, double-blind, placebo-controlled, parallel-group, dose-ranging	Intracoronary infusion	Safety acceptable – benefit with highest dose in 7 efficacy parameters

Abbreviations: FGF, fibroblast growth factor; VEGF, vascular endothelial growth factor; SERCA, sarcoplasmic reticulum calcium ATPase; Ad, adenovirus; AAV, adeno-associated virus; SPECT, single-photon emission computed tomography.

receiving a single intracoronary injection of AAV1/SERCA2a (34). A different gene therapy strategy using AAV6-SERCA2 is proposed in patients with advanced nonischemic HF undergoing left ventricular assist placement but the trial has not yet started active recruitment (http://data.linkedct.org/resource/trials/NCT00534703).

The CUPID trial has a staged study design with an open-label dose escalation portion including four sequential, appropriately spaced doses followed by a randomized double-blind phase aimed at identifying safe and effective doses of AAV1-SERCA2a in HF patients. The open-label portion of the study in nine patients confirmed safety and suggested evidence of biologic activity across a number of parameters important for assessing HF status (72). Of note, the latter effects were not observed in two patients with pre-existing anti-AAV1 neutralizing antibodies, recapitulating the important effect of preimmune status of the host in other gene therapy protocols (9).

In the subsequent double-blind, randomized, placebo-controlled study in 39 patients with HF (NYHA Class III/IV, ejection fraction <35%, and maximal oxygen uptake capacity <20 mL/min/kg), intracoronary infusion of the high dose of AAV1/SERCA2a was found to be superior over placebo in a predefined set of primary endpoint success criteria (34). The endpoint analysis differed markedly from all previous gene transfer studies as it combined seven efficacy parameters in four different domains, including symptoms (NYHA Class, Minnesota Living With Heart Failure Questionnaire), functional status (six-minute walk test, peak maximum oxygen consumption), biomarker (N-terminal prohormone B-type natriuretic peptide), and LV function/remodeling (ejection fraction, LV end-systolic volume). Success at the group-level was prespecified as a concordant improvement in all seven efficacy parameters and no clinically significant worsening in any parameter. Of note, of the 509 prescreened patients, 265 were excluded from the study because of pre-existing neutralizing antibodies to AAV1 gene vector and only 39 were finally randomized and followed for 12 months. The concomitant reduction of recurrent clinical events by 12 months and the reassuring safety profile with the high-dose AAV1/SERCA2a is promising, but restricted to antibody naïve HF patients. A larger scale phase 3 study is ongoing to determine the role of AAV1/SERCA2a gene transfer in HF treatment.

Hybrid Gene and Cell Therapy Studies

Finally, in an approved study in Canada a hybrid cell and gene transfer approach is proposed in postmyocardial infarction patients with depressed LV function. In these patients autologous endothelial progenitor cells will be transfected with the human NOS3 gene and bioengineered endothelial progenitor cells (EPCs) will be infused in the ischemic heart in a dose escalation safety and feasibility study (73). The rational for this hybrid strategy is the observation that genetically engineered EPCs overexpressing human NOS3 display significantly enhanced cell functionality when tested in vitro (74,75) and hence may be more effective in mediating a biologically relevant repair process in the dysfunctional heart in vivo.

CONCLUSIONS

Although a growing body of evidence indicates that angiogenic gene therapy is effective for myocardial ischemia in a variety of preclinical models, randomized controlled trials in patients appear much less convincing. It is currently not clear whether the lackluster results are related to suboptimal gene delivery procedures or whether they are attributable to intrinsically different pathophysiologic mechanisms involved in complex and multifactorial clinical diseases.

Paradigms applicable to older and atherosclerotic patients with advanced LV dysfunction do not hold in young and healthy animal models. We should therefore be cautious when extrapolating findings from murine or larger animal models to the human population. Experimental conditions vary significantly but more importantly, basic molecular mechanisms in human cardiomyopathies cannot always be recapitulated in "knockout" or "gain of function" mutations in mice. For the same reason, we cannot expect genetic interventions that correct abnormalities in calcium cycling or β-adrenergic receptor signaling in experimental HF models to predict a similar outcome in clinical trials involving patients with significant comorbidity. Further progress in our understanding of basic molecular defects in excitation–contraction coupling in patients with advanced HF will no doubt identify novel targets for HF treatment with equal or perhaps superior promise than those identified to date.

To take advantage of the full potential of gene-based therapies for clinical HF patients, remaining questions regarding the optimal delivery route, gene or vector type, copy number, and biodistribution need to be addressed in appropriately designed exploratory trials. To do so, we need to integrate specific noninvasive molecular imaging technologies that enable repeated tracking of the genetic material after in vivo administration. Basic scientists, imaging experts along with clinician-scientists should engage in such collaborative translational studies to maintain the momentum for HF gene therapy.

REFERENCES

1. Guerrero M, Athota K, Moy J, et al. Vascular endothelial growth factor-165 gene therapy promotes cardiomyogenesis in reperfused myocardial infarction. J Interv Cardiol 2008; 21: 242–51.
2. Giordano FJ, Ping P, McKirnan MD, et al. Intracoronary gene transfer of fibroblast growth factor-5 increases blood flow and contractile function in an ischemic region of the heart. Nat Med 1996; 2: 534–9.
3. Gao MH, Lai NC, McKirnan MD, et al. Increased regional function and perfusion after intracoronary delivery of adenovirus encoding fibroblast growth factor 4: report of preclinical data. Hum Gene Ther 2004; 15: 574–87.
4. Jones JM, Petrofski JA, Wilson KH, et al. Beta2 adrenoceptor gene therapy ameliorates left ventricular dysfunction following cardiac surgery. Eur J Cardiothorac Surg 2004; 26: 1161–8.
5. Byrne MJ, Power JM, Preovolos A, et al. Recirculating cardiac delivery of aav2/1serca2a improves myocardial function in an experimental model of heart failure in large animals. Gene Ther 2008; 15: 1550–7.
6. Chatterjee S, Stewart AS, Bish LT, et al. Viral gene transfer of the antiapoptotic factor bcl-2 protects against chronic postischemic heart failure. Circulation 2002; 106: I212–17.
7. Boekstegers P, von Degenfeld G, Giehrl W, et al. Myocardial gene transfer by selective pressure-regulated retroinfusion of coronary veins. Gene Ther 2000; 7: 232–40.
8. Boekstegers P, Kupatt C. Current concepts and applications of coronary venous retroinfusion. Basic Res Cardiol 2004; 99: 373–81.
9. Szelid Z, Sinnaeve P, Vermeersch P, et al. Preexisting antiadenoviral immunity and regional myocardial gene transfer: modulation by nitric oxide. Hum Gene Ther 2002; 13: 2185–95.
10. Wang Z, Zhu T, Qiao C, et al. Adeno-associated virus serotype 8 efficiently delivers genes to muscle and heart. Nat Biotechnol 2005; 23: 321–8.
11. Palomeque J, Chemaly ER, Colosi P, et al. Efficiency of eight different AAV serotypes in transducing rat myocardium in vivo. Gene Ther 2007; 14: 989–97.
12. Pacak CA, Mah CS, Thattaliyath BD, et al. Recombinant adeno-associated virus serotype 9 leads to preferential cardiac transduction in vivo. Circ Res 2006; 99: e3–9.
13. Muller OJ, Katus HA, Bekeredjian R. Targeting the heart with gene therapy-optimized gene delivery methods. Cardiovasc Res 2007; 73: 453–62.
14. Muller OJ, Leuchs B, Pleger ST, et al. Improved cardiac gene transfer by transcriptional and transductional targeting of adeno-associated viral vectors. Cardiovasc Res 2006; 70: 70–8.
15. Franz WM, Rothmann T, Frey N, Katus HA. Analysis of tissue-specific gene delivery by recombinant adenoviruses containing cardiac-specific promoters. Cardiovasc Res 1997; 35: 560–6.
16. Boecker W, Bernecker OY, Wu JC, et al. Cardiac-specific gene expression facilitated by an enhanced myosin light chain promoter. Mol Imaging 2004; 3: 69–75.

17. Jin Y, Pasumarthi KB, Bock ME, et al. Effect of "enhancer" sequences on ventricular myosin light chain-2 promoter activity in heart muscle and nonmuscle cells. Biochem Biophys Res Commun 1995; 210: 260–6.

18. Ray S, Paulmurugan R, Patel MR, et al. Noninvasive imaging of therapeutic gene expression using a bidirectional transcriptional amplification strategy. Mol Ther 2008; 16: 1848–56.

19. Barbash IM, Chouraqui P, Baron J, et al. Systemic delivery of bone marrow-derived mesenchymal stem cells to the infarcted myocardium: feasibility, cell migration, and body distribution. Circulation 2003; 108: 863–8.

20. Hofmann M, Wollert KC, Meyer GP, et al. Monitoring of bone marrow cell homing into the infarcted human myocardium. Circulation 2005; 111: 2198–202.

21. Liu X, Simpson JA, Brunt KR, et al. Preemptive heme oxygenase-1 gene delivery reveals reduced mortality and preservation of left ventricular function 1 yr after acute myocardial infarction. Am J Physiol Heart Circ Physiol 2007; 293: H48–59.

22. Hou D, Youssef EA, Brinton TJ, et al. Radiolabeled cell distribution after intramyocardial, intracoronary, and interstitial retrograde coronary venous delivery: implications for current clinical trials. Circulation 2005; 112: I150–6.

23. Rodriguez-Porcel M, Gheysens O, Chen IY, Wu JC, Gambhir SS. Image-guided cardiac cell delivery using high-resolution small-animal ultrasound. Mol Ther 2005; 12: 1142–7.

24. Kaplitt MG, Xiao X, Samulski RJ, et al. Long-term gene transfer in porcine myocardium after coronary infusion of an adeno-associated virus vector. Ann Thorac Surg 1996; 62: 1669–76.

25. Kaspar BK, Roth DM, Lai NC, et al. Myocardial gene transfer and long-term expression following intracoronary delivery of adeno-associated virus. J Gene Med 2005; 7: 316–24.

26. Hajjar RJ, Schmidt U, Matsui T, et al. Modulation of ventricular function through gene transfer in vivo. Proc Natl Acad Sci USA 1998; 95: 5251–6.

27. Kankkonen HM, Vahakangas E, Marr RA, et al. Long-term lowering of plasma cholesterol levels in ldl-receptor-deficient whhl rabbits by gene therapy. Mol Ther 2004; 9: 548–56.

28. Klages N, Zufferey R, Trono D. A stable system for the high-titer production of multiply attenuated lentiviral vectors. Mol Ther 2000; 2: 170–6.

29. Bonci D, Cittadini A, Latronico MV, et al. 'Advanced' generation lentiviruses as efficient vectors for cardiomyocyte gene transduction in vitro and in vivo. Gene Ther 2003; 10: 630–6.

30. Meier O, Greber UF. Adenovirus endocytosis. J Gene Med 2004; 6:S152–63.

31. Tripathy SK, Black HB, Goldwasser E, Leiden JM. Immune responses to transgene-encoded proteins limit the stability of gene expression after injection of replication-defective adenovirus vectors. Nat Med 1996; 2: 545–50.

32. Verma IM, Weitzman MD. Gene therapy: twenty-first century medicine. Annu Rev Biochem 2005; 74: 711–38.

33. Nakai H, Montini E, Fuess S, et al. Helper-independent and AAV-ITR-independent chromosomal integration of double-stranded linear DNA vectors in mice. Mol Ther 2003; 7: 101–11.

34. Jessup M, Greenberg B, Mancini D, et al. Calcium upregulation by percutaneous administration of gene therapy in cardiac disease (cupid): a phase 2 trial of intracoronary gene therapy of sarcoplasmic reticulum Ca2+-ATPase in patients with advanced heart failure. Circulation 2011; 124: 304–13.

35. Tilley DG, Rockman HA. Role of beta-adrenergic receptor signaling and desensitization in heart failure: new concepts and prospects for treatment. Expert Rev Cardiovasc Ther 2006; 4: 417–32.

36. Ungerer M, Bohm M, Elce JS, Erdmann E, Lohse MJ. Altered expression of beta-adrenergic receptor kinase and beta 1-adrenergic receptors in the failing human heart. Circulation 1993; 87: 454–63.

37. Williams ML, Koch WJ. Viral-based myocardial gene therapy approaches to alter cardiac function. Annu Rev Physiol 2004; 66: 49–75.

38. Rengo G, Lymperopoulos A, Zincarelli C, et al. Myocardial adeno-associated virus serotype 6-beta-arkct gene therapy improves cardiac function and normalizes the neurohormonal axis in chronic heart failure. Circulation 2009; 119: 89–98.

39. Lai NC, Roth DM, Gao MH, et al. Intracoronary adenovirus encoding adenylyl cyclase vi increases left ventricular function in heart failure. Circulation 2004; 110: 330–6.

40. Roth DM, Gao MH, Lai NC, et al. Cardiac-directed adenylyl cyclase expression improves heart function in murine cardiomyopathy. Circulation 1999; 99: 3099–102.

41. Hoshijima M, Ikeda Y, Iwanaga Y, et al. Chronic suppression of heart-failure progression by a pseudo-phosphorylated mutant of phospholamban via in vivo cardiac raav gene delivery. Nat Med 2002; 8: 864–71.

42. Iwanaga Y, Hoshijima M, Gu Y, et al. Chronic phospholamban inhibition prevents progressive cardiac dysfunction and pathological remodeling after infarction in rats. J Clin Invest 2004; 113: 727–36.

43. Kaye DM, Preovolos A, Marshall T, et al. Percutaneous cardiac recirculation-mediated gene transfer of an inhibitory phospholamban peptide reverses advanced heart failure in large animals. J Am Coll Cardiol 2007; 50: 253–60.

44. del Monte F, Williams E, Lebeche D, et al. Improvement in survival and cardiac metabolism after gene transfer of sarcoplasmic reticulum Ca(2+)-ATPase in a rat model of heart failure. Circulation 2001; 104: 1424–9.

45. Kawase Y, Ly HQ, Prunier F, et al. Reversal of cardiac dysfunction after long-term expression of ser-Ca2a by gene transfer in a pre-clinical model of heart failure. J Am Coll Cardiol 2008; 51: 1112–19.

46. Yamada M, Ikeda Y, Yano M, et al. Inhibition of protein phosphatase 1 by inhibitor-2 gene delivery ameliorates heart failure progression in genetic cardiomyopathy. FASEB J 2006; 20: 1197–9.

47. Yano M, Kobayashi S, Kohno M, et al. Fkbp12.6-mediated stabilization of calcium-release channel (ryanodine receptor) as a novel therapeutic strategy against heart failure. Circulation 2003; 107: 477–84.

48. Zhang R, Khoo MS, Wu Y, et al. Calmodulin kinase ii inhibition protects against structural heart disease. Nat Med 2005; 11: 409–17.

49. del Monte F, Harding SE, Schmidt U, et al. Restoration of contractile function in isolated cardiomyocytes from failing human hearts by gene transfer of serca2a. Circulation 1999; 100: 2308–11.

50. Hajjar RJ, Zsebo K, Deckelbaum L, et al. Design of a phase 1/2 trial of intracoronary administration of aav1/serca2a in patients with heart failure. J Card Fail 2008; 14: 355–67.

51. Chen Y, Escoubet B, Prunier F, et al. Constitutive cardiac overexpression of sarcoplasmic/endoplasmic reticulum ca2+-atpase delays myocardial failure after myocardial infarction in rats at a cost of increased acute arrhythmias. Circulation 2004; 109: 1898–903.

52. Hirsch JC, Borton AR, Albayya FP, et al. Comparative analysis of parvalbumin and serca2a cardiac myocyte gene transfer in a large animal model of diastolic dysfunction. Am J Physiol Heart Circ Physiol 2004; 286: H2314–21.

53. Nakamura H, Morishita R, Kaneda Y. Molecular therapy via transcriptional regulation with double-stranded oligodeoxynucleotides as decoys. In Vivo 2002; 16: 45–8.

54. Iida S, Chu Y, Francis J, et al. Gene transfer of extracellular superoxide dismutase improves endothelial function in rats with heart failure. Am J Physiol Heart Circ Physiol 2005; 289: H525–32.

55. Foo RS, Siow RC, Brown MJ, Bennett MR. Heme oxygenase-1 gene transfer inhibits angiotensin ii-mediated rat cardiac myocyte apoptosis but not hypertrophy. J Cell Physiol 2006; 209: 1–7.

56. Liu X, Pachori AS, Ward CA, et al. Heme oxygenase-1 (HO-1) inhibits postmyocardial infarct remodeling and restores ventricular function. FASEB J 2006; 20: 207–16.

57. Braudeau C, Bouchet D, Tesson L, et al. Induction of long-term cardiac allograft survival by heme oxygenase-1 gene transfer. Gene Ther 2004; 11: 701–10.

58. Okada H, Takemura G, Kosai K, et al. Combined therapy with cardioprotective cytokine administration and antiapoptotic gene transfer in postinfarction heart failure. Am J Physiol Heart Circ Physiol 2009; 296: H616–26.

59. Ren J, Zhang X, Scott GI, et al. Adenovirus gene transfer of recombinant endothelial nitric oxide synthase enhances contractile function in ventricular myocytes. J Cardiovasc Pharmacol 2004; 43: 171–7.

60. Bott-Flugel L, Weig HJ, Knodler M, et al. Gene transfer of the pancaspase inhibitor p35 reduces myocardial infarct size and improves cardiac function. J Mol Med 2005; 83: 526–34.

61. Yang ZJ, Chen B, Sheng Z, et al. Improvement of heart function in postinfarct heart failure swine models after hepatocyte growth factor gene transfer: comparison of low-, medium- and high-dose groups. Mol Biol Rep 2010; 37: 2075–81.

62. Cittadini A, Monti MG, Iaccarino G, et al. Adenoviral gene transfer of akt enhances myocardial contractility and intracellular calcium handling. Gene Ther 2006; 13: 8–19.

63. Nagoshi T, Matsui T, Aoyama T, et al. Pi3k rescues the detrimental effects of chronic akt activation in the heart during ischemia/reperfusion injury. J Clin Invest 2005; 115: 2128–38.

64. Xue T, Siu CW, Lieu DK, et al. Mechanistic role of i(f) revealed by induction of ventricular automaticity by somatic gene transfer of gating-engineered pacemaker (hcn) channels. Circulation 2007; 115: 1839–50.

65. Kashiwakura Y, Cho HC, Barth AS, Azene E, Marban E. Gene transfer of a synthetic pacemaker channel into the heart: a novel strategy for biological pacing. Circulation 2006; 114: 1682–6.

66. Cai J, Yi FF, Li YH, et al. Adenoviral gene transfer of hcn4 creates a genetic pacemaker in pigs with complete atrioventricular block. Life Sci 2007; 80: 1746–53.

67. Grines CL, Watkins MW, Mahmarian JJ, et al. A randomized, double-blind, placebo-controlled trial of ad5fgf-4 gene therapy and its effect on myocardial perfusion in patients with stable angina. J Am Coll Cardiol 2003; 42: 1339–47.

68. Hedman M, Hartikainen J, Syvanne M, et al. Safety and feasibility of catheter-based local intracoronary vascular endothelial growth factor gene transfer in the prevention of postangioplasty and in-stent

restenosis and in the treatment of chronic myocardial ischemia: phase ii results of the kuopio angiogenesis trial (kat). Circulation 2003; 107: 2677–83.

69. Kastrup J, Jorgensen E, Ruck A, et al. Direct intramyocardial plasmid vascular endothelial growth factor-a165 gene therapy in patients with stable severe angina pectoris a randomized double-blind placebo-controlled study: the euroinject one trial. J Am Coll Cardiol 2005; 45: 982–8.

70. Stewart DJ, Hilton JD, Arnold JM, et al. Angiogenic gene therapy in patients with nonrevascularizable ischemic heart disease: a phase 2 randomized, controlled trial of ADVEGF(121) (ADVEGF121) versus maximum medical treatment. Gene Ther 2006; 13: 1503–11.

71. Kukula K, Chojnowska L, Dabrowski M, et al. Intramyocardial plasmid-encoding human vascular endothelial growth factor a165/basic fibroblast growth factor therapy using percutaneous transcatheter approach in patients with refractory coronary artery disease (VIF-CAD). Am Heart J 2011; 161: 581–9.

72. Jaski BE, Jessup ML, Mancini DM, et al. Calcium upregulation by percutaneous administration of gene therapy in cardiac disease (cupid trial), a first-in-human phase 1/2 clinical trial. J Card Fail 2009; 15: 171–81.

73. Ward MR, Stewart DJ, Kutryk MJ. Endothelial progenitor cell therapy for the treatment of coronary disease, acute mi, and pulmonary arterial hypertension: current perspectives. Catheter Cardiovasc Interv 2007; 70: 983–98.

74. Kaur S, Kumar TR, Uruno A, et al. Genetic engineering with endothelial nitric oxide synthase improves functional properties of endothelial progenitor cells from patients with coronary artery disease: an in vitro study. Basic Res Cardiol 2009; 104: 739–49.

75. Ward MR, Thompson KA, Isaac K, et al. Nitric oxide synthase gene transfer restores activity of circulating angiogenic cells from patients with coronary artery disease. Mol Ther 2011; 19: 1323–30.

76. Shah AS, White DC, Emani S, et al. In vivo ventricular gene delivery of a beta-adrenergic receptor kinase inhibitor to the failing heart reverses cardiac dysfunction. Circulation 2001; 103: 1311–16.

77. Vinge LE, Raake PW, Koch WJ. Gene therapy in heart failure. Circ Res 2008; 102: 1458–70.

78. Hata JA, Williams ML, Koch WJ. Genetic manipulation of myocardial beta-adrenergic receptor activation and desensitization. J Mol Cell Cardiol 2004; 37: 11–21.

79. Davia K, Bernobich E, Ranu HK, et al. SERCA2a overexpression decreases the incidence of aftercontractions in adult rabbit ventricular myocytes. J Mol Cell Cardiol 2001; 33: 1005–15.

80. Hajjar RJ, del Monte F, Matsui T, Rosenzweig A. Prospects for gene therapy for heart failure. Circ Res 2000; 86: 616–21.

81. Carr AN, Schmidt AG, Suzuki Y, et al. Type 1 phosphatase, a negative regulator of cardiac function. Mol Cell Biol 2002; 22: 4124–35.

82. Most P, Pleger ST, Volkers M, et al. Cardiac adenoviral s100a1 gene delivery rescues failing myocardium. J Clin Invest 2004; 114: 1550–63.

83. Pleger ST, Most P, Boucher M, et al. Stable myocardial-specific AAV6-s100a1 gene therapy results in chronic functional heart failure rescue. Circulation 2007; 115: 2506–15.

84. Szatkowski ML, Westfall MV, Gomez CA, et al. In vivo acceleration of heart relaxation performance by parvalbumin gene delivery. J Clin Invest 2001; 107: 191–8.

85. Hammond HK. Adenylyl cyclase gene transfer in heart failure. Ann NY Acad Sci 2006; 1080: 426–36.

86. Okumura S, Takagi G, Kawabe J, et al. Disruption of type 5 adenylyl cyclase gene preserves cardiac function against pressure overload. Proc Natl Acad Sci USA 2003; 100: 9986–90.

Index

Abdomino-jugular reflex, 243
ACE inhibitors
    aspirin interaction, 325–326
    in post-myocardial infarction management,
        324–325
Acidosis, systolic heart failure, 212
Acquired cardiomyopathy, 150–153
Action potential, heartbeat, 52
    phases, 43–44
    ventricular cardiomyocyte, 44
Acute Decompensated Heart Failure National
        Registry (ADHERE), 265, 267, 284
Acute volume overload, 80
Adrenomedullin (ADM), 267
African American Heart Failure Trial
        (AHeFT), 130
African Americans
    beta blockers use in, 334–335
Alcohol
    systolic heart failure and, 212
Aldosterone, 181
    escape, 367–368
    pathophysiology of, 366–367
    physiology, 365–366
Aldosterone escape, 367–368
Allele, 11, 12
Amiodarone, 402–403
Amyloidosis, 285
Anemia, 226
Angiotensin II, in heart failure, 120, 131
Angiotensin-converting enzyme inhibitors,
        190–191
Angiotensin receptor antagonists, 381–382
Angiotensin receptor blockers, 341–352
    adverse effects of ARB therapy, 348–350
    ARBs as alternatives to ACE inhibitors,
        343–346
    ARBs in combination with ACE inhibitors,
        346
    clinical studies of ARBs, 343
    clinical trials of, 344–345
    role of ARBs in asymptomatic LV
        dysfunction, 348
    treatment of patients with, and preserved
        LVEF, 347, 349
    treatment of patients with, and reduced
        LVEF, 343–346, 349

treatment of patients with, post-myocardial
        infarction, 347–348
Animal models, 78–89
    chronic-pacing models, 84–85
    different animal species, 79
    dilated cardiomyopathy, 87
    drug-induced models, 87–88
    ischemia and infarction, 85–87
    large animal models, 79
    pressure overload, 80, 81–82
    rapid-pacing models, 82–85
    small animal models, 79
    specific models, 79–80
    volume overload, 80–81
Antiarrhythmic medications, 401–404
    with arrhythmias, 419
    beta-adrenergic blockers, antiarrhythmic
        effects of, 401
        amiodarone, 402–403
        class I sodium channel blocking
            antiarrhythmic medications, 401–402
        dofetilide, 403
        sotalol, 403
    interactions with implantable defibrillators,
        418–419
    sudden death, primary prevention of,
        413–419
        antiarrhythmic drug, interactions with
            ICDs, 418–419
        antiarrhythmic medication interactions
            with implantable defibrillators,
            418–419
        anxiolytics, 419
        bradycardia pacing, implantable
            defibrillators, 417
        continuing care, 418
        depression, 419
        heart failure severity, implantable
            defibrillators, 415
        implantable defibrillator implantation
            considerations, 417–418
        nonsustained VT, ventricular ectopic
            activity, 415–416
        psychological support, 419
        severity and ICDs, 416–417
    supraventricular tachycardias, 404–409
        atrial fibrillation, 404–408

Antiarrhythmic medications (*Continued*)
   atrial flutter, 408–409
  therapy with, 419
  ventricular arrhythmias, sudden cardiac
      death, 409–413
    monomorphic ventricular tachycardia,
      409–411
    syncope, 412–413
    torsades de pointes, 412
Anticoagulation in systolic heart failure,
    353–364
  drug-eluting stents, 359–360
    stroke, 360
  prothrombotic state, heart failure as, 353–354
  special populations/misconceptions, 357–359
    coronary arterial disease, 357–358
    stents, 358–359
  thromboembolism, 353–357
    aspirin use for prevention of, 357
    risk factors for, 254–355
    warfarin use for prevention of, 355–357
Anxiety
  with arrhythmias, 419
  with heart failure, 226, 227, 419
Anxiolytics medications, therapy with, 419
Aortic banding, 81, 82
  in guinea pigs, 82
  in rats, 81
Apical ballooning, 152
Apnea, in systolic heart failure, 212
Apoptosis, 101–103
Arginine vasopressin antagonists, 191
Arginine vasopressin, 181
Arrhythmias, 219–221
  atrial fibrillation, 219–221
  ventricular tachycardia, 221
Arrhythmic right ventricular cardiomyopathy/
    dysplasia (ARVC)
  clinical features, 144
  management, 144
  morphology, 144
  natural history, 144
  pathology, 144
Arrhythmogenic right ventricular
    cardiomyopathy (ARVC), 286
Arterial afterload, 378–379
ARVC. *See* Arrhythmic right ventricular
    cardiomyopathy/dysplasia
Ascites, 244
Aspirin
Aspirin, 353–361
Associated valvular dysfunction, 109
Asymptomatic left ventricular dysfunction beta
    blockers and, 336–337

Atria, formation, 3–4
Atrial arrhythmias, 401–426
Atrial fibrillation, 219–221
  with supraventricular tachycardias, 404–408
Atrial flutter, with supraventricular
    tachycardias, 408–409
Automated implantable cardiac
    defibrillators, 452

Bedside assessment, heart failure, 240–250
Beta-adrenergic antagonists, 382
Beta-adrenergic blockers, 330–340
  administration of, 336–337
  antiarrhythmic effects of, 401
    amiodarone, 402–403
      class I sodium channel blocking
        antiarrhythmic medications, 401–402
    dofetilide, 403
    sotalol, 403
  asymptomatic left ventricular dysfunction,
    336–337
  beneficial effects of, 330–332
    exercise tolerance, 330
    ventricular remodeling, 330–332
  cardiac pacemaker implantation, 337
  in class IV heart failure, 334
  clinical considerations in selection of,
    335–336
  clinical trials, 333
  contraindication to treatment, 337–339
  effects on mortality, 332–334
    bisoprolol, 333
    bucindolol, 334
    carvedilol, 333–334
    metoprolol, 332–333
  initiation of therapy, 337–339
  in special populations, 334–Beta-adrenergic
    signalling cascade, 464–466
  types of beta blockers, 332
Beta-blockers, 190–191
Biomarker-guided therapy, potential, 270–271
Biomarkers
  adrenomedullin (ADM), 267
  biomarker-guided therapy, potential, 270–271
  cardiac troponin, 267–268
  extracellular matrix remodeling, 268–269
  hemodynamic stress, 264–267
  inflammatory cytokines, 269
  neurohormonal activation, 268
  oxidative stress, 269–270
  research, limitations and future directions,
    271–272
Bisoprolol, 333
Body fluid compartments, 164

Bradycardia pacing, implantable defibrillators and, 417
Brain natriuretic peptide (BNP), 120, 129, 131
B-type natriuretic peptide (BNP), 191, 264–267, 270
Bucindolol, 334

Calcium channel antagonists, 383
Calcium cycling regulation, 466
Calcium signal, excitation-contraction coupling
    activation, 44–48
    effectors, 48–50
    inactivation, 50
Cardiac cachexia, 225–226
Cardiac computed tomography (CCT), 304–307
    cardiomyopathy, evaluation of, 306
    ischemic cardiomyopathy, exclusion of, 306–307
    nonischemic cardiomyopathies, 307
Cardiac crescent, formation, 1
Cardiac decompensation, cell biology, 36
Cardiac disease
    update on human gene herapy for, 467–470
Cardiac hypertrophy, molecular signaling
        networks, 31–38. See also
        Hypertrophic cardiomyopathy
Cardiac magnetic resonance (CMR), 293–304
    arrythmogenic right ventricular
        cardiomyopathy (ARVC), 301
    cardiac sarcoidosis, 299
    cardiomyopathy, other forms of, 303–304
    in cardiomyopathy evaluation, 294–295
    dilated cardiomyopathy, 297
    hypertrophic cardiomyopathy, 301–303
    infiltrative cardiomyopathy, 298–299
    iron overload cardiomyopathy, 300–301
    ischemic cardiomyopathy, 296–297
    myocarditis, 299–300
    noncompaction cardiomyopathy, 303
    pericardial disease, 304
    structural and functional evaluation, 295–296
Cardiac myocyte death, neurohormonal
        stimulation, 36–38
Cardiac pacemaker implantation, 337
Cardiac resynchronization therapy, 388–400
    candidates for, 397
    left ventricular filling time, increased, 389
    limitations of, 397
    mechanisms of action, 389–390
    mitral regurgitation, reduced, 390
    septal dyskinesis, decreased, 389–390
    trials of, 390–396
        CARE-HF study, 396
        COMPANION study, 396

CONTAK CD study, 394–396
MIRACLE ICD study, 394
MIRACLE study, 393–394
MUSTIC study, 392
PATH-CHF study, 392
    ventricular reverse remodeling, left, 390
Cardiac sarcoidosis, 285
Cardiac troponin, 267–268
Cardiomyocyte protection, 467
Cardiomyopathy
    ARVC, 144
    classification, 137
    conduction defects, 145
    dilated
        adult dilated cardiomyopathy loci, 16
        allele, 11
        clinical diagnosis, 12
        clinical evaluation, 15–18
        clinical genetics, 20
        cytoskeletal protein, 22
        definitions, 19–20
        diagnosis-history, 15
        disease models, 22–23
        dystrophin, 21
        etiology, 20
        familial aggregation, 10
        family-based diagnosis, 15
        genetic association studies, 13–14
        genetic linkage, 10–12
        genetic mapping, 12, 20–21
        genetic methods, 9–14
        genetics of, 9–26
        genetic terminology, 11
        genome, 11
        haplotype, 11
        hypertrophic cardiomyopathy loci, 17
        introns, 11
        locus, allelic heterogeneity, 14
        management, 19
        messenger RNA, 11
        molecular genetics, 21–22
        mutation, 11
        myotonic dystrophy, 22
        nuclear membrane proteins, 21
        phenotype, 11
        polymorphism, mutation discrimination, defining criteria, 12
        positional cloning, 13
        prognosis, 18
        proteome, 11
        simple trait modifiers, 14
        single nucleotide polymorphism, 11
        transcription, 11
        translation, 11

Cardiomyopathy (*Continued*)
  genetic testing, 25–26
  glycogen storage, 145
  hypertrophic
    adult dilated cardiomyopathy
        loci, 16
    allele, 11
    clinical diagnosis, 12
    clinical evaluation, 15–18
    clinical features, 23
    clinical genetics, 23–25
    in clinical practice, 14–19
    clinical presentation, 142
    definitions, 23
    diagnosis-history, 15
    dilated cardiomyopathy clinical features,
        19–20
      Duchenne and Becker muscular
          dystrophy, 21
      pathophysiology, 21–22
      sarcomeric protein, 22
    disease models, 25
    epidemiology, 140
    etiology, 140–142
    evaluation, 142–143
    familial aggregation, 10
    family-based diagnosis, 15
    family screening, 144
    genetic association studies, 13–14
    genetic linkage, 10–12
    genetic methods, 9–14
    genetics of, 9–26
    genetic terminology, 11
    genome, 11
    haplotype, 11
    introns, 11
    loci, 17
    management, 19, 143–144
    messenger RNA, 11
    molecular genetics, 25
    molecular signaling networks, 31–38
    morphology and pathology, 137–140
    mutation, 11
    phenotype, 11
    polymorphism, mutation discrimination,
        defining criteria, 12
    positional cloning, 13
    prognosis, 18
    proteome, 11
    simple trait modifiers, 14
    single nucleotide polymorphism, 11
    transcription, 11
    translation, 11
  ion channel disorders, 145

    left ventricular noncompaction (LVNC),
        144–145
    mitochondrial cardiomyopathies, 145
    primary cardiomyopathies, 137–144
Cardiopulmonary exercise testing, 223
"Cardiorenal" phenomena, 225
Cardiorenal syndrome, 160–193
    angiotensin-converting enzyme inhibitors,
        190–191
    arginine vasopressin antagonists, 191
    beta-blockers, 190–191
    B-type natriuretic peptide, 191
    diuretics and diuretic resistance, 184–190
    epidemiology, 161–162
    therapeutic strategies, 184–193
    treatment, acutely decompensated heart
        failure, 191–193
    ultrafiltration, 191
Cardiovascular reserve function, 379–380
CARE-HF study, cardiac resynchronization
        therapy, 396
Carvedilol, 333–334
Cell therapy studies, 469
Cellular effects of beta-adrenergic blockers, 331
Chemotherapy, systolic heart failure, 212
Chronic volume overload, 80
Chronic-pacing models, 84–85
Class I sodium channel blocking antiarrhythmic
        medications, 401–402
Clinical genetics, 14–19
    adult dilated cardiomyopathy loci, 16
    allelic heterogeneity, 14
    clinical evaluation, 15–18
    clinical genetics, 20
    cytoskeletal protein, 22
    definitions, 19–20
    disease models, 22–23
    dystrophin, 21
    etiology, 20
    in family-based diagnosis, 15
    genetic mapping, 12, 20–21
    hypertrophic cardiomyopathy loci, 17
    management, 19
    molecular genetics, 21–22
    myotonic dystrophy, 22
    nuclear membrane proteins, 21
    prognosis, 18
    trait modifiers, 14
Clinical profiles, heart failure
    disease progression, 240–241
Cocaine, systolic heart failure and, 212
Collagen vascular disease
    systolic heart failure, 212
Combination therapy, 372

COMPANION study, cardiac resynchronization therapy, 396

Conduction system, formation, 5–6

Congestion
primary therapeutic target in decompensated heart failure, 427
treatment of, 427–429
traditional approach to fluid overload, 427–428
ultrafiltration for, 428–429

Congestive heart failure (CHF), 78, 81–85, 87, 89

CONTAK CD study, cardiac resynchronization therapy, 394–396

Contraindication to treatment, beta-adrenergic blockers, 337–339

Conventional therapy, for chronic heart failure, 320–340. *See also under* specific therapeutic modality

Coronary arterial disease, 357–358

Coronary artery disease
systolic heart failure, 212
controlled gene therapy trials for, 468

Coronary vessels, formation, 4–5

Costs
of heart failure, 210

Coupling, excitation-contraction
calcium signal
activation, 44–48
effectors, 48–50
inactivation, 50
cardiac progenitor cells, 57–58
contractility, regulation, 50–52
electrical activity of the heart, 43–44
scheme, 45

C-reactive protein (CRP), 269

Cytokine activation, 125–128

Definitions of heart failure, 208, 209

Depression, 226, 227, 451
with arrhythmias, 419
with heart failure, 419

Developmental cardiogenesis, 6

Diabetes, 371–372

Diagnosis of heart failure, 216–219

Diastolic dysfunction, 377–378

Diastolic function, assessment, 284–289
cardiomyopathies, echo findings specific, 285–286
strain and strain rate imaging, 286–289
three-dimensional echocardiography, 289

Diastolic heart failure, 214–216, 370–371
abnormalities resulting in, 215
criteria for diagnosis of, 215

Digitalis, 326–328
clinical trials, 326
consensus guidelines on digoxin use, 328
digoxin dosing, 327–328
effects of mortality, 327

Digoxin
for chronic heart failure, 320–329
consensus guidelines on, 328
dosing, 327–328

Dilated cardiomyopathy
adult dilated cardiomyopathy loci, 16
allele, 11
clinical diagnosis, 12
clinical evaluation, 15–18
clinical genetics, 20
cytoskeletal protein, 22
definitions, 19–20
diagnosis-history, 15
disease models, 22–23
Duchenne and Becker muscular dystrophy, 21
dystrophin, 21
etiology, 20
familial aggregation, 10
family-based diagnosis, 15
genetic association studies, 13–14
genetic linkage, 10–12
genetic mapping, 12, 20–21
genetic methods, 9–14
genetics of, 9–26
genetic terminology, 11
genome, 11
haplotype, 11
hypertrophic cardiomyopathy loci, 17
introns, 11
large-breed dogs, 87
locus, allelic heterogeneity, 14
management, 19
messenger RNA, 11
molecular genetics, 21–22
mutation, 11
myotonic dystrophy, 22
nuclear membrane proteins, 21
pathophysiology, 21–22
phenotype, 11
polymorphism, mutation discrimination, defining criteria, 12
positional cloning, 13
prognosis, 18
proteome, 11
sarcomeric proteins, 22
simple trait modifiers, 14
single nucleotide polymorphism, 11
splicing factors, 22

Dilated cardiomyopathy (*Continued*)
  Syrian hamsters, 87
  transcription, 11
  translation, 11
Disease management programs, 453
Diuretics and diuretic resistance, 184–190
Diuretics, 320–323, 382–383
  for chronic heart failure, 320–329
  loop diuretics, 321–322
  potassium sparing diuretics, 322
  thiazide diuretics, 322
  tolerance, 322–323
Dofetilide, 403
Do-not-resuscitate orders, 451–452
Dose-response curves, loop diuretics, 186
Doxorubicin, 87–88
Drug-induced models, 87–88
  doxorubicin, 87–88
  monocrotaline, 88
  propranolol, 88
Duchenne and Becker muscular dystrophy, 21
Dyspnea, 242, 449–450

Echocardiography, 278–289
  diastolic function, assessment, 284–289
  left ventricular performance assessment,
    280–284
  left ventricular structure and function, 279
  right ventricular structure and function, 284
  systolic function, assessment, 280
  ventricular mass and volume, assessment,
    279–280
Economics of heart failure, 210
Edema, 244
EFFECT heart failure scoring system, 256
Elderly
  disproportionate economic burden of heart
    failure on, 210
Electrolyte disorders, systolic heart failure, 212
Endocrine
  disorders of, systolic heart failure, 212
Endomyocardial fibroelastosis, 286
Endothelin, 181
Endothelin-1, 130
Epicardium-derived cells (EPDCs), 4–5
Eplerenone, 372
Equilibrium multiple gated blood pool
    scintigraphy method, 291
Ergoreflexes, exercise capacity and, 222
Evaluation Study of Congestive Heart Failure
    and Pulmonary Artery Catheterization
    Effectiveness (ESCAPE), 314–317
Excitation-contraction coupling
  calcium signal

    activation, 44–48
    effectors, 48–50
    inactivation, 50
  cardiac progenitor cells, 57–58
  contractility, regulation, 50–52
  electrical activity of the heart, 43–44
  scheme, 45
Exercise
  capacity, 221–224
    cardiac, 221
    clinical assessment of, 223–224
    ergoreflexes, 222
    gene polymorphisms, effects on exercise
      capacity, 222
    lungs, 222
    mechanisms, 221
    peripheral blood flow, 222
    skeletal muscle, 222
  training, 224
Exons, 11
Expenditures on heart failure, annually, 210
Extracellular matrix degradation, 100
Extracellular matrix remodeling, 268–269

Failing myocardium, [ATP] and [Cr] in, 66
Familial hypertrophic cardiomyopathy
    (FHC)-associated missense
    mutations, 72
Familial/genetic cardiomyopathy, systolic heart
    failure, 212
Fetal gene program, 101
Fibrosis, 100–101
Financial burden of heart failure, 210
Functional limitations with heart failure,
    221–222
  cardiac, 221
  ergoreflexes, 222
  gene polymorphisms, effects on exercise
    capacity, 222
  lungs, 222
  mechanisms of, 221
  peripheral blood flow, 222
  skeletal muscle, 222

Gene polymorphisms, effects on exercise
    capacity, 222
Gene therapy studies, 467–469
Gene therapy, heart failure, 457–470
  human gene therapy, update on, 467–470
    cell therapy studies, 469
    gene therapy studies, 467–469
    hybrid gene, 469
  targeted, 458–459
    transcriptional targeting, 458–459

transductional targeting, 458
targets in heart failure, 463–467
    beta-adrenergic signalling cascade,
        464–466
    calcium cycling regulation, 466
    cardiomyocyte protection, 467
    impulse generation and conduction, 467
therapeutic delivery routes for, 459–460
    intracoronary delivery, 459–460
    intramyocardial delivery, 459
    intravenous delivery, 459
vectors for gene transfer, 460–463
    adeno-associated viral, 462–463
    adenoviral, 462
    nonviral, 461
    viral, 461–462
Genetic diversity, pharmacogenetics interac-
        tions, 123–125
Genetic primary cardiomyopathy, 137–140
Glomerular filtration rate (GFR), 160, 168,
        170–173

Heart development, 2
    atria, formation, 3–4
    cardiac crescent, formation, 1
    conduction system, formation, 5–6
    coronary vessels, formation, 4–5
    developmental cardiogenesis, 6
    outflow tract, formation, 4
    therapeutic implications, 6
    valves, formation, 5
    ventricles, formation, 2–3
Heart failure, 208–228
    action potential, 52
    and palliative care, 445–456
    anemia, 226
    angiotensin receptor blockers for, 341–352
    animal models, 78–89
    antiarrhythmic drug, interactions with ICDs,
        418–419
    anticoagulation in systolic, 353–364
    architectural changes, 57
    arrhythmias, 219–221
    ATP-synthesizing pathways, integration, 70
    atrial arrhythmias, 401–426
    basic concepts of, 31–32
    bedside assessment, 240–250
    biomarkers, 264–272
    bradycardia pacing with ICDs, 417
    calcium handling, activation and inactivation,
        52–55
    CAMKII signaling, 56
    cardiac cachexia, 225–226
    cardiac resynchronization therapy, 388–400

"cardiorenal" phenomena, 225
causes and consequences, 72–73
classification of, 208
clinical assessment, 241
clinical experience with ultrafiltration for
        (case studies), 430–432
clinical experience with ultrafiltration for
        (randomized controlled trials),
        433–434
clinical features, 219–227
clinical presentation
    classification, 218
    interpretation of, 218
clinical profiles, 240–250
clinical syndrome of, 208–228
complications of, 219–227
congestion and, 427–429
continuing care, 418
controlled trials in chronic, 429–435
controlled trials in decompensated,
        435–437
conventional therapy, 320–340
cytokine activation in, 119–131
definitions of, 208, 209
diagnosis of, 216–219
diagnostic consideration, 317
diagnostic laboratory modalities, 218–219
diastolic, 214–216
    abnormalities resulting in, 215
    criteria for diagnosis of, 215
different from cancer, 446
dilated cardiomyopathy, 87
disease progression, relevant profiles,
        240–241
drug-induced models, 87–88
economics of, 210
end effectors, contractile proteins, 55
epidemiology, 208–211
epidemiology, 445–446
ESCAPE trial, 314–317
excitation-contraction coupling, 43–58
exercise capacity, 223–224
    clinical assessment of, 223–224
    functional limitation and, 221–222
failing myocardium, rescue, 73–74
FHC-associated missense mutations,
        sarcomeric proteins, 72
force-frequency, 55
functional capacity, 223–224
    clinical assessment of, 223–224
gene therapy targets in, 463–467
    beta-adrenergic signalling cascade,
        464–466
    calcium cycling regulation, 466

Heart failure (*Continued*)
    cardiomyocyte protection, 467
    impulse generation and conduction, 467
  guidelines for, 447
  guiding management, 318
  hemodynamic profiles, 241–245
  historical perspectives, 313–314
  ICD implantation considerations, 417–418
  incidence, 209–210
  invasive monitoring in, 313–318
  ischemia and infarction, 85–87
  large animal models, 79
  late-stage disease, patient INTERMACS
      profiles, 248–250
  lower ATP concentration, 65–66
  lower PCr concentration, 65–66
  metabolic remodeling
    impaired energy reserve, 66
    transcriptional and post-transcriptional
      control, 70–72
  metabolic reserve, decreased
    via creatine kinase (CK), 66–67
    via glycolysis, 68–69
    via mitochondrial ATP synthesis, 69–70
  mineralocorticoid antagonists, 365–376
  mitral regurgitation, 224
  molecular signaling networks, 31–38
  mortality, 445–446
  myocardial energetics and metabolism,
      64–74
  neurohormonal activation in, 119–131
  noninvasive imaging modalities, 278–307
  normal integrated function of heart, 211
  pathophysiology of, 211–216
  patient evaluation, 220
  patients symptoms, 447–448
  perfusion, 245–247
  prediction of survival, 228
  pressure overload, 80, 81–82
  prevalence of, 209–210
  prognosis, 227–228
  prognosis, 252–259
  psychiatric issues with, 226–227
  psychological support, 419
  pulmonary artery catheters, 313–318
  rapid-pacing models, 82–85
  renal function and progression, 180–184
  repolarizing currents, 52
  risk factors for, 210–211
  risk stratification, 318
  secondary valvular dysfunction in, 95–110
  severity and ICDs, 416–417
  signs/symptoms, 216–218
  sleep apnea, 224–225
  small animal models, 79
  specific models, 79–80
  survival, prediction of, 228
  therapeutics, neurohormonal signaling,
      32–33
  treatment of patients with, and preserved
      LVEF, 347, 349
  treatment of patients with, and reduced
      LVEF, 343–346, 349
  treatment of patients with, post-myocardial
      infarction, 347–348, 349
  treatment, implications for, 57
  ultrafiltration, 427–444
  ventricular arrhythmias, 401–426
  ventricular remodeling, 95–110
  volume overload, 80–81
  b-receptor signaling, 56
  systolic, 213–214
    abnormalities resulting in, 214
    causes of, 212
  treatment of, with preserved ejection fraction,
      377–387
    future directions, 384
    putative therapeutic targets, 377–381
    role of agents, 381–384
  treatment of symptoms, 448–453
    depression, 451
    disease management programs, 453
    dyspnea, 449–450
    hospice criteria for, 452–453
    pain, 450–451
    standard treatment for, 448–449
    symptomatic treatment, 449
Heart failure preserved ejection fraction.
      See Diastolic heart failure
Heart failure reduced ejection fraction.
      See Systolic heart failure
Heart failure survival models, 258
Heart, normal integrated function of, 211
Hemodynamics
  with beta-adrenergic blockers, 331
Hemodynamic profiles, bedside assessment,
      241–245
  congestion, 242–245
  prevalence of, 248
  prognosis of, 248
Hemodynamic stress, 264–267
  natriuretic peptides, 264–266
  ST2, 266–267
Hospice criteria, for heart failure, 452–453
Human gene therapy, update on, 467–470
  cell therapy studies, 469
  coronary artery disease, controlled gene
      therapy trials for, 468

gene therapy studies, 467–469
hybrid gene, 469
Hybrid gene, 469
Hypertension, 371
systolic heart failure, 212
Hypertrophic cardiomyopathy (HCM)
adult dilated cardiomyopathy loci, 16
allele, 11
clinical diagnosis, 12
clinical evaluation, 15–18
clinical features, 23
clinical genetics, 23–25
in clinical practice, 14–19
clinical presentation, 142
definitions, 23
diagnosis-history, 15
dilated cardiomyopathy clinical features,
19–20
Duchenne and Becker muscular
dystrophy, 21
pathophysiology, 21–22
sarcomeric protein, 22
disease models, 25
epidemiology, 140
etiology, 140–142
evaluation, 142–143
familial aggregation, 10
family screening, 144
family-based diagnosis, 15
genetic association studies, 13–14
genetic linkage, 10–12
genetic mapping, 12
genetic methods, 9–14
genetic terminology, 11
genetics of, 9–26
genome, 11
haplotype, 11
introns, 11
loci, 17
management, 143–144
management, 19
messenger RNA, 11
molecular genetics, 25
mutation, 11
phenotype, 11
polymorphism, mutation discrimination,
defining criteria, 12
positional cloning, 13
prognosis, 18
proteome, 11
simple trait modifiers, 14
single nucleotide polymorphism, 11
transcription, 11
translation, 11

Hypertrophy, cardiac
basic concepts of, 31–32
cardiac myocyte death, neurohormonal
stimulation, 36–38
modifying signaling pathways, 35–36
neurohormonal signaling pathways, 33–35

ICD implantation, considerations, 417–418
Idiopathic restrictive cardiomyopathy, 149, 150
Implantable defibrillators
antiarrhythmic medication interactions with,
418–419
bradycardia pacing, 417
implantation considerations, 417–418
primary prevention trials, 414
sudden death, primary prevention of, 415
Impulse generation and conduction, 467
Index of myocardial performance (IMP),
283–284
Inflammatory cytokines, 269
Introns, 11
Invasive monitoring, heart failure, 313–318
Ion channel disorders, 145
Iron overload cardiomyopathy, 286
Ischemia and infarction models, 85–87
ameroid constrictors, 86–87
canine models, 86
coiling/gelfoam, 87
large animal models, 86
rat coronary ligation model, 85

Jugular venous distention, 243
Juxtaglomerular apparatus, 168

Left ventricular asymptomatic dysfunction beta
blockers and, 336–337
Left ventricular ejection fraction (LVEF),
252, 253
Left ventricular filling time, increased, cardiac
resynchronization therapy, 389
Left ventricular noncompaction (LVNC),
144–145, 285
Left ventricular performance assessment,
280–284
dP/dt, 283
E-point septal separation, 283
fractional shortening (FS), 280–283
index of myocardial performance (IMP),
283–284
Left ventricular remodeling. See also
Ventricular remodeling
assessment, multimodality imaging
techniques, 107
reversibility of, 106–107

Loop diuretics, 321–322
L-type Ca²⁺ channels (LTCC), 43–48, 51, 53, 56–58

Macula densa cells, 169
Medications, 320–329. *See also under* specific medication
  angiotensin receptor blockers, 341–352
  beta-adrenergic blockers, 330–340
  digitalis, 326–328
    clinical trials, 326
    consensus guidelines on digoxin use, 328
    digoxin dosing, 327–328
    effects of mortality, 327
  diuretics, 320–323
    loop diuretics, 321–322
    potassium sparing diuretics, 322
    thiazide diuretics, 322
    tolerance, 322–323
  mineralocorticoid antagonists, 365–376
  vasodilator therapy, 323–326
    ACE inhibitors
      aspirin interaction, 325–326
      postmyocardial infarction management, 324–325
    dosing, 324
Metabolic remodeling
  impaired energy reserve, 66
  transcriptional and post-transcriptional control, 70–72
Metabolic reserve, decreased
  via creatine kinase (CK), 66–67
  via glycolysis, 68–69
  via mitochondrial ATP synthesis, 69–70
Metoprolol, 332–333
Mineralocorticoid antagonists, 365–376, 383
  agents and their use, 372
    eplerenone, 372
    spironolactone, 372
  aldosterone physiology, 365–366
  clinical applications of, 368–372
    combination therapy, 372
    diabetes, 371–372
    diastolic heart failure, 370–371
    hypertension, 371
    renal disease, 371–372
    systolic heart failure, 368–370
  future studies, 373–374
  pathophysiology of aldosterone, 366–367
  renal pathology, 367
  precautions to use, 373
MIRACLE ICD study, cardiac resynchronization therapy, 394

MIRACLE study, cardiac resynchronization therapy, 393–394
Mitochondrial cardiomyopathies, 145
Mitral regurgitation
  reduced, cardiac resynchronization therapy, 390
Mixed genetic and acquired cardiomyopathy, 145–148
  Myocarditis, 150–152
Molecular signaling networks
  cardiac hypertrophy, 31–38
  heart failure, 31–38
Monocrotaline, 88
Monomorphic ventricular tachycardia, 409–411
MUSTIC study, cardiac resynchronization therapy, 392
Myocardial recovery, 106
Myocarditis, systolic heart failure, 212
Myocyte hypertrophy, 101
Myocyte necrosis, 101–103

Natriuretic peptides, 181
Nephron, salt and water transport, 162–168
Neurohormonal activation, 119–131, 268
Neurohormonal theory, 33
Nitrates, 382–383
Nitric oxide, 131, 171
Noninvasive imaging modalities, heart failure, 278–307
  cardiac computed tomography (CCT), 304–307
  cardiac magnetic resonance, 293–304
  echocardiography, 278–289
  radionuclide imaging methods, 289–293
Nonischemic dilated cardiomyopathy
  clinical presentation, 147
  epidemiology, 146
  etiology, 146–147
  evaluation, 147–148
  morphology and pathology, 145
  natural history, 146
  treatment, 148
Nonpharmacologic measures, 383–384
Nonsustained VT, ventricular ectopic activity, 415–416
Norepinephrine, 131

Outflow tract, formation, 4
Oxidative stress, 269–270

Pacemaker implantation, 337
Pain, 450–451
Palliative care

communication in, 451–452
    automated implantable cardiac
        defibrillators, 452
    do-not-resuscitate orders, 451–452
    and heart failure, 445–456
    and hospice, 445
PATH-CHF study, cardiac resynchronization
        therapy, 392
Periodic breathing, 245
Peripartum cardiomyopathy (PPCM),
        152–153
Pharmacologic neurohormonal activation, 32
Pharmacologic neurohormonal inhibition, 33
Plasma osmolality, 168–175
Plasma volume, 168–175
Plasma volume, regulation, 128–129
Pleural effusions, 245
Potassium sparing diuretics, 322
Pressure overload
    aortic banding, 81, 82
    in rabbits, 80
    in rats and mice, 81–82
    spontaneous hypertensive rats (SHR), 82
    systemic hypertension, rats, 81–82
Primary cardiomyopathies
    epidemiology, 140
    etiology, 140–142
    genetic primary cardiomyopathy, 137–140
    natural history, 140
Prognosis, heart failure, 252–259
    cardiac structure and function, 253–254
    clinical factors, 253
    clinical prognostic models, 255–259
    demographic and clinical factors, 252–253
    factors, systolic heart failure, 253
    functional capacity, 253, 254
    laboratory data, 253, 254–255
    medications/device, 253
    neurohormal activation, 254–255
Proportional pulse pressure, 247
Propranolol, 88
Prothrombotic state, heart failure as,
        353–354
Psychiatric issues with heart failure
    anxiety, 419
    depression, 419
Pulmonary artery catheters, heart failure,
        313–318
Putative therapeutic targets, 377–381
    arterial afterload, 378–379
    cardiovascular reserve function, 379–380
    diastolic dysfunction, 377–378
    systolic dysfunction, 380–381
    ventricular-vascular stiffening, 378–379

Radionuclide imaging methods, 289–293
    electrocardiogram (ECG)-gated SPECT
        (GSPECT) imaging, 289–290
    equilibrium multiple gated blood pool
        scintigraphy method, 291
    first-pass radionuclide angiography
        (FPRNA), 291
    meta-iodobenzylguanidine (MIBG), 292–293
    myocardial perfusion imaging (MPI), 290
    positron emission tomography (PET),
        291–292
    radionuclide cardiac neuronal imaging, 292
    radionuclide ventriculography, 290–291
    specific cardiomyopathies, perfusion
        imaging, 290
    ventricular function assessment, 289–290
Renal disease, 371–372
Renal nerves, 181
Renal pathology, 367
Renal prostaglandins, 181
Renal sodium and water handling
    in heart failure, 175–180
    principles, 162–168
Renin–angiotensin–aldosterone system
        (RAAS), 120–121, 181
Restrictive cardiomyopathy (RCM)
    clinical presentation, 149
    epidemiology, 149
    etiology, 149
    evaluation, 149–150
    management, 150
    morphology, 148–149
    natural history, 149
    pathology, 148–149
Right ventricle remodeling, 109
RNA Binding Motif protein 20 (RBM20), 22

Salt and water transport, nephron, 162–168
Seattle heart failure model calculator, 257, 259
Secondary cardiomyopathies
    cardiotoxic cancer chemotherapy, 154
    endomyocardial fibrotic conditions, 154
    infiltrative cardiomyopathies, 153
    storage diseases, 153
    toxicity, 154
Septal dyskinesis, decreased, cardiac
        resynchronization therapy, 389–390
Signaling
    beta-adrenergic, cascade, 464–466
Skin temperature, 247
Sotalol, 403
Special population heart failure
    beta blockers use in, 334–335
Spironolactone, 372

Spontaneous hypertensive rats (SHR), 82
Stents, 358–360
Stress-induced cardiomyopathy, 152
Stroke, 360
Sudden death
    primary prevention of, 413–419
        antiarrhythmic medication interactions
            with implantable defibrillators,
            418–419
        anxiolytics and antidepressant
            medications, therapy with, 419
        bradycardia pacing, implantable
            defibrillators, 417
        continuing care, 418
        depression and anxiety, 419
        heart failure severity, implantable
            defibrillators, 415
        implantable defibrillator implantation
            considerations, 417–418
        nonsustained VT, ventricular ectopic
            activity, 415–416
        psychological support, 419
        risk stratification, 413–415
Suffusion with socks, 242
Supraventricular tachycardias, 404–409
    atrial fibrillation, 404–408
    atrial flutter, 408–409
Systemic blood pressure, 168–175
Systemic hypertension, rats, 81–82
Systolic blood pressure, 246
Systolic dysfunction, 380–381
Systolic heart failure, 213–214
Systolic heart failure, 368–370
Sympathetic nerve activation, 121–122
    renin–angiotensin, interaction of, 122
Syncope
    with arrhythmia, 412–413

Tachycardia-induced cardiomyopathy, 153
Takotsubo cardiomyopathy, 152
Targeted gene therapy, 458–459
    transcriptional targeting, 458–459
    transductional targeting, 458
"Tei" Index, 283–284
Thiazide diuretics, 322
Therapeutic delivery routes, for gene therapy,
    459–460
    intracoronary delivery, 459–460
    intramyocardial delivery, 459
    intravenous delivery, 459
Three-dimensional echocardiography, 289
Thromboembolism, 353–357
    aspirin use for prevention of, 357

risk factors for, 354–355
    warfarin use for prevention of, 355–357
TNF-alpha, 131
Treatment of congestion, 427–429
    traditional approach to fluid overload,
        427–428
    ultrafiltration for, 428–429
Treatment of Symptoms, of heart failure,
    448–453
Trials of cardiac resynchronization therapy,
    390–396
    CARE-HF study, 396
    COMPANION study, 396
    CONTAK CD study, 394–396
    MIRACLE ICD study, 394
    MIRACLE study, 393–394
    MUSTIC study, 392
    PATH-CHF study, 392
Tubuloglomerular feedback, 170, 173

Ultrafiltration, 191, 427–444
    clinical experience with, 429–437
        case series, 429
        controlled trials in chronic heart failure,
            429–435
        controlled trials in decompensated heart
            failure, 435–437
    cost effectiveness of, 440
    future directions, 440
    other strategies of fluid removal, 440
    possible mechanisms of benefit, 437–438
        diuretic sparing, 437–438
        effective fluid removal, 437
        effective sodium removal, 438
        removal of inflammatory cytokines, 438
    prescription of, 438–439
        patient selection, 438
        treatment termination conditions, 439
        worsening renal function, 438
    risks of, 439
    treatment of congestion, 427–429
        traditional approach to fluid overload,
            427–428
        ultrafiltration for, 428–429

Valsalva maneuver, 245
Valves, formation, 5
Vascular reactivity, 129–130
Vasoconstrictor systems, 181
Vasodilator systems, 181
Vasodilator therapy, 323–326
    ACE inhibitors
        aspirin interaction, 325–326

postmyocardial infarction management, 324–325
    dosing, 324
Vasomotor center, 168
Vectors, for gene transfer, 460–463
    adeno-associated viral, 462–463
    adenoviral, 462
    nonviral, 461
    viral, 461–462
Ventricles, formation, 2–3
Ventricular arrhythmias, 401–426
    sudden cardiac death, 409–413
        monomorphic ventricular tachycardia, 409–411
        syncope, 412–413
        torsades de pointes, 412
Ventricular cardiomyocyte action potential, 44
Ventricular remodeling
    assessment, multimodality imaging techniques, 107
    and associated valvular dysfunction, 109
    with beta-adrenergic blockers, 330–332

changes, macroscopic level, 103–105
    functional changes, 105–106
    neurohormonal activation, 97–100
    pathogenesis, 96–97
    reversibility of, 106–107
    therapeutic targets, 109–110
Ventricular reverse remodeling, left, cardiac resynchronization therapy, 390
Ventricular-vascular stiffening, 378–379
Volume overload
    acute, 80
    chronic, 80
    in goats, 80–81
    in rabbits, 80

Warfarin, 353, 355–357
Warfarin and Aspirin for the Prevention of Recurrent Ischemic Stroke (WARSS), 360
Water excretion, control, 174–175
Women, heart failure in
    beta blockers use, 334–335

Milton Keynes UK
Ingram Content Group UK Ltd.
UKHW050456071024
449327UK00015B/408